Pocket Companion to
Accompany

OBSTETRICS

Normal and Problem Pregnancies

Pocket Companion to
Accompany

OBSTETRICS

Normal and Problem Pregnancies

Fourth Edition

STEVEN G. GABBE, M.D.
Dean, Vanderbilt University School of Medicine
Professor of Obstetrics and Gynecology
Vanderbilt University Medical Center
Nashville, Tennessee

JENNIFER R. NIEBYL, M.D.
Professor and Head
Department of Obstetrics and Gynecology
University of Iowa College of Medicine
Iowa City, Iowa

JOE LEIGH SIMPSON, M.D.
Ernst W. Bertner Professor and Chairman
Department of Obstetrics and Gynecology
Professor of Molecular and Human Genetics
Baylor College of Medicine
Houston, Texas

Illustrated by
Mikki Senkarik, M.S., A.M.I. and Michael Cooley, A.M.I.

CHURCHILL LIVINGSTONE
An Imprint of Elsevier Science
New York   Edinburgh   London   Philadelphia

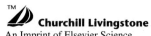

Churchill Livingstone
An Imprint of Elsevier Science

UNIVERSITY OF GREENWICH
18 AUG 2004
LIBRARY

The Curtis Center
Independence Square West
Philadelphia, PA 19106

Notice

Obstetrics is an ever-changing field. Standard safety precautions must be followed, but as new research and clinical experience broaden our knowledge, changes in treatment and drug therapy may become necessary or appropriate. Readers are advised to check the most current product information provided by the manufacturer of each drug to be administered to verify the recommended dose, the method and duration of administration, and contraindications. It is the responsibility of the treating physician, relying on experience and knowledge of the patient, to determine dosages and the best treatment for each individual patient. Neither the Publisher nor the editor assumes any liability for any injury and/or damage to persons or property arising from this publication.

The Publisher

First Edition 1999.

Library of Congress Cataloging-in Publication Data

Pocket companion to accompany Obstetrics: normal and problem pregnancies / [edited by] Steven G. Gabbe, Jennifer R. Niebyl, Joe Leigh Simpson.—4th ed.
     p. cm.
  Includes bibliographical references and index.
  Companion v. to: Obstetrics: normal and problem pregnancies. 4th ed.
  ISBN 0-443-06593-4 ✓ ᔕᴠᴏ
  1. Obstetrics—Handbooks, manuals, etc. 2.
Pregnancy—Complications—Handbooks, manuals, etc.
  DNLM: 1. Pregnancy—handbooks. 2. Pregnancy
Complications—handbooks. 3. Perinatal Care—handbooks.] I. Gabbe, Steven G. II. Niebyl, Jennifer R. III. Simpson, Joe Leigh
RG531 .P63 2002   618.2—dc21   2002018913

PIT / RDC

Printed in the United States of America.

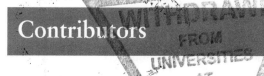
Contributors

THOMAS J. BENEDETTI, M.D., M.H.A.
Professor and Director, Division of Perinatal Medicine,
Vice-Chair Network Development and Operations,
Department of Obstetrics and Gynecology, University of
Washington School of Medicine, Seattle, Washington
Obstetric Hemorrhage

RICHARD L. BERKOWITZ, M.D.
Professor and Chairman, Department of Obstetrics,
Gynecology, and Reproductive Sciences, Mount Sinai
School of Medicine of New York University; Director
of Obstetrics and Gynecology, Mount Sinai Hospital, New York
Multiple Gestations

IRA BERNSTEIN, M.D.
Associate Professor, Department of Obstetrics and Gynecology,
University of Vermont College of Medicine; Attending Physician,
Fletcher Allen Health Care, Burlington, Vermont
Intrauterine Growth Restriction

WATSON A. BOWES, JR., M.D.
Emeritus Professor of Obstetrics and Gynecology,
University of North Carolina at Chapel Hill School of
Medicine, Chapel Hill, North Carolina
Postpartum Care and Breast-Feeding

D. WARE BRANCH, M.D.
Professor, Department of Obstetrics and Gynecology,
University of Utah School of Medicine, Salt Lake City, Utah
Alloimmunization in Pregnancy

PATRICK M. CATALANO, M.D.
Professor, Department of Reproductive Biology, Case Western
Reserve University; Chairman, Department of Obstetrics and
Gynecology, MetroHealth Medical Center, Cleveland, Ohio
Diabetes Mellitus

FRANK A. CHERVENAK, M.D.
Given Foundation Professor and Chairman,
Department of Obstetrics and Gynecology, Weill
Medical Center of Cornell University; Obstetrician and
Gynecologist In-Chief, Department of Obstetrics and
Gynecology, New York Presbyterian Hospital, New York
Obstetric Ultrasound: Assessment of Fetal Growth and Anatomy

DAVID H. CHESTNUT, M.D.
Alfred Habeeb Professor and Chairman of Anesthesiology,
and Professor of Obstetrics and Gynecology, University of
Alabama School of Medicine, Birmingham, Alabama
Obstetric Anesthesia

USHA CHITKARA, M.D.
Professor, Division of Maternal-Fetal Medicine,
Department of Gynecology and Obstetrics, Stanford
University School of Medicine, Stanford, California
Multiple Gestations

DAVID F. COLOMBO, M.D.
Assistant Professor, Division of Maternal-Fetal Medicine,
Department of Obstetrics and Gynecology, The Ohio State
University College of Medicine, Columbus, Ohio
Renal Disease

ROY COLVEN, M.D.
Assistant Professor of Medicine, Division of Dermatology, University
of Washington School of Medicine; Attending Physician, Harborview
Medical Center, Seattle, Washington
Dermatologic Disorders

LARRY J. COPELAND, M.D.
Professor and Chair, Department of Obstetrics and
Gynecology, William Greenville Pace III and Joann
Norris Collins-Pace Chair, The Ohio State University
College of Medicine and Public Health, and James
Cancer Hospital and Solove Research Institute, Columbus, Ohio
Malignant Diseases and Pregnancy

RICHARD DEPP, M.D.
Professor, Department of Obstetrics
and Gynecology, MCP Hahnemann University School
of Medicine, Philadelphia, Pennsylvania
Cesarean Delivery

MICHAEL Y. DIVON, M.D.

Professor of Obstetrics, Gynecology and Women's Health, Albert Einstein College of Medicine, Bronx; Chairman of Obstetrics and Gynecology, Lenox Hill Hospital, New York, New York
  Prolonged Pregnancy

MITCHELL P. DOMBROWSKI, M.D.

Professor, Division of Maternal-Fetal Medicine, Department of Obstetrics and Gynecology, Wayne State University School of Medicine, Hutzel Hospital, Detroit, Michigan
  Pulmonary Disease

MAURICE L. DRUZIN, M.D.

Professor of Gynecology and Obstetrics, Stanford University School of Medicine; Chief, Division of Maternal-Fetal Medicine, Director of the Perinatal Diagnostic Center, Stanford University Medical Center, Stanford, California
  Antepartum Fetal Evaluation

PATRICK DUFF, M.D.

Professor and Residency Program Director, Department of Obstetrics and Gynecology, University of Florida College of Medicine, Gainesville, Florida
  Maternal and Perinatal Infection

THOMAS R. EASTERLING, M.D.

Associate Professor, Division of Prenatal Medicine, Department of Obstetrics and Gynecology, University of Washington School of Medicine, Seattle, Washington
  Cardiac Disease and Critical Care

MARK I. EVANS, M.D.

Professor and Chairman of Obstetrics and Gynecology, Professor of Human Genetics, and Director, Fetal Therapy Program, MCP Hahnemann University, Philadelphia, Pennsylvania
  Fetal Therapeutic Intervention

ALAN W. FLAKE, M.D.

Associate Professor of Surgery, and Obstetrics and Gynecology, University of Pennsylvania; Director, Children's Institute for Surgical Science, Children's Hospital of Philadelphia, Philadelphia, Pennsylvania
  Fetal Therapeutic Intervention

PAMELA M. FOY, B.S., R.D.M.S.
Clinical Coordinator of Ultrasound Services,
Department of Obstetrics and Gynecology, The Ohio
State University College of Medicine, Columbus, Ohio
   Appendices: Obstetric Ultrasound Measurement Tables

STEVEN G. GABBE, M.D.
Dean, Vanderbilt University School of Medicine,
Professor of Obstetrics and Gynecology, Vanderbilt
University Medical Center, Nashville, Tennessee
   *Obstetric Ultrasound: Assessment of Fetal Growth
   and Anatomy; Antepartum Fetal Evaluation;
   Intrauterine Growth Restriction; Diabetes Mellitus*

THOMAS J. GARITE, M.D.
Professor and Chairman, Department of Obstetrics and Gynecology,
University of California, Irvine, School of Medicine, Irvine, California
   Intrapartum Fetal Evaluation

CHARLES P. GIBBS, M.D.
Professor Emeritus of Anesthesiology, University of
Colorado School of Medicine, Denver, Colorado
   Obstetric Anesthesia

MICHAEL R. HARRISON, M.D.
Professor of Surgery and Pediatrics, and Director, The Fetal Treatment
Center, Chief, Division of Pediatric Surgery, University of California,
San Francisco School of Medicine, San Francisco, California
   Fetal Therapeutic Intervention

JOY L. HAWKINS, M.D.
Director of Obstetric Anesthesia and Professor of Anesthesiology,
University of Colorado School of Medicine, Denver, Colorado
   Obstetric Anesthesia

JAY D. IAMS, M.D.
Frederick P. Zuspan Chair and Director, Division of Maternal-Fetal
Medicine, Department of Obstetrics and Gynecology, The Ohio State
University College of Medicine and Public Health, Columbus, Ohio
   Preterm Birth

MARC JACKSON, M.D.
Associate Professor, Department of Obstetrics and Gynecology, Temple
University School of Medicine, Philadelphia; Division of Maternal-Fetal
Medicine, Crozer-Chester Medical Center, Upland, Pennsylvania
   Alloimmunization in Pregnancy

MARK P. JOHNSON, M.D.

Associate Professor, Departments of Obstetrics and Gynecology, and Surgery, University of Pennsylvania School of Medicine; Director of Obstetrical Services, Center for Fetal Diagnosis and Treatment, Children's Hospital of Philadelphia, Philadelphia, Pennsylvania
Fetal Therapeutic Intervention

TIMOTHY R.B. JOHNSON, M.D.

Bates Professor of the Diseases of Women and Children, Professor and Chair of Obstetrics and Gynecology, Research Scientist, Center for Human Growth and Development, and Professor of Women's Studies, Medical School and College of Literature, Science and the Arts, University of Michigan, Ann Arbor, Michigan
Preconception and Prenatal Care: Part of the Continuum

VERN L. KATZ, M.D.

Clinical Assistant Professor, Department of Obstetrics and Gynecology, University of Oregon School of Medicine, Portland; Director of Perinatal Services, Sacred Heart Medical Center, Eugene, Oregon
Postpartum Care and Breast-Feeding

MARK B. LANDON, M.D.

Professor and Vice Chair, Department of Obstetrics and Gynecology, Division of Maternal-Fetal Medicine, The Ohio State University College of Medicine and Public Health, Columbus, Ohio
Diabetes Mellitus; Gastrointestinal Disease; Malignant Diseases and Pregnancy

SUSAN M. LANNI, M.D.

Assistant Professor of Obstetrics and Gynecology and Maternal Fetal Medicine, Virginia Commonwealth University, Medical College of Virginia Hospitals, Richmond, Virginia
Malpresentations

JACK LUDMIR, M.D.

Professor of Obstetrics and Gynecology, University of Pennsylvania School of Medicine; Chair, Department of Obstetrics and Gynecology, Pennsylvania Hospital, University of Pennsylvania Health System, Philadelphia, Pennsylvania
Surgical Procedures in Pregnancy

JORGE H. MESTMAN, M.D.

Professor of Medicine and Obstetrics and Gynecology, University of Southern California Keck School of Medicine, Los Angeles, California
Other Endocrine Disorders

EDWARD R. NEWTON, M.D.

Professor and Chairman, Department of Obstetrics and Gynecology, Brody School of Medicine, East Carolina University, Greenville, North Carolina
Postpartum Care and Breast-Feeding

JENNIFER R. NIEBYL, M.D.

Professor and Head, Department of Obstetrics and Gynecology, University of Iowa College of Medicine, Iowa City, Iowa
Preconception and Prenatal Care: Part of the Continuum; Occupational and Environmental Causes of Birth Defects; Drugs in Pregnancy and Lactation

ERROL R. NORWITZ, M.D., Ph.D.

Assistant Professor, Harvard Medical School; Attending Perinatologist, Division of Maternal-Fetal Medicine, Department of Obstetrics and Gynecology, Brigham and Women's Hospital, Boston, Massachusetts
Labor and Delivery

CATHERINE OTTO, M.D.

Professor, Division of Cardiology, Department of Medicine, University of Washington, Seattle, Washington
Cardiac Disease and Critical Care

KATHRYN L. REED, M.D.

Professor, Department of Obstetrics and Gyneology and Director of Ultrasound and Director of Maternal-Fetal Medicine, Arizona Health Sciences Center, Tucson, Arizona
Antepartum Fetal Evaluation; Intrauterine Growth Restriction

JOHN T. REPKE, M.D.

Chris J. and Marie A. Olson Professor of Obstetrics and Gynecology, and Chairman, Department of Obstetrics and Gynecology, University of Nebraska Medical Center, Omaha, Nebraska
Labor and Delivery

JULIAN N. ROBINSON, M.D.

Assistant Professor, and Attending Perinatologist, Division of Maternal-Fetal Medicine, Department of Obstetrics and Gynecology, Columbia-Presbyterian Medical Center, Columbia University, New York
Labor and Delivery

ADAM A. ROSENBERG, M.D.

Professor of Pediatrics, University of Colorado School of Medicine; Director of Nurseries, University of Colorado Hospital, Denver, Colorado
Delivery Room Management of the Neonate

PHILIP SAMUELS, M.D.

Associate Professor and Director of Residency Education Program, Department of Obstetrics and Gynecology, The Ohio State University College of Medicine and Public Health, Columbus, Ohio
  Renal Disease; Hematologic Complications; Collagen Vascular Diseases; Hepatic Disease; Neurologic Disorders

JOHN W. SEEDS, M.D.

Professor and Chairman, Department of Obstetrics and Gynecology, Virginia Commonwealth University, Medical College of Virginia Hospitals, Richmond, Virginia
  Malpresentations

BAHA M. SIBAI, M.D.

Professor and Chairman, Department of Obstetrics and Gynecology, University of Cincinnati College of Medicine; Chief of Obstetrics, University Hospital, Cincinnati, Ohio
  Hypertension in Pregnancy

JOE LEIGH SIMPSON, M.D.

Ernst W. Bertner Professor and Chairman, Department of Obstetrics and Gynecology, and Professor of Molecular and Human Genetics, Baylor College of Medicine, Houston, Texas
  Occupational and Environmental Causes of Birth Defects; Genetic Counseling and Prenatal Diagnosis; Fetal Wastage

ROXANNE STAMBUK, M.D., Ph.D.

Assistant Professor, Division of Dermatology, University of Southern California Keck School of Medicine; Attending Physician, Los Angeles County and University of Southern California Medical Center, Los Angeles, California
  Dermatologic Disorders

PHILLIP G. STUBBLEFIELD, M.D.

Professor and Chairman, Department of Obstetrics and Gynecology, Boston University School of Medicine; Director of Obstetrics and Gynecology, Boston Medical Center, Boston, Massachusetts
  Surgical Procedures in Pregnancy

JANICE E. WHITTY, M.D.

Associate Professor, Division of Maternal-Fetal Medicine, Department of Obstetrics and Gynecology, Wayne State University School of Medicine, Hutzel Hospital, Detroit, Michigan
  Pulmonary Disease

Preface

The second edition of our *Pocket Companion* has been written to accompany the fourth edition of our recently published textbook, *Obstetrics: Normal and Problem Pregnancies*. It has been prepared by the three editors to provide easy access to the most important clinical information contained in our textbook wherever patient care is being delivered. Readers of the first edition found it a valuable resource for review before seeing a complicated patient in the clinic, when writing admission orders on the antepartum unit, or discussing options for care during a telephone consultation. Like its predecessor, the second edition of our *Pocket Companion* includes a summary of important points at the end of each chapter, tables of ultrasound biometry, and the reference numbers from our textbook so that readers will be able to refer to the "big book" if they want to find the original sources. This second edition of the *Pocket Companion* does differ, however, in several ways. It contains three new chapters on fetal therapeutic interventions, surgical procedures in pregnancy, and endocrine diseases in pregnancy. It has also benefited from our experience with the first edition of the *Pocket Companion*. Each of us used the first edition in our own obstetric practices and made note of areas we thought needed more or less information. We also heard from readers who requested that additional material be included. Readers will note these changes, for example, in the chapters on labor and delivery, intrapartum fetal monitoring, prolonged pregnancy, and in a separate chapter on diabetes mellitus complicating pregnancy.

This second edition of our *Pocket Companion* would not have been possible without the outstanding chapters written by our contributors and the support of our publishers including Judith Fletcher and Ann Ruzycka at Elsevier Science.

Steven G. Gabbe, M.D.
Jennifer R. Niebyl, M.D.
Joe Leigh Simpson, M.D.

Notice about references

Please note that superscript reference numbers appearing throughout **Pocket Companion** refer to references in equivalent chapters of *Obstetrics: Normal and Problem Pregnancies* (fourth edition).

Contents

Prenatal Care

Chapter 1

Preconception and Prenatal Care: Part of the Continuum

TIMOTHY R. B. JOHNSON AND
JENNIFER R. NIEBYL

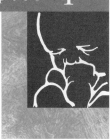

Prenatal care is an excellent example of preventive medicine. The goal of prenatal care is to help the mother maintain her well-being and achieve a healthy outcome for herself and her infant. Education about pregnancy, childbearing, and childrearing is an important part of prenatal care, as are detection and treatment of abnormalities. This process is best realized when begun even before pregnancy at a preconceptional visit. Another important component of prenatal care is establishment of gestational age.

PRENATAL CARE

The fetus has emerged as a patient in utero, and prevention of morbidity as well as mortality is now the goal. At the same time, pregnancy is basically a physiologic process, and the normal pregnant patient may not benefit from application of advanced technology.

There have been no prospective controlled trials demonstrating efficacy of prenatal care overall. However, many individual components have been shown to be effective (e.g., treatment with corticosteroids to prevent respiratory distress syndrome and screening for and treating asymptomatic bacteriuria for prevention of pyelonephritis).[27] In retrospective studies, however, patients with increased numbers of visits have improved maternal and fetal outcomes. This may be because of self-selection of patients for care who are motivated to take care of themselves in other ways, as women with no prenatal care often come from underprivileged socioeconomic groups.

PRECONCEPTIONAL EDUCATION

The best time to see a woman for prenatal care is when she is considering pregnancy. At gynecologic visits, patients should be asked about their plans for pregnancy. A visit with a negative pregnancy test should prompt scheduling a preconceptional visit. If there are questions about the history, such as family history of fetal anomaly or previous cesarean delivery, further details can be obtained from family members or the appropriate medical facility. This is the time to draw a rubella titer and immunize the susceptible patient. Varicella titers or immunization is recommended in women with no history of chickenpox. Toxoplasmosis screening may be indicated at this time. Hepatitis B immunization can be given to appropriate patients and human immunodeficiency virus (HIV) testing offered.

Before pregnancy is the time to screen appropriate populations for genetic disease carrier states such as Tay-Sachs disease, Canavan's disease, cystic fibroisis, or hemoglobinopathies.[34] Resolution of these issues is much easier and less hurried without the time limits placed by an advancing pregnancy. Medical conditions such as anemia, urinary tract infection, or hypothyroidism can be fully evaluated and the woman medically treated before pregnancy. If the patient is obese, weight reduction should be attempted before pregnancy.

For some conditions, such as diabetes mellitus and phenylketonuria, medical disease management before conception can positively influence pregnancy outcome. This is also the time to review drug usage and other practices, such as alcohol ingestion and smoking. Advice can be given about avoiding medications in the first trimester, and general advice can be given concerning diet, exercise, and occupational exposures.

Periconceptional supplements with folic acid can reduce the incidence of neural tube defects (NTDs). The CDC recommends that all women of childbearing age who are capable of becoming pregnant should consume 0.4 mg of folic acid daily, which is most easily achieved by taking a supplement. For women with a previously affected child, the recommendation is that the patient take 4 mg daily from 4 weeks before conception through the first 3 months of pregnancy.

THE INITIAL PRECONCEPTIONAL OR PRENATAL VISIT

Social and Demographic Risks

Extremes of age are obstetric risk factors. The pregnant teenager has particular nutritional and emotional needs. She is at special risk for sexually transmitted diseases; it has been shown that she benefits particularly from education in areas of childbearing and contraception. The pregnant woman over age 35 is at increased risk for a chromosomally abnormal child,[37] and she must be so advised. Patients should be asked about family histories of Down syndrome, neural tube defects, hemophilia, hemoglobinopathies, and other birth defects, as well as mental retardation. Consultation for genetic counseling and genetic testing, if desired, may be appropriate. The age of the father may be important, as there may be genetic risks to the fetus when the father is older than 55 years.[38] African-American patients should be screened for sickle cell disease; those of Jewish and French Canadian heritage should be screened for Tay-Sachs disease, Canavan's disease, and cystic fibrosis; and those of Mediterranean descent should be screened for β-thalassemia.

Low socioeconomic status should be identified and attempts to improve nutritional and hygienic measures undertaken. Appropriate referral to federal programs, such as that for women, infants, and children (WIC), and to public health nurses can have real benefits. If a patient has a history of previous neonatal death or stillbirth, records should be carefully reviewed so that the correct diagnosis is made and recurrence risk appropriately assessed.

Occupational hazards should be identified. Patients whose occupations require heavy physical exercise or excess stress should be informed that they may need to decrease such activity.

Tobacco, alcohol, and recreational drug use can all adversely affect pregnancy and are a critical part of the history. Specific questions concerning smoking, alcohol, and drugs (prescriptive, over-the-counter, and illicit) should be asked.[40] Screening for alcohol and substance use should be carried out using such tools as the T-ACE questionnaire (Table 1–1)[41]. Women should be urged to stop

Table 1–1. ALCOHOL ABUSE SCREENING: THE T-ACE QUESTIONNAIRE*

T	How many drinks does it take to make you feel "high" (can you hold)? (*tolerance*; a positive response consists of two or more drinks)
A	Have people *annoyed* you by criticizing your drinking?
C	Have you ever felt you ought to *cut down* on your drinking?
E	Have you ever had a drink first thing in the morning to steady your nerves or to get rid of a hangover (*eye-opener*)?

Scoring: The tolerance question has substantially more weight (2 points) than the three other questions (1 point each).

*These questions were found to be significant identifiers of risk drinking in pregnancy (i.e., alcohol intake potentially sufficient to damage the embryo/fetus).
From Sokol RJ, Martier SS, Ager JW: The T-ACE questions: practical prenatal detection of risk-drinking. Am J Obstet Gynecol 160:863, 1989, with permission.

smoking prior to pregnancy and to drink not at all or minimally once they are pregnant. Drug addiction confers a particularly high risk, and addicted mothers require specialized care throughout pregnancy.

Violence against women is increasingly recognized as a problem that should be addressed, with reports suggesting that abuse occurs during 3 to 8 percent of pregnancies. Questions addressing personal safety and violence should be included during the prenatal period.

Medical Risk

Family history of diabetes, hypertension, tuberculosis, seizures, hematologic disorders, multiple pregnancies, congenital abnormalities, and reproductive wastage should be elicited. A better history may be obtained if patients are asked to fill out a preinterview questionnaire or history form. Any significant maternal cardiovascular, renal, or metabolic disease should be defined. Infectious diseases such as urinary tract disease, syphilis, tuberculosis, or herpes genitalis should be identified. Surgical history with special attention to any abdominal or pelvic operations should be noted. A history of previous cesarean birth should include indication, type of uterine incision, and any complications. Allergies, particularly drug allergies, should be prominent on the problem list.

Obstetric Risk

Previous obstetric and reproductive history are essential to care in subsequent pregnancy, and the outcome for each prior pregnancy should be recorded in detail. Previous miscarriages not only confer risk and anxiety for another pregnancy loss but can increase the risk of genetic disease as well as preterm delivery.[44]

Previous preterm delivery is strongly associated with recurrence; it is important to delineate the events surrounding the preterm birth. Did the membranes rupture before labor? Were there painful uterine contractions? Was there bleeding? Were there fetal abnormalities? What was the neonatal outcome? Incompetent cervix and uterine anomalies are conditions that may be known from a previous pregnancy. Previous fetal macrosomia makes glucose screening essential.

After all the specific questions, it is recommended to ask the patient a few simple questions: What important items haven't I asked? What else about you and your pregnancy do I need to know? What problems and questions do you have? Leaving time for open-ended questions is the best way to complete the initial visit.

Physical and Laboratory Evaluation

Physical examination should include a general physical examination as well as a pelvic examination. Baseline height and weight as well as prepregnancy weight are recorded. Special attention should be given to the initial vital signs, cardiac examination, and reflexes, since many healthy young women have not had a physical examination immediately before becoming pregnant. Any physical finding that might have an impact on pregnancy (e.g., short cervix) or that might be affected by pregnancy (e.g., mitral valve prolapse) should be defined. It is particularly important to perform and record a complete physical examination at this initial visit, since less emphasis will be placed on nonobstetric portions of the examination as pregnancy progresses.

The pelvic examination should focus on the uterine size. Before 12 to 14 weeks, size can give a fairly accurate estimate of gestational age. Papanicolaou smear and culture for gonorrhea and chlamydia are done. The cervix should be carefully palpated, and any deviation from normal should be noted. Clinical pelvimetry should be performed and the clinical impression of adequacy noted. The pelvic examination is limited by examiner and patient variation as well as by obesity. If there is difficulty in examining the uterus, an ultrasound study is indicated.

Basic laboratory studies are routinely performed (Table 1–2).

Specific conditions will require further evaluation. A history of thyroid disease will lead to thyroid function testing. Anticonvulsant therapy requires blood level studies to determine adequacy of medication. Screening for varicella has been suggested for women with no known history of chickenpox.

The ACOG has recommended routine screening of all pregnant women for hepatitis B.[34] HIV screening should also be offered.

REPEAT PRENATAL VISITS

A plan of visits is outlined to the patient. This has been traditionally every 4 weeks for the first 28 weeks of pregnancy, every 2 to 3 weeks until 36 weeks, and weekly thereafter, if the pregnancy progresses normally. The Public Health Service[4] suggested that this number of visits can be decreased, especially in parous, healthy women. If there are any complications, the intervals can be decreased appropriately. For example, patients with hypertensive disease may require weekly visits.

If the patient is Rh negative and unsensitized, she should receive Rhesus immune globulin (RhIG) prophylaxis at 28 to 32 weeks. A glucose screening test for diabetes is also appropriately performed at this time (see Chapter 24),[48] and routine fetal movement counting can

Table 1–2. RECOMMENDATIONS FOR ALL WOMEN FOR PRENATAL CARE

	Preconception or First Visit	6–8*	14–16	24–28	32	36	38	39	40	41
Weeks										
History										
Medical, including genetic	X									
Psychosocial	X									
Update medical and psychosocial		X	X	X	X	X	X	X	X	X
Physical examination										
General	X									
Blood pressure	X	X	X	X	X	X	X	X	X	X
Height	X	X								
Weight	X	X	X	X	X	X	X	X	X	X
Height and weight profile	X									
Pelvic examination and pelvimetry	X	X								
Breast examination	X	X								
Fundal height			X	X	X	X	X	X	X	X
Fetal position and heart rate			X	X	X	X	X	X	X	X
Cervical examination	X									
Laboratory tests										
Hemoglobin or hematocrit	X	X		X		X				
Rh factor, type blood	X									
Antibody screen	X			X						

Pap smear	x				
Diabetic screen				x	
MSAFP, HCG, Estriol			x		
Urine					
Dipstick	x				
Protein	x				
Sugar	x				
Culture		x			
Infections					
Rubella titer	x				
Syphilis test	x				
Gonococcal culture	x	x			
Hepatitis B	x				
HIV (offered)	x	x			
Toxoplasmosis	x				
Illicit drug screen (offered)	x				
Genetic screen	x				x

*If preconception care has preceded.
MSAFP, maternal serum α-fetoprotein; HIV, human immunodeficiency virus.

begin using a organized system.[49] At 36 weeks, a repeat hematocrit, especially in those women with anemia or at risk for peripartum hemorrhage (multipara, repeat cesarean), may be performed. Also, appropriate cultures for sexually transmitted disease (gonorrhea, chlamydia) should be obtained as indicated in the third trimester.

After 41 weeks from the last menstrual period, the patient should be entered into a screening program for fetal well-being, which may include electronic monitoring tests or ultrasound evaluation (see Chapter 21).

INTERCURRENT PROBLEMS

It is the practice in prenatal care to evaluate the pregnant patient for the development of certain complications. If a patient shows a tendency to blood pressure elevation at 28 weeks, for example, she should be seen again in a week, not a month. Development of hypertension must be recognized and evaluation and hospitalization appropriately instituted.

Weight gain in pregnancy has been shown to be an important correlate of fetal weight gain and is therefore closely monitored. Too little weight gain should lead to an evaluation of nutritional factors and an assessment of associated fetal growth. Excess weight gain is one of the first signs of fluid retention, but it may also reflect increased dietary intake or decreased activity. Dependent edema is physiologic in pregnancy, but generalized or facial edema can be a first sign of disease.

Proteinuria reflects urinary tract disease, generally either infection or glomerular dysfunction, possibly the result of preeclampsia. Urinary tract infection should be looked for, and the degree of protein quantitated in a 24-hour urine collection.

Growth restriction and macrosomia can often be suspected clinically, usually on the basis of an abnormality in fundal growth.

Nutrition

One of the earliest purposes of prenatal care was to counsel and ensure that women received adequate nutrition for pregnancy. The health care provider may be influential in correcting inappropriate dietary habits.[50] Strict vegetarians may need supplemental vitamin B_{12}. Occasionally, consultation with a registered dietitian may be necessary when there is poor compliance or a special medical need such as diabetes mellitus.

The U.S. Department of Agriculture has published the food guide pyramid.[51] Americans are encouraged to eat 6 to 11 servings per day of bread, cereal, rice, and pasta; three to five servings per day of vegetables; two to four servings per day of fruit; two to three servings per day of milk, yogurt, and cheese; and two to three servings per day of meat, poultry, fish, beans, eggs, and nuts. Fats, oils, and sweets should be used sparingly. Pregnant women need three servings per day of dairy products, a serving being a cup of milk or yogurt, 1 1/2 oz of natural cheese, or 2 oz processed cheese.

Recommended dietary allowances (RDAs) for most substances increase during pregnancy. According to the 1989 RDAs, only the recommendations for iron, folic acid, and vitamin D double during gestation.[52] The RDA for calcium and phosphorus increase by one half; the RDA for pyridoxine and thiamine increase by about one third. The RDA for protein, zinc, and riboflavin increase by about one fourth. The RDA for all other nutrients except vitamin A increase by less than 20 percent and vitamin A not at all. All of these nutrients, with the exception of iron, are supplied by a well-balanced diet.

The National Academy of Sciences currently recommends that 30 mg of ferrous iron supplements be given to pregnant women daily, since the iron content of the habitual American diet and the iron stores of many women are not sufficient to provide the increased iron required during pregnancy. For those at high nutritional risk, such as some adolescents, those with multiple gestation, heavy cigarette smokers, and drug and alcohol abusers, a vitamin/mineral supplement should be given. Increased iron is needed both for the fetal needs and for the increased maternal blood volume. Thus, iron-containing foods should also be encouraged. Iron is found in liver, red meats, eggs, dried beans, leafy green vegetables, whole-grain enriched bread and cereal, and dried fruits. The 30-mg iron supplement is contained in approximately 150 mg of ferrous sulfate, 300 mg of ferrous gluconate, or 100 mg of ferrous fumarate. Taking iron between meals will facilitate its absorption.

Weight Gain

The total weight gain recommended in pregnancy is 25 to 35 lb for normal women.[54] Underweight women may gain up to 40 lb, and overweight women should limit weight gain to 15 to 25 lb.

If the patient does not show a 10-lb weight gain by midpregnancy, her nutritional status should be reviewed. Inadequate weight gain is associated with an increased risk of a low-birth-weight infant. Inadequate weight gain seems to have its greatest effect in woman who are of low or normal weight before pregnancy. Patients should be cautioned against weight loss during pregnancy. Total weight gain in the obese can be modified downward to 15 lb, but less weight gain is associated with an increased risk of intrauterine growth restriction.

When excess weight gain is noted, an assessment for fluid retention is also performed. In the assessment of edema, some dependent edema in the legs is normal as pregnancy advances because of venous compression by the weight of the uterus. Elevation of the feet and bed rest on the left side will help correct this problem. Turning the patient from her back to her left side increases venous return from the legs as the pressure on the vena cava is relieved. This maneuver increases the effective circulating blood volume, cardiac output, and thus the blood flow to the kidney. A diuresis will follow as well as increased blood flow to the uterus.

Activity and Employment

Most patients are able to maintain their normal activity levels in pregnancy. Mothers tolerate pregnancy with considerable physical activity, such as looking after small children, but heavy lifting and excessive physical activity should be avoided. Recreational exercises should be encouraged, such as those available in prenatal exercise classes. The patient should be counseled to discontinue activity whenever she experiences discomfort.

Healthy pregnant women may work until their delivery. Strenuous physical exercise, standing for prolonged periods, and work on industrial machines may be associated with increased risk of poor pregnancy outcome, and these should be modified.

Travel

The patient should be advised against prolonged sitting during car or airplane travel because of the risk of venous stasis and possible thromboembolism. The usual recommendation is stopping at least every 2 hours for 10 minutes to allow the patient to walk around and increase venous return from the legs.

The patient should be instructed to wear her seat belt during car travel, but under the abdomen as pregnancy advances. Most U.S. airlines allow flying up to 36 weeks of gestation.

Nausea and Vomiting in Pregnancy

Nonpharmacologic measures are usually recommended initially to treat nausea and vomiting in early pregnancy. Patients should avoid eating greasy or spicy foods. In addition, frequent small feedings in order to keep some food in the stomach at all times is helpful. A protein snack at night is advised, and the patient is instructed to keep crackers at her bedside so that she can have these before arising in the morning. Drug therapy for nausea in pregnancy is covered in Chapter 3.

Heartburn

Heartburn is a common complaint in pregnancy because of relaxation of the esophageal sphincter. The patient should be advised to save part of her meal for later if she is experiencing postprandial heartburn and also not to eat immediately before lying down. Liquid antacids coat the esophageal lining more effectively than do tablets.

Hemorrhoids

Hemorrhoids are varicose veins of the rectum. Since straining during bowel movements contributes to their aggravation, avoidance of constipation is preventive, and prolonged sitting should also be avoided. Hemorrhoids will often regress after delivery.

Constipation

Constipation is physiologic during pregnancy with decreased bowel transit time, and the stool may be hardened. Dietary modification with increased bulk such as with fresh fruit and vegetables and plenty of water can usually help this problem. Constipation is aggravated by the addition of iron supplementation; if dietary measures are inadequate, patients may require stool softeners. Additional dietary fibers such as Metamucil (psyllium hydrophilic muciloid) or surface-active agents such as Colace (docusate) are recommended. Laxatives are rarely necessary.

Urinary Frequency

Often during the first 3 months of pregnancy, the growing uterus places increased pressure on the bladder. Urinary frequency usually will improve as the uterus rises out of the pelvis by the second trimester. However, as the head engages near the time of delivery, urinary frequency may return as the head presses against the bladder. If the patient experiences pain with urination, it is appropriate to check for infection.

Round Ligament Pain

Frequently, patients will notice sharp groin pains caused by spasm of the round ligaments associated with movement. This is more frequently felt on the right side as a result of the usual dextrorotation of the uterus. The pain may be helped by local heat or acetaminophen. Modification of activity with gradual rising and sitting down and avoidance of sudden movement will decrease problems with this type of pain.

Syncope

Compression of the veins in the legs from the advancing size of the uterus places patients at risk of venous pooling associated with prolonged standing. Measures to prevent this possibility include wearing support stockings and exercising the calves to increase venous return. In later pregnancy, patients may have problems with supine hypotension, a distinct problem when undergoing a medical evaluation or an ultrasound examination. A left lateral tilt position with wedging below the right hip will help keep the weight of the pregnancy off the inferior vena cava.

Backache

Backache can be prevented to a large degree by avoidance of excessive weight gain. Exercises to strengthen back muscles can also be helpful. Posture is important, and sensible shoes, not high heels, should be worn.

Sexual Activity

No restriction need generally be placed on sexual intercourse. For women at risk for preterm labor or with a history of previous pregnancy loss avoidance of sexual activity may be recommended.

Breast-Feeding

During prenatal visits, the patient should be encouraged to breast-feed her infant (see Chapter 16). Human milk is the most appropriate nutrient for human infants and also provides significant immunologic protection against infection. Infants who are breast-fed have a lower incidence of infection and require fewer hospitalizations than do infants who are fed formula. The reasons a woman decides to bottle-feed should be explored, as they may be based on a misconception.

Working outside the home need not be a contraindication to breast-feeding. Many women with careers are now finding time to breast-feed their infants. Women should be aware that alternative ways of breast-feeding can be used to correspond with their work schedules. They can decrease the frequency of lactation to a few times a day in most cases and still continue to nurse. Other women may pump their breasts at work, leaving milk for the child's caretaker during the day and thus providing breast milk to the infant even more frequently. The milk may be refrigerated and is safe to use for 24 hours. For a longer duration, the milk should be frozen. Because freezing and thawing destroy the cellular content, fresh milk is preferred.

There is no need for specific nipple preparation during pregnancy. Soap and drying agents should not be used on the nipples, which should be washed only with water.

Preparation for Childbirth

Childbirth education and consumerism focus on the quality of the child and of the perinatal experience. Prepared childbirth can have a beneficial effect on performance in labor and delivery.[61,62]

ASSESSMENT OF GESTATIONAL AGE

The establishment of an estimated date of delivery and confirmation of that date by accumulation of supportive information remains one of the most important tasks of good prenatal care.

Human pregnancy has a duration of 280 days, measured from the first day of the last menstrual period (LMP) until delivery. The standard deviation is 14 days. Clinicians measure menstrual weeks (not conceptional weeks) with an assumption of ovulation and conception based on day 14 of a 28-day cycle. This gives pregnancy the 40-week gestational period in common clinical use. Confusion exists among patients who try to measure pregnancy in terms of 9 months (40/4 = 10) or who try to measure in conceptional weeks. It is helpful to explain to patients and their families that their pregnancy will be described in terms of weeks, rather than months, and that the pregnancy can be broken into three trimesters lasting 1 to 14 weeks, 14 to 28 weeks, and 28 weeks to delivery. The commonly used term "4 months pregnant" has no meaning (one does not know whether this is 16 or 20 weeks) and has no place on a contemporary prenatal record.

Clinical Dating

The most reliable clinical estimator of gestational age is an accurate LMP. Using Naegele's rule, the estimated date of confinement is calculated by subtracting 3 months and adding 1 week from the first day of the LMP. A careful history must be taken from the patient verifying that the date given is the first day of the period as well as whether the period was normal, heavy, or light. The date of the previous menstrual period will help ascertain the length of the cycle. History should also be taken about previous use of oral contraceptives, which might influence ovulation.

The size of the uterus on early pelvic examination, or by direct measurement of the abdomen from the pubic symphysis to the top of the uterine fundus (over the curve), provides useful information. Fundal height measurement in centimeters using the over-the-curve technique approximates the gestational age from 16 to 38 weeks within 3 cm.

In the first pregnancy, quickening, the first perception of fetal movement by the mother, occurs at about 19 weeks; in subsequent pregnancies, probably because of the experience of the observer, it tends to occur about 2 weeks earlier.[63]

Audible fetal heart tones, in addition to being absolute evidence of pregnancy, are another marker of gestational age. Using an unamplified Hillis-DeLee fetoscope, they are generally audible at 19 to 20 weeks.[48]

Use of the electronic Doppler device is widespread and permits detection of the fetal heart by 10 to 12 weeks. If fetal heart tones are not heard at the expected time, an ultrasound is appropriate.

Ultrasound

Ultrasound plays a major role in assessment of size and duration of pregnancy. The National Institutes of Health (NIH) consensus conference in 1984 concluded that in a low-risk pregnancy followed from the first trimester, routine ultrasound examination was not justified for determining gestational age. However, a long list of indications justify an ultrasound examination.[65]

A randomized trial has shown that the risk of being called overdue was reduced from 8 percent to 2 percent for patients who received early ultrasound.[66] Also, twins were detected more often and perinatal mortality was reduced in the ultrasound group. The Routine Antenatal Diagnostic Imaging with Ultrasound (RADIUS) study reported no improvement in perinatal outcome with use of routine ultrasound in normal, low-risk women.[67,68] However, 61 percent of women were excluded for many reasons such as an uncertain menstrual history, and only 35 percent of anomalies were detected in the ultrasound-screened group (only 17 percent before 24 weeks). A meta-analysis[69] indicated that routine scanning can detect many more anomalies. The authors' practice is to perform ultrasound at 16 to 20 weeks for a baseline gestational age measurement and as a screening for fetal abnormality or multiple gestation. If ultrasound is not done routinely, the caregiver must be vigilant in detecting problems that are indications for a scan.

Ultrasound is an accurate means of estimating gestational age in the first half of pregnancy.[70] The crown-rump length, biparietal diameter, and femur length in the first half of pregnancy correlate closely with age. As pregnancy progresses, fetal size varies considerably, and measurement of the fetus is a poor tool for estimation of gestational age, especially in the third trimester (see Chapter 5).

Key Points

➤ Preconceptional evaluation should include rubella testing, hepatitis testing, and possibly toxoplasmosis and HIV testing, in addition to medical and family history.

➤ Preconceptional supplementation with folic acid can reduce the incidence of NTDs and other defects. All women of childbearing age should consume 0.4 mg of folic acid daily. Women who have had a child previously affected by an NTD should take 4 mg daily from 4 weeks before conception through the first 3 months of pregnancy.

➤ The triple screen (α-fetoprotein, hCG, and estriol) can detect women younger than 35 years of age at increased risk for chromosomal abnormalities.

➤ The number of prenatal visits can be decreased safely in healthy parous women.

➤ The total weight gain recommended for healthy women is 25 to 35 lb. Underweight women may gain up to 40 lb, and overweight women should limit weight gain to 15 to 25 lb.

➤ Bed rest on the side increases venous return from the legs, as pressure on the vena cava is relieved. This maneuver increases the effective circulating blood volume, cardiac output and, thus, the blood flow to the kidney. A diuresis follows, as well as increased blood flow to the uterus.

Box continued on following page

Key Points *Continued*

➤ The pregnant woman should be advised against prolonged sitting during car or airplane travel because of the risk of venous stasis and possible thromboembolism.

➤ For infant nutrition, breast is best.

➤ Ultrasound evaluation between 16 and 20 weeks allows accurate assessment of gestational age and screening for fetal abnormality and multiple gestation.

Chapter 2

Occupational and Environmental Causes of Birth Defects

JOE LEIGH SIMPSON AND
JENNIFER R. NIEBYL

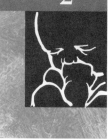

Prenatal environmental influences can act maternally and cause adverse fetal development. The focus in this chapter is on structural malformations (birth defects), but some attention is paid to aberrations in behavior and to other adverse reproductive outcomes. Agents that produce such deleterious effects are called teratogens. A teratogen is a substance, organism, or physical agent capable of causing abnormal development. A teratogen can cause abnormalities of structure or function, growth restriction, or death of the organism. Prior to surveying known environmental teratogen, it is important to consider the principles of abnormal development (teratogenesis).

BASIC PRINCIPLES OF TERATOLOGY

Six general principles of teratalogy can be delineated. These apply both to environmental toxins as well as medications (Chapter 3) and infectious agents.

Genotype and Interaction with Environmental Factors

The first principle is that susceptibility to a teratogen depends on the *genotype of the conceptus* and on the manner in which the genotype interacts with environmental factors.

Timing of Exposure

The second principle is that susceptibility of the conceptus to teratogenic agents varies with the developmental stage at the time of exposure. It is during the second to the eighth weeks of development after conception—the embryonic period—that most structural defects occur.

This chapter substantially reflects the contribution in the previous edition by Lowell E. Sever and Mary Ellen Mortensen.

Mechanisms of Teratogenesis

The third principle is that teratogenic agents act in specific ways *(mechanisms)* on developing cells and tissues in initiating abnormal embryogenesis (pathogenesis).

Manifestations

Irrespective of the specific deleterious agent, the final manifestations of abnormal development are death, malformation, growth restriction, and functional disorder. The observed effect is thought to depend largely on the stage of development at which exposure occurs; a teratogen may have one effect if exposure occurs during embryogenesis and another if the exposure is during the fetal period. Embryonic exposure is likely to lead to structural abnormalities or embryonic death; fetal exposure is likely to lead to functional deficits or growth restriction.

Agent

The fifth principle is that access of adverse environmental influences to developing tissues depends on the nature of the influence *(agent)*. This principle relates to such pharmacologic factors as maternal metabolism and placental passage. For an adverse effect to occur, an agent must reach the conceptus, by being transmitted indirectly through maternal tissues or by directly traversing the maternal body.

Dose Effect

Manifestations of abnormal development increase in degree from the no-effect level to the lethal level as *dosage* increases. Thus, the response (e.g., malformation, growth restriction) may be expected to vary according to the dose, duration, or amount of exposure. For most human teratogens, data regarding in utero exposure to ionizing radiation clearly show the importance of dose on observed effects.[6]

ANIMAL MODELS FOR THE STUDY OF HUMAN TERATOGENS

Premarket testing of drugs and food additives involves animal testing to determine potential teratogenicity. Although important in recognizing potential reproductive toxicants and teratogens, such studies have a number of significant limitations. Extrapolation from animal data may or may not be relevant to human exposures to an agent because of interspecies differences in metabolism, end-organ response, transport across the placenta, and sensitivity of fetal structures, to name a few. For example, humans and rabbits are sensitive to the teratogenic effect of thalidomide, but rats are relatively insensitive.[9] There are also problems extrapolating from high doses to low doses, as most teratologic experiments involve exposure at high doses. Human exposures typically involve lower doses. Yet the oft-made assumption that teratogenic risk is identical at high- and low-dose exposures (e.g., linearity of dose-response) may not be true. Thus, is not surprising that there is little or no evidence for human teratogenicity at low doses for many substances teratogenic in animals at high doses (e.g., arsenic and some solvents).[10]

While teratologic testing of drugs and chemicals in animals serves an extremely important public health function, it does not necessarily prevent exposure of pregnant women to teratogens. Two drugs shown to be human teratogens (isotretinoin [Accutane] and valproic acid [Depakene]) were known to be teratogenic based on animal studies, but it was only through human exposure that their teratogenicity in humans was established. Tens of thousands of chemicals have never been tested for reproductive toxicity or teratogenicity.[7] The limitations of animal testing and the immense number of potentially hazardous substances underscore the need for human studies, which often must be epidemiologic.

EPIDEMIOLOGIC APPROACHES TO THE STUDY OF BIRTH DEFECTS

There are three general categories of epidemiologic studies: descriptive, analytical, and experimental. The following discussion briefly considers some of the major features of these study designs, relating them to studies of birth defects and other adverse reproductive outcomes.

Descriptive Epidemiology

Case Reports

Most known teratogens and reproductive toxicants have been identified through case reports of an unusual number of cases or a constellation of abnormalities. These have often come from astute clinicians, who observed something out of the ordinary.[22-24] Although the importance of astute observations of abnormal aggregations of cases or patterns of malformations must be recognized, we cannot rely on such methods for identifying health hazards. Furthermore, etiologic speculations based on case reports or case series usually do not lead to a causal agent and are often false-positive speculations. Whereas case reports may identify a new teratogen, they can never provide an estimate of the risk of disease after exposure.

Descriptive Studies

Descriptive epidemiologic studies can be used to provide information about the distribution and frequency of some outcome of interest, resulting in rates of occurrence that can be compared among populations, places, or times.

Descriptive studies determine rates so that they can be compared. Possible differences in case ascertainment methods must be kept in mind.

Surveillance Programs

In surveillance programs, an at-risk population is identified and then followed over time to detect outcomes of interest. As they occur, cases are included in the database. Surveillance programs provide rates that can be examined for changes over time. They develop baseline data and subsequently permit early recognition of potential problems, based on ongoing data collection and analysis.

Birth defect surveillance (monitoring) systems (BDMSs) are designed to identify cases occurring in a defined population, usually by reviewing vital records or hospital record abstracts or charts. The defined population often is a sociopolitical unit, such as a state, but some monitoring programs have been based on discharge data from particular groups of hospitals or births to women residing in a specified metropolitan area.

In the last 20 years, there has been a dramatic increase in the number of state-based birth defect surveillance systems. Approximately half the states have some type of birth defect surveillance system.[28]

Analytical Epidemiology

Analytical epidemiologic studies are designed to generate or test hypotheses about associations between exposures and outcomes. Such associations can be examined at either the group or individual level.

Ecologic Studies

Ecologic studies are important for generating hypotheses about the causes of an outcome such as a birth defect. In such studies, occurrence rates for an outcome are compared between groups thought to differ in terms of some exposure. Studies of this type do not collect information about exposures of individuals and are often used in environmental epidemiology, where residence in a particular area is used as an indicator of exposure. Lack of specific individual exposure data can be a critical limitation of this study design.

Examples include studies of congenital malformations in communities with vinyl chloride production facilities[33,34] and in communities with solvent-contaminated drinking water.[35] Ecologic studies often lead to hypotheses that can be tested using other study designs.

Case-Control Studies

In a case-control study design groups of individuals with some outcome or disease of interest (cases) are compared to controls with regard to a history of one or more exposures, is the one most widely used in reproductive outcomes research. The controls are individuals as similar as possible to the cases, except that they are without the outcome of interest.

After cases and controls have been identified, the hypothesis to be tested is whether these two groups differ in exposure as well as outcome.

An advantage of case-control studies in testing etiologic hypotheses is that they are applicable to outcomes of infrequent occurrence, and can be conducted relatively rapidly and inexpensively. A disadvantage is that they have a potential for several important types of bias, including bias in recalling exposure, in selecting appropriate controls, and in ascertaining cases. The latter problem can be addressed in part by use of two control groups, one "normal" and the second "abnormal." Any of several abnormal controls seem equally useful, for example, infants with mendelian disorders as well as infants with no specific malformation.[36] In the former, mothers have incentive to recall but teratogenesis is not the etiology.

Most human studies of potential teratogens following descriptive studies have been case-control studies.

Cohort Studies

Cohort studies use the reverse approach from case-control studies; individuals who differ in exposure history are examined for differences in the occurrence of outcomes of interest. The groups are defined by the presence or absence of exposure to a given factor and then are followed over time and compared for rates of occurrence (i.e., incidence rates) of the outcome of interest.

Cohort studies have three advantages: (1) the cohort is classified by exposure before the outcome is determined, thereby eliminating the exposure recall bias; (2) incidence rates can be calculated among those exposed; and (3) multiple outcomes can be observed simultaneously.

Cohort studies, often called *prospective studies,* require that groups differing in exposure be followed through time, with outcomes observed. Therefore, these studies tend to be time consuming and expensive. In addition, since occurrence rates for many adverse reproductive outcomes, such as congenital malformations, are low, large samples must be followed for long periods of time. Two main types of cohort studies have been developed: (1) those that identify a cohort and follow it into the future (concurrent cohort study), and (2) those that identify a cohort at some time in the past and follow it to the present (nonconcurrent cohort study).

Numerous studies of reproductive outcome have been conducted by the noncurrent cohort approach. These studies, also known as *historical prospective studies,* begin by identifying groups who differ in terms of some past exposure and follow them to the present and determine outcomes; exposure groups are defined before outcomes are known. A major advantage is that despite the prospective time frame, investigators do not have to follow the cohort into the future, waiting for events to occur. A disadvantage is that these studies require the ability to determine exposure status retrospectively.

Cohort studies enable investigators to calculate incidence rates that provide a measure of the risk of an outcome after the exposure. Risk in the exposed group can be compared with the risk in an unexposed group. Most frequently, the ratio of the incidence rate among the exposed to the rate among the unexposed is determined. This ratio, referred to as *relative risk,* is a measure of how much the presence of exposure increases the risk of the outcome.

Experimental Epidemiology

Clinical Trials

The most common experimental study design in epidemiology is the clinical trial, in which the efficiency of a prevention or treatment regimen is evaluated. Ideally, subjects are randomly assigned to different treatment groups. The individuals must be as similar as possible in terms of unknown factors that may affect the response before they are randomly assigned to the treatment groups and receive the different regimens.[45]

Experimental studies in epidemiology involve intervention as well as observation. They are limited, however, in what can be ethically tested, namely, treatment or preventive measures, rather than etiologic hypotheses.

Exposure Assessment

As a prerequisite to evaluating the reproductive hazards associated with an occupational or environmental agent, one must be able to measure or estimate exposure to potential hazards. A number of investigators have recently addressed the problems associated with this exposure assessment.[20,51-54]

Concerns in assessing occupational exposure can be categorized into three areas: defining and determining amount of exposure, timing of exposure, and problems of mixed exposures.[20] First are problems determining what a particular worker is exposed to and determining the amount of exposure. Workers often may not be aware of the chemical substances to which they are exposed. It is particularly difficult to determine exposures in studies of the ambient environment.

Timing of exposure is crucial in studies of reproductive outcome. Exposures must occur within a limited period to produce teratogenic effects. However, exposures can also be associated with mutational events altering germ cells. An agent suspected of causing an NTD could not be implicated as the cause of an infant's neural tube's failing to close if the mother had been exposed to the agent after the tube should have closed. Third, employees may be exposed to a variety of potentially hazardous substances, leading to difficulty in demonstrating that a specific substance is a reproductive hazard. Most occupational exposures are to more than one substance, and it may not be possible to determine the reproductive effects of one agent—often occupational groups rather than specific exposures are studied.

EXPOSURES THAT MAY LEAD TO ADVERSE REPRODUCTIVE OUTCOMES

Known human teratogens number about 30. To date, only two have caused human maldevelopment (cerebral palsy and mental retardation) as a result of environmental contamination: high-dose ionizing radiation and methylmercury. Agents suspected of being teratogens on the basis of animal studies and limited epidemiologic studies are more numerous. When these agents are found to be polluting the environment, there is justifiable concern about potential prenatal exposure and adverse reproductive effects (Table 2–1). The difficulty of demonstrating an association between an environmental hazard and any adverse reproductive outcome must be appreciated.[63]

Table 2–1. OCCUPATIONAL AND ENVIRONMENTAL AGENTS
THAT MAY BE ASSOCIATED WITH HUMAN ADVERSE
REPRODUCTIVE OUTCOMES

Agent	Outcome
Ionizing radiation	
Acute high-dose	Microcephaly, mental retardation, growth restriction
Chronic low-dose or before pregnancy	?Down syndrome
Methylmercury	Mental retardation, cerebral palsy, deafness, blindness, seizures (abnormal neuronal migration)
Mercury vapor	Cranial defects, spontaneous abortion, ?stillbirth
Lead	
High-dose	Infertility, spontaneous abortion, growth restriction, psychomotor retardation, seizures, stillbirth
Chronic low-dose	Lower IQ, cognitive impairment in speech and language, attention deficit
Polychlorinated biphenyls	
High-dose	Spontaneous abortion, low birth weight, neuroectodermal dysplasia (skin staining, natal teeth, dysplastic nails, developmental and psychologic deficits), abnormal bone calcification
Chronic low-dose	Lower birth weight, smaller head circumference, ?cognitive impairment
Polybrominated biphenyls	
Chronic low-dose	?Lower birth weight, ?smaller head circumference, ?cognitive impairment
Anesthetic gases	
Chronic low-dose	Spontaneous abortion
Birth defects	
Organic solvents	
Chronic high-dose	Developmental impairment, facial dysmorphism, growth restriction (similar to fetal alcohol embryopathy)
Chronic low-dose	Spontaneous abortion, CNS malformations, orofacial clefts

Ionizing Radiation

Acute High Dose

During the 1920s and 1930s, ionizing radiation was used to treat women with pelvic disease; soon afterward, it was identified as the first known environmental human teratogen.[67] Systematic studies of atomic bomb survivors in Japan showed that in utero exposure to high-dose radiation increased the risk of microcephaly and mental and growth **restriction** in the offspring.[6,68-71]

Studies of the Japanese survivors clearly show that distance from the hypocenter—the area directly beneath the detonated bomb— and the gestational age at the time of exposure were directly related to microcephaly and mental and growth restriction in the infant. Nine and 20 years after exposure, the greatest number of children with microcephaly and mental retardation and growth restriction were in the group exposed at 15 weeks' gestation or earlier. These findings contrast with those of children exposed in utero during the third trimester and whose mothers were farthest from the hypocenter at the time of exposure. Although teratogenic effects have been found in several organ systems of animals exposed to acute, high-dose radiation, no structural malformations other than those mentioned above have been reported among humans exposed prenatally.

Using data from animals and from outcomes of reported human exposures at various times during pregnancy, DeKaban[72] constructed a timetable for extrapolating acute, high-dose radiation (> 250 rad) to various reproductive outcomes in humans. Similarities between animal and known human effects support DeKaban's proposal.

Chronic Low Dose

Effects of chronic low-dose radiation on reproduction have not been identified in animals or humans. Increased risk of adverse outcomes was not detected among animals with continuous low-dose exposure (<5 rad) throughout pregnancy.[73]

Mutagenesis

Children exposed in utero to radiation from the atomic bomb were studied over several years for evidence of genetic damage, with no evidence for effects using six indicators: congenital malformations, stillbirths and neonatal death rates, birth weight, sex ratio at birth, anthropomorphic measurements during the first year of life, and mortality in offspring (F1 generation).[67,79-81]

In contrast to the atomic bomb follow-up studies, other investigations have found that mutagenic effects may occur when women are exposed prenatally to diagnostic radiation. These effects include altered sex ratios among the offspring—slightly more females than expected[82]—and abnormal karyotypes in spontaneously aborted fetuses.[83]

Mutagenic effects in the offspring of irradiated women may be manifested years after the birth of the infant. Compared with non-irradiated controls, the estimated risk of leukemia was increased 50 percent for children exposed in utero to radiation during maternal pelvimetry examinations.[84-86] Although this increase seems considerable, it translates into an approximate risk of 1 in 2,000 for exposed versus 1 in 3,000 for unexposed children. As Brent[73] points out, if one were to recommend that pregnancies be terminated whenever exposure from diagnostic radiation occurred because of the increased probability of leukemia in the offspring, 1,999 exposed pregnancies would have to be terminated to prevent a single case of leukemia.

Questions have been raised about potential risks to children associated with parental (paternal) occupational exposure to low-dose radiation.[87] A case-control study by Gardner et al.[88,89] in the area around the Sellafield Nuclear Facility in the United Kingdom found a statistically significant association between paternal preconception radiation dose and childhood leukemia risk. A similar association had been observed between paternal preconception radiation and risk in workers at the Hanford Nuclear Facility in the United States.[90] The finding regarding childhood leukemia risk is a particularly contentious issue, contradicting studies of the children born to atomic bomb survivors who do not show genetic effects, such as increased risks of childhood cancers.[81] A study in the vicinity of nuclear facilities in Ontario also failed to demonstrate an association between childhood leukemia risk and paternal preconception dose (exposure).[91]

Video Display Terminals

In the 1980s, there was concern about video display terminals (VDTs) linked to adverse reproductive outcomes. Much of the early concern grew out of reports of spontaneous abortion clusters among groups of women who used VDTs at work, and some of the reported clusters also included birth defects.[92] While it was suggested that these "unexpected" clusters were actually expected based on the frequency of occurrence of spontaneous abortions (10 to 15 percent of recognized pregnancies) and the extremely large number of women working with VDTs,[93] several large epidemiologic studies were carried out to examine the association.[94,95] Numerous papers have been published on this topic, along with a number of reviews.[56,92,93] Our interpretation of these studies is that VDT use does not increase the risk of adverse reproductive outcomes.

Organic Mercury—Methylmercury

Organic mercury compounds, such as methyl- or ethylmercury, can definitely produce teratogenic effects. Exposures are no longer common, but in the United States, methylmercury was once used as a fungicide. In the 1960s, U.S. production was halted because of the compound's recognized toxicity and bioaccumulation. Today exposure mainly occurs through the consumption of contaminated fish. Fish may become contaminated when organomercurials are present in water or when bacteria in water convert inorganic mercury to organic mercury, part of a complex environmental mercury cycle.[96]

The prototypic cases of methylmercury teratogenicity were discovered in 1959 after an epidemic of poisoning in Minamata, Japan. Infants exposed in utero showed neurologic damage with psychomotor retardation, seizures, cerebral palsy, blindness, and deafness.[97] In 1972, similar fetal effects were observed in Iraq after an epidemic of methylmercury poisoning.[98] In both epidemics, breast-fed infants had additional exposure through maternal milk.[97]

Methylmercury crosses the placenta easily and accumulates in embryonic and fetal tissues, particularly brain tissues, at concentrations exceeding those in the mother.[103,104] Methylmercury does not cause obvious structural malformations in humans; thus, the devastating effects are not apparent at birth and are manifested only as the child ages. The developing nervous system of the conceptus and infant is more sensitive to the toxic effects of organic mercury than that of the adult or older child,[97] and the infant of an asymptomatic mother can be affected severely.[98,101,105]

Little is known of the human effects of methylmercury at *low levels* of *exposure*. Minor neurologic differences, mainly brisker deep tendon reflexes, were found among native Quebec boys exposed in utero compared with boys who had no such exposure.[106] Nonhuman primates chronically treated with low-dose methylmercury were more likely to experience reproductive failure (nonconception, spontaneous abortion) than nontreated controls.[108] Prenatal exposure of nonhuman primates resulted in offspring with impaired visual recognition.

Mercury is an unusual element. At room temperature it is liquid, with a high vapor pressure, and vapor concentrations can rise rapidly to toxic concentrations in closed or poorly ventilated areas. The vapor is odorless and colorless, making it virtually nondetectable without special equipment.

Women theoretically at risk for exposure to mercury vapor work primarily in health-related occupations such as nursing, medicine, dentistry, and dental hygiene. For example, exposure may occur when dental amalgams are prepared and when thermometers or manometers are broken or mercury is spilled. More recently, encapsulated amalgam preparations and electronic methods for measuring blood pressure and temperature have been developed, and mercury exposure in medicine and dentistry in the United States has probably decreased.

To protect the developing conceptus, the recommendations are that women of childbearing age should not be exposed to vapor concentrations exceeding 0.01 mg/m^3.

Rowland[121] reviewed the reproductive effects of mercury vapor and presented data from studies of female dental assistants in California. Women who prepared 50 or more dental amalgams per week had a statistically insignificantly increased risk for spontaneous abortion. Women who prepared 30 or more amalgams a week in offices with poor mercury hygiene showed evidence of reduced fecundity. A detailed analysis of fecundity, assessed as time to pregnancy in this cohort of dental assistants, was published recently.[122] To our knowledge, there are no published data on congenital malformations among births to dental assistants in the United States.

Lead

Exposure to high levels of lead is known to cause embryotoxicity, growth restriction and mental retardation, increased perinatal mortality, and developmental disability.[123] Originally observed in the 19th Century, these adverse reproductive effects were seen when women in occupational settings were exposed to concentrations of lead in air that far exceeded levels allowable today. As a matter of historic interest, unscrupulous vendors sold pills containing lead as an abortifacient at the turn of the century.[124]

Sources of nonoccupational lead exposure commonly encountered by U.S. women are unlikely to result in detectable effects. Regulatory and public health efforts are directed at reducing preconceptional and prenatal exposure in order to reduce maternal-to-fetal lead transmission. Twenty-five years of public health efforts have produced a striking reduction in lead exposure in the United States. The average blood lead level has decreased to less than 20 percent of levels measured in the 1970s.

High lead concentration in maternal blood is associated with an increased risk of delivery of a small-for-gestational-age infant.[126] The frequency of preterm birth was also almost three times higher among women who had umbilical cord levels greater than or equal to 5.1 μg/dl, compared with those who had levels below that cutoff.

Because the nervous system may be more susceptible to the toxic effects during the embryonic and fetal periods than at any other time of life[104] and because maternal and cord blood lead concentations are directly correlated,[132] lead concentrations in blood should not exceed 25 µg/dl in women of reproductive age.[133] Ideally, the maternal blood lead level should be less than 10 µg/dl to ensure that a child begins life with minimal lead exposure. A dose-response relationship is strongly supported by numerous epidemiologic studies of children showing a reduction in IQ with increasing blood lead concentrations above 10 µg/dl. Of note, these studies measured blood lead concentrations over time (often 2 years or more) and reported averaged values. Other neurologic impairments associated with increased blood lead concentrations include attention deficit disorder ("hyperactivity"), hearing deficits, learning disabilities, and shorter stature. Thus, for public health purposes, childhood lead poisoning has been defined as a blood lead level of 10 µg/dl or higher.[134]

In occupational settings, federal standards mandate that women should not work in areas where air lead concentrations can reach 50 µg/cm³, since this may result in blood concentrations above 25 to 30 µg/dl.[135]

Lead screening of pregnant women is highly controversial and not presently recommended. Lead is mobilized from the maternal skeleton during pregnancy and the postpartum period.[140] In the absence of excessive exposure, most of the lead in blood comes from bone stores, and no intervention is available to reduce the blood lead.[141] Chelation therapy is potentially hazardous, and some agents are teratogenic.[142] On the other hand, screening could identify women who may benefit from environmental or other interventions to reduce their lead exposure.

The Phenoxy Herbicide 2,4,5-Trichlorophenoxyacetic acid and Dioxins/Agent Orange

These compounds are considered together because 2,3,7,8-tetra-chlorodibenzodioxin (TCDD or dioxin) and other chlorinated dibenzodioxins were produced as contaminants during production of the herbicide 2,4,5-trichlorophenoxyacetic acid (2,4,5-T).[143] This herbicide is no longer marketed in the United States, largely because of concerns about possible teratogenic and fetotoxic effects (seen after high doses are administered to animals during critical periods of organogenesis).[144]

Agent Orange, a defoliant used in Vietnam, was a mixture of herbicides, including 2,4,5-T. During the later years of the Vietnam War, public opinion against the ecologic effects of Agent Orange was fueled by reports of birth defects in South Vietnamese babies born to mothers who lived in areas where Agent Orange had been sprayed. The ensuing debate about the potential human teratogenicity of Agent Orange involved numerous federal agencies, and the use of 2,4,5-T containing any chlorodioxin contaminants was cancelled in 1970.[145]

Because 2,4,5-T contained small amounts of TCDD and since long-term human effects were unknown, the U.S. Public Health Service began an immense follow-up of Vietnam veterans. One portion of the study evaluated Vietnam veterans' risks of fathering infants with birth defects. The investigators concluded that "Vietnam veterans who had greater estimated opportunities for Agent Orange exposure did not seem to be at greater risk for fathering babies with all types of defects combined."[146] In a subsequent follow-up study, Vietnam and non-Vietnam veterans were interviewed regarding congenital malformations in their offspring. Although Vietnam veterans were more likely to report birth defects in their offspring, hospital records showed similar rates of birth defects for children born to both veteran groups.[147] In contrast, increased central nervous system (CNS), skeletal, and cardiovascular malformations and disease were reported among Australian Vietnam veterans.[148] This study was less rigorous than its American counterparts, since it was an unconventional case-control design and relatively few children had diagnoses confirmed by medical record review.

Overall, the data appear inadequate to support allegations of adverse reproductive outcomes following human exposure to the dioxin-contaminated herbicide, although this is a topic of continuing discussion.[145] The 1996 Institute of Medicine report concluded that "limited/suggestive evidence exists of an association between dioxin exposure in veterans and offspring they sired with spina bifida."[150] The strength of even this tenuous statement seems arguable to us.

Polychlorinated Biphenyls

Polychlorinated biphenyls (PCBs) were widely used in industry because of their thermal stability and heat transfer properties.[151] PCBs are also extremely stable and resistant to metabolic or biologic degradation and have become ubiquitous in the environment because of past dumping or disposal in unregulated landfills and failure to recycle. PCBs are highly lipid soluble, accumulate in fat, and can be found at high concentrations in the breast milk of women despite low concentrations in their blood.[152]

Two epidemics of cooking oil contamination provide evidence that high-dose PCBs are hazardous to human reproduction. In these epidemics, adults consumed cooking oil tainted with thermally degraded PCBs and developed a disease termed "Yusho" (in Japan) and "Yu-cheng" (in Taiwan). The disease was characterized by chloracne (an acneform rash), eyelid swelling and discharge, and skin hyperpigmentation.[156] Although PCBs alone are usually blamed for these and subsequent health problems, it is clear that heat-degradation products of PCBs (polychlorodibenzofurans [PCDEs] and polychlorinated quarterphenyls [PCQs]) contributed significantly to toxicity.[157,158] A follow up in 1999 compared 795 subjects exposed postnatal to 693 controls.[159] Lifetime prevalences in the former were increased for chloracne, abnormal nails, hyperkeratosis, skin allergy, goiter, headache, gum pigmentation, broken teeth, anemia in women, arthritis, and herniated intervertebral disks in men. For other medical conditions no differences were observed.

A teratogenic effect was observed as well, as reviewed by Jacobson and Jacobson.[155] High-dose transplacental exposure to the cooking oil resulted in congenital anomalies and low birth weight.[160] Skin and mucosal hyperpigmentation were the most often noted abnormalities.[160] Other anomalies included natal teeth, gingival hyperplasia, exophthalmos, skull calcifications, and delayed bone age.[160]

Compared with unexposed children, those exposed children with prenatal and/or breast milk exposure to the PCB/PCDF/PCQ-contaminated oil demonstrated delayed developmental milestones, psychological deficits, and behavioral abnormalities. Physical abnormalities included shorter stature, lighter weight, and epidermal disorders such as acne, hyperpigmentation, deformed nails, gingival hypertrophy, and tooth chipping.[161] Developmentally, cognitive impairment persisted up to age 7 years.[162] In aggregate, these findings suggest a neuroectodermal dysplasia due to combined effects of the PCBs and contaminants.[161]

In addition to the teratogenic effects, the contaminated oils led to excessive reproductive losses among exposed women. Increased risks for spontaneous abortion, stillbirth, and infant mortality were documented in follow-up study of a group of Taiwanese women.[163] Women exposed in 1979 reported more stillbirths (4.2 percent vs. 1.7 percent controls), more abnormal menstrual bleeding (16 percent vs. 8 percent), and more offspring dying during childbirth (10.2 percent vs. 6.1 percent).[164]

Low-Level PCB Exposure

Effects of high-level cooking oil contamination should be distinguished from those of ambient or low-level exposure to PCBs. Low-level PCB maternal exposure can occur throughout life by consumption of fish from PCB-contaminated waters as well as other dietary sources. Transplacental transfer of PCBs occurs,[165] but the largest dose is delivered to the nursing infant via breast milk.[152,166] Maternal exposure and PCB tranfer to nursing infants has resulted in justifiable concern about reproductive and developmental effects.

Maternal PCB exposure via fish consumption (defined as 11.8 kg of Lake Michigan fish in the 6 years before delivery), was reported to be associated with a slight decrease in infant birth weight (160 to 190 g) and head circumference, relative to unexposed controls.[167] Neonatal assessment of the same infants provides some evidence that at low concentrations, PCBs may be behavioral teratogens.[168] Short-term memory impairment noted in infancy persisted at 4 years of age only in those children whose cord blood PCB concentrations were in the top 5 percent of values for the cohort.[166] A later study on the Lake Michigan–exposed cases also showed a small decrease in IQ in children exposed to in utero.[169] The difference was 6.2 points in the most highly exposed group, and only one child was mentally retarded. Others have criticized this conclusion on grounds of the small observed difference and the relatively small subset of the original exposed sample available for study (potential selection bias).[170,171]

A cohort of North Carolina children followed since birth, representative of the general population and without unusual PCB exposure, have not demonstrated a relationship between prenatal or postnatal (breast-feeding) PCB exposure.

A Dutch cohort of children exposed 42 months earlier in utero reported that scores on the Kaufman Assessment Battery for Children were lowered by 4 points.[172,173]

Overall, the developmental effect of *low-level* PCB exposure remains unclear. Any deleterious effect is not substantive and potentially explainable on the basis of confounding variables.

Polybrominated Biphenyls

Polybrominated biphenyl (PBB) compounds are structurally similar to PCBs and share characteristics of high lipid solubility and resistance to metabolic or biologic degradation.

PBBs were used as fire-retardants in the United States until 1974. In 1973 and 1974, cattle feed distributed in Michigan inadvertently became contaminated with PBBs. Before the contamination was recognized, people in the state consumed PBB-tainted meat and poultry.

Transplacental and breast milk exposure of infants was documented in the Michigan incident.[181] An early follow-up study reported that children with higher PBB body burdens scored lower on standardized tests of perceptual motor, attentional, and verbal abilities.[182] Later testing of these children showed that their overall developmental scores were within the normal range.[183] Fetal mortality in high- versus low-exposure regions of Michigan was not appreciably different after the PBB contamination.[179]

Nitrates and Nitrite

Nitrate contamination of drinking water supplies may result from agricultural (fertilizer) run-off, sewerage, or industrial waste. Nitrates and nitrite appear not to be teratogenic in animals.[184,185]

Despite claims, human epidemiologic studies overall provide no conclusive evidence that pregnant women who consume low levels of nitrates from drinking water are at increased risk for having a malformed baby. In South Australia, an excess of birth defects prompted a case-control study examining the relationship between maternal drinking water source (groundwater vs. rainwater) and risk of malformations.[187] The risk of having a malformed infant was increased among women who drank groundwater. Using estimated nitrate concentration, a dose–response relationship was found with a threefold increased risk at 5 to 15 mg/L nitrates and fourfold nitrates. Study strengths include case ascertainment and monitoring of water nitrate concentrations during the study period. Limitations include the assumption that water concentrations were constant during monitoring intervals and that subjects used the same source of drinking water throughout pregnancy, and most notably the assumption that nitrates rather than some unmeasured drinking water contaminant was responsible. In fact, the seasonal variation in malformation risks suggests that dietary, nutritional, or other environmental factors were more likely to have contributed to the increased malformation rates.

In conclusion, toxic effects of nitrates on pregnant women and fetuses have not been studied extensively, but no adverse effects have been found. The Iowa Health Department guidelines state that no toxicity exists under 10 parts per million of nitrates. Above this, infants under 6 months of age could be at risk of methemoglobinemia.

Organic Solvents

Many women are employed in industries that use organic solvents, and women also may be exposed through use of household products or drinking water contamination. Not surprisingly, concerns have arisen that such exposures may cause any of several adverse reproductive outcomes.

High-Level Exposure

Well known human health effects of high-dose solvent exposure include the central nervous system of cortical atrophy, cerebellar degeneration, and loss of intellectual functioning. These observations have been documented following chronic, high-dose solvent abuse ("sniffing" or "huffing").[188] Solvent intoxication is also an established occupational hazard in such diverse groups as painters and rubber, semiconductor, and dry-cleaning workers. Symptoms may follow inhalation, dermal, or ingestion exposure routes and may include headache, nausea, dizziness, and confusion progressing to CNS depression with loss of consciousness. Chronic exposure to low levels of solvents may lead to neuropsychiatric impairment and peripheral nerve damage.[189]

Analogous to the health effects described above, maternal solvent abuse by "sniffing" is reported to cause an embryopathy similar to the fetal alcohol syndrome (FAS).

Low-Level Exposure

At lower levels of maternal exposure there is no clear evidence of embryopathic, fetal, or neurobehavioral adverse effects. Most occupational studies of this subject are case-control studies, with exposure status based on job descriptions and no actual exposure data available (e.g., air concentrations or duration of exposure). Multiple solvent exposures often are likely.[196]

Studies have supported an association between semiconductor manufacturing and spontaneous abortion risk. In a study of IBM employees, investigators from Johns Hopkins University reported an association between spontaneous abortion risk and working with ethylene glycol ethers in "clean rooms" (R.H. Gray, personal communication, 1993). Similarly, a study by investigators at the University of California, Davis, carried out for the Semiconductor Industry Association, found a significant increase in spontaneous abortion risk among fabrication workers. This increase was suggested to be associated with exposure to glycol ethers.[200]

Occupational exposure to organic solvents in the first trimester of pregnancy is also associated with an increased risk of major fetal malformation[201] (relative risk, 13.0; 95 percent confidence interval, 1.8 to 99.5). The risk is increased in women with symptoms associated with the exposure.[201]

On numerous occasions, drinking water contamination by organic solvents has resulted from storage tank leaks or hazardous waste leachate. Affected communities may identify a temporal or geographic clustering of adverse reproductive effects, believing that the contamination has caused the epidemic. To date, there is no published evidence to support such a cause-and-effect relationship, but at least one study demonstrated an increased risk of spontaneous abortions among women during the time that their drinking water supply was contaminated with trichloroethane and other organic solvents.[35]

In conclusion, toluene and possibly other organic solvents are probably teratogenic at high exposure levels seen with solvent abuse. The risk for the "fetal solvent syndrome" is unknown, and no exposure threshold for effect can be identified at this time. Occupational exposure to organic solvents in the first trimester is also associated with an increased risk of major fetal malformations,[204] especially in women with symptoms.

In a similar vein, when a pregnant woman asks if it is safe for her to paint the baby's nursery, Scialli[204] wisely advises counseling to minimize exposure without giving the impression that paint is an established developmental toxicant. Similar advice can be offered to women who want to color their hair, (e.g., recommending a well-ventilated area).

Anesthetic Gases

Large numbers of women working in medical and dental professions may be exposed occupationally to anesthetic gases, raising serious concerns about the reproductive hazards of such exposures. There is evidence that chronic first-trimester exposure may increase the risk of spontaneous abortion.[205,206] Despite numerous studies, the question of whether or not a mother's exposure to anesthetic gas increases the risk of her bearing a congenitally malformed infant is still debated.

Virtually all epidemiologic studies of exposure to waste anesthetic gas and reproductive outcomes have design problems that affect the interpretation of reported results. Crude estimates of anesthetic gas exposure have been used because no actual measurements of gas concentrations were available. The specific gases were usually not identified, and exposure to mixtures of anesthetic agents is likely.[206] Many studies have been conducted by survey, with no validation of the responses and, often, poor response rates. In such studies, selection bias cannot be evaluated because there is no information about nonresponders. Study subjects may forget or inaccurately recall events that took place years before. Women who think they are exposed to an adverse environmental agent may be more likely to recall having a spontaneous abortion or a child with a minor malformation than are unexposed women.[219] One last problem pertains to the inherent difficulty of studying spontaneous abortions.

Despite problems in study design, epidemiologic evidence supports the view that it is prudent to minimize repeated maternal exposure to waste anesthetic gases during pregnancy. Women who work in areas with a potential for repeated anesthetic gas exposure (no gas scavenger system in place) should be aware of the possibility of adverse reproductive effects and decide whether they want to continue to work in the same area during pregnancy or request to be transferred. In settings where anesthetic gases are administered, a gas scavenger system should be used, and particular attention must be given to maintaining that system. A properly functioning gas scavenging system should provide adequate protection from exposure.[206,222,223] Given uncertainty about completely avoiding exposure to anesthetic gases, a woman with a history of pregnancy loss or having a child with congenital malformations may want to transfer to another work area.[211]

Environmental Contamination and Hazardous Waste Sites

The role of environmental contamination in causing birth defects is controversial and the data are equivocal. Much of the concern focused around specific hazardous waste sites such as Love Canal, New York, and Woburn, Massachusetts. Studies at Love Canal showed an effect on birth weight[224-226] but no increased risk of congenital malformations. A study at Woburn suggested increased risks of selected birth defects associated with consumption of water from specific wells that had been contaminated with volatile organic compounds.[227] The original Woburn study has been criticized on methodologic grounds,[228] and recently completed studies by the Massachusetts Department of Public Health failed to show elevated birth defect risks.[229]

Three recent studies examined residential proximity to hazardous waste sites, as surrogates for exposure, and the risk of birth defects. One of the studies received considerable press coverage.

This was the study of Geschwind et al.[31], who examined birth defect cases from the New York State Congenital Malformation Registry based on proximity to hazardous waste sites. Cases and controls came from 20 counties in upstate New York, and information on exposure to hazardous waste sites was based on geographic proximity to sites included in a large database. Statistically significant associations were observed between hazardous waste sites and all birth defects combined and several groups of birth defects (nervous system, musculoskeletal system, and skin). Statistically significant associations were also observed between specific types of contaminants and some types of birth defects: pesticides and musculoskeletal system; metals and nervous system; solvents and nervous system; and plastics and chromosomal anomalies. Notably, the observed increases in risk were for the most part small, control of confounding was minimal, there was considerable heterogeneity within the birth defect categories, and the methods used to assign exposure were subject to exposure misclassification.

Dolk et al.[231] generated systematic data from seven research centers in five European countries. The seven centers maintained population-based registries of congenital anomalies as part of the EUROCAT Network. Among those within 7 km of a landfill site a total of 1,089 pregnancies with nonchromosomal anomalies occurred; 2,366 control births occurred without malformation.

Next, the zone within 3 km was considered the exposed one, and in this zone there was a significantly increased risk for a congenital anomaly. The odds ratio (OR) for residence within 3 km of a landfill site was increased for neural-tube defects (OR, 1.86) cardiac septal defects (OR, 1.49), hypospadias (OR, 1.96), gastroschisis (OR, 3.19), and tracheoesophageal fistula (OR, 2.25); the former two were statistically significant. It was not possible to compare results among individual landfill sites, which obviously were heterogeneous as to composition.

CONCLUSION

Experimental studies in laboratory animals have identified a number of agents that are capable of causing abnormal development. While we know less about substances that are teratogenic in humans, a limited number of environmental and occupational agents have been identified as teratogens. There is increasing evidence that some chemicals found in the occupational setting or in the ambient environment may be reproductive or developmental toxicants. While some of this evidence is for associations between exposures and congenital malformations, our interpretation is that there is more evidence for spontaneous abortions associated with occupational exposures than for congenital malformations. Because spontaneous abortion is only one part of a spectrum of outcomes potentially associated with teratogenic exposures, agents that increase risks for spontaneous abortion could also increase risks for congenital malformations.

In the future it is hoped that refined exposure assessment and improved outcome ascertainment will enhance epidemiologic studies and help determine the extent to which occupational and environmental exposures may contribute to birth defects and other adverse reproductive outcomes. This is particularly the case for studies of environmental contamination in which residential location may be a poor surrogate for exposure. In the meantime, prenatal counseling about most occupational and environmental exposures requires reasoned judgment and interpretation of imperfect/imprecise animal and epidemiologic data.

Key Points

➤ Teratogens and high-dose occupational toxins cause not only structural birth defects but also intrauterine death, growth restriction, and functional abnormalities.

➤ Established principles of teratogenesis are recognized, and must be fulfilled in order to implicate an agent as a teratogen.

➤ Exposure to high-dose ionizing radiation during gestation causes microcephaly and mental retardation, but deleterious effects of low-dose exposures on the conceptus have not been identified.

➤ Prenatal exposure to metals, namely lead and mercury, has been shown to have adverse effects on the development and function of the central nervous system. Doses required for deleterious (teratogenic) effects are usually well above ambient exposures. Women in certain potential high-level exposure occupations may need to alter work practices during exposure.

➤ The herbicides dioxin and Agent Orange are unlikely to increase the frequency of birth defects in offspring subsequently sired by Vietnam war veterans exposed during combat, despite the politically charged nature of allegations.

➤ High doses of polychlorinated biphenyls (PCBs), once ingested in Taiwan through contaminated cooking oil, cause a recognizable pattern of abnormalities: postnatal and prenatal low birth weight, skin hyperpigmentation, and skull calcifications.

➤ Effects of low-dose PCB contamination, through environmental contamination (e.g., eating Great Lakes fish contaminated with PCBs) is uncertain; however, not even the largest alleged effect is more than a 6-point decrease in IQ.

➤ Organic solvent exposure in high doses (e.g., chronic "sniffing") causes teratogenic effects similar to the fetal alcohol syndrome; in lower level exposure (e.g., occupational), the risk is less, although some reports suggest an increased risk for spontaneous abortion.

Box continued on opposite page

Key Points *Continued*

➤ Occupational exposures to anesthetic gases have been associated with increased risks for spontaneous abortions and birth defects in some studies.

➤ Concerns have been raised about the reproductive and developmental effects of pregnancies near toxic waste sites. Reliable data are very difficult to generate, and the validity of claims for increased anomalies close to the site are still unclear.

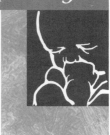

Chapter 3

Drugs in Pregnancy and Lactation

JENNIFER R. NIEBYL

Virtually all drugs cross the placenta to some degree, with the exception of large organic ions such as heparin and insulin. Approximately 25 percent of birth defects are known to be genetic in origin; drug exposure accounts for only 2 to 3 percent. Approximately 65 percent of defects are of unknown etiology but may be from combinations of genetic and environmental factors.

The incidence of major malformations in the general population is 2 to 3 percent.[1] A major malformation is defined as one that is incompatible with survival, requiring major surgery for correction, or producing major dysfunction. If minor malformations are also included, the rate is 7 to 10 percent. The risk of malformation after exposure to a drug must be compared with this background rate.

There is a marked species specificity in drug teratogenesis.[2] For example, thalidomide was not found to be teratogenic in rats and mice but is a potent human teratogen. On the contrary in mice certain drugs may produce defects although no studies have shown them to be teratogenic in humans. The Food and Drug Administration (FDA) lists five categories of labeling for drug use in pregnancy:

A. Controlled studies in women fail to demonstrate a risk to the fetus in the first trimester, and the possibility of fetal harm appears remote.
B. Animal studies do not indicate a risk to the fetus; there are no controlled human studies, or animal studies do show an adverse effect on the fetus, but well-controlled studies in pregnant women have failed to demonstrate a risk to the fetus.
C. Studies have shown the drug to have animal teratogenic or embryocidal effects, but no controlled studies are available in women, or no studies are available in either animals or women.
D. Positive evidence of human fetal risk exists, but benefits in certain situations (e.g., life-threatening situations or serious

43

diseases for which safer drugs cannot be used or are ineffective) may make use of the drug acceptable despite its risks.

X. Studies in animals or humans have demonstrated fetal abnormalities, or evidence demonstrates fetal risk based on human experience, or both, and the risk clearly outweighs any possible benefit.

The classic teratogenic period is from day 31 after the last menstrual period in a 28-day cycle to 71 days from the last period (Fig. 3–1). During this critical period, organs are forming, and teratogens may cause malformations that are usually overt at birth. The timing of exposure is important. Administration of drugs early in the period of organogenesis will affect the organs developing at that time, such as the heart or neural tube. Closer to the end of the classic teratogenic period, the ear and palate are forming and may be affected by a teratogen. Before day 31, exposure to a teratogen produces an all-or-none effect. With exposure around conception, the conceptus usually either does not survive or survives without anomalies.

Patients should be educated about avenues other than the use of drugs to cope with tension, aches and pains, and viral illnesses during pregnancy. The risk/benefit ratio should justify the use of a particular drug, and the minimum effective dose should be employed. As long-term effects of drug exposure in utero may not be revealed for many years, caution with regard to the use of any drug in pregnancy is warranted.

TERATOGEN INFORMATION SERVICES

An organization of teratology information services and several computer databases are available to physicians who counsel pregnant women (Table 3–1).

EFFECTS OF SPECIFIC DRUGS

Estrogens and Progestins

No teratogenic risk has been confirmed for oral contraceptives and progestins. A meta-analysis of first-trimester sex hormone exposure revealed no association between exposure and fetal genital malformations.[6]

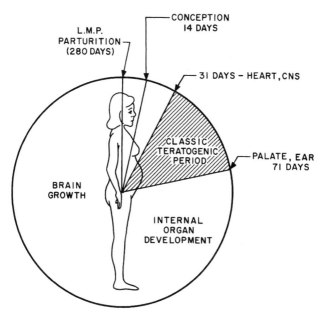

Figure 3–1. Gestational clock showing the classic teratogenic period. (From Blake DA, Niebyl JR: Requirements and limitations in reproductive and teratogenic risk assessment. *In* Niebyl JR (eds): Drug Use in Pregnancy, 2nd ed. Philadelphia, Lea & Febiger, 1988, p 1, with permission.)

Table 3–1. TERATOGEN INFORMATION SERVICES AND COMPUTER DATABASES

Organization of Teratogen Information Services:
  http://orpheus.ucsd.edu/ctis, Telephone 801-328-2229.
Computer databases:
  MICROMEDEX, Inc., 6200 South Syracuse Way, Suite 300, Englewood, CO 80111-4740.
  Reproductive Toxicology Center, REPROTOX, Columbia Hospital for Women Medical Center, 2440 M Street NW, Suite 217, Washington, DC 20037-1404.
  Teratogen Information Service, TERIS, University of Washington, Office of Technology Transfer, 4225 Roosevelt Way NE Suite 301, Seattle, WA 98105.

Androgenic Steroids

Androgens may masculinize a developing female fetus. Synthetic testosterone derivatives may cause clitoromegaly and labial fusion if given before 13 weeks of pregnancy.[7] Danazol (Danocrine) has been reported to produce mild clitoral enlargement and labial fusion when given inadvertently for the first 10 to 12 weeks after conception.

Anticonvulsants

Epileptic women taking anticonvulsants during pregnancy have approximately double the general population risk of malformations, especially cleft lip with or without cleft palate and congenital heart disease. Valproic acid (Depakene) and carbamazepine (Tegretol) each carry approximately a 1 percent risk of neural tube defects and possibly other anomalies.[12,13] A combination of more than three drugs or a high daily dose increases the chance of malformations.[14] Folic acid supplementation should be given to these mothers, and most authorities would recommend 4 mg/day folic acid for high-risk women.[16]

Fewer than 10 percent of offspring show the fetal hydantoin syndrome,[18] which consists of microcephaly, growth deficiency, developmental delays, mental retardation, and dysmorphic craniofacial features, hypoplasia of the nails and distal phalanges, and hypertelorism. Carbamazepine (Tegretol) is also associated with an increased risk of a dysmorphic syndrome.[20] Children exposed in utero to phenytoin scored 10 points lower on IQ tests than children exposed to carbamazepine or nonexposed controls.[24] After Lamotrigine (Lamictal) exposure during the first timester, eight of 123 infants (6.5 percent) were found to have congenital anomalies.[26]

Some women may have taken anticonvulsant drugs for a long period without reevaluation of the need for continuation of the drugs. For patients with idiopathic epilepsy who have been seizure free for 2 years and who have a normal electroencephalogram (EEG), it may be safe to attempt a trial of withdrawal of the drug before pregnancy.[29]

Most authorities agree that the benefits of anticonvulsant therapy during pregnancy outweigh the risks of discontinuation of the drug if the patient is first seen during pregnancy. The blood level of drug should be monitored to ensure a therapeutic level but minimize the dosage. Neonatologists need to be notified when a patient is on anticonvulsants, because this therapy can affect vitamin K–dependent clotting factors in the newborn. Vitamin K supplementation at 10 mg daily for these mothers has been recommended for the last month of pregnancy.[30]

Isotretinoin and Vitamin A Derivatives

Isotretinoin (Accutane) is a significant human teratogen. It is labeled as contraindicated in pregnancy (FDA category X) with appropriate warnings that a negative pregnancy test is required before therapy. The risk of structural anomalies in patients studied prospectively is now estimated to be about 25 percent. An additional 25 percent have mental retardation alone.[32] The malformed infants have a characteristic pattern of craniofacial, cardiac, thymic, and central nervous system anomalies. They include microtia/anotia (small/absent ears), micrognathia, cleft palate, heart defects, thymic defects, retinal or optic nerve anomalies, and central nervous system malformations including hydrocephalus.[31] Microtia is rare as an isolated anomaly yet appears commonly as part of the retinoic acid embryopathy.

Unlike vitamin A, isotretinoin is not stored in tissue. Therefore, a pregnancy after discontinuation of isotretinoin is not at risk, as the drug is no longer detectable in serum 5 days after its ingestion. Topical tretinoin (Retin-A) has not been associated with any teratogenic risk.[34]

Etretinate (tegison) is used for psoriasis and may well have a teratogenic risk similar to that of isotretinoin. Case reports of malformation, especially central nervous system,[35] have appeared, but the absolute risk is unknown. The half-life of several months makes levels cumulative, and the drug carries a warning to avoid pregnancy within 6 months of use.

There is no evidence that vitamin A itself in normal doses is teratogenic, nor is betacarotene. The levels in prenatal vitamins (5,000 IU/day orally) have not been associated with any documented risk. Eighteen cases of birth defects have been reported after exposure to levels of 25,000 IU of vitamin A or greater during pregnancy. Vitamin A in doses greater than 10,000 IU/day was shown to increase the risk of malformations in one study,[35] but not in another.[36]

Psychoactive Drugs

There is no clear risk documented for most psychoactive drugs with respect to overt birth defects. However, effects of chronic use of these agents on the developing brain in humans is difficult to study, and so a conservative attitude is appropriate. Lack of overt defects does not exclude the possibility of behavioral teratogenesis.

Lithium (Eskalith, Lithobid)

The risk of anomalies after lithium exposure is much lower than previously thought. A prospective study of 148 women exposed to lithium in the first trimester showed one fetus in the lithium-exposed group had Ebstein's anomaly, and one infant in the control group had a ventricular septal defect. As Ebstein's anomaly may increase after lithium exposure, we do recommend that exposed women be offered ultrasound and fetal echocardiography.

Perinatal effects of lithium have been noted, including hypotonia, lethargy, and poor feeding in the infant. Also, complications similar to those seen in adults on lithium have been noted in newborns, including goiter and hypothyroidism.

Two cases of polyhydramnios associated with maternal lithium treatment have been reported.[44,45] Because nephrogenic diabetes insipidus has been reported in adults taking lithium, the presumed mechanism of this polyhydramnios is fetal diabetes insipidus. Polyhydramnios may be a sign of fetal lithium toxicity.

It is usually recommended that drug therapy be changed in pregnant women on lithium to avoid fetal drug exposure. Tapering over 10 days will delay the risk of relapse.[46] However, discontinuing lithium is associated with a 70 percent chance of relapse of the affective disorder in 1 year as opposed to 20 percent in those who remain on lithium. Discontinuation of lithium may pose an unacceptable risk of increased morbidity in women who have had multiple episodes of affective instability. These women should be offered appropriate prenatal diagnosis with ultrasound, including fetal echocardiography.

Antidepressants

In the Michigan Medicaid study, 467 newborns had been exposed during the first trimester to amitriptyline (Elavil) with no increased risk of birth defects.[48] No increased risk of major malformations has been found after first trimester exposure to fluoxetine (Prozac) in over 500 pregnancies.[49,50] There has also been no increased risk of birth defects in 267 women exposed to fluvoxamine, paroxetine, and sertraline.

Anticoagulants

Warfarin (Coumadin) has been associated with chondrodysplasia punctata. This syndrome, occurring in about 5 percent of exposed pregnancies, includes nasal hypoplasia, bone stippling seen on radiologic examination, ophthalmologic abnormalities including bilateral optic atrophy, and mental retardation. The ophthalmologic abnormalities and mental retardation may occur[55] even with use only beyond the first trimester.

The alternative drug, heparin, does not cross the placenta, and it should be the drug of choice for patients requiring anticoagulation. Therapy with 20,000 units/day for greater than 20 weeks has also been associated with bone demineralization.[57] The risk of spine fractures was 0.7 percent with low-dose heparin and 3 percent with a high-dose regimen.[59] Heparin can also cause thrombocytopenia.

Low-molecular-weight heparins also do not cross the placenta.[61] The half-life is longer, allowing for once-daily administration. However, enoxaparin is cleared more rapidly during pregnancy, and so twice-daily dosing may be advised. There is a more predictable dose–response relationship, obviating the need for monitoring. There is less risk of heparin-induced thrombocytopenia.

The risks of heparin during pregnancy may not be justified in patients with only a single episode of thrombosis in the past.[64,65] Certainly, conservative measures should be recommended, such as elastic stockings and avoidance of prolonged sitting or standing.

In patients with cardiac valve prostheses, full anticoagulation is necessary, as low-dose heparin resulted in three valve thromboses (two fatal) in 35 mothers so treated.[66]

Thyroid and Antithyroid Drugs

Propylthiouracil (PTU) and methimazole (Tapazole) both cross the placenta and may cause mild fetal goiter. The goal of such therapy during pregnancy is to keep the mother slightly hyperthyroid to minimize fetal drug exposure.

The need for thyroxine increases in many women with primary hypothyroidism when they are pregnant, as reflected by an increase in serum thyroid-stimulating hormone (TSH) concentrations.[70] As hypothyroidism in pregnancy may adversely affect the fetus,[71] it is prudent to monitor thyroid function throughout pregnancy and to adjust the thyroid dose to maintain a normal TSH level.

Antineoplastic Drugs and Immunosuppressants

Methotrexate, a folic acid antagonist, causes multiple congenital anomalies, including cranial defects and malformed extremities. When low-dose oral methotrexate (7.5 mg/week) was used for rheumatoid disease in the first trimester, five full-term infants were normal, and three patients experienced spontaneous abortions.[81] The frequency of anomalies in 80 women treated with azathioprine (Imuran) in the first trimester was not increased.[82]

No increased risk of anomalies in 67 fetuses exposed to cyclosporine (Sandimmune) in utero has been reported.[83]

Eight malformed infants have resulted from first-trimester exposure to cyclophosphamide (Cytoxan), but these infants were also exposed to other drugs or radiation.[85]

Chloroquine (Aralen) is safe in doses used for malarial prophylaxis, and there was no increased incidence of birth defects among 169 infants exposed to 300 mg once weekly.[86] However, after exposure to larger anti-inflammatory doses (250 to 500 mg/day), two cases of cochleovestibular paresis were reported.[87]

When cancer chemotherapy is used during embryogenesis there is an increased rate of spontaneous abortion and major birth defects. Later in pregnancy there is a greater risk of stillbirth and intrauterine growth restriction, and myelosuppression is often present in the infant.[89]

Antiasthmatics

Isoproterenol (Isuprel) and Metaproterenol (Alupent)

When isoproterenol and metaproterenol are given as topical aerosols for the treatment of asthma, the total dose absorbed is usually not significant. With oral or intravenous doses, however, the cardiovascular effects of the agents may result in decreased uterine blood flow. No teratogenicity has been reported.[73]

Cromolyn Sodium (Intal)

Cromolyn sodium may be administered in pregnancy, and the systemic absorption is minimal. Teratogenicity has not been reported in humans.

Corticosteroids

When prednisone or prednisolone are maternally administered, the concentration of active compound in the fetus is less than 10 percent of that in the mother. Therefore, these agents are the drugs of choice for treating medical diseases such as asthma. Inhaled corticosteroids are also effective therapy, and very little drug is absorbed. When steroid effects are desired in the fetus, for example, to accelerate lung maturity, betamethasone (Celestone) and dexamethasone (Decadron) are preferred, as these readily cross the placenta.

Antiemetics

Faced with a self-limited condition occurring at the time of organogenesis, the clinician is well advised to avoid the use of medications whenever possible and to encourage supportive measures initially.

Vitamin B$_6$

Vitamin B$_6$ (pyridoxine) 10 to 25 mg three times a day has been reported in two randomized placebo controlled trials to be effective for treating the nausea and vomiting of pregnancy.[91,92] There is no evidence of teratogenicity.

Doxylamine

Doxylamine (Unisom) is an effective antihistamine for nausea in pregnancy and can be combined with vitamin B_6. Vitamin B_6 (25 mg) and Unisom (25 mg) at bedtime, and one half of each in the morning and afternoon, is an effective combination.

Meclizine (Bonine)

In one randomized, placebo-controlled study, meclizine gave significantly better results than placebo.[94] Prospective clinical studies have provided no evidence that meclizine is teratogenic in humans.

Dimenhydrinate (Dramamine)

No teratogenicity has been noted with dimenhydrinate, but a 29 percent failure rate and a significant incidence of side effects, especially drowsiness, has been reported.[96]

Diphenhydramine (Benadryl)

In 595 patients treated in the Collaborative Perinatal Project, no teratogenicity was noted with diphenhydramine.[73] Drowsiness can be a problem.

Trimethobenzamide (Tigan)

For trimethobenzamide, an antihistaminic phenothiazine, the data collected from a small number of patients are conflicting. In 193 patients in the Kaiser Health Plan study[95] there was a suggestion of increased congenital anomalies but no concentration of specific anomalies. In 340 patients in the Collaborative Perinatal Project,[73] no evidence for an association between this drug and malformations was found.

Phenothiazines

Chlorpromazine (Thorazine) and prochlorperazine (Compazine) have been shown to be effective in hyperemesis gravidarum. Teratogenicity does not appear to be a problem.

Ondansetron (Zofran)

Ondansetron is no more effective than promethazine (Phenergan), and has not been evaluated for teratogenicity.

Methylprednisolone

Forty patients with hyperemesis admitted to the hospital were randomized to oral methylprednisolone or oral promethazine, and methylprednisolone was more effective.[99] Corticosteroids may act centrally in the brain stem to exert an antiemetic effect.

Acid-Suppressing Drugs

The use of cimetidine, omeprazole, and ranitidine has not been found to be associated with any teratogenic risk in 2,261 exposures.[100]

Antihistamines and Decongestants

No increased risk of anomalies has been associated with most of the commonly used antihistamines, such as chlorpheniramine (Chlor-Trimeton).

Terfenadine (Seldane) has been associated in one study with an increased risk of polydactyly.[101] Astemizole (Hismanal) did not increase the risk of birth defects in 114 infants exposed in the first trimester.[102]

An association between exposure to antihistamines during the last 2 weeks of pregnancy in general and retrolental fibroplasia in premature infants has been reported.[103]

In the Collaborative Perinatal Project,[73] an increased risk of birth defects was noted with phenylpropanolamine (Entex LA) exposure in the first trimester. In one retrospective study, an increased risk of gastroschisis was associated with first-trimester pseudoephedrine (Sudafed) use.[104]

Patients should be educated that antihistamines and decongestants are only symptomatic therapy for the common cold and have no influence on the course of the disease. Other remedies should be recommended, such as use of a humidifier, rest, and fluids.

Antibiotics and Anti-infective Agents

Penicillins

Penicillin, ampicillin, and amoxicillin (Amoxil) are safe in pregnancy.

Cephalosporins

In a study of 5,000 Michigan Medicaid recipients, there was a suggestion of possible teratogenicity (25 percent increased birth defects) with cefaclor, cephalexin, and cephradine, but not other cephalosporins.[106] Because other antibiotics that have been used extensively (e.g., penicillin, ampicillin, amoxicillin, erythromycin) have not been associated with an increased risk of congenital defects, they should be first-line therapy when such treatment is needed in the first trimester.

Sulfonamides

Among 1,455 human infants exposed to sulfonamides during the first trimester, no teratogenic effects were noted.[73]

Sulfonamides cause no known damage to the fetus in utero, as the fetus can clear free bilirubin through the placenta. Sulfonamides compete with bilirubin for binding sites on albumin, thus raising the levels of free bilirubin in the serum and increasing the risk of hyperbilirubinemia in the neonate. Although this toxicity occurs with direct administration to the neonate, kernicterus in the newborn following in utero exposure has not been reported.[107]

Sulfasalazine (Azulfidine)

Sulfasalazine is used for treatment of ulcerative colitis and Crohn's disease because of its relatively poor oral absorption. However, it does cross the placenta, leading to fetal drug concentrations approximately the same as those of the mother, although both are low. No neonatal jaundice has been reported following maternal use of sulfasalazine even when the drug was given up to the time of delivery.[109]

Sulfamethoxazole with Trimethoprim (Bactrim, Septra)

Two published trials including 131 women failed to show any increased risk of birth defects after first-trimester exposure to trimethoprim.[110,111] However, one unpublished study of 2,296 Michigan Medicaid recipients suggested an increased risk of cardiovascular defects after exposure in the first trimester.[112] In a retrospective study of trimethoprim with sulfamethoxazole, the odds ratio for birth defects was 2.3.[113]

Nitrofurantoin (Macrodantin)

No reports have linked the use of nitrofurantoin with congenital defects.

Tetracyclines

The tetracyclines readily cross the placenta and are firmly bound by chelation to calcium in developing bone and tooth structures. This produces brown discoloration of the deciduous teeth, hypoplasia of the enamel, and inhibition of bone growth.[116] The staining of the teeth takes place in the second or third trimesters of pregnancy, First-trimester exposure to doxycycline is not known to carry any risk.[17] Alternate antibiotics are currently recommended during pregnancy.

Aminoglycosides

Streptomycin and kanamycin have been associated with congenital deafness in approximately 2% of the offspring of mothers who took these drugs during pregnancy. Neuromuscular blockade may be potentiated by the combined use of aminoglycosides and curariform drugs; therefore, the dosages should be reduced appropriately. Potentiation of magnesium sulfate–induced neuromuscular weakness has also been reported in a neonate exposed to magnesium sulfate and gentamicin (Garamycin).[121]

No known teratogenic effect other than ototoxicity has been associated with the use of aminoglycosides in the first trimester.

Antituberculosis Drugs

There is no evidence of any teratogenic effect of isoniazid (INH), para-aminosalicylic acid (PAS), rifampin (Rifadin), or ethambutol (Myambutol).

Erythromycin

No teratogenic risk of erythromycin has been reported. The transplacental passage is unpredictable, and so it is not an adequate therapy for syphilis in pregnancy. Of 122 first-trimester exposures to clarithromycin there was no significant risk of birth defects.[127]

Clindamycin (Cleocin)

Of 647 infants exposed to clindamycin in the first trimester, no increased risk of birth defects was noted.[128]

Quinolones

The quinolones (e.g., ciprofloxacin [Cipro], norfloxacin [Noraxin]) have a high affinity for bone tissue and cartilage and may cause arthralgia in children. However, no malformations or musculoskeletal problems were noted in 38 infants exposed in utero in the first trimester.[129]

Metronidazole (Flagyl)

Studies have failed to show any increase in the incidence of congenital defects among the newborns of mothers treated with metronidazole during early or late gestation.

Acyclovir (Zovirax)

The Acyclovir Registry has recorded 581 first-trimester exposures during pregnancy, with no increased risk of abnormalities in the infants.[26] The Centers for Disease Control and Prevention recommends that pregnant women with disseminated infection (e.g., herpetic encephalitis or hepatitis, or varicella pneumonia) be treated with acyclovir.[134]

Antifungal Agents

The imidazoles are absorbed in only small amounts from the vagina. Clotrimazole (Lotrimin) or miconazole (Monistat) in pregnancy is not known to be associated with congenital malformations.

An increased risk of limb deformities was reported in fetuses exposed to 400 to 800 mg/day of fluconazole in the first trimester.[137] In 460 who received a single 150-mg dose of fluconazole, no increased risk of defects was observed.[138,139]

Drugs for Induction of Ovulation

In more than 2,000 exposures, no evidence of teratogenic risk of clomiphene (Clomid) has been noted.[140] Although infants are often exposed to bromocriptine (Parlodel) in early pregnancy, no teratogenic effects have been observed in more than 1,400 pregnancies.[141]

Mild Analgesics

Aspirin

There is no evidence of any teratogenic effect of aspirin taken in the first trimester.[73,142] Aspirin does have significant perinatal effects, however, as it inhibits prostaglandin synthesis. Uterine contractility is decreased, and patients taking aspirin in analgesic doses have delayed onset of labor, longer duration of labor, and an increased risk of a prolonged pregnancy.[143]

Aspirin also decreases platelet aggregation, which increases the risk of bleeding before as well as at delivery. Platelet dysfunction has been described in newborns within 5 days of ingestion of aspirin by the mother.[144]

Acetaminophen (Tylenol, Datril)

Acetaminophen has also shown no evidence of teratogenicity.[150] The bleeding time is not prolonged with acetaminophen in contrast to aspirin,[151] and the drug is not toxic to the newborn.

Other Nonsteroidal Anti-inflammatory Agents

No evidence of teratogenicity has been reported for other nonsteroidal anti-inflammatory drugs (e.g., ibuprofen[153] [Motrin, Advil], or naproxen[154] [Naprosyn]), Chronic use may lead to oligohydramnios, and constriction of the fetal ductus arteriosus or neonatal pulmonary hypertension, as has been reported with indomethacin, might occur.

Propoxyphene (Darvon)

Propoxyphene is an acceptable alternative mild analgesic with no known teratogenicity.[73] It carries potential for narcotic addiction similar to codeine.

Codeine

In the Collaborative Perinatal Project, no increased relative risk of malformations was observed in 563 codeine uses.[73] Codeine can cause addiction and newborn withdrawal symptoms.

Sumatriptan

Of 183 exposures in the first trimester,[26] seven infants (3.8 percent) had birth defects, not significantly different from the nonexposed population.

Smoking

Smoking has been associated with a fourfold increase in small size for gestational age as well as an increased prematurity rate.[156] The spontaneous abortion rate is up to twice that of nonsmokers. Abortions associated with maternal smoking tend to have a higher percentage of normal karyotypes and occur later than those with chromosomal aberrations.[157] The higher perinatal mortality rate associated with smoking is attributable to an increased risk of abruptio placentae, placenta previa, premature and prolonged rupture of membranes, and intrauterine growth restriction. The risks of complications and of the associated perinatal loss rise with the number of cigarettes smoked. Discontinuation of smoking during pregnancy can reduce the risk of both pregnancy complications and perinatal mortality.

Smoking Cessation during Pregnancy

Tobacco smoke contains nicotine, carbon monoxide, and thousands of other compounds. Although nicotine is the mechanism of addiction to cigarettes, other chemicals may contribute to adverse pregnancy outcome. Carbon monoxide decreases oxygen delivery to the fetus, whereas nicotine decreases uterine blood flow.

Nicotine withdrawal may first be attempted with nicotine fading, switching to brands of cigarettes with progressively less nicotine over a 3-week period. Exercise may also improve quitting success rates.[160] Nicotine medications are indicated for patients with nicotine dependence, defined as greater than one pack per day smoking, smoking within 30 minutes of getting up in the morning, or prior withdrawal symptoms.[161] Nicotine medications are available as patches, gum, or inhalers. Although one might question the propriety of prescribing nicotine during pregnancy, if the patient can stop smoking she eliminates many other toxins, including carbon monoxide, and nicotine blood levels are similar to that of smokers.[162] There are no studies of bupropion (Zyban) in human pregnancy for smoking cessation.

Alcohol

The fetal alcohol syndrome (FAS) has been reported in the offspring of alcoholic mothers and includes the features of gross physical retardation with onset prenatally and continuing after birth. The diagnosis of FAS requires[164] at least one characteristic from each of the following three categories.

1. Growth retardation before and/or after birth
2. Facial anomalies
3. Central nervous system dysfunction.

Among alcoholic mothers, perinatal deaths are about eight times more frequent. Growth restriction, microcephaly, and IQ below 80 are considerably more frequent than among the controls.

Heavy drinking remains a major risk to the fetus, and reduction even in midpregnancy can benefit the infant. An occasional drink during pregnancy carries no known risk, but no level of drinking is known to be safe.

Marihuana

No teratogenic effect of marihuana has been documented. One study suggested a mean 73-g decrease in birth weight associated with marihuana use when urine assays were performed rather than relying on self-reporting.[171]

Cocaine

A serious difficulty in determining the effects of cocaine on the infant is the frequent presence of many confounding variables in the population using cocaine. These mothers often abuse other drugs, smoke, have poor nutrition, fail to seek prenatal care, and live under poor socioeconomic conditions. The neural systems likely to be affected by cocaine are involved in neurologic and behavioral functions that are not easily quantitated by standard infant development tests.

Cocaine-using women have a higher rate of spontaneous abortion than controls.[172] Studies have suggested an increased risk of congenital anomalies after first-trimester cocaine use,[173-175] particularly microcephaly.

Cocaine is a central nervous system stimulant and has local anesthetic and marked vasoconstrictive effects. Abruptio placentae has been reported to occur immediately after nasal or intravenous administration.[172] Several studies have also noted increased stillbirths, preterm labor, premature birth, and small-for-gestational-age infants with cocaine use.[171-173,176,177]

Cocaine has been reported to cause fetal disruption[181] presumably due to interruption of blood flow to various organs. Bowel infarction has been noted with unusual ileal atresia and bowel perforation. Limb infarction has resulted in missing fingers and central nervous system bleeding in utero may result in porencephalic cysts.

Narcotics

The goal of methadone maintenance is to bring the patient to a level of approximately 20 to 40 mg/day. The dose should be individualized at a level sufficient to minimize the use of supplemental illicit drugs, since they represent a greater risk to the fetus than do the higher doses of methadone required by some patients. Manipulation of the dose in women maintained on methadone should be avoided in the last trimester because of an association with increased fetal complications and in utero deaths attributed to fetal withdrawal in utero.[182]

The infant of the narcotic addict is at increased risk of abortion, prematurity, and growth restriction. Withdrawal should be watched for carefully in the neonatal period.

Caffeine

There is no evidence of teratogenic effects of caffeine in humans. There is still some conflicting evidence concerning the association between heavy ingestion of caffeine and increased pregnancy complications. Early studies suggested that the intake of greater than seven to eight cups of coffee per day was associated with low-birth-weight infants, spontaneous abortions, prematurity, and stillbirths.[183] However, these studies were not controlled for the concomitant use of tobacco and alcohol. In one report controlled for smoking, other habits, and medical history, no relationship was found between either low birth weight or short gestation and heavy coffee consumption.[184] When pregnant women consumed over 300 mg of caffeine per day, one study suggested an increase in term low-birth-weight infants,[185] less than 2,500 g at greater than 36 weeks.

Concomitant consumption of caffeine with cigarette smoking may increase the risk of low birth weight.[186] Maternal coffeine intake decreases iron absorption and may contribute to maternal anemia.[187]

A prospective cohort study found no evidence that moderate caffeine use increased the risk of spontaneous abortion or growth retardation.[189] Measurement of serum paraxanthine, a caffeine metabolite, revealed that only extremely high levels are associated with spontaneous abortions.[190]

Aspartame (NutraSweet)

The major metabolite of aspartame is phenylalanine,[191] which is concentrated in the fetus by active placental transport. Sustained high blood levels of phenylalanine in the fetus as seen in maternal phenylketonuria (PKU) are associated with mental retardation in the infant. Within the usual range of aspartame ingestion, peak phenylalanine levels do not exceed normal postprandial levels, and even with high doses phenylalanine concentrations are still very far below those associated with mental retardation. These responses have also been studied in women known to be carriers of PKU, and the levels are still normal. Thus, it seems unlikely that use of aspartame in pregnancy would cause any fetal toxicity.

Drugs in Breast Milk

The dose to the infant of drugs in breast milk is approximately 1 to 2 percent of the maternal dose. This amount is usually so trivial that no pharmacologic effects are noted. In the case of toxic drugs, however, any exposure may be inappropriate. Short-term effects of most maternal medications on breast-fed infants are mild and pose little risk to the infants. As the benefits of breast-feeding are well known, the risk of drug exposure must be weighed against these benefits.

The American Academy of Pediatrics has reviewed drugs in lactation[194] and categorized the drugs as listed below.

Drugs Commonly Listed as Contraindicated during Breast-Feeding

Cytotoxic Agents

Cyclosporine (Sandimmune), doxorubicin (Adriamycin), and cyclophosphamide (Cytoxan) might cause immune suppression in the infant, although data are limited with respect to these and other cytotoxic agents.

After oral administration to a lactating patient with choriocarcinoma, methotrexate was found in milk in low levels. Most individuals would elect to avoid any exposure of the infant to this drug. However, in environments in which bottle feeding is rarely practiced and presents practical and cultural difficulties, therapy with this drug would not in itself appear to constitute a contraindication to breast-feeding.[195]

Bromocriptine (Parlodel)

This ergot alkaloid derivative has an inhibitory effect on lactation. However, in one report, a mother taking 5 mg/day for a pituitary tumor was able to nurse her infant.[197]

Ergotamine (Ergomar)

This medication has been reported to be associated with vomiting, diarrhea, and convulsions in the infant in doses used in migraine medications. However, short-term ergot therapy in the postpartum period for uterine atony is not a contraindication to lactation.

Lithium (Eskalith, Lithobid)

Lithium reaches one third to one half the therapeutic blood concentration in infants, who might develop lithium toxicity, with hypotonia and lethargy.[198]

Amphetamines

One report of 103 cases of exposure to amphetamines in breast milk noted no insomnia or stimulation in the infants.[199] However, amphetamines are concentrated in breast milk.

Radioactive Compounds That Require Temporary Cessation of Breast-Feeding

Radiopharmaceuticals require variable intervals of interruption of nursing to ensure that no radioactivity is detectable in the milk. Intervals generally quoted are, for ^{67}Ga, 2 weeks; ^{131}I, 5 days; radioactive sodium, 4 days; and ^{99}Tc, 24 hours. For reassurance, the milk may be counted for radioactivity before nursing is resumed.[200]

Drugs Whose Effects on Nursing Infants Are Unknown but May Be of Concern

Psychotropic drugs such as antianxiety, antidepressant, and antipsychotic agents are sometimes given to nursing mothers for long periods. Although there are no data about adverse effects in infants exposed to these drugs via breast milk, they could theoretically alter central nervous system function.[194] Fluoxetine (Prozac) is excreted in breast milk at low levels. Sertraline causes a decline in 5-hydroxytryptamine levels in mothers, but not in their breast-fed infants.[203] This implies that the small amount of drug the infant ingests in breast milk is not enough to have a pharmacologic effect.

Temporary cessation of breast-feeding after a single dose of metronidazole (Flagyl) may be considered. Its half-life is such that interruption of lactation for 12 to 24 hours after single-dose therapy usually results in negligible exposure to the infant.

Drugs Usually Compatible with Breast-Feeding

Narcotics, Sedatives, and Anticonvulsants

In general, no evidence of adverse effect is noted with most of the sedatives, narcotic analgesics, and anticonvulsants. Patients may be reassured that, in normal doses, carbamazepine (Tegretol),[204] phenytoin (Dilantin), magnesium sulfate, codeine, morphine, and meperidine (Demerol) do not cause any obvious adverse effects in the infants.[205] Phenobarbital and diazepam (Valium) are slowly eliminated by the infant, however, and so accumulation may occur. Women consuming barbiturates or benzodiazepines should observe the infants for sedation.

Analgesics

Aspirin is transferred into breast milk in small amounts. The risk is related to high dosages (e.g., >16 300-mg tablets per day in the mother, when the infant may get sufficiently high serum levels to affect platelet aggregation or even cause metabolic acidosis). No harmful effects of acetaminophen (Tylenol, Datril) have been noted.

Antihistamines and Decongestants

No harmful effects have been noted from antihistamines or decongestants. Less than 1 percent of a pseudoephedrine dose or tripolidine dose ingested by the mother is excreted in the breast milk.[211]

Antihypertensives

β-BLOCKERS. Propranolol (Inderal) is excreted in breast milk, at approximately 1 percent of the maternal dose, which is unlikely to cause any adverse effect.[216] As milk accumulation can occur with atenolol, propranolol is a safer alternative.

ACE inhibitors, e.g., Captopril (Capoten) and **calcium channel blockers**, e.g., nifedipine, are excreted into breast milk in low concentrations.

Anticoagulants

Most mothers requiring anticoagulation may continue to nurse their infants with no problems. Heparin does not cross into milk and is not active orally.

At a maternal dose of warfarin (Coumadin) of 5 to 12 mg/day, no warfarin was detected in infant breast milk or plasma. Thus, with monitoring of neonatal prothrombin times to ensure lack of drug accumulation, warfarin may be safely administered to nursing mothers.

Corticosteroids

In one patient requiring corticosteroids, breast milk was obtained 2 hours after an oral dose of 10 mg of prednisone (Deltasone). The levels in the milk were 0.1 μg/dl of prednisolone and 2.67 μg/dl of prednisone. Thus, an infant taking 1 L of milk would obtain 28.3 μg of the two steroids, an amount not likely to have any deleterious effect.[227] In another study of seven patients,[228] 0.14 percent of a sample was secreted in the milk in the subsequent 60 hours, a negligible quantity. Breast-feeding is allowed in mothers taking corticosteroids, as the nursing infant would ingest less than 0.1 percent of the maternal dose.

Antibiotics

Penicillin derivatives are safe in nursing mothers. In susceptible individuals or with prolonged therapy, diarrhea and candidiasis are theoretical concerns.

Dicloxacillin (Pathocil) is 98 percent protein bound. If this drug is used to treat breast infections, very little will get into the breast milk, and nursing may be continued.

Cephalosporins appear only in trace amounts in milk, and the infant is exposed to less than 1 percent of the maternal dose.

Tooth staining or delayed bone growth from tetracyclines have not been reported after the drug was taken by a breast-feeding mother, due to the high binding of the drug to calcium and protein, limiting its absorption from the milk. The amount of free tetracycline available is too small to be significant.

Sulfonamides only appear in small amounts in breast milk and are ordinarily not contraindicated during nursing. However, the drug is best avoided in premature infants or ill infants when hyperbilirubinemia may be a problem, as the drug may displace bilirubin from binding sites on albumin. When a mother took sulfasalazine (Azulfidine) 500 mg every 6 hours, the drug was undetectable in all milk samples.

Gentamicin (Garamycin) is transferred into breast milk, and half of nursing newborn infants have the drug detectable in their serum.

The low levels detected would not be expected to cause clinical effects.[232]

Nitrofurantoin (Macrodantin) is excreted into breast milk in very low concentrations. In one study the drug could not be detected in 20 samples from mothers receiving 100 mg four times a day.[233]

Erythromycin and azithromycin (Zithromax) appear in breast milk in low concentrations.[234] Clindamycin (Cleocin) is excreted into breast milk in low levels, and nursing is usually continued during administration of these drugs.

There are no reported adverse effects on the infant of isoniazid (INH) administered to nursing mothers, and its use is considered compatible with breast-feeding.[194]

H_2-Receptor Blockers

In theory, H_2-receptor antagonists (e.g., ranitidine, cimetidine) might suppress gastric acidity and/or cause central nervous system stimulation in the infant, but these effects have not been confirmed in published studies. The American Academy of Pediatrics now considers H_2-receptor antagonists to be compatible with breast-feeding.[194] Famotidine, nizatidine, and roxatidine are less concentrated in breast milk and may be preferable in nursing mothers.[244]

Caffeine

Caffeine has been reported to have no adverse effects on the nursing infant, even after the mother consumes several cups of strong coffee.[243] In one study, the milk level contained 1 percent of the total dose 6 hours after coffee ingestion, which is not enough to affect the infant. In another report, no significant difference in 24-hour heart rate or sleep time was observed in nursing infants when their mothers drank coffee for 5 days or abstained for 5 days.[245]

Smoking

Nicotine and its metabolite cotinine enter breast milk. Infants of smoking mothers achieve significant serum concentrations of nicotine even if they are not exposed to passive smoking, and exposure to passive smoking further raises the levels of nicotine.[246] Women who smoke should be encouraged to stop smoking during lactation as well as during pregnancy.[247]

Key Points

➤ Infants of epileptic women taking anticonvulsants have double the rate of malformations of unexposed infants; the risk of fetal hydantoin syndrome is less than 10 percent.

➤ The risk of malformations after in utero exposure to isotretinoin is 25 percent, and an additional 25 percent of infants have mental retardation.

➤ Heparin is the drug of choice for anticoagulation during pregnancy, although there is some risk of osteoporosis from its use.

➤ Angiotensin-converting enzyme inhibitors can cause fetal renal failure in the second and third trimesters, leading to oligohydramnios and hypoplastic lungs.

➤ Vitamin B_6 10 to 25 mg three times a day is a safe and effective therapy for first-trimester nausea and vomiting; doxylamine (Unisom) 12.5 mg three times a day is also effective in combination with B_6.

➤ Most antibiotics are generally safe in pregnancy. Trimethoprim may carry an increased risk in the first trimester, and tetracyclines cause tooth discoloration in the second and third trimesters. Aminoglycosides can cause fetal ototoxicity.

➤ Aspirin in analgesic doses inhibits platelet function and prolongs bleeding time; thus, alternate analgesics are preferred in pregnancy.

➤ Fetal alcohol syndrome occurs in infants of mothers drinking heavily during pregnancy. A safe level of alcohol intake during pregnancy has not been determined.

➤ Cocaine has been associated with increased risk of spontaneous abortions, abruptio placentae, and congenital malformations, in particular, microcephaly.

➤ Most drugs are safe during lactation, as subtherapeutic amounts appear in breast milk, approximately 1 to 2 percent of the maternal dose.

Genetic Counseling and Prenatal Diagnosis

JOE LEIGH SIMPSON

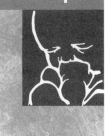

Approximately 3 percent of liveborn infants have a major congenital anomaly. Genetic factors are usually responsible. In addition, more than 50 percent of first-trimester spontaneous abortions and at least 5 percent of stillborn infants show chromosomal abnormalities. Given such an important role for genetic factors, knowledge of medical genetics clearly becomes integral to the practice of modern obstetrics.

This chapter first considers the principles of genetic counseling and genetic screening. Thereafter, disorders amenable to genetic screening and prenatal diagnosis are discussed.

FREQUENCY OF GENETIC DISEASE

Phenotypic variation—normal or abnormal—may be considered in terms of several etiologic categories: (1) chromosomal abnormalities, numerical or structural; (2) single-gene or mendelian disorders; (3) polygenic and multifactorial disorders, polygenic implying an etiology resulting from cumulative effects of more than one gene and multifactorial implying interaction as well with environmental factors; and (4) teratogenic disorders, caused by exposure to exogenous factors (e.g., drugs) that deleteriously affect an embryo otherwise destined to develop normally. Principles of these mechanisms are reviewed elsewhere.[1]

Chromosomal Abnormalities

The incidence of chromosomal aberrations is 1 in 160. Table 4–1 shows the incidences of individual abnormalities.[2]

Table 4-1. CHROMOSOMAL ABNORMALITIES IN LIVEBORN INFANTS

Type of Abnormality	Incidence
Numerical aberrations	
Sex chromosomes	
47,XYY	1/1,000 MB
47,XXY	1/1,000 MB
Other (males)	1/1,350 MB
47,X	1/10,000 FB
47,XXX	1/1,000 FB
Other (females)	1/2,700 FB
Autosomes	
Trisomies	
13-15 (D group)	1/20,000 LB
16-18 (E group)	1/8,000 LB
21-22 (G group)	1/800 LB
Other	1/50,000 LB
Structural aberrations	
Balanced	
Robertsonian	
t(Dq;Dq)	1/1,500 LB
t(Dq;Gq)	1/5,000 LB
Reciprocal translocations and insertional inversions	1/7,000 LB
Unbalanced	
Robertsonian	1/14,000 LB
Reciprocal translocations and insertional inversions	1/8,000 LB
Inversions	1/50,000 LB
Deletions	1/10,000 LB
Supernumeraries	1/5,000 LB
Other	1/8,000 LB
Total	1/160 LB

LB, live births; MB, male births; FB, female births.
Pooled data tabulated by Hook and Hamerton.[2]

Single-Gene Disorders

Approximately 1 percent of liveborns are phenotypically abnormal as a result of a single-gene mutation. Several thousand single-gene (mendelian) disorders have been recognized, and many more are suspected.[3] However, even the most common mendelian disorders (cystic fibrosis in whites, sickle cell anemia in blacks, β-thalassemia in Greeks and Italians, α-thalassemia in Southeast Asians, Tay-Sachs disease in Ashkenazi Jews) are individually rare. In aggregate, however, mendelian disorders account for 40 percent of the congenital defects seen in liveborn infants.

Polygenic/Multifactorial Disorders

Another 1 percent of neonates are abnormal but possess a normal chromosomal complement and have not undergone mutation at a *single* genetic locus. It can be deduced that several different genes are involved (polygenic/multifactorial inheritance).[1]

Disorders in this etiologic category include most common malformations limited to a single organ system. These include hydrocephaly, anencephaly, and spina bifida (neural tube defect [NTDs]); facial clefts (cleft lip and palate); cardiac defects; pyloric stenosis; omphalocele; hip dislocation; uterine fusion defects; and club foot (see the box, Polygenic/Multifactorial Traits). After the birth of one child with such anomalies, the recurrence risk in subsequent progeny is usually 1 to 5 percent.[1] This frequency is less than would be expected if only a single gene were responsible but greater than

---

Polygenic/Multifactorial Traits*

Hydrocephaly (excepting some forms of aqueductal stenosis and Dandy-Walker syndrome)
Neural tube defects (anencephaly, spina bifida, encephalocele)
Cleft lip, with or without cleft palate
Cleft lip (alone)
Cardiac anomalies (most types)
Diaphragmatic hernia
Pyloric stenosis
Omphalocele
Renal agenesis (unilateral or bilateral)
Ureteral anomalies
Posterior urethral values
Hypospadias
Müllerian fusion defects
Müllerian aplasia
Limb reduction defects
Talipes equinovarus (clubfoot)

---

*Relatively common traits considered to be inherited in polygenic/multifactorial fashion. For each, normal parents have recurrence risks of 1 to 5 percent after one affected child. After two affected offspring, the risk is higher.

that for the general population. The recurrence risks for malformations are also 1 to 5 percent for offspring of affected parents. That recurrence risks are similar for both siblings and offspring diminishes the likelihood that environmental causes are the exclusive etiologic factor because it is unlikely that households in different generations would be exposed to the same teratogen. Further excluding environmental factors as sole etiologic agents are observations that monozygotic twins are much more often concordant (similarly affected) than are dizygotic twins, despite both types of twins sharing a common intrauterine environment.

The above observations are best explained on the basis of polygenic/multifactorial inheritance. Although more than one gene is involved, only a few genes are necessary to produce the number of genotypes necessary to explain recurrence risks of 1 to 5 percent. That is, large numbers of genes and complex mechanisms need *not* be invoked. Polygenic/multifactorial etiology can thus plausibly be assumed responsible for most liveborns who have an anomaly of a single organ system and who have neither a chromosomal abnormality nor a mendelian mutation.

Teratogenic Disorders

Perhaps 20 proved teratogens are known, as reviewed in Chapter 3. Although many other agents are suspected teratogens, the quantitative contribution of known teratogens to the incidence of anomalies seems relatively small (with the possible exception of alcohol).

GENETIC HISTORY

All obstetrician-gynecologists must attempt to determine whether a couple, or anyone in their family, has a heritable disorder or is at increased risk for abnormal offspring. To address this question, some obstetricians find it helpful to elicit genetic information through the use of questionnaires or check lists that are often constructed in a manner that requires action only to positive responses. Figure 4–1 reproduces a form that has been modified from that recommended by the American College of Obstetricians and Gynecologists (ACOG).

One should inquire into the health status of first-degree relatives (siblings, parents, offspring), second-degree relatives (nephews, nieces, aunts, uncles, grandparents), and third-degree relatives (first cousins, especially maternal). Adverse reproductive outcomes such as repetitive spontaneous abortions, stillbirths, and anomalous liveborn infants should be pursued. Couples having such histories should undergo chromosomal studies in order to exclude balanced

Prenatal Genetic Screen

Name _____ Patient# _____ Date _____

1. Will you be 35 years or older when the baby is due?   Yes ___ No ___
2. Have you, the baby's father, or anyone in either of your families ever had any of the following disorders?

   Down syndrome (mongolism)   Yes ___ No ___
   Other chromosomal abnormality   Yes ___ No ___
   Neural tube defect, i.e., spina bifida (meningomyelocele or open spine), anencephaly   Yes ___ No ___
   Hemophilia   Yes ___ No ___
   Muscular dystrophy   Yes ___ No ___
   Cystic fibrosis   Yes ___ No ___
   If yes, indicate the relationship of the affected person to you or to the baby's father:
   _____

3. Do you or the baby's father have a birth defect?   Yes ___ No ___
   If yes, who has the defect and what is it? _____

4. In any previous marriages, have you or the baby's father had a child born, dead or alive, with a birth defect not listed in question 2 above?   Yes ___ No ___

5. Do you or the baby's father have any close relatives with mental retardation?   Yes ___ No ___
   If yes, indicate the relationship of the affected person to you or to the baby's father:
   _____
   Indicate the cause, if known: _____

6. Do you, the baby's father, or a close relative in either of your families have a birth defect, any familial disorder, or a chromosomal abnormality not listed above?   Yes ___ No ___
   If yes, indicate the condition and the relationship of the affected person to you or to the baby's father:
   _____

Figure 4-1. Questionnaire for identifying couples having increased risk for offspring with genetic disorders. (Modified from a form recommended by the American College of Obstetricians and Gynecologists: Antenatal Diagnosis of Genetic Disorders. Technical Bulletin No. 108. Washington, DC, ACOG, 1987.)

Illustration continued on following page

69

7. In any previous marriage, have you or the baby's father had a stillborn child or three or more first-trimester spontaneous pregnancy losses?   Yes____ No____

Have either of you had a chromosomal study?   Yes____ No____

8. If you or the baby's father is of Jewish ancestry, have either of you been screened for Tay-Sachs disease, Canavan disease, or cystic fibrosis?   Yes____ No____

If yes, indicate who and the results: _____

9. If you or the baby's father is black, have either of you been screened for sickle cell trait?   Yes____ No____

If yes, indicate who and the results: _____

10. If you or the baby's father is of Italian, Greek, or Mediterranean background, have either of you been tested for β–thalassemia?   Yes____ No____

If yes, indicate who and the results: _____

11. If you or the baby's father is of Philippine or Southeast Asian ancestry, have either of you been tested for α–thalassemia?   Yes____ No____

If yes, indicate who and the results: _____

12. Irrespective of ethnic group, have you or the baby's father been screened for cystic fibrosis?   Yes____ No____

13. Excluding iron and vitamins, have you taken any medications or recreational drugs since becoming pregnant or since your last menstrual period? (include nonprescription drugs)

If yes, give name of medication and time taken during pregnancy: _____

14. Have you currently been taking folic acid supplements?   Yes____ No____

Figure 4–1. *Continued*

translocations. Genetic counseling may prove sufficiently complex to warrant referral to a clinical geneticist, or it may prove simple enough for the well-informed obstetrician to manage. If a birth defect exists in a second-degree relative (uncle, aunt, grandparent, nephew, niece) or third-degree relative (first cousin), the risk for that anomaly will usually not prove substantially increased over that in the general population. For example, identification of a second- or third-degree relative with an autosomal recessive trait places the couple at little increased risk for an affected offspring, an exception being if the patient and her husband are consanguineous. However, a maternal first cousin with an X-linked recessive disorder would identify a couple at increased risk for a similar occurrence.

Parental ages should also be recorded. Advanced maternal age (Table 4–2) warrants discussion irrespective of a physician's personal convictions regarding pregnancy termination, as knowledge of an abnormality may affect obstetric management. Ethnic origin should be recorded. The above applies for both gamete donors as well as couples achieving pregnancy by natural means.

ANTENATAL GENETIC SCREENING

Genetic screening implies routine monitoring for the presence or absence of a given condition in apparently normal individuals. Screening is now offered routinely for (1) all individuals of certain ethnic groups to identify those individuals heterozygous for a given autosomal recessive disorder (Table 4–3), (2) all pregnant women to detect elevated maternal serum α-fetoprotein for diagnosis of fetal neural tube defects, (3) all pregnant women 35 years of age and above to undergo invasive tests and to detect Down syndrome, and (4) all pregnant women *under* age of 35 years to undergo maternal serum screening to detect Down syndrome.

Neonatal Screening

Population screening for Tay-Sachs disease, α- and β-thalassemia, and sickle cell anemia is reasonable in order to determine whether they are heterozygous for autosomal recessive disorders amenable to prenatal diagnosis. Table 4–3 lists disorders for which screening is currently recommended. The most well-known example in the United States is Tay-Sachs disease, an autosomal recessive disorder for which Ashkenazi Jews are at increased risk (heterozygote frequency, 1 in 27). In the United States, Jewish individuals may be uncertain whether they are of Ashkenazic or Sephardic descent (90 percent are Ashkenazi); thus, obstetricians should screen all

Table 4-2. MATERNAL AGE AND CHROMOSOMAL ABNORMALITIES (LIVE BIRTHS)*

Maternal Age	Risk for Down Syndrome	Risk for Any Chromosome Abnormalities[†]
20	1/1,667	1/526[†]
21	1/1,667	1/526[†]
22	1/1,429	1/500[†]
23	1/1,429	1/500[†]
24	1/1,250	1/476[†]
25	1/1,250	1/476[†]
26	1/1,176	1/476[†]
27	1/1,111	1/455[†]
28	1/1,053	1/435[†]
29	1/1,100	1/417[†]
30	1/952	1/384[†]
31	1/909	1/385[†]
32	1/769	1/322[†]
33	1/625	1/317[†]
34	1/500	1/260
35	1/385	1/204
36	1/294	1/164
37	1/227	1/130
38	1/175	1/103
39	1/137	1/82
40	1/106	1/65
41	1/82	1/51
42	1/64	1/40
43	1/50	1/32
44	1/38	1/25
45	1/30	1/20
46	1/23	1/15
48	1/18	1/12
48	1/14	1/10
49	1/11	1/7

*Because sample size for some intervals is relatively small, confidence limits are sometimes relatively large. Nonetheless, these figures are suitable for genetic counseling.
[†]47,XXX excluded for ages 20 to 32 (data not available).
Data from Hook[112] and Hook et al.[113]

Table 4–3. GENETIC SCREENING IN VARIOUS ETHNIC GROUPS

Ethnic Group	Disorder	Screening Test	Definitive Test
Ashkenazi Jews	Tay-Sachs disease	Decreased serum hexosamidase-A, possibly molecular analysis	Chorionic villus sampling (CVS) or amniocentesis for enzymatic assay or molecular analysis to detect affected fetus
	Canavans disease	DNA analysis to detect most common alleles	CVS or amniocentesis for molecular analysis to detect affected fetus
African-Americans	Sickle cell anemia	Presence of sickle cell hemoglobin, confirmatory hemoglobin, electrophoresis	CVS or amniocentesis for genotype determination (direct molecular analysis)
Mediterranean people	β-Thalassemia	Mean corpuscular volume (MCV) <80%, followed by hemoglobin electrophoresis	CVS or amniocentesis for genotype determination (direct molecular analysis or linkage analysis)

Table continued on following page

Table 4–3. GENETIC SCREENING IN VARIOUS ETHNIC GROUPS *Continued*

Ethnic Group	Disorder	Screening Test	Definitive Test
Southeast Asians and Chinese(Vietnamese, Laotian, Cambodian, Filipino)	α-Thalassemia	MCV < 80%, followed by hemoglobin electrophoresis	CVS or amniocentesis for genotype determination; (direct molecular studies) (direct linkage analysis)
All ethnic groups	Cystic fibrosis	DNA analysis of specified panel of 25 CFTR mutations (those present in ≥ 0.1% of the general U.S. population)	CVS or amniocentesis for genotype determination; definitive diagnosis on all fetuses is not possible, sensitivity varying by ethnic group.
	In Caucasians and Ashkenazi Jews shouldbe offered; in other ethnic groups (Asians, Hispanics) African-Americans should be made available		80% Caucasians, 97% Ashkenazi Jews; 57% Hispanics; 69% African-Americans

Jewish couples, and possibly also couples in which only one partner is Jewish. The most recent conditions for which genetic screening can be considered standard are cystic fibrosis (see below) and Canavans disease. Ashkenazi Jews may also benefit from screening for Gaucher disease and Nieman-Pick disease (as well as Tay-Sachs, Canavans, and cystic fibrosis [CF]).[5] In aggregate, the likelihood of an Ashkenazi Jewish individual being heterozygous for one of these five autosomal recessive disorders is 1 in 7. Heterozygote detection for β-thalassemia in Italians and Greeks relies on measurement of mean corpuscular volume (MCV), as does screening for α-thalassemia in Southeast Asians and Filipinos. Greater than 80 percent excludes heterozygosity for α- or β-thalassemia. Values less than 80 percent are more likely to reflect iron deficiency anemia than heterozygosity, so additional confirmatory tests are indicated to exclude heterozygosity for the thalassemias. Genes for all the above disorders have been isolated and cloned. However, molecular heterogeneity is enormous for all except sickle cell anemia (see below for further discussion). Thus, screening preferentially still utilizes the methods listed in Table 4–3. Possible exceptions include sickle cell anemia and Tay-Sachs disease. In the latter, molecular testing is equal but not superior to enzyme testing in the Ashkenazi Jewish population.[6]

Routine screening is now standard for cystic fibrosis. Recommendations have recently become available as a result of a joint effort of ACOG, the American College of Medical Genetics (ACMG), and the National Institutes of Health (NIH) Genome Center. The gene is large (27 exons) and its gene product is a chloride channel. About 75 percent of the cystic fibrosis mutations are caused by deletion of amino acid 508 (ΔF508), resulting in loss of a phenylalanine residue. About 50 percent of couples at risk for cystic fibrosis offspring can be identified by screening solely for this mutation, offering unequivocal prenatal diagnosis. However, screening only for ΔF508 would uncover couples in which one parent has the ΔF508 mutation but the other does not. If one parent has ΔF508 but the other does not, the actual risk of that couple having an affected child is 1 in 400. Amniotic fluid analysis for the cystic fibrosis gene product (protein) is not yet available, meaning prenatal diagnosis is not possible except to exclude the fetus who inherited the ΔF508 from the known heterozygous parent.

The obvious solution is to detect other mutations within the cystic fibrosis locus. Unfortunately, except for one specific mutation (W1282X) in Ashkenazi Jews, all other mutations are individually rare. As increasing numbers of CF-causing alleles are sought sensitivity reaches an asymptote, not exceeding 90 to 97 percent in the European Caucasians and Ashkenazi Jews, respectively. Thus, not all at-risk pregnancies will be identified.

The recommendations by the ACOG, the American College of Medical Genetics, and NIH[7] are "to offer" CF heterozygote screening to non-Jewish Caucasians and Ashkenazi Jews, both of which show carrier frequencies of 1 in 25 to 30. In other ethnic group (Asian-Americans, Hispanics, African-Americans) the carrier frequency is lower; thus, it is recommended CF carrier screening be "made available" and that couples "be informed of their detectability through educational brochures." In Caucasians and Ashkenazi Jews, the overall heterozygote detection rates are 90 and 97 percent, respectively, whereas in the three other ethnic groups rates approximate 70 percent even using a panel of ethnic-specific markers to maximize detection.[8-10] At present it is recommended that a panethnic mutation panel be used that includes all mutant CF alleles having a frequency of 0.1 percent in the general U.S. population. This encompasses 25 mutations at present (Table 4–4) and is subject to yearly review. Screening for other alleles is not discouraged (e.g., as part of ethnic-specific panels); however, screening for more than the 25 alleles is optional.

If a couple has already had a child with cystic fibrosis, or recounts an affected close relative, screening as described above is not germane. Rather, case detection strategies become appropriate. The index case, or the couple if the proband is unavailable, should be screened not just for the panel in Table 4–4 but, if uninformative, for a larger panel totaling up to 70 CF mutations. If the mutation is still not evident, family studies to identify polymorphic loci informative for linkage analysis should be considered if prenatal genetic diagnosis is planned (see Disorders Detectable by Molecular Methods, below).

The complexity engendered in cystic fibrosis screening will be repeated for most mendelian disorders because molecular heterogeneity is the rule rather than the exception for single-gene disorders.

Maternal Serum α-Fetoprotein Screening for Neural Tube Defects

Relatively few (5 percent) NTDs occur in families who have had previously affected offspring. Thus, a method other than a positive family history is needed to identify couples in the general population at risk for an NTD. Maternal serum α-fetoprotein (MSAFP) serves this purpose, identifying couples with a negative family history who nonetheless have sufficient risk to justify amniocentesis.

MSAFP is greater than 2.5 multiples of the median (MOM) in 80 to 90 percent of pregnancies in which the fetus has an NTD. Because considerable overlap exists between MSAFP in normal pregnancies and MSAFP in pregnancies characterized by a fetus with an NTD, systematic protocols for evaluating elevated MSAFP values are necessary. Elevated MSAFP occurs for reasons other

Table 4–4. RECOMMENDED PANEL OF MUTATIONS IN THE CYSTIC FIBROSIS TRANSMEMBRANE REGULATORY (CFTR) GENE THAT SHOULD BE SOUGHT IN CARRIER DETECTION PROGRAMS*

ΔF508	ΔI507	G542X	G551D	W1282X	N1303K
R553X	621 + 1G > T	R117H	1717 – 1G > A	A455E	R560T
R1162X	G85E	R334W	R347P	711 + 1G > T	1898 + 1G > A
2184delA	1078delT	3849 + 10kbC > T	2789 + 5G > A	3659delC	I148T
3120 + 1G > A					

*The panel is applicable in all ethnic groups. If R117H is detected, status of the 5T-7T-9T polymorphism should be determined.

than an NTD: (1) underestimation of gestational age, inasmuch as MSAFP increases as gestation progresses; (2) multiple gestation (60 percent of twins and almost all triplets having MSAFP values that would be elevated if judged on the basis of singleton values); (3) fetal demise, presumably caused by fetal blood extravasating into the maternal circulation; (4) Rh isoimmunization, cystic hygroma, and other conditions associated with fetal edema; and (5) anomalies other than NTD, usually characterized by edema or skin defects.

Maternal serum values above either 2.0 or 2.5 MOM are usually considered elevated. The precise value above which MSAFP is considered elevated is less important than setting a consistent policy per program. In twin gestations MSAFP is judged abnormal only at 4.5 to 5.0 MOM or greater.

The initial MSAFP assay should be performed at 15 to 20 weeks' gestation. Corrections for maternal weight and some other factors are necessary, using various algorithms that provide a weight-adjusted MSAFP appropriate for gestational age. (Without weight adjustment, dilutional effects can result in heavier women having a spuriously low value when in fact MSAFP might actually be elevated for women of their weight.)

Approximately 5 percent of women will have an elevated MSAFP value. If not already performed, ultrasound is obviously required to exclude erroneous gestational age, multiple gestations, or fetal demise. Amniocentesis for AFP and acetylcholinesterase (AChE) is necessary if no explanation for elevated MSAFP is evident on ultrasound. The presence of AChE indicates an open NTD or other anomalies.

MSAFP screening identifies 90 percent anencephaly and 80 to 85 percent of spina bifida, at the cost of 1 to 2 percent of all pregnant women undergoing amniocentesis. Approximately 1 in 15 women having an unexplained elevated serum AFP will prove to have a fetus with an NTD. Sensitivity of detecting an NTD in twin gestations is less than in singleton gestations, being only about 30 percent for spina bifida given a threshold of 4.5 MOM. Lower sensitivity exists because twins are usually discordant for an NTD. Liberal use of comprehensive ultrasound is recommended in twin gestations.

Maternal Serum Screening for Detecting Fetal Trisomy

Soon after maternal serum screening for the detection of NTDs was introduced, it became clear that a low MSAFP level was associated with trisomy 21.[13] The possibility arose that maternal serum screening could be offered to women under the age of 35 for detection of Down syndrome. Low serum values could confer a risk sufficiently high that women who are not otherwise candidates for invasive procedures like amniocentesis or chorionic villus sampling (CVS) might wish to undergo such. This proposition is attractive because only 25 percent of infants with Down syndrome are born to women aged 35 and above. Thus, decreasing the population incidence requires identifying younger women at sufficient risk to justify an invasive procedure. However, screening for Down syndrome is more complicated than screening for NTDs because the risk of Down syndrome is age specific. A slightly low MSAFP value might raise the age-associated risk of a 34-year-old high enough to justify amniocentesis, but the same value would not necessarily increase the risk similarly for a 25-year-old woman. The preferable way to identify couples with sufficient risk to justify invasive procedures is to utilize likelihood ratios. For example, a maternal serum value for AFP of 0.4 MOM carries a likelihood ratio of 3.81 for having a child with Down syndrome. If the a priori (age-specific) risk is 1 in 581 (for a 25-year-old woman), the recalculated risk after taking into account MSAFP is 1 in 148.

In addition to the association between low MSAFP and Down syndrome, an association exists for other maternal serum analytes. The analyte having the greatest discriminatory value is human chorionic gonadotropin (hCG), which is elevated in Down syndrome pregnancies.[14] In the second trimester, either intact hCG or free β-hCG will suffice for assay. Irrespective, the combination of hCG, AFP, and maternal age, when analyzed with appropriate software to derive likelihood ratios, allows detection of some 60 to 65 percent of cases of Down syndrome at an amniocentesis rate of 5 percent.[15] Other analytes offer slight added value, in particular, inhibin A and unconjugated estriol (uE$_3$) are most widely added.

Importantly, for accurate counseling, sensitivity of detecting Down syndrome is age dependent; thus, not all cohort studies will show identical results. Detection rates are 90 percent for women aged 35 and above, but much lower for those in their early third decade. Women should be given *precise* answers as to the sensitivity of detecting trisomy in their pregnancy; 65 percent detection is not the correct information to impart to a 25-year-old who inquires about her own detection rate. Confounding factors can affect serum screening. Corrections for maternal weight and ethnic group are routine, but adjustments for other confounding variables are not. Maternal weight affects AFP, uE$_3$ and hCG levels, all of which decrease with increasing weight. Insulin-dependent diabetes in mothers results in slightly decreased uE$_3$ and hCG levels. Maternal serum screening to detect Down syndrome in twin gestations has become available. Down syndrome occurs more frequently (20 percent) in twin pregnancies than in singleton pregnancies, which is predictable given the known positive correlation between twinning and maternal age. Unfortunately, Down syndrome screening using multiple serum markers is not as sensitive in twin pregnancies as it is for singleton pregnancies. Using singleton cutoffs, 73 percent of monozygotic twin pregnancies but only 43 percent of dizygotic twin pregnancies with Down syndrome should be detected, with a 5 percent false-positive rate.[18] The lower sensitivity in dizygotic twins reflects the blunting effect of the concomitant presence of one normal and one aneuploid fetus. Thus, patients should be informed that the detection rate is less than in singleton pregnancies. It may simply be preferable to perform invasive procedures in women 33 years or older.[19] Younger women may still wish to avail themselves of noninvasive screening despite its lower sensitivity.

Despite different policies in other venues (e.g., Europe), the ACOG continues to recommend that women aged 35 years or older be offered invasive procedures without prior serum screening. In twin questations the cutoff is 33 years of age. Women under 35 years of age should be counseled about serum screening. If older women insist on maternal serum screening in lieu of an invasive procedure, they must appreciate that detection is not 100 percent but only 90 percent at best.

Screening for Trisomy 18

Trisomy 18 can be detected by triple-marker through decreased hCG, AFP, and uE_3 levels, a pattern that differs from trisomy 21, in which hCG is elevated. One recommendation is to offer invasive prenatal diagnosis whenever serum screening shows each of these three markers to fall below certain thresholds (MSAFP $\leq$ 0.6 MOM; hCG $\leq$ 0.55 MOM; uE_3 $\leq$ 0.5 MOM).[20] Screening for trisomy 18 by simply using these thresholds would detect 60 to 80 percent of trisomy 18 fetuses, with a 0.4 percent amniocentesis rate.[21] Calculating individual risk estimation on the basis of three markers and maternal age, Palomaki and colleagues reported that 60 percent of trisomy 18 pregnancies can be detected with an amniocentesis (false-positive) rate of about 0.2 percent[20] One in nine pregnencies identified as being at increased risk for trisomy 18 by serum screening would be expected to be affected.

First-Trimester Screening

Screening in the first trimester would be highly desirable because patients at increased risk can be offered CVS, avoiding the increased late-pregnancy terminations if fetal abnormalities are detected. Associations exist between Down syndrome and low MSAFP, low pregnancy- associated placental protein A (PAPP-A), and elevated free β-hCG. Using PAPP-A and free β-hCG for first-trimester Down syndrome screening gives a 62 percent detection rate with a 5 percent false-positive rate.[25]

A second approach is to measure nuchal translucency thickening.[26] Risk of trisomy is derived by multiplying the background maternal age and gestational-related risk by a likelihood ratio that reflects the deviation of nuchal translucency from the normal mean for gestation. In one study of 96,127 pregnant women of median age 31 years, a risk of 1 in 300 or higher for Down syndrome was observed in 8.3 percent. Detection rate was 82.2 percent for trisomy 21 and 77.9 percent for other chromosomal abnormalities. A few of these may have aborted spontaneously had not intervention occurred, but sensitivity is still well over 70 percent.

First-trimester screening with maternal serum analytes (PAPP-A) and free β-hCG can be combined with fetal nuchal translucency screening to further refine risks for fetal trisomies.[27] Sequential first-trimester (PAPP-A and β-hCG; nuchal translucency) and second-trimester (maternal serum so-called integrated test) screening is also possible. This approach theoretically detects nearly 90 percent, with a false-positive rate of 5 percent.[28] Alternatively, one can accept a detection rate of 80 percent for a lower (1 percent) rate of amniocentesis. Sequential screeners has the advantage of maximum sensitivity but the disadvantage of requiring that first-trimester results be withheld until second-trimester results are obtained. In addition to failing to disclose information in a timely fashion, termination would be deferred until the second trimester, when risks are higher.

DIAGNOSTIC PROCEDURES FOR PRENATAL GENETIC DIAGNOSIS

Prenatal genetic diagnosis usually requires obtaining fetal tissue, necessitating an invasive procedure like amniocentesis or CVS. In this section we shall consider common techniques and their safety.

Traditional Amniocentesis

Technique

In amniocentesis, amniotic fluid is aspirated, often for the purpose of genetic diagnosis at 15 to 16 weeks' gestation (menstrual weeks). While the procedure has traditionally been performed at 15 to 16 weeks, it can be performed earlier (especially 12 to 14 weeks).[27] A 22-gauge spinal needle with stylet is usually used. Ultrasound examination is obligatory in order to determine gestational age, placental position, location of amniotic fluid, and number of fetuses. Ultrasound should be performed concurrently with amniocentesis. Rh-immune globulin should be administered to the Rh-negative, Du-negative, unsensitized patient.

In multiple gestations, amniocentesis can usually be performed on all fetuses. Following aspiration of amniotic fluid from the first sac, 2 to 3 ml of indigo carmine, diluted 1:10 in bacteriostatic water, is injected before the needle is withdrawn. A second amniocentesis is then performed at a site determined after visualizing the membranes separating the two sacs. It is important to note the locations of each sac in case selective termination is later required. Aspiration of clear fluid confirms that the second (new) sac was entered. Triplets and other multiple gestations can be managed similarly, sequentially injecting dye into successive sacs. Although cross-contamination of cells in multiple gestations appears to be rare, confusion may sometimes arise in interpreting amniotic fluid AChE or AFP results. Some obstetricians aspirate the second sac without dye injection or use a single-puncture technique; however, I still prefer dye injection for confirmation.

After amniocentesis, the patient may resume all normal activities. Common sense dictates that strenuous exercise such as jogging or "aerobic" exercise be deferred for a day or so. The patient should report persistent uterine cramping, vaginal bleeding, leakage of amniotic fluid, or fever; however, physician intervention is almost never required, unless overt abortion occurs.

If only one fetus in a multiple gestation is abnormal, parents should be prepared to choose between aborting all fetuses or continuing the pregnancy with one or more normal and one abnormal fetus. Selective termination in the second trimester is possible, but success of this procedure is greater in the first trimester.[30]

Safety of Traditional Amniocentesis

Any procedure that involves entering the pregnant uterus logically carries risk to the fetus. Amniocentesis is no exception. Amniocentesis carries potential danger to both mother and fetus. Maternal risks are quite low, with symptomatic amnionitis occurring only rarely (0.1 percent). Minor maternal complications such as transient vaginal spotting or minimal amniotic fluid leakage occur in 1 percent or fewer of cases, but almost always these are self-limited in nature. Other very rare complications include intra-abdominal viscus injury or hemorrhage.

Older studies cited above were used to provide the traditional risk figure of 1 miscarriage per 200 procedures. These were not conducted with high-quality ultrasonography as defined by today's standards, nor was concurrent ultrasonography even universally applied. A 1986 Danish study was a true randomized, controlled study of 4,606 women aged 25 to 34 years who were without known risk factors for fetal genetic abnormalities;[33] a control group underwent no procedure. The spontaneous abortion rate after 16 weeks was 1.7 percent in the amniocentesis study group compared with 0.7 percent in controls ($p < 0.01$); a 2.6-fold relative risk of spontaneous abortion was observed if the placenta was traversed.

Studies conducted within the past decade have universally shown little to no statistical difference between outcomes following amniocentesis groups and controls. In British Columbia, children delivered of women who had second-trimester amniocentesis and were identified by a population-based database of congenital anomalies showed disabilities at the same rate as matched controls (i.e., offspring of women who had not undergone amniocentesis).[34] In Thailand, a randomized study found no statistically significant difference between women undergoing and not undergoing amniocentesis between 15 and 24 weeks.

In conclusion, it still seems wise to continue to counsel that the risk of pregnancy loss secondary to amniocentesis is low, probably 1 in 400 or 500, but in some hands potentially up to 0.5 percent. Serious maternal complications and fetal injuries are stated to be "remote" risks. Concurrent ultrasound is essential.

Safety of Early Amniocentesis

Amniocentesis prior to 13 weeks cannot be recommended. Preliminary work had been encouraging,[38,39] but the definitive study by the Canadian Early and Mid-Trimester Amniocentesis Trial (CEMAT) cohort showed this.[40] The salient comparison involved 1,916 women having an amniocentesis before 13 gestational weeks versus 1,775 having amniocentesis after 15 gestational weeks. Total fetal loss rates were 7.5 percent versus 5.9 percent ($p = 0.012$). Talipes equinovarus occurred in 1.3 percent in the early amniocentesis group, compared to the expected population incidence of 0.1 percent in the traditional amniocentesis group. Technical factors associated with these adverse results were difficult-to-perform procedures (e.g., multiple needle insertions) and post procedure amniotic fluid leakage.[41] The ACOG and others recommend that amniocentesis not be performed prior to 12 gestational weeks.[42]

Chorionic Villus Sampling

CVS allows prenatal diagnosis in the first trimester to permit pregnancy termination early in gestation and also protect patient privacy. Both chorionic villi analysis and amniotic fluid cell analysis offer the same information concerning chromosomal status, enzyme levels, and DNA patterns. The one major difference is that assays requiring amniotic fluid, specifically AFP, necessitate amniocentesis.

Technique

CVS can be performed by transcervical, transabdominal, or transvaginal approaches. *Transcervical* CVS is usually performed with a flexible polyethylene catheter that encircles a metal obturator extending just distal to the catheter tip. The outer diameter is usually about 1.5 mm. Introduced transcervically under simultaneous ultrasonographic visualization (Fig. 4–2), the catheter/obturator is directed toward the trophoblastic tissue surrounding the gestational sac. After withdrawal of the obturator, 10 to 25 mg of villi are aspirated by negative pressure into a 20-or 30-ml syringe containing tissue culture media. The optimal time for transcervical sampling is 10 to 12 completed gestational weeks.

In *transabdominal* chorionic villus sampling (Fig. 4–3), concurrent ultrasound is used to direct an 18- or 20-gauge spinal needle into the long axis of the placenta. After removal of the stylet, villi are aspirated into a 20-ml syringe containing tissue culture media. Unlike transcervical CVS, transabdominal CVS can be performed throughout pregnancy, therefore serving as an alternative to cordocentesis (percutaneous umbilical blood sampling [PUBS]) later in pregnancy. If oligohydramnios is present, transabdominal CVS is preferable to PUBS. The former is widely utilized in Europe in lieu of amnioinfusion techniques prior to PUBS.

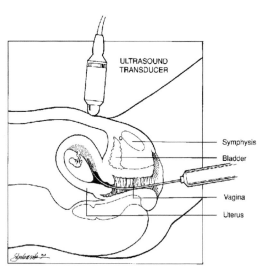

Figure 4–2. Transcervical chorionic villus sampling.

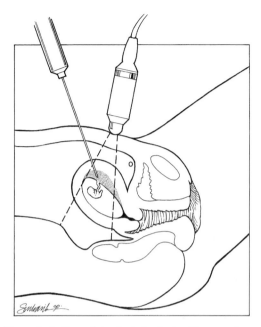

Figure 4–3. Transabdominal chorionic villus sampling.

Pregnancy Losses

The U.S. Cooperative Clinical Comparison of Chorionic Villus Sampling and Amniocentesis study[43] and the Canadian Collaborative CVS-Amniocentesis Trial Group study[44] have reported that pregnancy loss rates after CVS are no different from loss rates after amniocentesis.

Transcervical CVS and transabdominal CVS appear to be equally safe procedures.[46] In a second U.S. NICHD collaborative study, 1,194 patients were randomized to transcervical CVS and 1,929 patients to transabdominal CVS. The loss rates of cytogenetically normal pregnancies through 28 weeks were 2.5 percent and 2.3 percent, respectively.[47] Of considerable interest, the overall loss rate (i.e., background plus procedure-related) following CVS decreased by about 0.8 percent compared with rates observed during the earlier (1985 to 1987) transcervical versus amniocentesis self-selection study. This decrease in procedure-related loss rate probably reflects increasing operator experience as well as availability of both transcervical and transabdominal approaches. In a small randomized trial conducted in Italy, Brambati et al.[48] also found no difference between transabdominal and transcervical CVS.

CVS is widely used prior to selective reduction in multiple gestation. It is desirable to test the inferior fetus (destined to remain to minimize risk of ascending infection) and at least two or three other fetuses to maximize normalcy in the requisite number.

Limb Reduction Defects

Controversy about the safety of CVS has more recently shifted focus from concerns about the risk of fetal loss to its being the possible cause for congenital abnormalities. In 1991, Firth and colleagues[51] reported that 5 of 289 (1.7 percent or 17 of 1,000) infants exposed to CVS between 56 and 66 days of gestation (i.e., 42 to 50 days after fertilization) had severe limb reduction deformities (LRDs). In the United States, Burton et al.[56] reported a second cluster among 394 infants whose mothers had undergone CVS.

In an effort to quantify the risk for LDR associated with CVS, Olney et al.[61] conducted a case-control study in the United States. Case subjects consisted of 131 infants with nonsyndromic limb deficiency, identified in seven population-based birth defects surveillance programs. Controls consisted of 131 infants with other birth defects, matched to case subjects by the infant's year of birth, mother's age, race, and state of residence. The odds ratio for limb deficiency after CVS from 8 to 12 weeks' gestation was 1.7. This was not significantly increased because the 95 percent confidence limit crosses 1 (95 percent CI, 0.4 to 6.3); however, subsequent analysis by anatomic subtypes revealed a significant association for transverse digital deficiency (OR, 6.4; 95 percent CI, 1.1 to 38.6), an observation that was widely promulgated. It was concluded that the absolute risk for such defects was approximately 1 in 3,000, a figure that can be considered the upper limit of risk. By contrast, the World Health Organization (WHO) Committee on Chorionic Villus Sampling has for years collected and failed to find increased LRD. In addition pattern analysis of the types of limb defects and calculation of overall incidences failed to reveal a difference between the CVS and background populations. The 1999 WHO[64] report continued to confirm these results.

In 1995, the Committee on Genetics of the American College of Obstetricians and Gynecologists[67] reached these conclusions.

1. Transcervical CVS and transabdominal CVS performed at 10 to 12 weeks of gestation are relatively safe and accurate procedures that may be considered acceptable alternatives to second-trimester genetic amniocentesis.

2. CVS should not be performed before 10 weeks' gestation.
3. Chorionic villus sampling requires appropriate counseling before the procedure, an experienced operator, and a laboratory experienced in processing the specimen and interpreting the results. Counseling should contrast the risks and benefits of amniocentesis and CVS.
4. Although further studies were stated as needed to determine whether there is truly an increased risk of transverse digital deficiency following CVS performed at 10 to 12 weeks of gestation, it was considered prudent to counsel patients that such a complication is possible; the estimated risk may be on the order of 1 in 3,000 births.

Fetal Blood Sampling

Cordocentesis (PUBS) is usually performed from perhaps 18 weeks onward, although successful procedures have been reported as early as 12 weeks.[68,69] Preliminary ultrasonographic examination of the fetus is performed to assess fetal viability, placental and umbilical cord location, fetal position, and presence or absence of fetal or placental anomalies. Maternal sedation is not usually required, but oral benzodiazepine given before the procedure may be of benefit to the anxious patient.

There are various potential sampling sites, but given its fixed position the placental cord root is the optimal site. Free loops of cord or the intrahepatic vein are alternatives.[70] The spinal needle is percutaneously inserted into the fetal blood vessel under direct ultrasound guidance, and a small amount of blood is aspirated.

Maternal complications are rare, but include amnionitis and transplacental hemorrhage.[71,72] Fetal risks are more substantive. Data from several large perinatal centers estimate the risk of in utero death or spontaneous abortion to be 3 percent or less following PUBS.[73-77] Other collaborative data from 14 North American centers sampling 1,600 patients at varying gestational ages for a variety of indications revealed an uncorrected fetal loss rate of 1.6 percent.[79] In selected fetal diagnosis and treatment units in the United States and Japan, the procedure-related fetal loss rate in 1,260 cases was 0.9 percent; excluding diagnoses other than chromosomal abnormalities and severe growth restriction, the procedure-related fetal loss rate was only 0.2 percent. Overall, loss rates for patients undergoing PUBS varies greatly by procedure indication, far more so than in amniocentesis or CVS.

INDICATIONS FOR PRENATAL GENETIC STUDIES

Cytogenetic Disorders

Every chromosomal disorder is potentially detectable in utero. It is not appropriate, however, to perform amniocentesis or CVS in every pregnancy because for many couples the risk of an invasive procedure outweighs diagnostic benefits. In addition to couples tested as a result of positive findings in population screening programs (see above), certain indications are considered standard.

Advanced Maternal Age

For approximately 20 years it has been standard medical practice in the United States to offer invasive chromosomal diagnosis to all women who at their expected delivery date will be 35 years or older. This is the most common indication for antenatal cytogenetic studies is advanced maternal age. The incidence of trisomy 21 is 1 per 800 liveborn births in the United States, but the frequency increases with age (see Table 4–2). Trisomy 13, trisomy 18, 47,XXX, and 47,XXY also increase with advanced age.

The choice of age 35 is largely arbitrary, however, having been chosen during an interval when risk figures were available only in 5-year intervals (i.e., 30 to 34 years, 35 to 39 years, 40 to 44 years). Flexibility is thus appropriate when answering inquiries from women younger than 35 years for, indeed, increasing numbers of women aged 33 or 34 years seek prenatal diagnosis.

The risk figures shown in Table 4–2 are applicable only for liveborns. The prevalence of abnormalities at the time when CVS or amniocentesis is performed is somewhat higher.[79,80] Some abnormal fetuses would have died in utero had iatrogenic intervention not occurred in the second trimester. In fact, 5 percent of stillborn infants show chromosomal abnormalities. (see Chapter 22)

Recall that maternal serum screening is recommended by the ACOG and other groups for women under age 35 years, the goal being identifying couples at sufficient risk for fetal trisomy to justify an invasive procedure. The logical corollary might be that a normal or slightly elevated MSAFP level decreases the risk of aneuploidy for older women to the extent that amniocentesis could be avoided. Most U.S. authorities do not agree because of the potential litigious hazard and because detection rates are not 100 percent but 90 percent. Still, noninvasive screening may be desired by some women, particularly if difficulty has occurred in becoming pregnant. This is most likely to be applicable for women ages 35 to 37; almost all women older than that will prove "screen positive" by maternal serum screening and still eventually require amniocentesis anyway.

Previous Child with Chromosomal Abnormality

After the occurrence of one child or abortus with autosomal trisomy, the likelihood that subsequent progeny will also have autosomal trisomy is increased, even if parental chromosomal complements are normal. Recurrence risks are perhaps 1 percent.[81]

Recurrence risk data following the birth of a liveborn infant trisomic for a chromosome other than 21 are limited. Counseling that the risk is 1 percent for either the same or for a different chromosomal abnormality seems appropriate. Thus, antenatal studies will usually be necessary.

Parental Chromosomal Rearrangements

An uncommon but important indication for prenatal cytogenetic studies is the presence of a parental chromosomal abnormality. A balanced translocation is the usual indication, but inversions and other chromosomal abnormalities exist. Empirical data invariably show that theoretical risks for abnormal (unbalanced) offspring are greater than empirical risks. Empirical risks approximate 12 percent for offspring of either male or female heterozygotes having reciprocal translocations.[82] For robertsonian (centric fusion) translocations, risks vary according to the chromosomes involved. For t(14q;21q), risks are 10 percent for offspring of heterozygous mothers and 2 percent for offspring of heterozygous fathers (Fig. 4–4).[82] For other nonhomologous robertsonian translocations, empirical risks for liveborns are less than 1 percent. For homologous translocations (e.g., 21q;21q), all liveborn offspring should have trisomy 21. For other homologous robertsonian translocations (13q;13q or 22q;22q), almost all pregnancies result in abortions.

De Novo Structural Chromosomal Abnormalities

If a phenotypically normal parent carries the same balanced translocation as the fetus, reassurance is usually appropriate. On the other hand, if an ostensibly balanced inversion or translocation is detected in the fetus but in neither parent (de novo rearrangement), the likelihood is increased that the neonate will be phenotypically abnormal at birth. Presumably, the inversion or translocation is not actually balanced, appearances to the contrary. The risk for the fetus being abnormal has been calculated at 6 percent for de novo reciprocal inversion and 10 to 15 percent for de novo translocation.[89] These risks are not chromosome specific but represent pooled date involving many chromosomes. These risks apply only to structurally anatomic abnormalities evident at birth and do not take into account developmental delay (mental retardation) that would be evident only later in life.

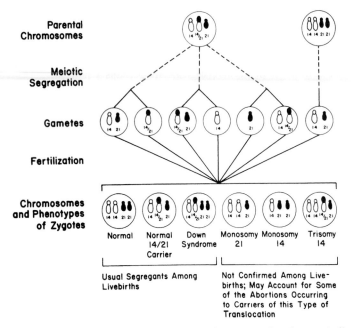

Figure 4–4. Diagram of possible gametes and progeny of a phenotypically normal individual heterozygous for a robertsonian translocation between chromosomes 14 and 21 (a form of D/G translocation). Three of the six possible gametes are incompatible with life. The likelihood that an individual with such a translocation would have a child with Down syndrome is theoretically 33 percent. However, the empirical risk is considerably less. (From Gerbie AT, Simpson JL: Antenatal diagnosis of genetic disorders. Postgrad Med 59:129, 1976, with permission.)

Marker chromosomes, also called supernumerary chromosomes, are those that by definition cannot be fully characterized on the basis of standard cytogenetic analyses. These small chromosomes usually contain a centromere, and a high proportion derive from the short arms of the acrocentric chromosomes (13, 14, 15, 21, and 22). Marker chromosomes are observed in approximately 0.06 percent of the population.[90]

Fluorescence In Situ Hybridization (FISH) in Prenatal Diagnosis

FISH merges molecular genetics with cytogenetics. Using DNA sequences unique to the chromosome in question, chromosome-specific probes (e.g., chromosomes 13, 18, 21, the X, or the Y) can be created. The probe is then labeled with a fluorochrome and used to challenge unknown DNA. Disomic cells (metaphase or interphase) should show two separate signals; trisomic cells should show three signals. Because of geometric vicissitudes, not every trisomic cell will show three signals; however, the modal count readily indicates probes permitting simultaneous assessment of multiple chromosomes. The appeal of FISH is that its use in interphase cells permits rapid (same day) diagnosis of aneuploidy. This is particularly important when a rapid diagnosis is needed to aid in the management of a high-risk fetus (e.g., with ultrasound findings of multiple anomalies).

Mendelian Disorders

Increasing numbers of mendelian disorders are now detectable in utero. Initially, only metabolic disorders were detectable on the basis of enzyme analysis. Antenatal diagnoses of hemoglobinopathies and hemophilia were later accomplished with fetal blood, originally obtainable only by fetoscopic sampling. DNA analysis now permits many diagnoses using any available nucleated cell (chorionic villi, amniotic fluid cells). The nature of the mutant or absent gene product need not necessarily even be known. We can predict confidently that in the foreseeable future all common mendelian disorders will be detectable. The rapid progress and increasing complexity required to diagnose mendelian traits dictate close liaison between the obstetrician-gynecologist and geneticist. Tabulated lists of detectable disorders should be considered suspect for timeliness.

Inborn Errors of Metabolism

Antenatal diagnosis is possible for approximately 100 inborn errors of metabolism. Most are transmitted in autosomal recessive fashion, although a few display X-linked recessive or autosomal dominant inheritance. Couples at increased risk will usually be identified because they previously had an affected child.

Detection of a metabolic error by enzyme analysis requires that the enzyme be expressed in amniotic fluid cells or chorionic villi. This requirement is fulfilled by most metabolic disorders, a prominent exception being phenylketonuria (PKU). All metabolic disorders detectable in amniotic fluid have proved detectable as well in chorionic villi. Cultured cells are usually necessary for diagnosis, but occasionally one can arrive at a diagnosis on the basis of a product in amniotic fluid. The most prominent example is 17α-hydroxyprogesterone, an elevated value of which indicates adrenal 21-hydroxylase deficiency (congenital adrenal hyperplasia).

Disorders Detectable by Molecular Methods

The power of molecular prenatal diagnosis is that any available nuclear cell can be utilized for diagnosis. All cells contain the same DNA, and the gene need not be expressed, unlike the situation when a gene product (enzyme protein) must be analyzed. Thus, molecular techniques are now widely applicable. Duchenne, muscular dystrophy, CF, adult-onset polycystic kidney disease, Huntington disease, and most other undetectable disorders have become diagnosable.

Diagnosis When the Molecular Basis Is Known

It is convenient for heuristic purposes to divide mendelian disorders into those in which the molecular basis (i.e., precise nucleotide abnormality) is known and those in which the gene is localized to a given chromosomal region but in which the molecular basis is not known. Known causes of mendelian disorders include absence of the gene or point mutations. If a disorder is known to be characterized by absence of DNA, one can determine whether a probe does or does not hybridize with the relevant sequence of DNA from an individual of unknown genotype (Fig. 4–5). Failure of amplification (by PCR) or hybridizaton (by ASO) indicates that the individual lacks the DNA sequence in question; thus, the disorder is assumed present. This approach is currently used to diagnose all forms of α-thalassemia, many cases of Duchenne-Becker muscular dystrophy, some cases of β-thalassemia, and some forms of hemophilia.

A second general approach becomes applicable if the molecular basis involves a point mutation whose nucleotide sequence is known. Sometimes, the mutation to be sought is obvious, and clinical diagnosis by molecular means is very straightforward. A clear example is sickle cell anemia, in which the triplet (codon) designating the sixth amino acid has undergone a mutation from adenine to guanine. As a result, codon 6 connotes valine rather than glutamic acid, leading to the abnormal protein (β^s). Several different molecular approaches can be exploited to make a diagnosis. For example, restriction enzymes recognize the normal but not the mutant DNA sequence at codons 5, 6, and 7. One could also construct ASOs designed to hybridize only if every single nucleotide is present. Use of a β^s oligonucleotide probe will confirm the specific mutant DNA sequence. Diagnosis with limited amounts of DNA can be achieved by the use of PCR amplification. A hybridized ASO usually appears as a "dot blot" (Fig. 4–6) or "slot blot."

Sickle cell anemia is very atypical for mendelian disorders in that its molecular basis is homogeneous. Far more commonly, many different molecular mutations are responsible (heterogeneity), as illustrated by cystic fibrosis.

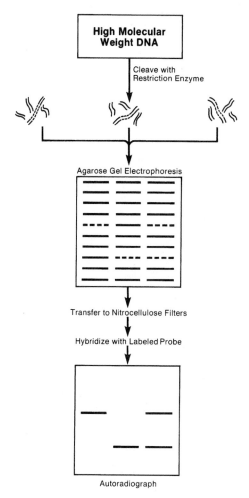

Figure 4–5. Southern blotting cuts DNA at a specific sequence of nucleotides. After DNA is cleaved with restriction enzymes, the cleaved DNA is separated by size using agarose gel electrophoresis. The gel is then laid on a piece of nitrocellulose and buffer allowed to flow through the gel into the nitrocellulose. DNA fragments migrate out of the gel and bind to the filter. A replica of the gel's DNA fragment pattern is thus made on the filter. The filter can then be hybridized to a suitable radioactivity-labeled probe, with DNA fragments hybridizing to the probe identified after autoradiography

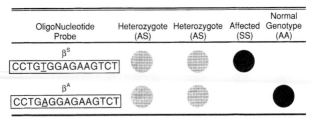

OligoNucleotide Probe	Heterozygote (AS)	Heterozygote (AS)	Affected (SS)	Normal Genotype (AA)
β^S CCTG**T**GGAGAAGTCT			●	
β^A CCTG**A**GGAGAAGTCT				●

Figure 4–6. Dot blot analysis. Oligonucleotides are constructed for sequences complementary to normal DNA (β^A) and mutant DNA (β^S). DNA challenged by the oligonucleotide probe will be hybridized if and only if the DNA contains all nucleotides connoted by the probe. Thus, AS individuals will respond to both AA and SS probes, whereas AA or SS individuals will respond only to one of the two probes (β^A and β^S, respectively). Homozygous individuals respond with a stronger (darker) signal than heterozygous individuals.

Diagnosis When the Molecular Basis Is Not Known

The molecular approaches described above are applicable only when the precise molecular basis of a disorder is known. This requirement is fulfilled less often than one would desire. Certain genes are not yet cloned and isolated. Even if the chromosomal location is known, an interval passes before the sequence is determined. A second reason is the considerable heterogeneity noted previously to exist at the molecular level. Mutations at multiple nucleotide sites within the gene can all produce a dysfunctional product. Given that genes are often very large, diagnostic complexities may be daunting. Sequencing the entire gene for every diagnostic situation is not practical, and even then the mutation might not be detected if it were located in a promoter region or involved in translation.

The problem cited above can be addressed by linkage analysis, taking advantage of the ostensibly innocuous differences in DNA that exist among individuals in the general population. These differences are called *polymorphisms* and are analogous to such well-known polymorphisms as the ABO blood group locus. The initial molecular approach utilized restriction fragment length polymorphisms (RFLPs). The approach was initially possible because of the existence among normal individuals of clinically insignificant differences in DNA fragment lengths following exposure to a given restriction endonuclease, thus the term "restriction fragment length polymorphisms."

More recently, commonly used markers are dinucleotide or trinucleotide polymorphisms. Throughout the genome there exist polymorphisms in which the number of nucleotide repeats (e.g., the dinucleotides cytosine and adenine [CA]) vary among individuals at a given locus. For example, some individuals may show 6 CA repeats, others 8, others 10 at a given locus. The almost innumerable number of such polymorphisms underlies the scientific basis of DNA analysis being used for forensic pathology. In linkage analysis, a diagnosis is made not on the basis of analyzing the mutant gene per se but rather on the basis of the presence or absence of a nearby marker. In RFLPs, the marker is a DNA variant capable of being recognized following exposure to a given endonuclease.

Figure 4–7 illustrates a simple example using RFLPs. The principle would be exactly the same using dinucleotide or trinucleotide repeats as the DNA polymorphic marker.

Pitfalls exist in linkage analysis using RFLP or nucleotide repeats. First, the marker may or may not be informative in a given family. If all family members show identical DNA fragment patterns at a given locus, that locus is obviously useless because affected and unaffected individuals cannot be distinguished from each other. If a given marker is uninformative, one searches for another marker that may prove informative. Second, the distance between the mutant gene and the marker is crucial because the likelihood of meiotic recombination is inversely related to this distance. Recombination can occur even between closely linked loci; thus, prenatal diagnosis based on linkage analysis is never 100 percent accurate.

Despite these caveats, linkage analysis permits prenatal diagnosis in many situations not otherwise possible. Linkage analysis is particularly applicable to the increasing numbers of single-gene (mendelian) disorders with considerable molecular heterogeneity.

Polygenic/Multifactorial Disorders

Amniotic Fluid α-Fetoprotein

Failure of the neural tube to close during embryogenesis leads to anencephaly, spina bifida (myelomeningocele or meningocele), encephalocele, and other less common midline defects (e.g., lipomeningocele). Anencephaly is almost never compatible with long-term survival. Spina bifida is compatible with long-term survival, although it is frequently associated with hemiparesis, urinary incontinence, and hydrocephalus.

Anencephaly and spina bifida represent different manifestations of the same pathogenic process and reflect the same genetic etiology. Couples who have had a child with an NTD have approximately a 1 percent risk for any subsequent offspring having spina bifida and a 1 percent risk for subsequent offspring having anencephaly (2 percent for any NTD).[96] This holds true irrespective of the type of NTD present in the index case (proband). If a prospective parent has an NTD, the risk is also about 2 percent. Second-

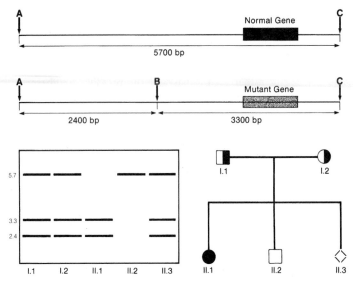

Figure 4–7. Restriction fragment length polymorphisms (RFLPs), which are invaluable for certain prenatal diagnoses. Suppose one mutant gene is linked to another gene (B) that governs whether or not a restriction site (B) is present. If the restriction site is present, DNA is cut by a certain restriction enzyme *(arrow)* to produce 3,300- and 2,400-bp-long fragments. If the segment conferring the restriction site is not present, the total fragment is 5,700 bp long. The different lengths can serve as markers to allow genotypes to be deduced. Suppose two obligate heterozygotes I.1 and I.2 have one affected child. Suppose further that a probe for the gene hybridizes to the region A to C. The probe can thus identify three fragments (2,400, 3,300, and 5,700 bp). If the affected child shows only the 2,400-and 3,300-bp fragments, it can be deduced that the mutant allele is in association (i.e., on the same chromosome) with the gene-conferring restriction site B and thus is producing both 2,400-and 3,300-bp fragments. The normal allele must be in association with the allele not conferring restriction B and thus is designated by the 5,700-bp fragment. Genotypes can thus be predicted from DNA analysis of chorionic villi and amniotic fluid cells. Fetus II.3 can be assumed to be heterozygous because all three fragments (2,400, 3,300, and 5,700 bp) are present.

degree relatives (nieces, nephews, grandchildren) and third-degree relatives (first cousins) are less likely to be affected.

Antenatal diagnosis of an NTD is best accomplished by amniotic fluid α-fetoprotein (AF-AFP) assay. Through AF-AFP analysis, diagnosis of an NTD is possible in all anencephaly cases and in all spina bifida cases except the 5 to 10 percent in which skin covers the lesion. Closed lesions are somewhat more common in encephaloceles. Ultrasonography by experienced physicians should readily exclude anencephaly, and spina bifida theoretically can be detected by serial views of the vertebral column, shape of the cranium, ventricles, cerebellum, and cisternal magna. Unfortunately, few ultrasonographers know the sensitivity or specificity for detecting NTDs. Until such data are available, AF-AFP analysis should be considered the standard method for detecting an NTD despite frequent hopes and statements to the contrary.

Elevated AFP is also associated with certain other polygenic/multifactorial anomalies (e.g., omphalocele, gastroschisis, cystic hygroma). In these disorders, AChE may or may not be elevated. With certain mendelian traits (e.g., congenital nephrosis), AFP is elevated but AChE is not. Ultrasonographic studies should therefore be undertaken to corroborate elevated AF-AFP and to determine the nature of any defect present. On the other hand, failure to detect an anomaly by ultrasound does not necessarily indicate that elevated AF-AFP was spurious. If AF-AFP is elevated and AChE is present, the fetus should be considered abnormal irrespective of ultrasound findings.

Folic acid deficiency is a major cause of NTD. This conclusion has been accepted for a decade, after a prospective, randomized study that found that folic acid supplementation decreased the recurrence rate of NTD, by 71 percent in women who had a previous child with an NTD.[97] The ACOG recommends 0.4 mg folate daily, beginning at least 1 month prior to conception.[97] In women who have had a child with a prior NTD, 4 mg daily is recommended.

Disorders Detectable Only by Ultrasound

Anomalies inherited in polygenic/multifactorial fashion usually carry recurrence risks of 1 to 5 percent for first-degree relatives (siblings, offspring, parent), a risk sufficiently high to justify prenatal diagnosis for many couples. Except for the few conditions amenable to AF-AFP analysis, the principal method of assessment involves visualization of fetal anatomy by ultrasound.

The typical couple at risk already has had a child with the anomaly in question, thus incurring a 1 to 5 percent risk for another affected child. To alter clinical management, a diagnosis should be made by 20 to 24 weeks' gestation. This is sufficiently early to weigh the alternative options of termination, fetal surgery, or preterm delivery followed by neonatal surgery. PUBS and second-trimester transabdominal CVS can exclude chromosomal abnormalities if either of the latter options are contemplated. A careful search for other defects is also necessary. For some anomalies (e.g., hydrocephaly), an isolated anomaly is rare, but for others (e.g., posterior urethral values), only a single malformation may be present.

Antenatal ultrasonography for anomaly detection should be performed only by highly experienced physicians. Physicians scanning obstetric patients only for fetal viability, multiple gestations, and placental location should explicitly inform their patients that anomaly assessment is not being attempted. Casual reassurance of fetal normalcy should be eschewed.

Key Points

- ➤ The frequency of major birth defects is 2 to 3 percent. Major etiologic categories include chromosomal abnormalities (1 per 160 live births), single-gene or mendelian disorders, polygenic/multifactorial disorders, and teratogenic disorders. Of the chromosomal abnormalities, approximately half represent autosomal trisomy and half sex chromosomal abnormalities.

- ➤ Genetic screening for heterozygote detection in the nonpregnant and, if not already evaluated, pregnant population is appropriate for only selected autosomal recessive disorders: Tay-Sachs disease in Jewish populations, α-thalassemia in Asians, β-thalassemia in Mediterranean peoples (Greek and Italian), sickle cell in African-American blacks.

- ➤ The ACOG and major genetic organizations have recently recommended that screening for cystic fibrosis be offered to Caucasian and Ashkenazi Jewish individuals, and made available to other ethnic populations. Detection rates are 80 to 95 percent in the two former groups, and 70 percent or lower in African-Americans, Hispanics, and Asians. Screening for a defined panel of alleles is considered the minimal standard.

- ➤ In all pregnancies, genetic screening should be performed for chromosomal abnormalities and NTDs. All women aged 35 years and above at delivery should be offered prenatal cytogenetic diagnosis. For younger women, maternal serum screening should be offered to detect autosomal trisomies. The profile of decreased MSAFP, elevated hCG, and decreased unconjugated serum estriol favors Down syndrome. Maternal serum analyte screening in combination with maternal age can detect 60 percent of Down syndrome cases, but the frequency varies

Box continued on following page

Key Points *Continued*

according to maternal age (90 percent over age 35 but about 25 percent in the early third decade). Screening for NTDs involves elevated MSAFP followed by amniotic fluid analysis; approximately 80 to 90 percent of NTDs can be detected at a cost of 5 percent amniocentesis.

➤ All invasive procedures carry risks. Amniocentesis at 15 weeks and above carries a procedure-related risk of perhaps 0.2 to 0.5 percent loss. Amniocentesis before 13 weeks is not recommended because of the unacceptable 1 to 2 percent risk of clubfoot. If experienced hands, CVS is considered equal to amniocentesis in terms of loss rates and diagnostic accuracy. Transcervical and transabdominal CVS are equivalent in safety.

➤ Controversy exists concerning LRDs associated with CVS. If a risk exists, it appears to be greatest below 10 weeks' gestation, for which reason, in general, the procedure should generally be available at 10 weeks and beyond. A maximum limb reduction risk of 1 in 3,000 has been reported, and many believe that the risk is not greater than that of the general population.

➤ The complication rate associated with fetal blood sampling is uncertain, but appears to be 1 to 2 percent. The rate varies according to the diagnosis being assessed.

➤ Many single-gene disorders are detectable by enzymatic analysis,whereas others can be recognized only through molecular methodologies.

➤ Two principal types of molecular analysis are employed. Direct analysis is possible if the gene sequence is known. Linkage analysis is necessary if the gene has been localized but not yet sequenced. Linkage analysis takes advantage of markers lying close to the gene in question; accuracy is not 100 percent because recombination can occur between the marker and the mutant gene.

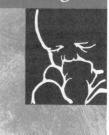

Chapter 5

Obstetric Ultrasound: Assessment of Fetal Growth and Anatomy

FRANK A. CHERVENAK AND
STEVEN G. GABBE

Diagnostic ultrasound has emerged as an important tool for antepartum fetal surveillance. This technology has permitted the most accurate assessment of gestational age and has enabled the obstetrician to follow fetal growth serially and to detect fetal growth disorders.

BIOPHYSICS OF ULTRASOUND

To use ultrasound most effectively, the obstetrician should understand the basic biophysics of the technique.[1] Sound is a waveform of energy that causes small particles in a medium to oscillate. The frequency of sound refers to the number of peaks or waves that traverse a given point per unit of time and is expressed in hertz. Sound with a frequency of one cycle or one peak per second would have a frequency of 1 Hz. Ultrasound applies to high-frequency sound waves exceeding 20,000 Hz. Diagnostic ultrasound instruments operate in a higher range of frequencies, varying from 2 to 10 million Hz, or 2 to 10 MHz.

Ultrasound energy is produced by a transducer containing crystal structures that convert electrical energy to ultrasound waves and the returning echoes to electrical energy. Therefore, each crystal in the transducer acts as both a transmitter and a receiver.

Diagnostic ultrasound equipment generates a sound pulse every 1 msec, and the duration of the pulse is 1 μsec. The time the sound pulse is off is 1,000 times greater than the time it is on. During a 15-minute diagnostic evaluation, the fetus is exposed to only 1 second of ultrasound energy.

PRINCIPLES OF IMAGING

A two-dimensional picture is created when the returning ultrasound echoes are displayed on an oscilloscope screen.[1] The ultrasound signal returning to the transducer is converted to an electrical impulse, and the strength of that electrical impulse is directly proportional to the strength of the returning echo. The density of the medium into which the sound wave has been transmitted and through which it is reflected will determine the strength of the signal. The velocity of the reflected sound wave will be faster and its signal on the oscilloscope brighter after reflection off bone than off tissues that are less dense, such as muscle, fat, brain, or water. Air greatly decreases the transmission of sound waves. For this reason, a coupling medium or gel is applied between the surface of the transducer and the skin or vaginal mucosa.

Ultrasound can be used to produce diagnostic images in several ways. B mode (brightness modulation) converts the strength of the returning echoes into signals of varying brightness that are proportional to the amplitude of the returning echoes. A storage oscilloscope is used to create a compounded image of the target and, in this way, produce a two-dimensional picture. Real-time array transducer systems create these images within a fraction of a second. The standard transducer used in these systems is 3.5 MHz. The higher the frequency of the sound the better the reproduction and resolution, but the shallower the depth of penetration.

Doppler ultrasound differs significantly from the imaging techniques that have been described. In this application of ultrasound, used in Doppler velocimetry and antepartum and intrapartum fetal heart rate monitoring, the receiver detects shifts in the frequency of the returning sound waves rather than in the amplitude of these reflected echoes.

SAFETY OF ULTRASOUND

Studies of clinical outcomes of infants exposed to ultrasound have failed to demonstrate any significant effects. In 1993, the American Institute of Ultrasound in Medicine (AIUM) Bioeffects Committee concluded[10]:

No confirmed biological effects on patients or instrument operators caused by exposure at intensities typical of the present diagnostic ultrasound instruments have ever been reported. Although the possibility exists that such biological effects may be identified in the future, current data indicate that the benefits to patients of the prudent use of diagnostic ultrasound outweigh the risks, if any, that may be present.

In considering the safety of any diagnostic procedure, one must also consider the skill with which the examination is conducted and the way in which the results are interpreted and utilized. False-positive and false-negative diagnoses appear to be the greatest risk for the patient undergoing an obstetric ultrasound examination.

TRANSVAGINAL ULTRASOUND

Transvaginal ultrasound, with its ability to use higher frequency transducers, can result in better visualization of the early pregnancy.[15-17]

A gestational sac can be seen with transvaginal ultrasound as early as 4.5 menstrual weeks[18]. The normal gestational sac is located in the upper uterine body and has a smooth contour and a round shape. Once seen, the gestational sac grows at a fairly constant rate of 1 mm in mean diameter per day.[19]

The yolk sac is visualized when the gestational sac is 10 mm or larger. Between the 7th and the 13th menstrual weeks, the yolk sac gradually increases in diameter from about 3 mm to 6 mm (Fig. 5–1).[20,21]

The amnion develops about the same time as the yolk sac but, because it is thinner, the amnion is more difficult to visualize. It surrounds the embryo and is opposite the yolk sac. The amnion

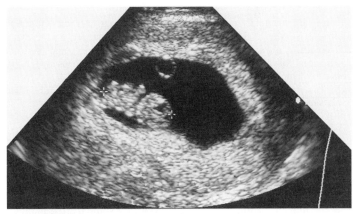

Figure 5–1. Sonogram demonstrating crown–rump length (between crosses) of 8-week fetus. Yolk sac is in the near field.

grows rapidly during early pregnancy, and fusion with the chorion is usually complete by the 16th week.

Cardiac activity is usually the first manifestation of the embryo at about 6 menstrual weeks. Once the embryo is 5 mm, cardiac activity should be present; its absence is indicative of early demise.[22-24] If cardiac activity is absent and the embryo is less than 5 mm, the findings are not conclusive. Embryonic movements can be seen between 7 and 8 menstrual weeks.

Although the gestational sac can be used to date an early pregnancy, the most accurate sonographic measure is the crown–rump length.[23] During the first trimester, this method is accurate to within 4 to 5 days. As this is the single best tool to assess gestational age at any time in pregnancy, it should be considered for patients at risk for growth restriction and other complications of pregnancy.

The embryonic pole, a flat, echogenic structure, can be visualized when it is 2 to 4 mm during the seventh menstrual week. During the eighth week, a large head with a posterior cystic space, representing the rhombencephalon, can be visualized, together with the spinal column and the lower and upper extremities. By the 9th week, the falx cerebri and the choroid plexus can be seen, and, by the 11th week, the echogenic choroid plexus fills the prominent ventricles. The cerebellum may not be visualized until after 12 weeks.[15-17]

Between the 8th and 12th weeks, there is a normal midgut herniation. This should not be confused with an omphalocele, which can be diagnosed with certainty after that time. The liver can be seen at 9 to 10 weeks; the stomach, at 10 to 12 weeks; the bladder, at 11 to 13 weeks; and the four chambers of the heart, at about 12 weeks.[15-17]

Many of the fetal anomalies identified during a transabdominal anatomic survey at 18 to 20 weeks can be diagnosed earlier with transvaginal ultrasound. The anomalies with the most serious disruptions of anatomy, such as anencephaly, holoprosencephaly, cystic hygroma, and conjoined twins, may be detected.[15-17] However, first-trimester ultrasound should not be used as a substitute for a second-trimester evaluation of anatomy.

An important aspect of first-trimester ultrasound is the evaluation of nuchal translucency (Fig. 5–2) to predict chromosomal aberrations. Nuchal translucency when combined with maternal age and/or serum analytes such as free β-human chorionic gonadotropin and pregnancy-associated plasma protein A have a combined sensitivity exceeding 90 percent in detecting chromosomal abnormalities including Down syndrome.[27-30] It is essential that the nuchal translucency be measured in a standardized manner.

Although the main value of vaginal ultrasound is in early pregnancy, it may also be of clinical use later in gestation. Vaginal

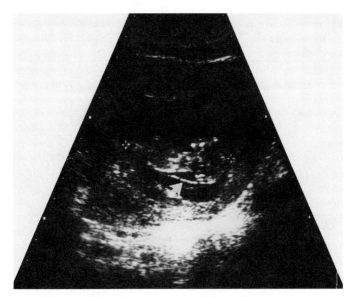

Figure 5-2. Sonogram demonstrating nuchal translucency *(arrow)* greater than 3 mm in 10-week embryo.

ultrasound permits direct visualization of the internal cervical os and allows accurate assessment of the location of the placenta and its distance from the internal os. Vaginal ultrasound may identify early signs of preterm labor or incompetent cervix, such as funneling or shortening of the cervical length.[32,33]

SECOND TRIMESTER

Assessment of Gestational Age

When performed during the first trimester, ultrasound permits an extremely accurate assessment of gestational age. The fetal crown–rump length, a measurement from the top of the fetal head to its rump, can define gestational ages between 6 and 10 weeks with an error of ± 3 to 5 days (Table 5-1).[35] In general, the gestational age of the pregnancy in weeks is equal to 6.5 plus the crown–rump length of the fetus in centimeters. When performing a crown–rump length measurement, care must be taken to avoid confusing the yolk sac with the fetal head. Beyond 12 weeks, the fetus begins to curve and the crown–rump length loses its accuracy.

Table 5–1. ULTRASONOGRAPHIC ASSESSMENT OF FETAL AGE

Measurement	Gestational Age (Menstrual Weeks)	Range (Days)
Crown-rump length	5–12	± 3
Biparietal diameter	12–20	± 8
	20–24	± 12
	24–32	± 15
	>32	± 21
Femur length	12–20	± 7
	20–36	± 11
	>36	± 16

From Gabbe SG, Iams JD: Intrauterine growth retardation. *In* Iams JD, Zuspan FP (eds): Manual of Obstetrics and Gynecology. St. Louis, CV Mosby, 1990, p 169.

The biparietal diameter (BPD) is the measurement most often used for establishing fetal gestational age. The BPD is the most accurate predictor of the estimated date of confinement (EDC) when performed between 12 and 18 weeks' gestation. The transaxial or transverse BPD is best obtained at the level of the thalami and cavum septum pellucidum (Fig. 5–3). The BPD measurement is made from the outer edge of the skull to the inner edge of the opposite side.

Gestational age assessment by ultrasound has recently been assessed in populations of patients with precisely dated pregnancies that resulted from in vitro fertilization (IVF).[37,38] The clinical practice in many units has been that, when gestational age by last menstrual period disagrees by more than 10 or 14 days from that derived from fetal biometry in the second trimester, the last menstrual period is superseded by fetal biometry. Data derived from an IVF population suggest that, in the face of a discrepancy of more than 7 days (2 SD), the sonographic biometric prediction should be given preference, provided there is no anomaly or severe growth delay. Other authorities would recommend that the biometric prediction should be given preference in every case.[38,39]

From 12 to 28 weeks' gestation, the relationship between BPD and gestational age is linear.[40] However, late in gestation, growth of the fetal head slows, and errors of several weeks may be made in estimating gestational age. In addition, later in gestation, the fetal head becomes more elongated in its anterior posterior plane. Such dolichocephaly may be assessed by measuring the cephalic index, the ratio of the BPD divided by the occipital frontal diameter. This

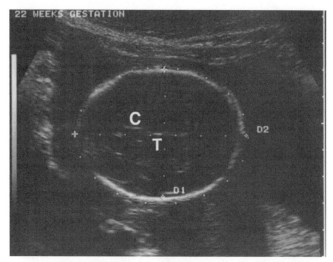

Figure 5-3. A determination of the BPD at the level of the thalami (T) and cavum septum pellucidum (C). The BPD measurement is made from the outer edge of the skull to the opposite inner edge (D1) and on a line perpendicular to the midline. The occipitofrontal diameter (D2) is also shown. The electronic calipers *(dots)* have been placed to obtain a measurement of the HC.

ratio should normally be 0.75 to 0.85. If the ratio falls outside this range, the BPD should not be used to estimate gestational age. Femur length may be applied in such cases.

Assessment of Fetal Viability

Real-time ultrasound can be used to confirm the presence of fetal death in utero. The absence of fetal cardiac motion as well as the presence of fetal scalp edema and overlapping of the fetal cranial bones confirms fetal death.

THIRD TRIMESTER

Evaluation of Fetal Growth

When establishing gestational age and evaluating fetal growth, it is best to evaluate a variety of parameters, including the BPD, long bones, especially the femur and humerus, as well as the abdominal circumference (AC) (Fig. 5-4), and transcerebellar diameter. The

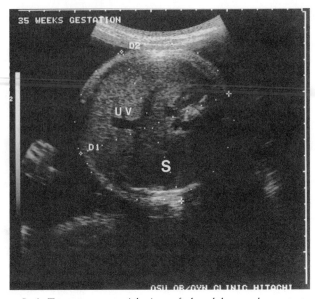

Figure 5–4. Transverse or axial view of the abdomen demonstrates the fetal stomach (S) and umbilical vein (UV). Note that the abdomen is round and the umbilical vein is well within the substance of the liver. This is the proper level for determination of the fetal AC; electronic calipers (*dots*) have been placed to make this measurement. The AC may also be calculated using measurements of the anteroposterior (D1) and transverse (D2) abdominal diameters using the following formula: $AC = D1 + D2 \times 1.57$.

uniformity of fetal growth that characterizes early gestation is lost after 20 weeks. Therefore, a single ultrasound study performed late in pregnancy cannot accurately establish gestational age (Table 5–1). The fetal AC measured at the level of the umbilical vein has been used not only to assess gestational age, but to detect the presence of intrauterine growth restriction (IUGR) and macrosomia. Composite tables estimating fetal weight have been constructed by several authors and are usually based on a combination of (1) head size, as measured by BPD or head circumference (HC); (2) femur length (FL); and (3) AC.[41] The BPD and fetal AC may be combined to calculate estimates of fetal weight that are likely to be within 10 percent of actual weight.

Abnormal Fetal Growth

Fetal growth restriction is discussed in Chapter 20.

Fetal Macrosomia (see Chapters 11 and 21)

Macrosomia has been defined by some investigators as a birth weight in excess of 4,000 to 4,500 g.[44] Other studies categorize infants with a birth weight above the 90th percentile as large for gestational age (LGA). Excessive fetal growth resulting in macrosomia has long been recognized as an important cause of perinatal morbidity and mortality, especially in the pregnancy complicated by diabetes mellitus. At delivery, the macrosomic fetus is more likely to suffer shoulder dystocia, traumatic injury, and asphyxia.

Macrosomia in the infant of the diabetic mother (IDM) is characterized by selected organomegaly, with increases in both fat and muscle mass resulting in a disproportionate increase in the size of the abdomen and shoulders. However, brain growth is not altered, and, therefore, the HC is usually normal. Thus, the macrosomia of the IDM is asymmetric. The macrosomic infant of an obese woman without glucose intolerance will demonstrate excessive growth of *both* the AC and HC, or symmetric macrosomia.

Antenatal sonographic detection of the LGA fetus could allow optimal selection of the route of delivery to reduce the likelihood of birth trauma. Unfortunately, our clinical ability to evaluate fetal size at term remains poor, with only 35 percent of large infants being identified by excessive symphysis–fundal height measurements.[45]

Several studies have emphasized the limited predictive value of ultrasound to identify the macrosomic fetus and the unnecessary interventions that may be undertaken for suspected macrosomia.[47-51] Overall, both the sensitivity and positive predictive value in these reports range between 50 and 60 percent. It must be remembered that formulas for estimation of fetal weight are associated with a 95 percent confidence range of at least 10 to 15 percent.[42] Thus, the predicted weight using ultrasonography would have to exceed 4,700 g for all fetuses with weights in excess of 4,000 g to be accurately identified!

In summary, detection of the macrosomic infant using both clinical *and* ultrasonographic techniques remains challenging. In patients at risk for fetal macrosomia—women who have diabetes mellitus, are obese, or whose pregnancies go beyond 41 weeks—a "growth profile" including ultrasound measurements of estimated fetal weight and the HC/AC ratio may improve the identification of excessive fetal growth.[55] In patients at low risk for macrosomia, a fundal height measurement of 4 cm or more than expected for gestational age should signal the need for an ultrasound study.

Assessment of Amniotic Fluid Volume

Ultrasound has proved valuable in the evaluation of amniotic fluid volume. Early application of this technology included measurements of the largest vertical pocket of fluid. Oligohydramnios, a reduction in amniotic fluid volume, was diagnosed when the largest pocket of amniotic fluid measured in two perpendicular planes was less than 1 cm. Hydramnios or excessive amniotic fluid was diagnosed when the largest pocket of amniotic fluid exceeded 8 cm in two perpendicular planes.[57] Fetal structural anomalies are significantly increased in pregnancies complicated by oligo- or polyhydramnios.

The amniotic fluid index (AFI) has improved the reproducibility and quantitation of amniotic fluid volume. The AFI measurement is performed with the patient in the supine or semi-Fowler's positive position. The maternal abdomen is divided into quadrants (Fig. 5–5). The umbilicus is used as one reference point to divide the uterus into upper and lower halves, and the linea nigra is used as the midline to divide the uterus into right and left halves. The ultrasound transducer head is then placed on the maternal abdomen along the longitudinal axis. The transducer head is maintained perpendicular to the floor, and the vertical diameter of the

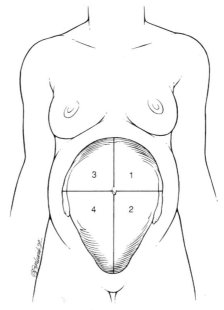

Figure 5–5. The AFI measurement utilizes ultrasound to assess the depth of fluid pockets in each quadrant of the uterus. Note that the umbilicus divides the uterus into upper and lower halves, and the linea nigra divides the uterus into right and left halves.

largest amniotic fluid pocket in each quadrant is identified and measured. The total of each of these measurements is summed to obtain the AFI in centimeters. If a fetal extremity or portion of the umbilical cord is observed in the quadrant to be measured, the transducer head is moved slightly to exclude these structures. A linear array, sector, or curvilinear transducer may be used to determine the AFI.[52] Care must be taken to avoid excessive pressure on the transducer, as this might decrease the AFI.[63] Only those amniotic fluid pockets completely clear of cord or extremities should be measured. The technique is extremely reproducible. When the AFI is determined in a patient at 20 weeks' gestation or less, the uterus is divided into halves using the linea nigra, and the largest pocket identified in each half is added to produce an AFI.

Using this technique, the mean AFI in over 350 pregnancies at 36 to 42 weeks was 12.9 ± 4.6 cm. Patients with an AFI less than 5.0 cm at term were considered to have oligohydramnios, and those with an AFI of 20 cm or greater were considered to have polyhydramnios. When the AFI fell below 5 cm, the frequency of nonreactive nonstress tests, fetal heart rate decelerations, meconium staining, cesarean sections for nonreassuring heart rate patterns, and low Apgar scores increased.

SONOGRAPHIC EVALUATION OF FETAL AND PLACENTAL ANATOMY

Evaluation of fetal and placental anatomy is an integral part of ultrasound examinations during the second and third trimesters. A basic ultrasound examination that documents fetal life, fetal number, fetal presentation, gestational age and growth, amniotic fluid volume, and placental localization without an evaluation of fetal anatomy, therefore, should be considered incomplete. The following is meant to represent the examination of fetal anatomy that should be part of the basic study. A comprehensive sonographic examination of fetal anatomy is often more detailed when it is targeted to look for a certain anomaly.[72-74]

The fetal skull should be elliptical, with the cranium ossified and intact. The ventricular system should be evaluated by assessment of the width of the atrium (Fig. 5–6), and the cerebellum should be visualized. (Fig. 5–7). An attempt should be made to visualize the face, especially to rule out a facial cleft. The spine is easier to evaluate in its entirety in the second trimester than in the third. A sagittal sonogram should be complemented by a series of transverse sonograms to identify normal anterior and normal posterior ossification elements (Figs. 5–8 and 5–9). A four-chambered view of the heart should be obtained.[75] Ventricles and atria of equal

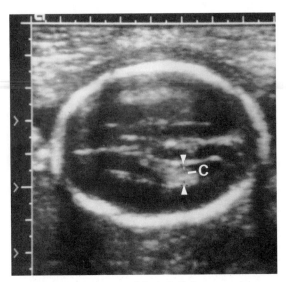

Figure 5–6. Transverse sonogram of fetal skull demonstrating normal ovoid contour. Arrowheads define width of the atrium of the lateral ventricle. C, choroid plexus.

and appropriate sizes and an intact ventricular septum should be observed (Fig. 5–10). Evaluation of outflow tracts should be attempted. The fetal bladder, stomach, and kidneys (Fig. 5–11) should be visualized. The abdominal wall should be intact (Fig. 5–12). The long bones of at least the lower extremities should be visualized (Fig. 5–13).

In addition to the assessment of placental location, ultrasound can provide an evaluation of placental anatomy[76,77] (Fig. 5–14). Although difficult during the first trimester, the location of the placenta can be clearly established by the second trimester. Placental thickness can be directly related to gestational age, with the thickness of the placenta in millimeters corresponding approximately to the weeks of gestation. For example, at 20 weeks' gestation, the placenta will be approximately 20 mm thick.

ULTRASOUND DIAGNOSIS OF FETAL ANOMALIES

Antenatal ultrasound scanning at about 18 to 20 weeks of gestation permits the detection of most major fetal structural anomalies.[80–82] It is important to appreciate, however, that even

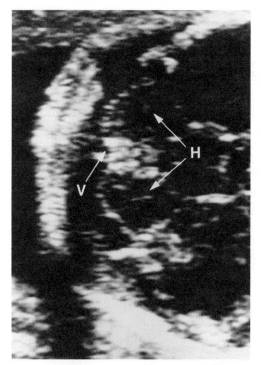

Figure 5-7. Sonogram demonstrating cerebellar hemispheres (H). V, cerebellar vermis.

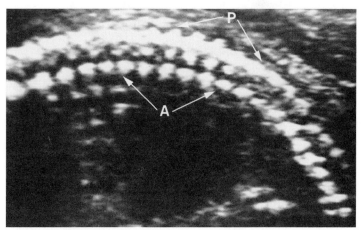

Figure 5-8. Longitudinal view of the spine demonstrating anterior (A) and posterior (P) ossification elements.

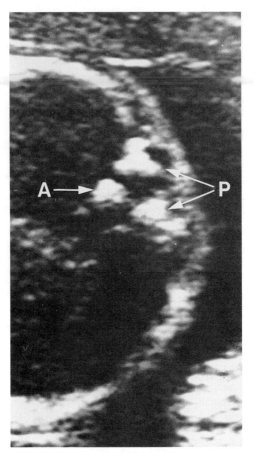

Figure 5–9. Transverse view of the spine demonstrating anterior (A) and posterior (P) ossification elements.

a thorough ultrasound evaluation during the second trimester will not detect all structural malformations. Anomalies such as hydrocephalus caused by aqueductal stenosis, duodenal atresia, microcephaly, achondroplasia, and polycystic kidneys may not manifest until the third trimester, when the degree of anatomic distortion is sufficient to be sonographically detectable.

What fetal malformations should be identified during a basic ultrasound examination? The anomalies believed to be observable in the majority of cases included anencephaly, hydranencephaly, ventriculomegaly of greater than 15 mm, alobar holoprosencephaly,

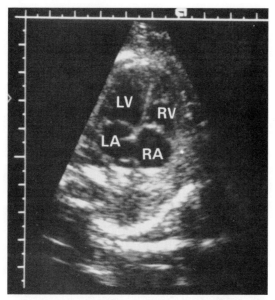

Figure 5–10. Four-chamber view of the heart. LA, left atrium; LV, left ventricle; RA, right atrium; RV, right ventricle.

open spina bifida, a large amount of ascites, bilateral hydronephrosis greater than 20 mm, omphalocele, gastroschisis, and hydrothorax with a mediastinal shift. A useful classification of fetal anomalies is based on the nature of the dysmorphology that permits sonographic detection.

Absence of a Normally Present Structure

A dramatic example of the absence of a structure normally detected by ultrasound is anencephaly, the absence of calvaria and forebrain (Fig. 5–15).

The kidneys are normally visualized as bilateral, ovoid, paraspinal masses with echospared renal pelves. When no visualized, the diagnosis of renal agenesis should be suspected. Severe oligohydramnios and the inability to visualize the bladder support the diagnosis of renal agenesis.

Presence of an Additional Structure

Masses that distort normal fetal anatomy can be readily identified with ultrasound.

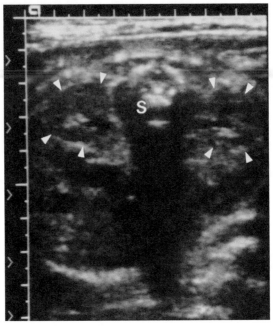

Figure 5–11. Sonogram demonstrating fetal kidneys outlined by *arrowheads*. S, fetal spine.

Fetal cystic hygromas are fluid-filled masses of the fetal neck that arise from abnormal lymphatic development. They are generally anechoic, with scattered septations and the presence of a midline septum arising from the nuchal ligament. (Fig. 5–16).

Fetal hydrops may be identified by the distortion of the normal fetal surface by skin edema. Ascites, pleural effusions, and pericardial effusions also may be identified. (Fig. 5–17).

Herniation Through Structural Defects

A common theme in the development of the fetus is the formation of compartments containing vital structures by folding and midline fusion. Incomplete fusion in a variety of locations can lead to defects and herniations of contained structures.[93]

Incomplete closure of the neural tube at the rostral end produces cephaloceles, with herniations of meninges and, frequently, of brain substance through a defect in the cranium.[94] Failed fusion at the caudal end produces spina bifida with protruding meningoceles and meningomyeloceles (Fig. 5–18). Sonographic diagnosis of each of

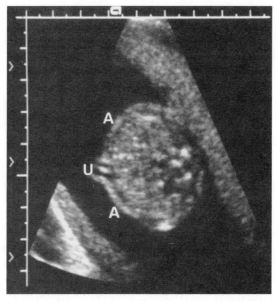

Figure 5–12. Sonogram demonstrating intact abdominal wall (A) and umbilical cord insertion (U).

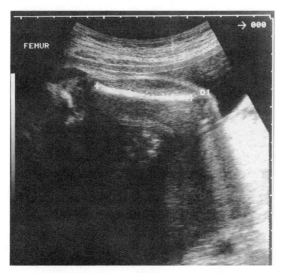

Figure 5–13. Sonogram demonstrating femur.

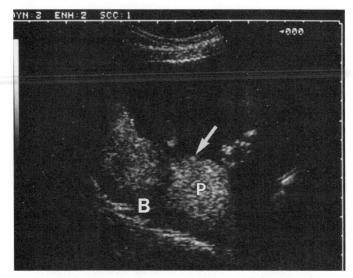

Figure 5–14. Ultrasound of a normal placenta at 24 weeks' gestation, demonstrating homogeneous placenta substance (P), smooth chorionic plate *(arrow)*, and hypoechoic basal layer (B).

these anomalies depends on the demonstration of a defect in the normal structure of the cranium or spine and of a protruding sac, often containing tissue.[95,96]

Most, if not all, cases of spina bifida are complicated by the Arnold-Chiari malformation.[97] The Arnold-Chiari malformation can serve, therefore, as an important marker for spina bifida. Two characteristic sonographic signs (the "lemon" and the "banana") of the Arnold-Chiari malformation have been described.[98] A scalloping of the frontal bones can give a lemon-like configuration, in axial section, to the skull of an affected fetus during the second trimester. The cerebellar hemispheres are centrally curved in a banana-like sonographic appearance. These characteristic cranial signs are valuable adjuncts to the sonographer in the search for spina bifida (Fig. 5–19).[98]

Omphaloceles result from failure of the intestines to retract from their temporary location in the umbilical cord and the subsequent herniation of other abdominal contents, including both hollow and solid structures contained within a peritoneal sac. Insertion of the umbilical cord into the sac helps to differentiate an omphalocele from gastroschisis, which has no covering membrane. Nonetheless, distinguishing these two entities may be difficult[99] (Figs. 5–20 and 5–21).

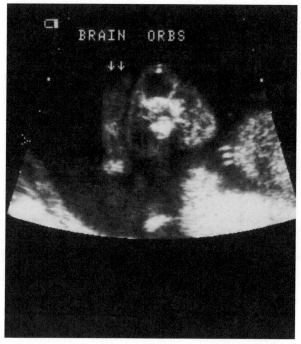

Figure 5–15. Coronal sonogram of fetal head demonstrating anencephaly.

Dilatation Behind an Obstruction

In this class of anomalies, the structural defect itself is rarely seen. Rather, what is observed is the distention of structures behind a defect. Such dilatation is caused by obstruction to the normal flow of cerebrospinal fluid, urine, or swallowed amniotic fluid.

Abnormal Fetal Biometry

Several fetal anomalies are best diagnosed not by observing alterations in shape or consistency, but by determining abnormalities in size. The science of fetal biometry has generated many nomograms defining normal values for parts of the fetal anatomy at various gestational ages.[109] (See Appendix; Obstetric Ultrasound Measurement Tables.)

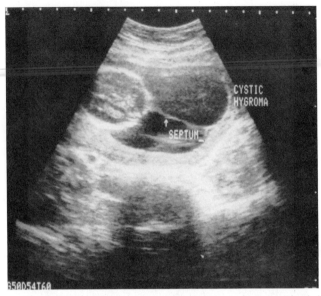

Figure 5–16. Sonogram demonstrating nuchal cystic hygroma divided by midline septum. (From Chervenak FA, Isaacson G, Lorber J: Anomalies of the Fetal Head, Neck and Spine: Ultrasound Diagnosis and Management. Philadelphia, WB Saunders Company, 1988, with permission.)

Absent or Abnormal Fetal Motion

Abnormalities in fetal motion may suggest a malformation that cannot itself be seen. Although the fetus normally can assume contorted positions in utero, the persistence of such an unusual posture over time may suggest an orthopedic or neurologic anomaly such as clubfoot or arthrogryposis.[119]

The fetal heart is the most conspicuously dynamic part of the fetus. Real-time ultrasound is invaluable in diagnosing most fetal cardiac anomalies. An attempt should be made to obtain a four-chamber view of the heart in any obstetric ultrasound examination in which fetal anatomy is surveyed.[75] Examination of the fetal outflow tracts increases the detection of heart anomalies. In cases of a suspected fetal arrhythmia, atrial and ventricular rates can be determined.[120,121]

Ultrasound Detection of Chromosomal Abnormalities in the Second Trimester

Ultrasound examination can suggest a chromosomal aberration. Sonographic markers for the most serious karyotype abnormalities

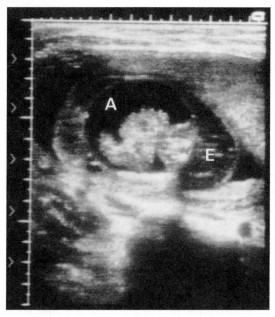

Figure 5–17. Transverse sonogram through fetal abdomen demonstrating fetal hydrops. E, edema of abdominal wall; A, ascites.

are often present. Holoprosencephaly, facial clefts, hypotelorism, omphalocele, polydactyly, and heart defects are associated with trisomy 13, whereas growth restriction, micrognathus, overlapping fingers, omphalocele, horseshoe kidney, and heart defects are associated with trisomy 18. Early-onset severe growth restriction, large head, syndactyly, and heart defects suggest triploidy. Turner's syndrome (45,X) is classically associated with nuchal cystic hygroma, but this ultrasound finding can occur in a wide variety of genetic disorders.[122]

Major structural malformations, including hydrops, duodenal atresia, and heart defects, are associated with trisomy 21. Nuchal skin thickness, defined as 6 mm or more, is a useful screening tool for trisomy 21 and other chromosomal malformations (Fig. 5–22).[121,125,126] Other sonographic signs used to screen for Down syndrome include short femur, short humerus, pyelectasis, mild cerebral ventriculomegaly, clinodactyly with hypoplastic middle phalanx of the fifth digit, widely spaced first and second toes, lowset ears, echogenic bowel, and a single palmar crease.[123,124,127] Scoring systems have been developed to include these sonographic markers, maternal age, and serum markers to achieve a reported sensitivity of 90 percent.[128-131]

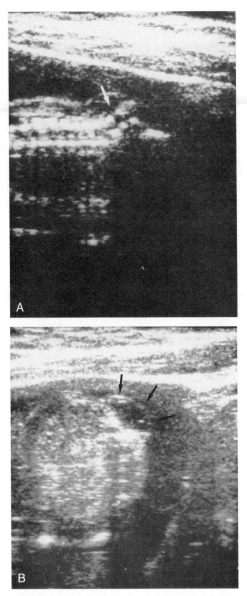

Figure 5–18. *A,* Longitudinal sonogram of fetal spine with *arrow* pointing to meningomyelocele. *B,* Transverse sonogram through fetal spine with *arrows* pointing to meningomyelocele. (From Chervenak FA, Isaacson G, Lorber J: Anomalies of the Fetal Head, Neck and Spine: Ultrasound Diagnosis and Management. Philadelphia, WB Saunders Company, 1988, with permission.)

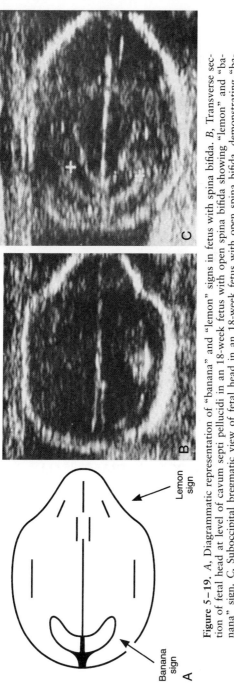

Figure 5–19. *A,* Diagrammatic representation of "banana" and "lemon" signs in fetus with spina bifida. *B,* Transverse section of fetal head at level of cavum septi pellucidi in an 18-week fetus with open spina bifida showing "lemon" and "banana" sign. *C,* Suboccipital bregmatic view of fetal head in an 18-week fetus with open spina bifida, demonstrating "banana" sign (+). (From Nicolaides KM, Campbell S, Gabbe SG, Guidetti R: Ultrasound screening for spina bifida: cranial and cerebellar signs. Lancet 2:72, 1986. Copyright 1986 The Lancet Ltd, with permission.)

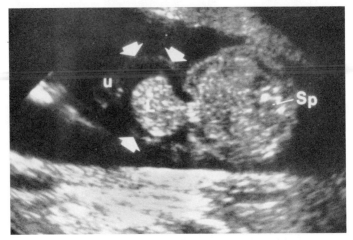

Figure 5–20. Omphalocele. The surrounding membrane (*arrowheads*), cord insertion into the apex of the omphalocele (u), liver (L) herniated into the omphalocele sac, and spine (Sp) can be seen. (Courtesy of Dr. Harbhajan Chawla.)

Choroid plexus cysts can occur in about 1 percent of fetuses and, although most are closely associated with trisomy 18, can be a marker for other chromosomal abnormalities[132,133] (Fig. 5–23). The need for a karyotype determination when the only structural abnormality seen is a choroid plexus cyst remains controversial.[134,135]

In summary, if a major structural malformation is detected with ultrasound, karyotype determination should be considered.

MANAGEMENT OF A PREGNANCY COMPLICATED BY AN ULTRASONICALLY DIAGNOSED FETAL ANOMALY

If a fetal anomaly is diagnosed by obstetric ultrasound, the fetus should be carefully evaluated for other anomalies before management options can be considered. Echocardiography and karyotype determination should usually be part of this evaluation.

WHO SHOULD HAVE AN OBSTETRIC ULTRASOUND EXAMINATION?

Routine performance of obstetric ultrasound examinations, the performance of an ultrasound study on every obstetric patient at

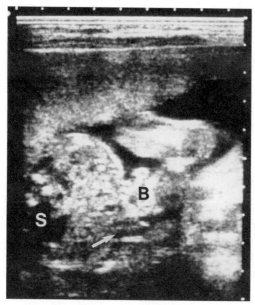

Figure 5–21. Loops of bowel (B) without a surrounding membrane are characteristic of gastroschisis. The *arrow* points to the insertion of the umbilical cord. Since the stomach (S) is on the left of the fetus, the site of the bowel herniation is to the right of the umbilical cord. (Courtesy of Dr. Harbhajan Chawla.)

approximately 18 weeks' gestation, remains controversial. A routine obstetric ultrasound examination describes what the American College of Obstetricians and Gynecologists (ACOG) has called a *basic* ultrasound examination, which would include the following information: fetal number, fetal presentation, documentation of fetal life, placental location, assessment of amniotic fluid volume, assessment of gestational age, survey of fetal anatomy for gross malformations, and an evaluation for maternal pelvic masses.[171,176] When the findings of a basic ultrasound examination suggest a fetal abnormality or in patients at greater risk of a fetal abnormality, a comprehensive ultrasound examination may be indicated. As noted by the ACOG, the comprehensive ultrasound study should be conducted by an individual experienced in these evaluations.

Routine obstetric ultrasound has become widely used in the United States. This practice offers at least six advantages: accurate dating of all pregnancies; accurate evaluation of maternal serum levels of α-fetoprotein, human chorionic gonadotropin, and unconjugated estriol (triple screening); early detection of multiple pregnancies; placental localization to rule out placenta previa; detection of structural abnormalities of the fetus; and psychological benefit to the parents.[177,178]

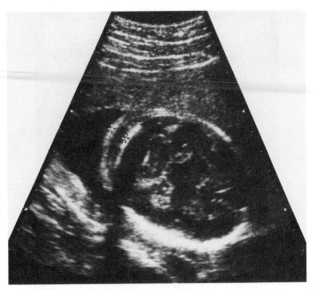

Figure 5–22. Sonogram demonstrating nuchal skin thickness greater than 6 mm.

The ideal timing for a routine ultrasound study would appear to be approximately 18 weeks' gestation. At this gestational age, the pregnancy can be accurately dated and fetal anatomy well visualized. Should a fetal abnormality be identified, sufficient time is available to perform a comprehensive ultrasound, obtain a fetal karyotype if necessary, and counsel the patient and her partner.

An ultrasound performed at 18 weeks' gestation will reveal that approximately 10 percent of placentas overlie the cervical os, allowing the obstetrician to exclude placenta previa in the remaining 90 percent of cases. Of patients with a low-lying placenta at 18 weeks, only those women in whom the placenta completely covers the os are at risk for a placenta previa in the third trimester. The risk of placenta previa in this group is 41 percent, and a repeat ultrasound evaluation should be performed in these cases.[176–185]

One of the most important benefits of routine ultrasound appears to be the identification of major congenital malformations. Major anomalies occur in 2 to 3 percent of all births, and are a leading cause of infant mortality, accounting for 22 percent of all infant deaths in 1995. Systematic examination of fetal structure as part of the basic ultrasound study outlined by the ACOG can identify a significant proportion of these abnormalities. Recent data from 61 European obstetric units participating in the Eurofetus

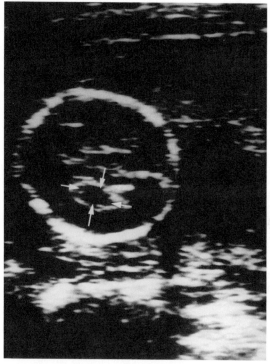

Figure 5–23. Sonogram demonstrating choroid plexus cyst outlined by *arrows*.

study demonstrate a sensitivity of 61.4 percent for the detection of 3,685 malformed fetuses.[187] Similar sensitivities and predictive values have been reported by experienced groups in this country.[188,189]

In the summary of its recent Practice Pattern on routine ultrasound in low-risk pregnancy, the ACOG concluded[208]:

- The specificity of a fetal anatomic survey in detecting fetal anomalies can be anticipated to exceed 99 percent.
- The sensitivity of a fetal anatomic survey in detecting fetal anomalies cannot be estimated with precision; rather, it should be acknowledged that sensitivity may vary in different clinical settings and with different levels of skill of professionals performing the examination.
- It is uncertain whether an improvement in the survival of fetuses with life-threatening anomalies can be expected from routine ultrasound in low-risk pregnancy.

- In a population of women with low-risk pregnancy, neither a reduction in perinatal morbidity and mortality nor a lower rate of unnecessary interventions can be expected from routine diagnostic ultrasound. Thus ultrasound should be performed for specific indications in low-risk pregnancy.

CONCLUSION

In summary, studies of routine ultrasound have failed to demonstrate any associated adverse effects on the mother or fetus. Routine ultrasound has a high positive predictive value for conditions known to be associated with poor perinatal outcome such as twins, placenta previa, and congenital malformations. To date, several large, prospective, randomized studies have evaluated the benefits of routine ultrasound in obstetric practice.[199–202] One, performed in Finland,[199] demonstrated a reduction in perinatal mortality, resulting from the identification of major fetal anomalies. The RADIUS trial,[201,202] performed in the United States, failed to show an improvement in perinatal outcome. Nevertheless, a large clinical experience from centers both in the United States and in Europe has repeatedly found that routine ultrasound screening at 18 weeks can improve gestational dating in approximately 10 to 25 percent of patients, detect nearly all multiple gestations, exclude placenta previa in most patients and recognize those at greatest risk for this condition, detect one third to one half of major fetal malformations, and reduce parental anxiety and increase compliance with the recommendations of health care providers. The cost of routine ultrasound screening must be compared with the costs created by false-positive diagnoses, which may lead to unnecessary patient anxiety and further intervention,[210] and to the cost savings resulting from reduction in the rate of inductions for suspected prolonged pregnancy, a decrease in the rate of preterm delivery for twins, and the identification of a fetus with an anomaly likely to survive but with a poor quality of life. Finally, like any analytic technique, the value of ultrasound screening is dependent on the skill with which the study is performed and the manner in which the results are interpreted and used in clinical care.[178]

Key Points

➤ Ultrasound energy is produced by a transducer containing crystal structures that convert electrical energy to ultrasound waves and the returning echoes to electrical energy.

➤ No deleterious effects on the pregnant woman or fetus caused by exposure to ultrasound at the intensities used for imaging have ever been reported.

➤ Although the gestational sac can be used to date an early pregnancy, measurement of the crown–rump length is the single best method to assess gestational age at any time in pregnancy.

➤ From 12 to 28 weeks' gestation, the relationship between the biparietal diameter and gestational age is linear.

➤ Formulas for estimation of fetal weight are associated with a 95 percent confidence range of at least 10 to 15 percent.

➤ Measurement of the fetal abdominal circumference is probably the most reliable sonographic parameter for the detection of macrosomia.

➤ At term, an AFI less than 5.0 cm indicates oligohydramnios and greater than 20 cm polyhydramnios.

➤ The thickness of the placenta in millimeters corresponds to the number of weeks gestation.

➤ The "lemon" and "banana" signs are important cranial markers for spina bifida.

➤ Major structural malformations, including hydrops, duodenal atresia, and cardiac anomalies, are observed in 30 percent of cases of Down syndrome (trisomy 21).

Chapter 6

Fetal Therapeutic Intervention

MARK I. EVANS, MICHAEL R. HARRISON,
ALAN W. FLAKE, AND MARK P. JOHNSON

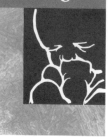

When structural and functional fetal anomalies[1] are severe or lethal, pregnancy termination may provide a reasonable management option for couples. In less severe cases, obstetric care can be tailored to optimize outcomes and prevent secondary complications. In certain situations, prenatal correction of the underlying problem has become possible. Structural malformations can sometimes be approached surgically, while metabolic disorders may benefit from pharmacologic or genetic therapy. Over the past decade, fetal therapy has evolved into four major areas: open surgical approaches, "closed" endoscopic surgical approaches, pharmacologic therapy, and stem cell/gene therapy.

If a disorder can be treated effectively and safely postnatally, there is no justification for prenatal intervention. However, for some conditions discussed, profound and irreparable damage occurs before birth, making fetal intervention the best, or sometimes only, way to ameliorate the damage. With improvements and increasing utilization of prenatal diagnosis, more women will chose to avail themselves of opportunities to treat fetuses with discernable problems.

SURGICAL THERAPY

In Utero "Closed" Fetal Surgery

The most efficacious percutaneous in utero fetal surgery has been for the evaluation and treatment of obstructive uropathy. Lower urinary tract obstruction (LUTO) is a heterogeneous entity that affects 1 in 5,000 to 1 in 8,000 newborn males. Posterior urethral valves (PUV) or urethral atresias are the most common causes for LUTO, although other causes have been observed. LUTO can result in massive distention of the bladder with compensatory hypertrophy and hyperplasia of the smooth muscle within the bladder wall, leading to a loss of compliance and elasticity, and poor postnatal function generally requiring surgical reconstruction.[2] Elevated intravesicular pressures prevent urine inflow from the ureters; distortion of the ureterovesical angles contributes to eventual reflux hydronephrosis. Progressive pyelectasis and calycectasis compress the delicate renal parenchyma within the encasing serosal capsule, leading to functional abnormalities within the medullary and eventually the cortical regions. Focal compressive hypoxia likely contributes to the progressive fibrosis and perturbations in tubular function resulting in the urinary hypertonicity that is observed. Obstructive processes can lead to type IV cystic dysplasia and renal insufficiency.

The effects are not limited to the genitourinary (GU) tract. Progressive oligo-/anhydramnios leads to compressive deformations as seen in Potter sequence, including extremity contractures and facial dysmorphology. Absence of normal amniotic fluid volume also interferes with pulmonary growth and development. Constant compressive pressure on the fetal thorax leads to restriction of expansion of the chest through normal physiologic "breathing movements." Babies born with LUTO generally die due to pulmonary complications and not renal failure.

Ruling out other congenital anomalies such as cardiac and neural tube defects is necessary before intervention can be considered. Karyotyping is essential to confirm a normal male chromosomal status, as cases of LUTO have an increased incidence of aneuploidy. Female fetuses almost always represent more complex syndromes of cloacal malformations, which do not benefit from in utero shunt therapy.

Perhaps the most important aspect of the prenatal work-up is the evaluation of underlying renal status in the fetus. A multicomponent approach to the analysis of fetal urine evaluates proximal tubular and possible glomerular status using sodium, chloride, osmolality, calcium, β_2-microglobulin, albumin, and total protein concentrations.[4] Using such an approach, one can directly correlate the degree of impaired renal function and damage with the extent of urinary hypertonicity and proteinuria. As such, the ability to counsel patients about the renal status of their fetus and the long-term prognosis has been dramatically improved.

The function of the vesicoamniotic catheter is to bypass the urethral obstruction, diverting urine into the amniotic space to allow appropriate drainage of the upper urinary tract and prevention of pulmonary hypoplasia and physical deformations. In fetuses with isolated LUTO, a normal male karyotype, and progressively improving urinary profile that meet threshold parameters (Table 6–1), succeses are accepted in salvaging fetuses using percutaneous vesicoamniotic shunt therapy.

Although vesicoamniotic shunting has certainly improved survival and renal function in cases of early obstructive uropathy, complications of this procedure remain unacceptably high. In

Table 6–1. UPPER THRESHOLD VALUES FOR SELECTING FETUSES THAT MIGHT BENEFIT FROM PRENATAL INTERVENTION

Sodium	<100 mg/dl
Chloride	<90 mg/dl
Osmolality	<190 mOsm/L
Calcium	<8 mg/dl
β_2-Microglobulin	<6 mg/L
Total protein	<20 mg/dl

48 percent of our cases the shunts have become physically displaced into the amniotic or intraperitoneal space, or have become obstructed with loss of drainage function, necessitating replacement. Concerns persist about the physiologic consequences of chronic shunt drainage on the normal development process of the lower urinary tract, given the presence of this foreign body and absence of normal filling and emptying cycles in the bladder.

Because of these concerns alternate ways to approach LUTO are being sought. One promising approach is using thin, fiberoptic endoscopes to perform in utero fetal cystoscopy and antegrade urethroscopy using simple needle systems and techniques similar to vesicocentesis.

However, on balance, intervention for LUTO has saved fetuses who would otherwise have surely died. Many have normal to moderately impaired renal function. A carefully balanced approach in counseling is required for patients to determine what is right for them.

Shunts for Thoracic Abnormalities

The other use of percutaneously placed shunts has been for thoracic abnormalities. The macrocystic form of congenital cystic adenomatous malformation can present with a large, dominant macrocyst that causes mediastinal shift with its potential hemodynamic changes, as well as pulmonary compression and risk of lung hypoplasia. Such dominant cysts can be approached using pleuroamniotic shunts to chronically drain these structures, reducing their volume, and diminishing their space-occupying effects.

Isolated pleural effusions can also accumulate, causing mediastinal hemodynamic changes and onset of generalized hydrops as well as pulmonary compression, which interferes with normal lung development, increasing the risk of hypoplasia. Small, unilateral effusions do not usually warrant intervention, but have the potential for rapid progression and initiation of generalized hydrops.[8]

Prenatal evaluation prior to intervention is critical for appropriate case selection, as isolated effusions may be the first sign of a cardiac malformation, aneuploidy, anemia, or an infectious process.

Positioning of the thoracoamniotic shunt is critical for success, and great care must be taken to avoid mediastinal structures. Shunts have the potential for displacement and obstruction, so continued ultrasound surveillance throughout the remainder of the pregnancy is necessary.[8] In most cases, postnatal management involves simple removal of the shunt in the nursery, as most of these cases represent transient chylothorax that require no additional therapy.

OPEN SURGICAL APPROACHES

Open fetal surgery has been performed for a limited number of indications for over 15 years. Its application has been limited by the appropriate concern for maternal risk, rigorous selection criteria, and somewhat frustrating results.

The Fetal Operation—General Considerations

Opening the Gravid Uterus

Open fetal surgery is performed through a maternal hysterotomy, preferentially performed in the lower uterine segment. The uterine incision must provide optimal exposure of a specific fetal part or region, avoid the placenta, and provide hemostasis with absolute control of the fetal membranes. Complete uterine relaxation facilitates fetal version when necessary and is essential for hysterotomy and the entire period of the fetal operation. Various regimens have proven effective, including a combination of preoperative indomethacin, with intraoperative isoflurane and nitroglycerin, supplemented with intravenous terbutaline or magnesium sulfate as required.

After adequate uterine relaxation is confirmed by palpation, the hysterotomy is initiated by placement of full-thickness, monofilament, absorbable traction sutures on large needles, under ultrasound guidance at the anticipated midpoint of the planned hysterotomy. Traction sutures are then used to elevate the uterine wall, which is grasped and compressed to assist in hemostasis. A large metal trocar is inserted under ultrasound guidance through this area into the amniotic space. The myometrium and membranes are then incised over the trocar for a distance of 2 to 4 cm. The full thickness of the uterus and membranes is grasped on each side with broad Allis clamps. This results in a circumferentially controlled, full-thickness puncture site in the uterine wall. A commercially available uterine stapler is then passed through the opening and fired once in each direction. The absorbable staples hemostatically compress and divide the layers of the uterus, including the membranes, with each application.[10,11]

Fetal Monitoring and Homeostasis

At this time, the use of intraoperative ultrasound remains the most reliable method of assessing fetal status, providing information on fetal heart rate, volume status, and contractility.

Fetal homeostasis is maintained by protection of uteroplacental blood flow through continued uterine relaxation and careful monitoring, and control of maternal volume status and blood pressure. Care is taken to avoid umbilical cord compression, which may occur at the margins of the hysterotomy or if inadequate amniotic fluid surrounds the fetus. Intra-amniotic volume is maintained by exteriorization of only the necessary part of the fetus, and by continuous high-volume perfusion of the amniotic space with warm lactated Ringer's solution. Without such high-volume flow, loss of uterine volume could initiate uterine contractions.

Congenital Diaphragmatic Hernia

Definitive repair of congenital diaphragmatic hernia (CDH) by reduction of viscera from the chest, diaphragmatic patch placement, and abdominal silo construction to reduce intra-abdominal pressure proved to have unacceptable mortality, particularly when the liver was herniated into the chest. Now, in utero tracheal occlusion is utilized. Tracheal occlusion induces lung growth through accumulation of pulmonary secretions, which reduces the herniated viscera from the chest and alleviates lung hypoplasia. The tracheal occlusion procedure is relatively simple, consisting of exposure of the fetal neck in hyperextension, dissection of the trachea circumferentially taking care to avoid the recurrent laryngeal nerves, and placement of occlusive hemoclips. The fetus is then gently placed back into the uterus, and the uterine incision close, paying careful attention to hemostasis.

One approach involves an open surgical approach, whereas the other favors the more technically difficult endoscopic surgical approach to minimize the complications of open fetal surgery. Published data on the two methods so far have been somewhat comparable.

After such surgical procedures as tracheal ligation, the EXIT procedure is employed. The underlying principle of the EXIT procedure is maintenance of uteroplacental perfusion until the fetal airway is secured and ventilation is established. In contrast to cesarean section, in which uterine contraction for hemostasis is encouraged, uterine relaxation is maintained by active tocolysis.

Clips can be removed, bronchoscopy performed, and stable airway access established in otherwise difficult circumstances. Only when the fetus is ready for transport to the nursery or operating suite is the cord is clamped and cut and the cesarean delivery completed.

Congenital Cystic Adenomatoid Malformation

Congenital cystic adenomatoid malformation (CCAM) is a space-occupying congenital cystic lesion of the lung that may grow and induce hydrops by causing mediastinal shift and compromising venous return to the heart. Fetuses with CCAM who develop hydrops have a mortality approaching 100 percent. Fetal resection of CCAM reverses hydrops and has improved survival dramatically.[15] The fetal operation is performed by exposure of the arm and chest wall on the side of the lesion through the maternal hysterotomy. A large thoracotomy is performed through midthorax of the fetus and the lobe containing the CCAM is exteriorized. The attachments of the lobe to adjacent lung tissue are bluntly divided and the lobar hilum is divided by application of a stapler or a bulk ligature.

Sacrococcygeal Teratoma

Fetal sacrococcygeal teratoma (SCT) arises from the presacral space and may grow to massive proportions. In some fetuses, high-output cardiac failure results from tumor vascular steal. Fetal SCT and high-output failure with associated placentomegaly or hydrops uniformly result in fetal demise. Ligation of vessels to the SCT may reduce the vascular steal and high-output failure. The fetal operation is performed by exteriorization of the fetal buttocks with the attached tumor.[16] Every attempt is made to keep the head, torso, and lower extremities of the fetus in the uterus. Since the tumor can sometimes be larger than the fetus, significant loss of uterine volume occurs, and the uterus may contract. After exteriorization of the fetus, the anus is identified, and the fetal skin incised posterior to the anorectal sphincter complex to avoid injury to the continence mechanism. A tourniquet is then applied to the base of the tumor and gradually compressed. The vascular pedicle is ligated with suture ligatures or stapled depending on the width of the pedicle. The entire fetal procedure can be performed in less than 15 minutes with minimal blood loss. Because of the increase in afterload following ligation of the low-resistance tumor circuit, fetal hemodynamic status must be monitored by ultrasound closely during and in the immediate period following the ligation.

Meningomyelocele

It has long been appreciated that babies with meningomyeloceles have impaired motor function and loss of bowel and bladder control. A significant percentage develop obstructive hydrocephalus, which requires ventriculoperitoneal shunting which, in and of itself, is fraught with complications. Experience from the 1970s and 1980s has shown that babies with meningomyeloceles delivered atraumatically by cesarean section maintain a better level of motor function for the given level of anatomic defect than those babies delivered through the vaginal canal.[17] Such data suggest that compression of the cord in the delivery process can have permanent long-term sequelae on motor function. It therefore follows that trauma to the spinal cord in utero, either from the uterine wall, or perhaps even the amniotic fluid could be detrimental to the function of the spinal cord. It was generally believed that an abnormally developed spinal cord prevented the normal proper development of the bony spinal column, leading to a meningomyelocele. It is now understood that the primary defect is likely to be the bony spinal column, which exposes a perfectly normal spinal cord, that is then damaged by the trauma of amniotic fluid and the uterine environment. Thus, the rationale was formed for attempts to patch over, or at least to protect the spinal cord in utero to minimize these sequelae.[18]

Several groups have attempted to repair meningomyeloceles in utero (Fig. 6-1), both as an open surgical procedure and endoscopically.[19,21] The principal benefit of the surgery is secondary (i.e., significant reduction in the number of babies requiring ventriculoperitoneal shunting for obstructive hydrocephalus has been

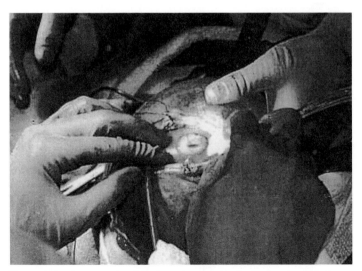

Figure 6-1. Open repair of fetal meningomyelocele. Uterus is opened over open meningomyelocele. (Courtesy of Dr. N. Scott Adzick.)

observed). Whether or not there will be significant improvements in long-term lower motor function is uncertain.

MEDICAL THERAPY

Congenital Adrenal Hyperplasia

The 21-hydroxylase enzyme defect most commonly present in congenital adrenal hyperplasia (CAH) impairs the metabolism of cholesterol to cortisol, generating excessive 17-hydroxyprogesterone. Alternate metabolism of this precursor shifts to androstenedione and other androgens (Fig. 6–2). Consequently, genetic females are exposed to high levels of androgens and can become masculinized. The resulting abnormal differentiation can vary from mild clitoral hypertrophy to formation of a phallus with labial fusion, giving rise to an apparent scrotum and misclassification of the newborn's sex.

The clinical spectrum of disease associated with CAH ranges from a severe salt-wasting variety to milder forms with simple

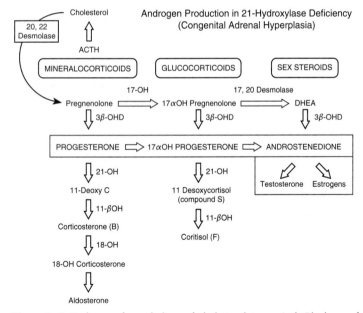

Figure 6–2. Pathway of metabolism of cholesterol to cortisol. Blockage of 21-hydroxylase leads to excess 17α-hydroxyprogesterone.

precocious virilization in males or genital ambiguity in females. Since virilization of the female fetus was thought to occur during weeks 10 to 16 of gestation, prenatal in utero therapy aimed at preventing these changes must be started prior to determination of gender or disease status.[21,24] Prenatal treatment for this problem has been aimed at pharmacologically suppressing the fetal adrenal by giving the mother dexamethasone, which readily crosses the placenta.

The fundamental principles addressed in attempts to prevent masculinization of the female fetus with CAH are logically extended to other fetal therapies. The concepts of a thorough informed consent for innovative treatments as well as detailed documentation of obstetric management and outcomes have generally been followed by investigators in this field.

Smith-Lemli-Opitz Syndrome

Smith-Lemli-Opitz syndrome (SLOS) was first reported in 1964.[29] In 1993, an inborn error of cholesterol biosynthesis in a patient with SLOS was confirmed to be a deficiency of the hepatic enzyme 7-dehydrocholesterol (7-DHC) reductase.[30-32]

Characteristic features of SLOS include facial phenotype; growth and mental retardation; and anomalies of the heart, kidneys, central nervous system, and limbs. Cleft palate, postaxial polydactyly, syndactyly of the toes 2 and 3, and cataracts are often seen in affected patients.

Patients with SLOS are deficient in cholesterol, and therefore also most likely have low levels of the steroid hormones necessary for masculinization of the male genitalia. The ambiguous genitalia seen in SLOS are the result of undermasculinization of male genitalia. Prenatal diagnosis is possible by either amniocentesis at or after 15 weeks' gestation or chorionic villus sampling (CVS) at 10 to 12 weeks.

Fetal treatment could theoretically involve providing cholesterol to the mother or to the fetus.[32-35] The former is not possible because cholesterol does not easily cross the placenta in the third trimester. Cholesterol is available only in a crystalline form that cannot be given intravenously or intramuscularly it cannot be placed in the amniotic fluid because it would precipitate. However, cholesterol can be administered to the fetus in the form of low-density lipoprotein (LDL) cholesterol in fresh frozen plasma. Early investigation is underway in patients late in pregnancy.[34]

Neural Tube Defects

In 1980, Smithells et al. suggested that vitamin supplementation containing 0.36 mg folate can reduce the frequency of NTD recurrence by sevenfold in women with one or more prior affected children.[36,37] In 1991, a randomized double-blinded trial designed by the MRC Vitamin Study Research Group demonstrated that preconceptional folate reduced the risk of recurrence in high-risk patients.[41] Subsequently, it was shown that preparations containing folate and other vitamins also reduced the occurrence of first-time NTDs.[42] In response to these findings, the Centers for Disease Control (CDC) issued guidelines calling for consumption of 4.0 mg/day folic acid by women with a prior child affected with an NTD, for at least 1 month prior to conception through the first 3 months of pregnancy. Lower amounts (0.4 mg/day folic acid) are recommended preconceptionally for *all women* of reproductive age. (Over half of all pregnancies in the United States are not planned.) As of January 1998, the U.S. Food and Drug Administration has mandated that breads and grains be supplemented with folic acid. The majority of experts believe that the primary incidence of NTDs could be cut by perhaps half by folic acid supplementation.

PRENATAL HEMATOPOIETIC STEM CELL TRANSPLANTATION

Hematopoietic stem cell (HSC) therapy for the treatment of congenital disease has tremendous theoretical appeal. The replacement of defective cells with normal cells during specific periods of organ development and cellular ontogeny may have significant advantages over postnatal transplantation.

The engraftment and clonal proliferation of a relatively small number of normal HSCs can sustain normal hematopoiesis for a lifetime. This observation provides the compelling rationale for bone marrow transplantation (BMT) and is now supported by thousands of long-term survivors of BMT who otherwise would have succumbed to lethal hematologic disease. Realization of the full potential of BMT, however, continues to be limited by a critical shortage of immunologically compatible donor cells, the inability to control the recipient or donor immune response, and the requirement for recipient myeloablation to achieve engraftment. The price of HLA mismatch remains high: the greater the mismatch, the higher the incidence of graft failure, graft-versus-host disease (GVHD), and delayed immunologic reconstitution. These problems remain prohibitive for most patients who might theoretically benefit from BMT. An attractive alternative that could address many of the limitations of BMT is in utero transplantation of HSC. This approach may be applicable to any congenital hematopoietic disease that can be diagnosed prenatally and can be cured or improved by engraftment of normal HSCs.

Rationale for In Utero Transplantation

The rationale for in utero transplantation is to take advantage of the window of opportunity created by normal ontogeny of hematopoietic cell lines. There is a period, prior to population of the bone marrow and prior to thymic processing of self-antigen, when the fetus theoretically should be receptive to engraftment of foreign HSC without rejection and without the need for myeloablation. In the human fetus, the ideal window would appear to be prior to 14 weeks' gestation, before release of differentiated T lymphocytes into the circulation and while the bone marrow is just beginning to develop sites for hematopoiesis. The window may extend beyond that in immunodeficiency states, particularly when T-cell development is abnormal. Technical advances in fetal intervention make transplantation feasible by 12 to 14 weeks' gestation. The ontologic window of opportunity falls well within these diagnostic and technical constraints, making application of this approach a realistic possibility.

With prenatal HSC transplantation there would be no requirement for HLA matching, resulting in expansion of the donor pool. Transplanted cells would not be rejected, and space would be available in the bone marrow, eliminating the need for toxic immunosuppressive and myeloablative drugs. The mother's uterus may also prove to be the ultimate sterile isolation chamber, eliminating the high risk and costly 2 to 4 months of isolation required after postnatal BMT and prior to immunologic reconstitution.

The source of donor cells may prove to be critical for the success of engraftment. The most obvious advantage of the use of fetal HSCs is the minimal number of mature T cells in fetal liver-derived populations prior to 14 weeks' gestation. This alleviates any concern about GVHD and avoids the necessity of T-cell depletion processes, which can negatively impact potential engraftment.

There are practical and ethical advantages to the use of cord blood or postnatal HSC sources, but efficacy especially for the latter is not proved.

Several diseases Amenable to Prenatal Treatment by HSC

Sickle cell anemia and thalassemia syndromes make up the largest patient groups potentially treatable. Both groups can be diagnosed within the first trimester. Both have been cured by postnatal BMT, but BMT is not recommended routinely because of its prohibitive morbidity and mortality and the relative success of modern postnatal medical management.

In SCD, erythrocytes have a circulating half-life of 10 to 20 days (normal half-life, 120 days) prior to destruction. In thalassemia, most cells (80 percent) never leave the bone marrow and also have shortened survival in the periphery. Engraftment of even a relatively small number of normal HSCs could result in significantly increased levels of peripheral donor cell expression.

Immunodeficiency diseases are a second indication. These heterogeneous groups of diseases differ in their likelihood of cure, based on their capacity to develop hematopoietic chimerism. Once again, the most likely to benefit from even low levels of donor cell engraftment are those diseases in which a survival advantage exists for normal cells. The best example of this situation is severe combined immunodeficiency disease (SCID). Several different molecular causes of SCID have been identified, with approximately two thirds of cases being of X-linked recessive inheritance (X-SCID). The genetic basis of X-SCID has been defined recently[48] as a mutation of the gene encoding the common -γ chain (-γc), which is a common component of several members of the cytokine receptor superfamily, including those for interleukin-2 (IL-2), IL-4, IL-7, IL-9, IL-15, and possibly IL-13. Children affected with X-SCID have simultaneous disruption of multiple cytokine systems, resulting in a block in thymic T-cell development and diminished T-cell response. Although present in normal or even increased numbers, B cells are dysfunctional, secondary to either the lack of helper T-cell function or an intrinsic defect in B-cell maturation. Another form of SCID arises secondary to adenosine deaminase (ADA) deficiency. Transfer of ADA-gene-corrected cells versus uncorrected cells from the same SCID patient into an immunodeficient BNX mouse results in survival of the corrected cells and death of the uncorrected cells, confirming a survival advantage for ADA-producing cells even when there is normal ADA production in the surrounding environment.

Flake et al. successfully treated a fetus with X-linked SCID in a family where a previously afflicted child died at 7 months of age. For this couple, abortion was not an option. Paternal bone marrow was harvested, T cells depleted, and enriched stem cell populations injected intraperitoneally into the fetus beginning at about 16 weeks' gestation. Subsequent injections were performed at 17 and 18 weeks. The baby presently shows a split chimerism with all of his T cells being his father's, whereas the majority of B cells are his. He has achieved normal milestones and immune progress through 2 years of age.[45]

A final group of diseases that could benefit from prenatal HSC are inborn errors of metabolism, caused by a deficiency of a specific lysosomal hydrolase, which results in the accumulation of substrates such as mucopolysaccharide, glycogen, or sphingolipid. Depending on the specific enzyme abnormality and the compounds that accumulate, certain patterns of tissue damage and organ failure occur. BMT or HSC transplantation in these diseases could provide HSC-derived mononuclear cells to repopulate various organs in the body, including the liver (Kupffer cells), skin (Langerhans' cells), lung (alveolar macrophages), spleen (macrophages), lymph nodes, tonsils, and the brain (microglia). Patients with disorders that have been corrected by postnatal BMT, such as Gaucher disease or Maroteaux-Lamy syndrome (minimal CNS involvement), are certainly reasonable candidates for prenatal treatment. In many cases, postnatal BMT has corrected the peripheral manifestations of the disease and has arrested the neurologic deterioration. However, postnatal BMT has not reversed neurologic injury that is present in such disorders. Neurologic injury may begin well before birth. Postnatal maturation of the blood-brain barrier restricts access to the CNS of transplanted cells or the deficient enzyme, but prenatal treatment could be more efficacious. The unanswered question is whether donor HSC-derived microglial elements would populate the CNS, providing the necessary metabolic correction inside the blood-brain barrier.

Key Points

➤ Fetal therapy is possible for a few anomalies, but only after proper diagnosis and informed consent.

➤ Diaphragmatic hernia can be treated in utero by tracheal occlusion, which leads to lung expansion. Postnatal surgical correction can then be undertaken.

➤ Extirpative in utero surgery for congenital cystadenomatoid malformation and sacrococcygeal teratomas has reduced mortality in these conditions.

➤ Surgery for meningomyelocele is showing promise, but will require many cases for proper evaluation.

➤ Prenatal medical therapy with dexamethasone can prevent external genital masculinization in 21-hydroxylase deficiency congenital adrenal hyperplasia.

➤ Folic acid supplementation of diet can reduce both the recurrence risk and the primary incidence of neural tube defects, but must begin preconceptionally.

➤ Stem cell transplantation can achieve engraftment and correction of immunodeficiencies, such as SCID, but has not yet been effective in nonimmunodeficiency disorders.

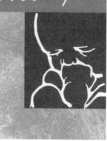

Chapter 7

Antepartum Fetal Evaluation

MAURICE L. DRUZIN, STEVEN G. GABBE, AND KATHRYN L. REED

Antepartum fetal deaths now account for almost half of all perinatal mortality in the United States.[2] The obstetrician must be concerned not only with prevention of this mortality, but with the detection of fetal compromise and the timely delivery of such infants in an effort to maximize their future potential.[3]

THE ETIOLOGY OF PERINATAL MORTALITY

The perinatal mortality rate (PMR) has been defined by the National Center for Health Statistics (NCHS) as the number of late fetal deaths (fetal deaths of 28 weeks' gestation or more) plus early neonatal deaths (deaths of infants 0 to 6 days of age) per 1,000 live births plus fetal deaths.[4] According to the NCHS, the neonatal mortality rate is defined as the number of neonatal deaths (deaths of infants 0 to 27 days of age) per 1,000 live births; the postneonatal mortality rate, the number of postneonatal deaths (the number of infants 28 to 365 days of age) per 1,000 live births; and the infant mortality rate, the number of infant deaths (deaths of infants under 1 year of age) per 1,000 live births. The American College of Obstetricians and Gynecologists (ACOG) has recommended that only deaths of fetuses and infants weighing 500 g or more at delivery be used to compare data among states in the United States.[5] For international comparisons, only deaths of fetuses and infants weighing 1,000 g or more at delivery should be included.[5]

Since 1965, the PMR in the United States has fallen steadily. Using the NCHS definition, the PMR reported in 1997 was 7.3 per 1,000.[2] The neonatal mortality rate was 3.8 per 1,000, with fetal deaths at 3.5 per 1,000. The PMR for blacks, 13.2 per 1,000, was more than twice that of whites, 6.3 per 1,000. The significantly greater PMR in blacks results from higher rates of *both* neonatal and fetal deaths.

145

Although the majority of fetal deaths occur before 32 weeks' gestation, fetuses at 40 to 41 weeks are at a threefold greater risk and those at 42 or more weeks are at a 12-fold greater risk for intrauterine death than fetuses at 28 to 31 weeks.

The infant mortality rate has fallen progressively from 47.0 per 1,000 in 1940 to 26.0 per 1,000 in 1960, 12.6 per 1,000 in 1980, 9.2 per 1,000 in 1990, and 7.2 per 1,000 in 1997.[9] Birth defects have been the single most important contributor to infant mortality for the past 20 years. In 1995, malformations were responsible for 22 percent of all infant deaths, with one third caused by cardiac abnormalities and respiratory, central nervous system, and chromosomal defects each contributing approximately 15 percent.[11]

Fetal deaths may be divided into those that occur during the antepartum period and those that occur during labor, intrapartum stillbirths. From 70 to almost 90 percent of fetal deaths occur before the onset of labor.[12] Antepartum deaths may be divided into four broad categories: (1) chronic asphyxia of diverse origin; (2) congenital malformations; (3) superimposed complications of pregnancy, such as Rh isoimmunization, placental abruption, and fetal infection; and (4) deaths of unexplained cause. If it is to succeed, a program of antenatal surveillance must identify malformed fetuses and recognize those at risk for asphyxia.

Recent data describing the specific etiologies of fetal deaths in the United States are not available. Fretts and colleagues[14,15] have analyzed the causes of deaths in fetuses weighing more than 500 g in 94,346 births at the Royal Victoria Hospital in Montreal from 1961 to 1993. Overall, the fetal death rate declined by 70 percent, from 11.5 per 1,000 in the 1960s to 3.2 per 1,000 during 1990 to 1993.[15] The decline in the fetal death rate may be attributed to the prevention of Rh sensitization, antepartum fetal surveillance, improved detection of intrauterine growth restriction (IUGR) and fetal anomalies with ultrasound, and improved care of maternal diabetes mellitus and preeclampsia. Whereas fetal mortality resulting from IUGR fell 60 percent, 17.9 to 7.0 per 1,000 births, the growth-restricted fetus still had a more than 10-fold greater risk for fetal death than an appropriately grown fetus.

Most of these deaths occurred between 28 and 36 weeks' gestation and that the diagnosis of IUGR was rarely identified before death. In addition to IUGR, leading causes of fetal death after 28 weeks' gestation included abruption and unexplained antepartum losses. Unexplained fetal deaths, were responsible for more than 25 percent of all stillbirths. Fetal–maternal hemorrhage may occur in 10 to 15 percent of cases of unexplained fetal deaths. Fetal deaths caused by infection, most often associated with premature rupture of the membranes before 28 weeks' gestation, did not decline over the 30 years of the study. After controlling for risk factors such as multiple gestation, hypertension, diabetes mellitus, placenta previa and abruption, previous abortion, and prior fetal death, women 35 years of age or older had a nearly twofold greater risk for fetal death than women under 30.

In summary, based on available data, approximately 30 percent of antepartum fetal deaths may be attributed to asphyxia (IUGR, prolonged gestation), 30 percent to maternal complications (placental abruption, hypertension, preeclampsia, and diabetes mellitus), 15 percent to congenital malformations and chromosomal abnormalities, and 5 percent to infection. At least 20 percent of stillbirths will have no obvious etiology.

Clinical experience has demonstrated that antepartum fetal assessment can have a significant impact on the frequency and causes of antenatal fetal deaths. The perinatal mortality rate in high-risk patients evaluated with the contraction stress test and nonstress test is significantly lower than in nontested patients. Most stillbirths within 7 days of testing are due to congenital malformations and placental abruption. In obstetric populations in which high-risk patients are monitored, the majority of stillbirths now occur in what had previously been considered normal pregnancies.

APPLICATION OF ANTEPARTUM FETAL TESTING

The information one might predict from an antepartum fetal test is listed in the first box. While the second box lists those aspects of obstetric management that might be influenced by antepartum testing.

Aspects of Fetal Condition That Might Be Predicted by Antepartum Testing

Perinatal death
Intrauterine growth restriction (IUGR)
Nonreassuring fetal status, intrapartum
Neonatal asphyxia
Postnatal motor and intellectual impairment
Premature delivery
Congenital abnormalities
Need for specific therapy

Adapted from Chard T, Klopper A: Introduction. *In* Placental Function Tests. New York, Springer-Verlag, 1982, p 1.

Testing can be initiated at early gestational ages, 25 to 26 weeks, to identify the fetus at risk. Maternal and fetal interventions can then be considered. Obviously, prolongation of intrauterine life is the primary goal, and better understanding of the pathophysiology of the premature fetus and the use of combinations of tests will allow this to be accomplished.

In selecting the population of patients for antepartum fetal evaluation, one would certainly include those pregnancies known to be at high risk of uteroplacental insufficiency (see the box "Indications for Antepartum Fetal Monitoring").[27]

Routine antepartum fetal evaluation would be necessary to detect most infants dying in utero as the result of hypoxia and asphyxia.[22] It would seem reasonable, therefore, to consider extending some

---

Obstetric Management That Might Be Influenced by Antepartum Testing

Preterm delivery
Route of delivery
Bed rest
Observation
Drug therapy
Operative intervention in labor
Neonatal intensive care
Termination of pregnancy for a congenital anomaly

Adapted from Chard T, Klopper A: Introduction. *In* Placental Function Tests. New York, Springer-Verlag, 1982, p 1.

Indications for Antepartum Fetal Monitoring

1. Patients at high risk of uteroplacental insufficiency
   Prolonged pregnancy
   Diabetes mellitus
   Hypertension
   Previous stillbirth
   Suspected IUGR
   Advanced maternal age
   Multiple gestation with discordant growth
   Antiphospholipid syndrome
2. When other tests suggest fetal compromise Suspected IUGR
   Decreased fetal movement
   Oligohydramnios
3. Routine antepartum surveillance

form of antepartum fetal surveillance to all obstetric patients. As described below, assessment of fetal activity by the mother may be an ideal technique for this purpose.

STATISTICAL ASSESSMENT OF ANTEPARTUM TESTING

To determine the clinical application of antepartum diagnostic testing, the predictive value of the tests must be considered.[36,37] The sensitivity of the test is the probability that the test will be positive or abnormal when the disease is present. The specificity of the test is the probability that the test result will be negative when the disease is not present. Note that the sensitivity and specificity refer not to the actual numbers of patients with a positive or abnormal result, but to the proportion or probability of these test results. The predictive value of an abnormal test would be that fraction of patients with an abnormal test result who have the abnormal condition, and the predictive value of a normal test would be the fraction of patients with a normal test result who are normal.

The prevalence of the abnormal condition has great impact on the predictive value of anterpartum fetal tests. When the prevalence of the disease is low, as it is for intrauterine fetal deaths, even tests with a high sensitivity and specificity are associated with many false predictions.

For most antepartum diagnostic tests, a cut-off point used to define an abnormal result must be arbitrarily established.[38] The cut-off point is selected to maximize the separation between the normal and diseased populations.

BIOPHYSICAL TECHNIQUES OF FETAL EVALUATION

Fetal State

When interpreting tests that monitor fetal biophysical characteristics, one must appreciate that, during the third trimester, the normal fetus may exhibit marked changes in its neurologic state.[39,40] Four fetal states have been identified. The near-term fetus spends approximately 25 percent of its time in a quiet sleep state (state 1F) and 60 to 70 percent in an active sleep state (state 2F). Active sleep is associated with rapid eye movement (REM), regular breathing movements and intermittent abrupt movements of its head, limbs, and trunk. The fetal heart rate in active sleep exhibits increased variability and frequent accelerations with movement. During quiet, or non-REM, sleep, the fetal heart rate slows and heart rate variability is reduced. The fetus may make infrequent breathing movements. Near term, periods of quiet sleep may last 20 minutes, and those of active sleep approximately 40 minutes.[40]

When evaluating fetal condition using the nonstress test or the biophysical profile, one must ask whether a fetus that is not making breathing movements or shows no accelerations of its baseline heart rate is in a quiet sleep state or is neurologically compromised. In such circumstances, prolonging the period of evaluation will usually allow a change in fetal state, and more normal parameters of fetal well-being will appear.

Maternal Assessment of Fetal Activity

Maternal assessment of fetal activity may be ideal for routine antepartum fetal surveillance.

During the third trimester the human fetus spends 10 percent of its time making gross fetal body movements, approximately 30 movements per hour.[41] Periods of active fetal body movement last approximately 40 minutes, whereas quiet periods last about 20 minutes. The longest period without fetal movements in a normal fetus is 75 minutes. The mother is able to appreciate about 70 to 80 percent of gross fetal movements. Fetal movement appears to peak between 9:00 P.M. and 1:00 A.M., a time when maternal glucose levels are falling.[34] Of note, the normal fetus does not decrease its activity in the week before delivery.

Maternal evaluation of fetal activity may reduce fetal deaths caused by asphyxia. A small fall in fetal PO_2 is associated with a cessation of limb movements in the fetal lamb.

Several methods have been used to monitor fetal activity in clinical practice. In general, the presence of fetal movements is a reassuring sign of fetal health. However, the absence of fetal activity requires further assessment before one can conclude that fetal compromise exists. Pearson and Weaver[48] advocated the use of the Cardiff Count-to-Ten chart. They found that only 2.5 percent of 1,654 daily movement counts recorded by 61 women who subsequently delivered healthy infants fell below 10 movements per 12 hours. Therefore, they accepted 10 movements as the minimum amount of fetal activity the patient should perceive in a 12-hour period. The patient is asked to start counting the movements in the morning and to record the time of day at which the 10th movement has been perceived. Should the patient not have 10 movements during 12 hours, or should it take longer each day to reach 10 movements, the patient is told to contact her obstetrician.

Moore and Piacquadio[60] demonstrated an impressive reduction in fetal deaths resulting from a formal program of fetal movement counting. Patients used the Count-to-Ten approach but were told to monitor fetal activity in the evening, a time of increased fetal movement. Most women observed 10 movements in an average of 21 minutes, and compliance was greater than 90 percent. Patients who did not perceive 10 movements in 2 hours, a level of fetal activity slightly more than 5 SD below the mean, were told to report immediately for further evaluation.

Whatever technique is used must be carefully explained to the patient. While there will be a wide but normal range in fetal activity, with fetal movement counting, each mother and her fetus serve as their own control.[7] Fetal and placental factors that decrease maternal assessment of fetal activity include an anterior placental location, short duration of fetal movements, an increased amniotic fluid volume, and fetal anomalies.[52] Approximately 80 percent of all mothers will be able to comply with a program of counting fetal activity.[7,55] Maternal factors that influence the evaluation of fetal movement include maternal activity, obesity, and medications.

In conclusion, there appears to be a clearly established relationship between decreased fetal activity and fetal death. Therefore, it would seem prudent to request that *all* pregnant patients, regardless of their risk status, monitor fetal activity starting at 28 weeks' gestation. The Count-to-Ten approach developed by Moore and Piacquadio[61] seems ideal.

Contraction Stress Test

The CST, also known as the oxytocin challenge test (OCT), was the first biophysical technique widely applied for antepartum fetal surveillance. Analyses of intrapartum fetal heart rate monitoring had demonstrated that a fetus with inadequate placental respiratory reserve would demonstrate late decelerations in response to hypoxia (see Chapter 9). The CST extended these observations to the antepartum period. The response of the fetus at risk for uteroplacental insufficiency to uterine contractions formed the basis for this test.

Performing the CST

The CST may be conducted in the labor and delivery suite or in an adjacent area, although the likelihood of fetal distress requiring immediate delivery in response to uterine contractions or hyperstimulation is extremely small. The patient is placed in the semi-Fowler's position at a 30- to 45-degree angle with a slight left tilt to avoid the supine hypotensive syndrome. The fetal heart rate is recorded using a Doppler ultrasound transducer, and uterine contractions are monitored with the tocodynamometer. Maternal blood pressure is determined every 5 to 10 minutes to detect maternal hypotension.[62] Baseline fetal heart rate and uterine tone are first recorded for a period of approximately 10 to 20 minutes. In some cases, adequate uterine activity will occur spontaneously, and additional uterine stimulation will not be necessary. An adequate CST requires uterine contractions of moderate intensity lasting approximately 40 to 60 seconds with a frequency of three in 10 minutes. These criteria were selected to approximate the stress experienced by the fetus during the first stage of labor. If uterine activity is absent or inadequate, nipple stimulation is used to initiate contractions or intravenous oxytocin is begun. Oxytocin is administered by an infusion pump at 0.5 mU/min. The infusion rate is doubled every 20 minutes until adequate uterine contractions have been achieved.[27] One does not usually need to exceed 10 mU/min to produce adequate uterine activity. After the CST has been completed, the patient should be observed until uterine activity has returned to its baseline level. With nipple stimulation, the test may take approximately 30 minutes. If oxytocin is needed, 90 minutes may be required to perform the CST.

Contraindications to the test include those patients at high risk for premature labor, such as patients with premature rupture of the membranes, multiple gestation, and cervical incompetence, although the CST has not been associated with an increased incidence of premature labor.[63] The CST should also be avoided in conditions in which uterine contractions may be dangerous, such as placenta previa and a previous classical cesarean section or uterine surgery.

Interpreting the CST

Most clinicians utilize the definitions proposed by Freeman to interpret the CST[63,64] (Table 7–1). A positive test would be any 10-minute segment of the tracing that includes three contractions, associated with consistent and persistent late decelerations. A negative test is one in which there are three uterine contractions in 10 minutes with no late decelerations (Figs. 7–1 and 7–2). The term *equivocal* rather than *suspicious* is preferred for a CST with an occasional late deceleration.

Variable decelerations that occur during the CST may indicate cord compression often associated with oligohydramnios. In such cases, ultrasonography should be performed to assess amniotic fluid volume.

A negative CST has been consistently associated with good fetal outcome. A negative result therefore permits the obstetrician to prolong a high-risk pregnancy safely. Only one preventable fetal death was reported in 1,337 high-risk patients within 7 days after a negative CST.

Table 7-1. INTERPRETATION OF THE CONTRACTION STRESS TEST

Interpretation	Description	Incidence (%)
Negative	No late decelerations appearing anywhere on the tracing with adequate uterine contractions (three in 10 minutes)	80
Positive	Late decelerations that are consistent and persistent, present with the majority (>50 percent) of contractions without excessive uterine activity; if persistent late decelerations seen before the frequency of contractions is adequate, test interpreted as positive	3-5
Suspicious	Inconsistent late decelerations	5
Hyperstimulation	Uterine contractions closer than every 2 minutes or lasting >90 seconds, or five uterine contractions in 10 minutes; if no late decelerations seen, test interpreted as negative	5
Unsatisfactory	Quality of the tracing inadequate for interpretation or adequate uterine activity cannot be achieved	5

Fetal deaths after a negative CST can be attributed to cord accidents, malformations, placental abruption, and acute deterioration of glucose control in patients with diabetes. Thus, the CST, like most methods of antepartum fetal surveillance, cannot predict acute fetal compromise. If the CST is negative, a repeat study is usually scheduled in 1 week. Changes in the patient's clinical condition may warrant more frequent studies.

A positive CST has been associated with an increased incidence of intrauterine death, late decelerations in labor, low 5-minute Apgar scores, IUGR, and meconium-stained amniotic fluid (Fig. 7-3).[74] The likelihood of perinatal death after a positive CST has ranged from 7 to 15 percent. There is a significant incidence of

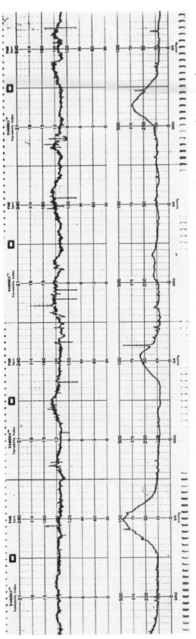

Figure 7–1. A reactive and negative CST. With this result, the CST would ordinarily be repeated in 1 week.

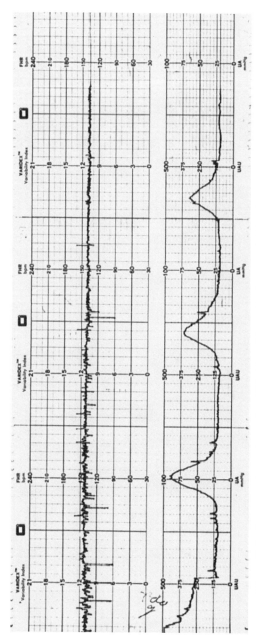

Figure 7–2. A nonreactive and negative CST. After this result, the test would ordinarily be repeated in 24 hours.

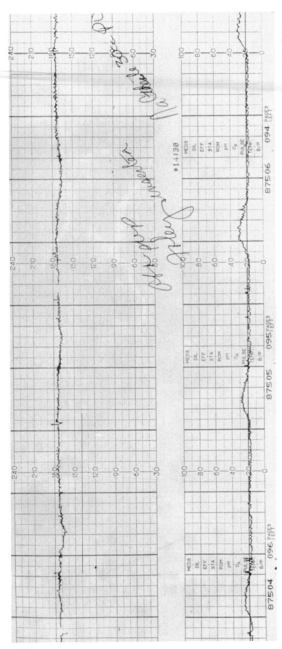

Figure 7–3. A nonreactive and positive CST with fetal tachycardia. At 34 weeks, a poorly compliant patient with type 1 diabetes mellitus, reported decreased fetal activity. The NST revealed a fetal tachycardia of 170 bpm and was nonreactive. The CST was positive, and a BPP score was 2. The patient's cervix was unfavorable for induction. The patient underwent a low transverse cesarean delivery of a 2,200-g male infant with Apgar scores of 1 and 3. The umbilical arterial pH was 7.21.

false-positive CSTs that, depending on the endpoint used, will average approximately 30 percent.[76] The positive CST is more likely to be associated with fetal compromise if the baseline heart rate lacks accelerations or "reactivity" and the latency period between the onset of the uterine contractions and the onset of the late deceleration is less than 45 seconds.[77,78]

The high incidence of false-positive CSTs is one of the greatest limitations of this test, as such results could lead to unnecessary premature intervention. False-positive CSTs may be attributable to misinterpretation of the tracing; supine hypotension, which decreases uterine perfusion; uterine hyperstimulation, which is not appreciated using the tocodynamometer; or an improvement in fetal condition after the CST has been performed. The high false-positive rate also indicates that a patient with a positive CST need not necessarily require an elective cesarean delivery. If a trial of labor is to be undertaken after a positive CST, the cervix should be favorable for induction so that direct fetal heart rate monitoring and careful assessment of uterine contractility with an intrauterine pressure catheter can be performed. False-positive results are not increased when the CST is used early in the third trimester.[76]

A suspicious or equivocal CST should be repeated in 24 hours. Most of these tests will become negative.

The Nipple Stimulation CST

Many centers utilize nipple stimulation to produce the uterine contractions needed for the CST. With nipple stimulation, the CST can generally be completed in less time, and an intravenous infusion is not required. Therefore, this approach would appear to be an ideal first step in performing a CST.

The patient may first apply a warm moist towel to each breast for 5 minutes. If uterine activity is not adequate, the patient is asked to massage one nipple for 10 minutes.

With intermittent nipple stimulation, the patient gently strokes the nipple of one breast with the palmar surface of her fingers through her clothes for 2 minutes and then stops for 5 minutes. This cycle is repeated only as necessary to achieve adequate uterine activity. Intermittent rather than continuous nipple stimulation is important in avoiding hyperstimulation. Defined as contractions lasting more than 90 seconds or five or more contractions in 10 minutes, hyperstimulation has been reported in approximately 2 percent of tests when intermittent nipple stimulation is employed.[87,88]

The Nonstress Test

Accelerations of the fetal heart rate in response to fetal activity, uterine contractions, or stimulation reflect fetal well-being and are the basis for the NST, the most widely applied technique for antepartum fetal evaluation.

In late gestation, the healthy fetus exhibits an average of 34 accelerations above the baseline fetal heart rate each hour.[90] These accelerations, require intact neurologic coupling between the fetal CNS and the fetal heart.[90] Fetal hypoxia will disrupt this pathway. Fetal heart rate accelerations may be absent during periods of quiet fetal sleep. The longest time between successive accelerations in the healthy term fetus is approximately 40 minutes. However, the fetus may fail to exhibit heart rate accelerations for up to 80 minutes and still be normal.

While an absence of fetal heart rate accelerations is most often attributable to a quiet fetal sleep state, CNS depressants such as narcotics and phenobarbital, as well as the β-blockers, can reduce heart rate reactivity.[91,92] Fetal heart rate accelerations are also decreased in smokers.[93]

The NST is usually performed in an outpatient setting. In most cases, only 10 to 15 minutes are required to complete the test. It has virtually no contraindications, and few equivocal test results are observed. The patient may be seated in a reclining chair, with care being taken to ensure that she is tilted to the left to avoid the supine hypotensive syndrome.[27,94] The patient's blood pressure should be recorded before the test is begun and then repeated at 5- to 10-minute intervals. Fetal heart rate is monitored using the Doppler ultrasound transducer, and the tocodynamometer is applied to detect uterine contractions or fetal movement. Fetal activity may be recorded by the patient using an event marker or noted by the staff performing the test. The most widely applied definition of a reactive test requires that at least two accelerations of the fetal heart rate of 15 bpm amplitude and 15 seconds' duration be observed in 20 minutes of monitoring (Fig. 7–4).[94] Since almost all accelerations are accompanied by fetal movement, fetal movement need not be recorded with the accelerations for the test to be considered reactive. However, fetal movements do provide another index of fetal well-being.

If the criteria for reactivity are not met, the test is considered nonreactive (Fig. 7–5). The most common cause for a nonreactive test will be a period of fetal inactivity or quiet sleep. The test may be extended for an additional 20 minutes with the expectation that fetal state will change and reactivity will appear. If the test has been extended for 40 minutes, and reactivity has not been seen, a biophysical profile (BPP) or CST should be performed. Of those fetuses that exhibit a nonreactive NST, approximately 25 percent will have a positive CST on further evaluation.[94,98,99] Reactivity that occurs during preparations for the BPP or CST has proved to be a reliable index of fetal well-being.

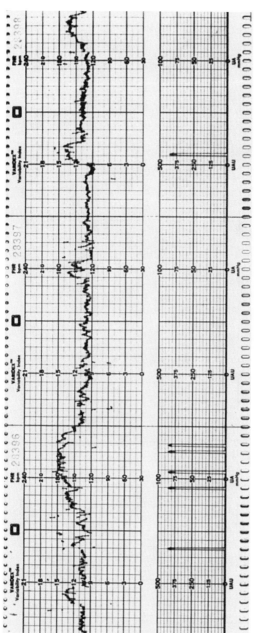

Figure 7-4. A reactive NST. Accelerations of the fetal heart that are greater than 15 bpm and last longer than 15 seconds can be identified. When the patient appreciates a fetal movement, she presses an event marker on the monitor, creating the arrows on the lower portion of the tracing.

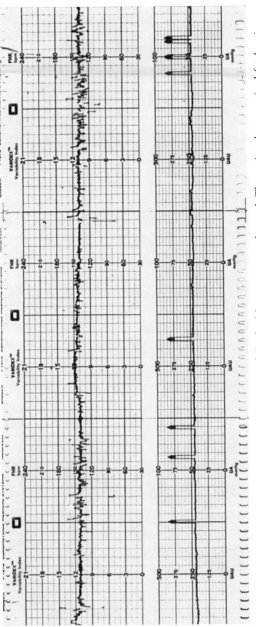

Figure 7–5. A nonreactive NST. No accelerations of the fetal heart rate are observed. The patient has perceived fetal activity as indicated by the arrows in the lower portion of the tracing.

Overall, on initial testing, 85 percent of NSTs will be reactive and 15 percent will be nonreactive.[94] Fewer than 1 percent of NSTs will prove unsatisfactory because of inadequately recorded fetal heart rate data. On rare occasions, a sinusoidal heart rate pattern may be observed as described in Chapter 9. This undulating heart rate pattern with virtually absent variability has been associated with fetal anemia, fetal asphyxia, congenital malformations, and medications such as narcotics.

The NST is most predictive when normal or reactive. Overall, a reactive NST has been associated with a perinatal mortality of approximately 5 per 1,000.[94,101] At least one half of the deaths of babies dying within 1 week of a reactive test may be attributed to placental abruption or cord accidents. The perinatal mortality rate associated with a nonreactive NST, 30 to 40 per 1,000, is significantly higher, for this group includes those fetuses who are truly asphyxiated. On the other hand, when considering perinatal asphyxia and death as endpoints, a nonreactive NST has a considerable false-positive rate. Most fetuses exhibiting a nonreactive NST will not be compromised but will simply fail to exhibit heart rate reactivity during the 40-minute period of testing. Malformed fetuses also exhibit a significantly higher incidence of nonreactive NSTs.[102] Overall, the false-positive rate associated with the nonreactive NST is approximately 75 to 90 percent.[94] However, if the NST is extended for 80 minutes and remains nonreactive, the fetus is likely to be severely compromised.

The likelihood of a nonreactive test is substantially increased early in the third trimester.[103] Between 24 and 28 weeks' gestation, approximately 50 percent of NSTs are nonreactive.[104] Fifteen percent of NSTs remain nonreactive between 28 and 32 weeks.[105,106] After 32 weeks, the incidences of reactive and nonreactive tests are comparable to those seen at term. In summary, when accelerations of the baseline heart rate are seen during monitoring in the late second and early third trimesters, the NST has been associated with fetal well-being.

Vibroacoustic stimulation (VAS) may be utilized to change fetal state from quiet to active sleep and shorten the length of the NST. Most clinicians use an electronic artificial larynx. With VAS, the incidence of nonreactive NSTs is halved.[115,116] VAS significantly increases the incidence of reactive NSTs in the preterm fetus as well.[119]

In most centers that use VAS, the baseline fetal heart rate is first observed for 5 minutes.[112] If the pattern is nonreactive, a stimulus of 3 seconds or less is applied near the fetal head. If the NST remains nonreactive, the stimulus is repeated at 1-minute intervals up to three times. If there continues to be no response to VAS, further evaluation should be carried out with a BPP or CST. VAS may be helpful in shortening the time required to perform an NST and may be especially useful in centers where large numbers of NSTs are done. Studies have confirmed the safety of VAS use during pregnancy with no long-term evidence of hearing loss in children followed in the neonatal period and up to 4 years of age.[122,123]

Significant fetal heart rate bradycardias defined as a fetal heart rate of 90 bpm or a fall in the fetal heart rate of 40 bpm below the baseline for 1 minute or longer have been observed in 1 to 2 percent of all NSTs. These bradycardias have been associated with increased perinatal morbidity and mortality, particularly antepartum fetal death, cord compression, IUGR, and fetal malformations.[130] Clinical management decisions should be based on the finding of bradycardia, *not* on the presence or absence of reactivity. Bradycardia has a higher positive predictive value for fetal compromise (fetal death or fetal intolerance of labor) than does the nonreactive NST. In this setting, antepartum fetal death is most likely because of a cord accident.[124,128,129]

If a bradycardia is observed, an ultrasound examination should be performed to assess amniotic fluid volume and to detect the presence of anomalies such as renal agenesis. Expectant management in the setting of a bradycardia has been associated with a perinatal mortality rate of 25 percent. Several reports have therefore recommended that delivery be undertaken if the fetus is mature. When the fetus is premature, one might elect to administer corticosteroids to accelerate fetal lung maturation before delivery. Continuous fetal heart rate monitoring is necessary if expectant management is followed.

In most cases, mild variable decelerations are not associated with poor perinatal outcome. When mild variable decelerations are observed, even if the NST is reactive, an ultrasound examination should be done to rule out oligohydramnios. A low amniotic fluid index and mild variable decelerations increase the likelihood of a cord accident.

In selected high-risk pregnancies, the false-negative rate associated with a weekly NST may be unacceptably high.[132,133] It appears that the frequency of the NST should be increased to *twice* weekly in pregnancies complicated by diabetes mellitus, prolonged gestation, and IUGR.[134]

Which antepartum heart rate test is best? The NST has proved to be an ideal screening test and remains the primary method for antepartum fetal evaluation at most centers. It can be quickly performed in an outpatient setting and is easily interpreted. In contrast, the CST is usually performed near the labor and delivery suite, may require an intravenous infusion of oxytocin, and may be more difficult to interpret. In initial studies, a reactive NST appeared to be as predictive of good outcome as a negative CST. Nevertheless, as more data have been gathered, it appears that the ability of the CST to stress the fetus provides an earlier warning of fetal compromise.

In most centers, the NST or modified BPP are used as the primary method for fetal evaluation with more frequent testing in higher risk pregnancies. The complete BPP or CST are utilized to evaluate the fetus with a nonreactive NST. The type of test and its application should be "condition" or diagnosis specific in which a similar basic screening approach is used, adding different types of evaluation and increased frequency of testing as appropriate for the clinical situation.

The healthy fetus should exhibit a reactive baseline heart rate with no late decelerations when a CST is performed. However, as the fetus deteriorates, one will first observe late decelerations, and, finally, the most ominous fetal heart rate pattern, the nonreactive NST and positive CST[72,78,139] (Fig. 7–3). When a nonreactive NST is followed by a positive CST, the incidence of perinatal mortality has been approximately 10 percent, a nonreassuring fetal heart rate pattern has occurred in most laboring patients, and IUGR has been reported in 25 percent of cases. The unusual combination of a reactive NST and a positive CST has been associated with a higher incidence of IUGR and late decelerations in labor than that seen with a negative CST.[140] The likelihood of fetal death is increased in patients demonstrating a nonreactive NST followed by a negative CST.[73,141,142] Consequently, repeating the NST in 24 hours appears the prudent course in such cases.

Fetal Biophysical Profile

The use of real-time ultrasonography to assess antepartum fetal condition has enabled the obstetrician to perform an in utero physical examination and evaluate dynamic functions reflecting the integrity of the fetal CNS.[143]

With real-time ultrasonography, fetal breathing movement (FBM) is evidenced by downward movement of the diaphragm and abdominal contents and by an inward collapsing of the chest. FBMs, when present, demonstrate intact neurologic control. Although the absence of FBMs may reflect fetal asphyxia, this finding may also indicate that the fetus is in a period of quiet sleep.[39,40]

The evaluation of FBM has been used to distinguish the truly positive CST from a false-positive CST. Those fetuses that displayed FBM but had a positive CST were unlikely to exhibit fetal distress in labor. However, when a fetus failed to show FBM and demonstrated late decelerations during the CST, the likelihood of fetal compromise was great. A pattern emerged from these studies that as long as one antepartum biophysical test was normal, the likelihood that the fetus would have a normal outcome was high.[148,149] As the number of abnormal tests increased, however, the likelihood that fetal asphyxia was present increased as well.

The BPP score combines the NST with four parameters that can be assessed using real-time ultrasonography: FBM, fetal movement, fetal tone, and amniotic fluid volume. FBM, fetal movement, and fetal tone are mediated by complex neurologic pathways and should reflect the function of the fetal CNS at the time of the examination. Amniotic fluid volume should provide information about the presence of chronic fetal asphyxia. The ultrasound examination performed for the BPP has the added advantage of detecting previously unrecognized major fetal anomalies.

A nonreactive NST and absent FBM are the earliest signs of fetal compromise. In most cases, the ultrasound-derived BPP parameters and NST can be completed within a relatively short time, each requiring approximately 10 minutes. Use of VAS for an equivocal BPP does not increase the false negative rate and may reduce the likelihood of unnecessary intervention.

In calculating the BPP score, the presence of a normal parameter, such as a reactive NST, was awarded 2 points, whereas the absence of that parameter was scored as 0. The highest score a fetus can receive is 10, and the lowest score is 0. The BPP may be used as early as 26 to 28 weeks' gestation. Of all patients tested, almost 97 percent had a score of 8, which means that only 3 percent required further evaluation for scores of 6 or less. A significant inverse linear relationship has been observed between the last BPP score and both perinatal morbidity and mortality.[152] The false-positive rate, depending on the endpoint used, ranges from 75 percent for a score of 6 to less than 20 percent for a score of 0. In eight investigations using the BPP for fetal evaluation, the corrected perinatal mortality rate, excluding lethal anomalies, was 0.77 per 1,000. Twice-weekly testing is recommended in pregnancies complicated by IUGR, diabetes mellitus, prolonged gestation, and hypertension with proteinuria. The scoring criteria and the clinical actions recommended in response to these scores, are presented in Tables 7–2 and 7–3.

Recent studies have demonstrated that antenatal corticosteroid administration may have an effect on the BPP, decreasing the profile score. Because corticosteroids are used in cases of anticipated premature delivery (24 to 34 weeks), any false-positives on biophysical testing may lead to inappropriate intervention and delivery. The most commonly affected variables have been FBM and the NST.[157] These changes are transient and return to normal by 48 to 96 hours after corticosteroid treatment. This effect must be considered at institutions where daily BPPs are used to evaluate the fetus in cases of preterm labor or preterm premature rupture of the membranes.

Several drawbacks of the BPP should be considered. Unlike the NST and CST, an ultrasound machine is required, and, unless the BPP is videotaped, it cannot be reviewed. If the fetus is in a quiet sleep state, the BPP can require a long period of observation. The present scoring system does not consider the impact of hydramnios.

Table 7–2. TECHNIQUE OF BIOPHYSICAL PROFILE SCORING

Biophysical Variable	Normal (Score = 2)	Abnormal (Score = 0)
Fetal breathing movements	At least one episode of > 30 seconds' duration in 30 minutes' observation	Absent or no episode of ≥ 30 seconds' duration 30 minutes
Gross body movement	At least three discrete body/limb movements in 30 minutes (episodes of active continuous movement considered a single movement)	Up to two episodes of body/limb in movements 30 minutes
Fetal tone	At least one episode of active extension with return to flexion of fetal limb(s) or trunk; opening and closing of hand considered normal tone	Either slow extension with return to partial flexion or movement of limb in full extension or absent fetal movement
Reactive fetal heart rate	At least two episodes of acceleration of ≥ 15 bpm and 15 seconds' duration associated with fetal movement in 30 minutes	Fewer than two accelerations or acceleration < 15 bpm in 30 minutes
Qualitative amniotic fluid volume	At least one pocket of amniotic fluid pocket measuring 2 cm in two perpendicular planes	Either no amniotic fluid pockets or a pocket < 2 cm in two perpendicular planes

Adapted from Manning FA: Biophysical profile scoring. *In* Nijhuis J (ed): Fetal Behaviour. New York, Oxford University Press, 1992, p 241.

Table 7-3. MANAGEMENT BASED ON BIOPHYSICAL PROFILE

Score	Interpretation	Management
10	Normal infant; low risk of chronic asphyxia	Repeat testing at weekly intervals; repeat twice weekly in diabetic patients and patients at ≥ 41 weeks' gestation
8	Normal infant; low risk of chronic asphyxia	Repeat testing at weekly intervals; repeat testing twice weekly in diabetics and patients at ≥ 41 weeks' gestation; oligohydramnios is an indication for delivery
6	Suspect chronic asphyxia	If ≥ 36 weeks' gestation and conditions are favorable, deliver; if at > 36 weeks and L/S < 2.0, repeat test in 4–6 hours; deliver if oligohydramnios is present
4	Suspect chronic asphyxia	If ≥ 36 weeks' gestation, deliver; if < 32 weeks' gestation, repeat score
0–2	Strongly suspect chronic asphyxia	Extend testing time to 120 minutes; if persistent score ≤ 4, deliver regardless of gestational age

Adapted from Manning FA, Harman CR, Morrison I, et al: Fetal assessment based on fetal biophysical profile scoring. Am J Obstet Gynecol 162:703, 1990; and Manning FA: Biophysical profile scoring. *In* Nijhuis J (ed): Fetal Behaviour. New York, Oxford University Press, 1992, p 241.

DOPPLER ULTRASOUND

Doppler ultrasound can provide a noninvasive assessment of the fetal, maternal, and placental circulations. The Doppler principle is based on changes in the frequency of sound produced by a changing relationship between two objects. Ultrasound waves beamed with a particular frequency will return to a receiver at a lower frequency when the target is moving away from the transducer, and at a higher frequency when the target is moving towards the transducer. By convention, information received from objects moving away from the transducer is recorded below a zero line, and information received from objects moving toward the transducer is recorded above a zero line (Figs. 7–6 and 7–7). The frequency of the reflected sound is proportional to the velocity of the moving red blood cells. Information about blood flow velocity provides an indirect assessment of changes in blood flow. Calculation of flow velocity is derived from the equation

$$f_d = 2 f_0 \frac{V_{\cos\theta}}{c},$$

where f_d is the change in ultrasound frequency or Doppler shift, f_0 is the transmitted frequency of the ultrasound beam, V is the

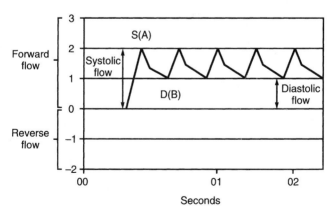

Figure 7–6. Diagram of a normal umbilical artery flow velocity waveform. Note the forward flow during both systole and diastole, the latter indicating low resistance in the placental bed. (Adapted from Warsof SL, Levy DL: Doppler blood flow and fetal growth retardation. *In* Gross TL, Sokol RJ (ed): Intrauterine Growth Retardation, A Practical Approach. Chicago, Year Book, 1989, p 158.)

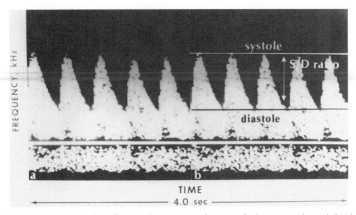

Figure 7–7. Doppler flow velocity waveforms of the normal umbilical artery. Note that umbilical arterial flow velocities are recorded above the baseline, whereas nonpulsatile umbilical vein flow in the opposite direction is found below the baseline (a). Measurement of the S/D ratio is also illustrated (b). (From Bruner JP, Gabbe SG, Levy DW, et al: Doppler ultrasonography of the umbilical cord in normal pregnancy. J South Med Assoc 86:52, 1993, with permission.)

velocity of the red blood cells, θ is the angle between the beam and the direction of movement of the reflector or red blood cells, and c is the velocity of sound in the medium (Fig. 7–8). The speed of sound in tissues is 1,540 m/sec. The number 2 in the equation accounts for the time spent from the transmission of the sound signal at its origin to its return. Volume flow may be calculated by multiplying the mean velocity by the cross-sectional area of the vessel. Velocities are measured in meters per second.

The combination of real-time ultrasound imaging with pulsed wave Doppler allows the identification of a specific area or vessel for sampling. A vessel can be identified, and the ultrasound beam placed across that vessel using range gating.

Given the difficulty of estimating the angle between the Doppler ultrasound beam and the direction of blood flow in a particular vessel, a variety of angle-independent indices have been developed to characterize flow velocity waveforms produced. Indices rely on systolic, diastolic, and mean velocities. Systolic velocities are peak velocities that result from cardiac contraction. Diastolic velocities result from an interaction between peak flows, vessel compliance, heart rate, and the vascular impedance of the sites perfused. These indices do not measure the volume of blood flow. A commonly used index is the systolic (S)/diastolic (D) velocity ratio, the S/D ratio (Figs. 7–6 and 7–7). The greater the diastolic flow, the lower the ratio. As resistance to flow increases, diastolic flow falls, and the S/D ratio increases.

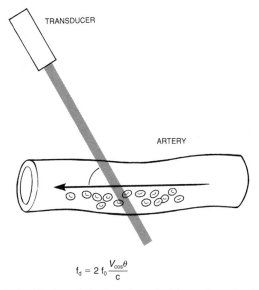

$$f_d = 2\,f_0\,\frac{V_{\cos}\theta}{c}$$

Figure 7–8. Application of the Doppler principle to determine blood flow velocity. The frequency (f_0) of the ultrasound beam directed at a moving column of red blood cells with velocity V will be increased to f_d in proportion to V and the cosine of the angle of intersection of the vessel by the beam (θ).

Values of normal umbilical artery flow velocity waveforms during pregnancy reveal that as the normal pregnancy progresses, there is proportionately more blood flow during diastole, and indices decrease. The normal decrease in umbilical artery velocity indices (Fig. 7–9) is consistent with a decrease in placental resistance with advancing gestational age.[176]

The main application of umbilical artery Doppler flow velocity measurements has been in the pregnancy at risk for or demonstrating IUGR (see Chapter 20).[177] IUGR is seen more often in fetuses with umbilical artery velocity indices that are elevated for their gestational age.[178] In some cases, end-diastolic flow is absent or reversed (Figs. 7–10 and 7–11).

The most extreme abnormalities in umbilical artery waveforms are those in which the velocities are absent or reversed.[183] Absence of end-diastolic velocities is associated with an increase in perinatal morbidity and mortality. Reverse flow is even more predictive of poor perinatal outcome than absent diastolic flow. In addition to an association with IUGR, markedly abnormal Doppler studies have been reported in fetuses with congenital malformations,

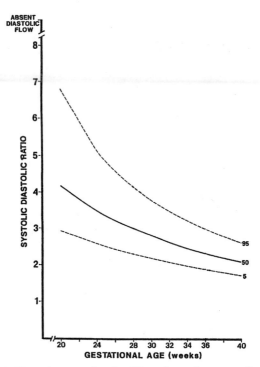

Figure 7–9. Normal ranges for the S/D ratio used to quantify the flow velocity waveform patterns of the umbilical artery during pregnancy. (Derived from Thompson et al.[173])

including chromosomal abnormalities. In 904 fetuses with absent or reversed end-diastolic flow,[183] the perinatal mortality was 36 percent, IUGR was observed in 80 percent, abnormal karyotypes were found in 6 percent, and malformations in 11 percent. The average duration from diagnosis to delivery was 6 to 8 days. Therefore, absence or reversal of end-diastolic flow velocities in the umbilical artery, although not an indication for immediate delivery, is considered an indication for immediate and intensive ongoing fetal surveillance. Delivery is usually based on the results of fetal heart rate monitoring or the BPP, with consideration of maternal condition and gestational age.

In summary, Doppler ultrasound is useful in high-risk pregnancies especially those complicated by conditions predisposing to IUGR such as hypertension, and can decrease perinatal mortality without increasing maternal or neonatal morbidity in these cases. Studies in which Doppler ultrasound of the umbilical artery has

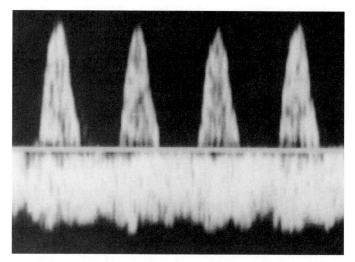

Figure 7-10. Umbilical arterial waveforms with absent end-diastolic velocities. In this case, venous velocities also demonstrate variation with the arterial waveforms.

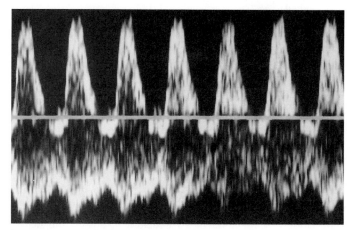

Figure 7-11. Umbilical arterial waveforms with reverse flow at end-diastole. Umbilical venous velocities have marked pulsations.

been used to screen low-risk pregnancies have not demonstrated a benefit from this approach.[192]

THE ASSESSMENT OF FETAL PULMONARY MATURATION

Available methods for evaluating fetal pulmonary maturity can be divided into three categories: (1) quantitation of pulmonary surfactant, such as the lecithin/sphingomyelin (L/S) ratio; (2) measurement of surfactant function including the shake test; and (3) evaluation of amniotic fluid turbidity.[196,197]

With the exception of amniotic fluid specimens obtained from the vaginal pool, the evaluation of fetal pulmonary maturation requires that a sample of amniotic fluid be obtained by amniocentesis. Ultrasound guidance for third-trimester amniocentesis has significantly decreased the risks of this procedure. In over 4,000 third-trimester amniocenteses, the frequency of complications was 3 percent for rupture of the membranes within 24 hours, 7 percent for a bloody tap, 4.4 percent for failed amniocentesis, 3.3 percent for labor within 24 hours, 1 percent for fetal trauma, and 0.05 percent for fetal death.[198] A bloody tap warrants careful observation.[199] Maternal complications, though rare, have included hemorrhage, in some cases from perforation of the uterine vessels, abdominal wall hematomas, Rh sensitization, and infection.

Quantitation of Pulmonary Surfactant

Lecithin/Sphingomyelin Ratio

The amniotic fluid concentration of lecithin increases markedly at approximately 35 weeks' gestation, whereas sphingomyelin levels remain stable or decrease. Amniotic fluid sphingomyelin exceeds lecithin until 31 to 32 weeks, when the L/S ratio reaches 1. Lecithin then rises rapidly, and an L/S ratio of 2.0 is observed at approximately 35 weeks. A ratio of 2.0 or greater has been reliably associated with pulmonary maturity, predicting the absence of respiratory distress syndrome (RDS) in 98 percent of neonates.[202] The L/S ratio, like most indices of fetal pulmonary maturation, rarely errs when predicting fetal pulmonary maturity, but is frequently incorrect when predicting subsequent RDS.[203] Many neonates with an immature L/S ratio will not develop RDS.

Several important variables must be considered in interpreting the predictive accuracy of the L/S ratio. A prolonged interval between the determination of an immature L/S ratio and delivery will necessarily increase the number of falsely immature results. It is probably best to discard amniotic fluid samples heavily contaminated by blood or meconium, because the effects of these compounds on the determination of the L/S ratio are quite unpredictable.[204,205] The presence of phosphatidy/glycerol (PG) in a bloody or meconium-stained amniotic fluid sample remains a reliable indicator of pulmonary maturity.[206] Finally, it is essential that the obstetrician know the analytic technique used and the predictive value of a mature L/S ratio in his or her laboratory.

Many perinatal processes alter the final interpretation of the L/S ratio. Surfactant deficiency, immaturity, and intrapartum complications are the prime factors in determining the pathogenesis of RDS.[209] Birth asphyxia may lead to RDS despite an L/S ratio greater than 2.0.

Slide Agglutination Test for PG

PG, which does not appear until 35 weeks' gestation and increases rapidly between 37 to 40 weeks, is a marker of completed pulmonary maturation.[212] Most infants who lack PG but have a mature L/S ratio fail to develop RDS. However, PG may provide further insurance against the onset of RDS despite intrapartum complications.

A rapid immunologic semiquantitative agglutination test (Amniostat-FLM) can be used to determine the presence of PG.[213] The test takes 20 to 30 minutes to perform, while the L/S ratio may require 1 to 3 hours. No cases of RDS have been observed when the Amniostat-FLM assay demonstrates PG. This technique can be applied to samples contaminated by blood and meconium.

Fluorescence Polarization

TDx Test (Surfactant Albumin Ratio)

The TDx analyzer, an automated fluorescence polarimeter, has been utilized to assess surfactant content in amniotic fluid.[215-217] The test requires 1 ml of amniotic fluid and can be run in less than 1 hour. The surfactant albumin ratio (SAR) is determined with amniotic fluid albumin used as an internal reference. A value of 70 was considered mature with the original assay, whereas with the newer FLM-II test, 55 is the mature cut-off.[196] A mature value reliably predicts the absence of RDS requiring intubation in infants of diabetic mothers.[218] The TDx test correlates well with the L/S ratio and has few falsely mature results, making it an excellent screening test.[219] The TDx assay proved to be reliable in predicting fetal lung maturity in vaginal pool specimens in patients with preterm premature rupture of the membranes at 30 to 36 weeks.[220] Approximately 50 percent of infants with an immature TDx result will develop RDS.

Measurement of Surfactant Function

Foam Stability Index

The test is based on the manual foam stability index (FSI), and is a variation of the shake test.[221] The kit currently available contains test wells with a predispensed volume of ethanol. The amniotic fluid/ethanol mixture is first shaken, and the FSI value is read as the highest value well in which a ring of stable foam persists.[222] This test appears to be a reliable predictor of fetal lung maturity.[223] Subsequent RDS is very unlikely with an FSI value of 47 or higher. The assay appears to be extremely sensitive, with a high proportion of immature results being associated with RDS, as well as moderately specific, with a high proportion of mature results predicting the absence of RDS. Contamination of the amniotic fluid specimen by blood or meconium invalidates the FSI results. The FSI can function well as a screening test.

Evaluation of Amniotic Fluid Turbidity

Visual Inspection

During the first and second trimesters, amniotic fluid is yellow and clear. It becomes colorless in the third trimester. By 33 to 34 weeks' gestation, cloudiness and flocculation are noted, and, as term approaches, vernix appears. Amniotic fluid with obvious vernix or fluid so turbid it does not permit the reading of newsprint through it will usually have a mature L/S ratio.[224]

Lamellar Body Counts

Lamellar bodies are the storage form of surfactant released by fetal type II pneumocytes into the amniotic fluid. Because they have the same size as platelets, the amniotic fluid concentration of lamellar bodies may be determined using a commercial cell counter.[225–228] The test requires less than 1 ml of amniotic fluid and takes only 15 minutes to perform. A lamellar body count greater than 30,000 to 55,000/μl is highly predictive of pulmonary maturity, whereas a count below 10,000/μl suggests a significant risk for RDS. The cut-off used to predict fetal pulmonary status will depend on the type of cell counter used and the speed of centrifugation of the amniotic fluid specimen. Neither meconium nor lysed blood has a significant effect on the lamellar body count.

Determination of Fetal Pulmonary Maturation in Clinical Practice

A large number of techniques are now available to assess fetal pulmonary maturation.[196] Several rapid screening tests, including the

TDx test, Amniostat-FLM, and lamellar body count appear to be highly reliable when mature. In an uncomplicated pregnancy, when a screening test such as the TDx demonstrates fetal pulmonary maturation, one can safely proceed with delivery.[217,229] This sequential approach is also extremely cost effective.[196,197,230,231] However, when the screening test is immature, the L/S ratio should be used. Similarly, in complicated pregnancies such as those with diabetes mellitus, IUGR, and Rh isoimmunization, the L/S ratio should be determined to assess fetal pulmonary maturation.

A PRACTICAL APPROACH TO TESTING

How can one most efficiently use all the techniques available for antepartum fetal surveillance? Obstetricians should take a "diagnosis-specific" approach to testing. That is, they must consider the pathophysiology of the disease process that will be evaluated and then select the best method or methods of testing for that problem. In a pregnancy complicated by diabetes mellitus, careful monitoring of maternal glucose levels should accompany antepartum heart rate testing. In contrast, in a pregnancy complicated by suspected IUGR, one might utilize Doppler ultrasound measurements of the S/D ratio as well as serial evaluations of amniotic fluid volume with ultrasound.

In a prolonged pregnancy, one would use a parallel testing scheme. In this situation, the obstetrician is not concerned with fetal maturity, but rather with fetal well-being. Several tests are performed at the same time, such as antepartum fetal heart rate testing and the BPP. It is acceptable in this high-risk situation to intervene when a single test is abnormal. One is willing to accept a false-positive test result to avoid the intrauterine death of a mature and otherwise healthy fetus.

In most other high-risk pregnancies, such as those complicated by diabetes mellitus or hypertension, it is preferable to allow the fetus to remain in utero as long as possible. In these situations, a branched testing scheme is used. To decrease the likelihood of unnecessary premature intervention, the obstetrician uses a series of tests and, under most circumstances, would only deliver a premature infant when all parameters suggest fetal compromise. In this situation, one must consider the likelihood of neonatal RDS as predicted by the evaluation of amniotic fluid indices and review these risks with colleagues in neonatology.

Maternal assessment of fetal activity would appear to be an ideal first-line screening test for both high-risk and low-risk patients. The use of this approach may decrease the number of unexpected intrauterine deaths in so-called normal pregnancies. Although a negative CST has been associated with fewer intrauterine deaths than a reactive NST, the NST appears to have significant advantages in screening high-risk patients. It can be easily and rapidly performed in an outpatient setting. Most clinicians use the BPP or CST to assess fetal condition in patients exhibiting a persistently nonreactive NST. This sequential approach may be particularly valuable in avoiding unnecessary premature intervention.

Figure 7–12 presents a practical testing scheme that has been utilized successfully by several centers.[112,143,233,234] The NST, an indicator of present fetal condition, may be combined with the amniotic fluid index (AFI) (see Appendix), a marker of long-term status, in a modified BPP. In this setting, an AFI greater than 5 cm is usually considered normal.[235] VAS may be used to shorten the time required to achieve a reactive NST. While most patients are evaluated weekly, patients with diabetes mellitus, IUGR, or a

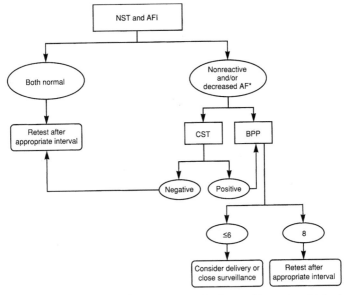

Figure 7–12. Flow chart for antepartum fetal surveillance in which the NST and AFI are used as the primary methods for fetal evaluation. A nonreactive NST and/or decreased AF are further evaluated using either the CST or the BPP. Further details regarding the use of the BPP are provided in Table 7–3. *If the fetus is mature and amniotic fluid volume is reduced, delivery should be considered before further testing is undertaken. (Adapted from Finberg HJ, Kurtz AB, Johnson RL, et al: The biophysical profile: a literature review and reassessment of its usefulness in the evaluation of fetal well-being. J Ultrasound Med 9:583, 1990.)

prolonged gestation are tested twice weekly. If the NST is nonreactive despite VAS or extended monitoring, or if the AFI is abnormal, either a full BPP or CST is performed. The low false-negative rate and ease of performance of the modified BPP make it an excellent approach for the evaluation of large numbers of high-risk patients.

STRATEGIES TO REDUCE ANTEPARTUM FETAL DEATHS

What strategies can be utilized to reduce antepartum fetal deaths?[239] (See the box "Strategies to Reduce Antepartum Fetal Deaths.") First, it is important to determine the cause of a fetal death so that the patient and her partner can be counseled, the risk of recurrence described, and a plan of care for subsequent pregnancies developed. The obstetrician should write a detailed note describing the stillborn fetus, amniotic fluid, umbilical cord, placenta, and membranes. If the infant is malformed, growth restricted, or hydropic, chromosomal studies should be obtained. An autopsy should be requested.[239,240] Tests for syphilis, antiphospholipid antibodies, and lupus anticoagulant should be done. If the patient has not been screened for diabetes mellitus during gestation, a fasting glucose should be ordered. Because significant fetal– maternal hemorrhage has been observed in approximately 5 percent of all fetal deaths, a Kleihauer-Betke test should be obtained.

To prevent antepartum deaths, routine fetal movement counting should be considered in all pregnancies, starting at 28 weeks' gestation. The modified Count-to-Ten method developed by Moore and Piacquadio is a simple and valuable technique.[60] To reduce fetal

---

Strategies to Reduce Antepartum Fetal Deaths

Determination of the cause of fetal death
Antepartum fetal evaluation in all pregnancies with routine fetal movement counting
Surveillance for fetal malformations in all pregnancies with a triple screen and routine ultrasound at 18–20 weeks
Surveillance for detection of IUGR with fundal height measurements and ultrasound at 30–32 weeks in high-risk patients and patients with lagging growth
Programs to identify and treat cocaine abuse in pregnancy

From Gabbe SG: Prevention of antepartum fetal deaths. OB/GYN Clinical Alert, April 1998, p 94, with permission.

deaths resulting from fetal malformations, a triple analyte screen should be offered and routine ultrasound performed at 18 to 20 weeks (see Chapters 4 and 5). To detect IUGR, careful serial measurements of fundal height should be performed with an ultrasound examination at 30 to 32 weeks in high-risk patients including those with vascular disease and in patients with lagging uterine growth (see Chapter 20). Finally, to reduce fetal deaths caused by placental abruption, patients who are known to be abusing cocaine should be counseled and enrolled in treatment programs.

Key Points

➤ The prevalence of an abnormal condition (i.e., fetal death) has great impact on the predictive value of antepartum fetal tests.

➤ The near-term fetus spends approximately 25 percent of its time in a quiet sleep state (state 1F) and 60 to 70 percent in an active sleep state (state 2F).

➤ Approximately 5 percent of women monitoring fetal movement will report decreased fetal activity.

➤ The incidence of perinatal death within 1 week of a negative CST is less than 1 in 1,000.

➤ The observation that accelerations of the fetal heart rate in response to fetal activity, uterine contractions, or stimulation reflect fetal well-being is the basis for the NST.

➤ The frequency of the NST should be increased to twice weekly in pregnancies complicated by diabetes mellitus, prolonged gestation, and IUGR.

➤ Use of VAS for an equivocal BPP does not increase the false-negative rate and may reduce the likelihood of unnecessary obstetric intervention.

➤ Reversed end-diastolic flow in the umbilical artery flow velocity waveform has been associated with an increased perinatal mortality rate.

➤ Most amniotic fluid indices of fetal pulmonary maturation rarely err when predicting maturity, but are frequently incorrect when predicting subsequent RDS.

➤ The NST, an indicator of present fetal condition, and the amniotic fluid index, a marker of long-term fetal status, have been combined in the modified BPP.

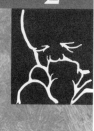

Intrapartum Care

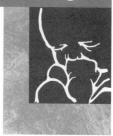

Chapter 8

Labor and Delivery

ERROL R. NORWITZ,
JULIAN N. ROBINSON,
AND JOHN T. REPKE

DEFINITIONS

Labor is defined as a switch in the myometrial contractility pattern from "contractures" (long-lasting, low-frequency activity) to regular "contractions" (frequent, high-intensity, high-frequency activity),[1] resulting in effacement and dilatation of the uterine cervix. These events usually occur before rupture of the membranes. Spontaneous rupture of the fetal membranes prior to the onset of uterine activity is seen in only 8 percent of term pregnancies.[2]

"Term" is defined as the period from 36 completed (37.0) to 42.0 weeks of gestation. "Preterm" (premature) labor refers to the onset of labor prior to 36 completed weeks' gestation (see Chapter 18). "Postterm" (prolonged) pregnancy refers to pregnancies continuing beyond 42.0 weeks' gestation (see Chapter 21).

Diagnosis

The classic diagnosis of labor includes regular painful uterine contractions and progressive cervical effacement and dilatation. Cervical dilatation in the absence of uterine contractions is seen most commonly in the second trimester and is suggestive of cervical incompetence. Similarly, the presence of uterine contractions in the absence of cervical change does not meet criteria for the diagnosis of labor.

MECHANICS OF LABOR

Mechanics of Normal Labor at Term

The ability of the fetus to successfully negotiate the pelvis during labor and delivery is dependent on the complex interaction of three variables: the powers, the passenger, and the passage.

181

The Powers

The powers refer to the forces generated by the uterine musculature. Uterine activity is characterized by the frequency, amplitude
(intensity), and duration of contractions. External tocodynamometry measures the change in shape of the abdominal wall as a function of uterine contractions and, as such, is qualitative rather than
quantitative. Although it permits graphic display of uterine activity
and allows for accurate correlation of fetal heart rate patterns with
uterine activity, external tocodynamometry does not allow measurement of contraction intensity or basal intrauterine tone. The most
precise method for determination of uterine activity is the direct
measurement of intrauterine pressure. Such techniques require
insertion of a pressure transducer directly into the uterine cavity
usually through the cervix after rupture of the fetal membranes.
A risk of uterine injury (perforation) exists during placement of the
catheter.

Classically, three to five contractions in 10 minutes has been used
to define adequate labor, and is seen in around 95 percent of
women in spontaneous labor at term. In the active management
of labor protocols, seven contractions in 15 minutes is regarded as
adequate.[24,25] Various units have been devised to objectively measure uterine activity, the most common of which is *Montevideo
units* (the average strength of contractions in millimeters of mercury multiplied by the number of contractions per 10 minutes),
which is a measure of average frequency and amplitude above
basal tone. Two hundred to 250 Montevideo units defines adequate
labor.[26,27] The ultimate measure of uterine activity is a clinical one.
If uterine contractions are "adequate" to effect vaginal delivery,
one of two things will happen. Either the cervix will efface and
dilate and the fetal head will descend, or there will be worsening
caput succedaneum (scalp edema) and/or moulding of the fetal
head (overlapping of the skull bones) without cervical effacement
and dilatation. The latter situation suggests the presence of
cephalopelvic disproportion (CPD), which can be either absolute (in
which a given fetus is simply too large to negotiate a given pelvis)
or relative (in which delivery of a given fetus through a given pelvis
would be possible under optimal conditions but is precluded by
malposition or abnormal attitude of the fetal head).

The Passenger

There are several fetal variables that influence the course of labor
and delivery. These are summarized below.

1. Absolute fetal *size* can be estimated both clinically by abdominal palpation or with ultrasound, but both are subject
   to a large degree of error. Fetal macrosomia (defined by the

American College of Obstetricians and Gynecologists (ACOG) as an absolute fetal size $\geq$ 4,500 g[28]) may be associated with failure to progress in labor.

2. *Lie* refers to the longitudinal axis of the fetus relative to the longitudinal axis of the uterus. Fetal lie can be either longitudinal, transverse, or oblique

3. *Presentation* refers to the fetal part that directly overlies the pelvic inlet. In a fetus presenting in the longitudinal lie, the presentation can be either cephalic (vertex), breech, or (rarely) shoulder. Compound presentation refers to the presence of more than one fetal part overlying the pelvic inlet. Funic presentation refers to presentation of the umbilical cord. In a cephalic fetus, the presentation is classified according to the leading bony landmark of the skull, which can be either the occiput, the mentum (chin), or the brow. *Malpresentation* refers to any presentation that is not cephalic with the occiput leading, and is seen in around 5 percent of all term labors (see Chapter 11).

4. *Attitude* refers to the position of the head with regard to the fetal spine (i.e., the degree of flexion and/or extension of the fetal head). Flexion of the head is important to facilitate *engagement* of the head in the maternal pelvis.

5. *Position* of the fetus refers to the relationship of a nominated site of the presenting part to a denominating location on the internal pelvis, and can be assessed most accurately on transvaginal examination. In a cephalic presentation, the nominated site is the occiput (e.g., right occiput anterior [ROA]). The various positions of a cephalic presentation are illustrated in Figure 8–1. *Malposition* refers to any position in labor which is not ROA, OA, or LOA.

6. *Station* is a measure of descent of the presenting part of the fetus through the birth canal (Fig. 8–2). The old classification was an arbitrary subjective assignment of seven stations (-3 to $+3$), whereas the new classification (-5 to $+5$) is an attempt to quantitate in centimeters the distance of the leading bony edge from the ischial spines. In both classifications, the midpoint (0 station) is defined as the plane of the maternal ischial spines.

The Passage

The passage consists of the bony pelvis and the resistance provided by the soft tissues. The pelvis can be broadly classified into the pelvic inlet, midcavity and outlet. Clinical pelvimetry involves assessment of three parameters of the pelvic inlet, midcavity, and outlet.

The shape of the female bony pelvis can be classified into one or more of four broad categories: gynecoid, anthropoid, android, and

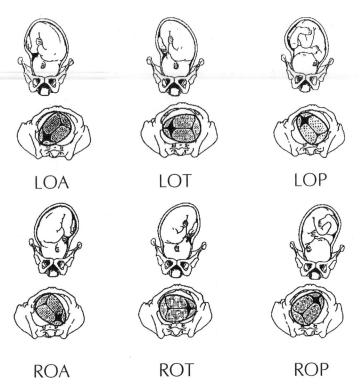

Figure 8-1. Fetal presentations and positions in labor. LOA, left occiput anterior; LOT, left occiput transverse; LOP, left occiput posterior; OA, occiput anterior; OP, occiput posterior; ROA, right occiput anterior; ROT, right occiput transverse; ROP, right occiput posterior. (Adapted from Norwitz ER, Robinson J, Repke JT: The initiation and management of labor. *In* Seifer DB, Samuels P, Kniss DA [eds]: The Physiologic Basis of Gynecology and Obstetrics. Baltimore, Lippincott Williams & Wilkins, 2001.)

platypelloid. Although the assessment of fetal size along with pelvic shape and capacity is useful to predict women at risk of CPD in labor, it is an inexact science. An adequate trial of labor is the only way to determine whether a given fetus will be able to safely negotiate a given pelvis.

Stages of Labor

Labor has traditionally been divided into three stages, with the first stage further subdivided into three phases.

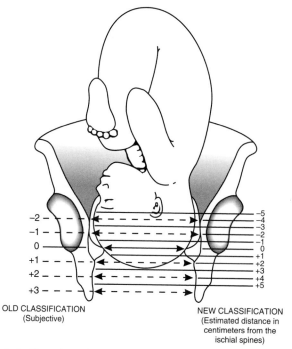

OLD CLASSIFICATION
(Subjective)

NEW CLASSIFICATION
(Estimated distance in
centimeters from the
ischial spines)

Figure 8–2. The relationship of the leading edge of the presenting part of the fetus to the plane of the maternal ischial spines determines the station. Station +1/+3 (old classification) or +2/+5 (new classification) is illustrated.

First Stage

The first stage of labor is the interval between the onset of labor and full cervical dilatation, subdivided into three phases according to the rate of cervical dilatation (Fig. 8–3). The *latent phase* is defined as the period between the onset of labor and a point at which a change in the slope of the rate of cervical dilatation is noted.[35,36] It is characterized by slow cervical dilatation and is of variable duration. The *active phase* is associated with a greater rate of cervical dilatation and usually begins at around 2 to 3 cm dilatation.[35–37] The active phase is further subdivided into an acceleration phase, a phase of maximum slope, and a deceleration phase. A *descent phase* usually coincides with the second stage of labor. There are significant differences between the labor curve of primigravid and multiparous women. Friedman[35,36] has described averages and a statistical maximum (2 SD greater than the mean) for each phase (Table 8–1). The minimum rate of cervical

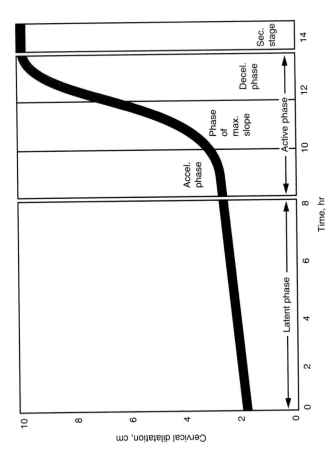

Figure 8-3. Characteristics of the average cervical dilatation curve for nulliparous labor. (Adapted from Friedman EA: Labor: Clinical Evaluation and Management, 2nd ed. Norwalk, CT, Appleton-Century-Croft, 1978.)

Table 8–1. PROGRESSION OF SPONTANEOUS LABOR AT TERM

Parameter	Mean	5th Percentile
Nulliparas		
Total duration of labor	10.1 h	25.8 h
Stage of labor		
Duration of the first stage	9.7 h	24.7 h
Duration of the second stage	33.0 min	117.5 min
Duration of latent phase	6.4 h	20.6 h
Rate of cervical dilatation during active phase	3.0 cm/h	1.2 cm/h
Duration of the third stage	5.0 min	30.0 min
Multiparas		
Total duration of labor	6.2 h	19.5 h
Stage of labor		
Duration of the first stage	8.0 h	18.8 h
Duration of the second stage	8.5 min	46.5 min
Duration of latent phase	4.8 h	13.6 h
Rate of cervical dilatation during active phase	5.7 cm/h	1.5 cm/h
Duration of the third stage	5.0 min	30.0 min

Data from Friedman EA: Labor: Clinical Evaluation and Management, 2nd ed. Norwalk, CT, Appleton-Century-Crofts, 1978.

dilatation of 1.2 cm/h for a nulliparous patient represents 2 SD from the mean, and not the average rate of dilatation. For any individual patient, the clinician responsible for managing the labor should have a sense at any point in time of where on the normal labor curve the patient is. This task can be facilitated by the use of the partogram,[39] a graphical representation of the labor curve against which a patient's progress in labor is plotted.

Second Stage

The second stage of labor is the interval between full cervical dilatation (10 cm) and delivery of the infant. It is characterized by descent of the presenting part through the maternal pelvis culminating in expulsion of the fetus. In modern obstetric practice, the nulliparous patient is recommended to push for a maximum of 2 hours without regional anesthesia (or 3 hours with regional anesthesia). The multiparous patient is recommended to push for a maximum of 1 hour without regional anesthesia (or 2 hours with regional anesthesia).[40] Descent can commence during the first stage, but no active intervention (either maternal expulsive efforts or obstetric intervention) should be attempted until full cervical dilatation has been achieved.

Third Stage

The third stage of labor is the interval between the delivery of the infant and the delivery of the placenta and fetal membranes. The third stage usually lasts less than 10 minutes, but up to 30 minutes may be allowed before manual removal of the placenta is performed, as long as blood loss is not excessive.

Cardinal Movements in Labor

The mechanisms of labor, also known as the cardinal movements, refer to the changes in position of fetal head during its passage through the birth canal. Seven discrete cardinal movements of the fetus are described: engagement, descent, flexion, internal rotation, extension, external rotation or restitution, and expulsion.

Engagement

Engagement refers to passage of the widest diameter of the presenting part to a level below the plane of the pelvic inlet. In the cephalic presentation with a well-flexed head, the largest transverse diameter of the fetal head is the biparietal diameter. Engagement is achieved when the presenting part is at 0 station (at the level of the maternal ischial spines) on bimanual examination. Engagement is considered an important clinical parameter as it demonstrates that, at least at the level of the pelvic inlet, the maternal bony pelvis is sufficiently large to allow descent of the fetal head. In nulliparas, engagement of the fetal head usually occurs by 36 weeks' gestation, but in multiparas, engagement can occur later in gestation or even during labor.

Descent

Descent of the fetus is not continuous, with the greatest rate of descent occurring during the deceleration phase of the first stage of labor and during the second stage of labor.

Flexion

Although flexion of the fetal head onto the chest is present to some degree in most fetuses before labor, complete flexion usually only occurs during the course of labor. The result of complete flexion is to present the smallest diameter of the fetal head for optimal passage through the pelvis.

Internal Rotation

Internal rotation refers to rotation of the presenting part from its original position (usually transverse with regard to the birth canal) to the anteroposterior position as it passes through the pelvis. The pelvic floor musculature, including the coccygeus and ileococcygeus muscles, form a V-shaped hammock. As the head descends, the occiput of the fetus rotates towards the symphysis pubis (or, less commonly, towards the hollow of the sacrum), thereby allowing the widest portion of the fetus to negotiate the pelvis at its widest dimension.

Extension

Extension occurs once the fetus has descended to the level of the introitus. At this point, the birth canal curves upwards. The fetal head is delivered by extension and rotates around the symphysis pubis.

External Rotation

External rotation, also known as restitution, refers to the return of the fetal head to the correct anatomic position in relation to the fetal torso. This is a passive movement resulting from a release of the forces exerted on the fetal head by the maternal bony pelvis and its musculature.

Expulsion

Expulsion refers to delivery of the rest of the fetus. Further descent brings the anterior shoulder to the level of the symphysis pubis. The anterior shoulder is delivered in much the same manner as the head, with rotation of the shoulder under the symphysis pubis. After the shoulder, the rest of the body is usually delivered without difficulty.

MANAGEMENT OF NORMAL LABOR AND DELIVERY

Initial Assessment in Labor

Initial assessment in labor should include a review of the patient's prenatal information, a focused history (including the time of onset of contractions, status of fetal membranes, presence or absence of vaginal bleeding,) physical examination, and laboratory testing as indicated. Physical examination should include documentation of the patient's vital signs; notation of fetal position and presentation;

an assessment of fetal well-being; and an estimation of the frequency, duration, and quality of uterine contractions. The size, presentation, and lie of the fetus can be assessed by abdominal palpation. Although abdominal examination has several limitations (small fetus, maternal obesity, multifetal pregnancies, polyhydramnios), it may add valuable information in the management of labor. Palpation is divided into four separate Leopold's maneuvers (Fig. 8–4).

Leopold's maneuver #1. The gravid uterus is slightly dextrorotated (deviated to the right) because of the position of the sigmoid colon. With the patient lying supine and her knees comfortably flexed, the examiner corrects for dextrorotation of the uterus with the back of one hand and delineates the fundus of the uterus with the other. The "fundal height" refers to a midline measurement from the symphysis pubis to the top of the uterine fundus.

Leopold's maneuver #2. The examiner runs his/her hands down the maternal abdomen on either side of the fetus to determine the fetal lie, and uses the fingers to locate the fetal spine and small parts (extremities).

Leopold's maneuver #3. Also known as Pawlik's grip, this maneuver involves the examiner firmly grasping the upper and lower poles of the fetus by placing their fingers laterally above the symphysis pubis and at the fundus. In this way, the characteristics of the two fetal poles can be determined and compared, and the presentation documented. The fetal breech is often larger, softer, less well defined, and less ballottable than the cranium.

Leopold's maneuver #4. In this maneuver, the examiner faces the patient's feet and moves his/her hands in bilaterally from the anterior superior iliac crests to determine whether or not the presenting part of the fetus is engaged in the maternal pelvis. In a cephalic presentation, the head is regarded as unengaged if the examiner's hands are seen to converge below the fetal head. If the examiner's hands are noted to diverge as they trace the fetal head into the pelvis, the vertex is regarded as engaged.

Intrapartum Management

After the patient has been admitted in labor, she and her family should be introduced to the members of the health care team responsible for her care. The patient and her family should be consulted and involved in such decisions as the use of oxytocin to

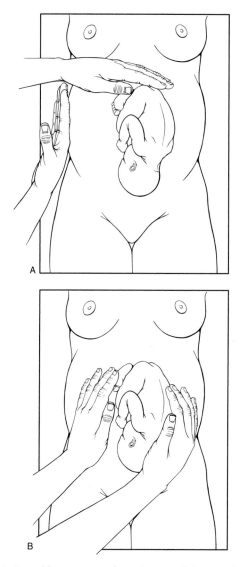

Figure 8–4. Leopold's maneuvers for palpation of the gravid abdomen.

Illustration continued on following page

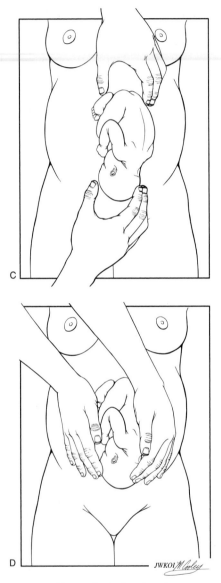

Figure 8-4 *Continued*

augment labor, the choice of agent for intrapartum pain management, and the need for assisted vaginal delivery. Emotional support of the patient during the birthing process has been shown repeatedly to lower intrapartum analgesia requirements, and to decrease intrapartum complications.

Assessment of the quality of the uterine contractions as well as cervical examinations at appropriate intervals should be performed in order to follow the progress of labor. Vaginal examinations should be kept to a minimum to avoid promoting intra-amniotic infection. During the first stage of labor, the fetal heart rate should be recorded at least every 30 minutes and should be auscultated during and immediately after a contraction. During the second stage of labor, the fetal heart should be auscultated at least every 15 minutes, and after each uterine contraction.

The goals of clinical assistance at spontaneous delivery are the reduction of maternal trauma, prevention of fetal injury, and initial support of the newborn if required. When the fetal head crowns and delivery is imminent, pressure from the accoucheur's hand is used to hold the head flexed and to control delivery, thereby preventing precipitous expulsion, which has been associated with perineal tears as well as intracranial trauma. If there is a delay in delivery of the fetal head, a modified Ritgen's maneuver may be attempted. Using a sterile towel, the fetal chin is palpated through the perineum or rectum, and upward pressure is applied to facilitate extension of the fetal head. Once the fetal head is delivered, external rotation (restitution) is allowed to occur. If the cord is around the neck, it should be looped over the head or, if not reducible, doubly clamped and transected. Mucus can then be gently suctioned from the fetal mouth, oropharynx, and nares using a bulb syringe. In the presence of meconium, aspiration with a DeLee suction catheter may reduce the risk of meconium aspiration syndrome. However, care should be taken not to suction too vigorously, as posterior pharyngeal stimulation can cause a vagal response and fetal bradycardia. Once the fetal airway has been cleared, a hand is placed on each parietal eminence and the anterior shoulder is delivered with the next contraction by downward traction towards the mother's sacrum in concert with maternal expulsive efforts. In this way, the anterior shoulder is encouraged to slip under the symphysis pubis. The posterior shoulder is then delivered by upward traction. After delivery, there is a net transfer of blood from the placenta to the fetus. Spasm of the umbilical artery occurs within approximately 1 minute of birth. However, the remaining communication between the neonate and placenta, the umbilical vein, permits passage of blood for up to 3 minutes after birth. Delay in clamping of the cord will allow an increase in the volume of transfusion.

Delivery of the Placenta and Fetal Membranes

The three classic signs of placental separation are: (1) lengthening of the umbilical cord, (2) a gush of blood from the vagina signifying separation of the placenta from the uterine wall, and (3) a change in the shape of the uterine fundus from discoid to globular with elevation of the fundal height.

After delivery, the placenta, umbilical cord, and fetal membranes should be examined. Abnormally large placentae are associated with such conditions as fetal hydrops fetalis and congenital syphilis. Inspection and palpation of the placenta should include the fetal and maternal surfaces and may reveal areas of fibrosis, infarction, or calcification. Although each of these conditions may be seen in the normal term placenta, excessive loss of surface area can result in impairment of exchange between mother and fetus. Abnormalities of lobulation (a missing placental cotyledon or a membrane defect suggesting a missing succenturiate lobe) may suggest retention of a portion of placenta, which can lead to postpartum hemorrhage or infection. The classic hallmark of placental abruption is a depressed area on the maternal side of the placenta with an attached blood clot. The absence of such a finding, however, does not exclude the diagnosis. The site of insertion of the umbilical cord into the placenta should be noted. Abnormal insertions include marginal insertion (in which the cord inserts into the edge of the placenta) and membranous insertion (in which the vessels of the umbilical cord course through the membranes prior to attachment to the placental disk). The cord itself should be inspected for length, the correct number of umbilical vessels (normally two arteries and one vein), true knots, hematomas, and strictures. A single umbilical artery is associated with other structural anomalies in 20 percent of cases.[49] The fetal membranes should also be examined for meconium staining and for opacification of the membranes, which may suggest chorioamnionitis.

Following delivery of the placenta, the cervix, vagina, and perineum should be carefully examined for evidence of birth injury. If a laceration is seen, its length and position should be noted and repair initiated. Adequate analgesia (either regional or local) is essential for repair.

The need for manual and/or surgical exploration of the uterus after delivery is controversial. Adequate analgesia is essential for any such procedure. Although it has been proposed by some investigators that manual exploration be performed after all deliveries,[50] it is usually reserved for women in whom there is suspicion of retained products of conception, where there is excessive vaginal bleeding, and in cases of premature delivery or vaginal birth after cesarean (VBAC).[51] If a transmural defect in a prior cesarean scar is palpated following delivery, it should be repaired only if there is excessive bleeding.

ABNORMAL PATTERNS OF LABOR

Abnormalities of the First Stage

Abnormalities of the first stage of labor imply a deviation from the normal pattern of cervical dilatation (Fig. 8–3). The abnormality may be either protraction or arrest, and may occur during the latent or active phases of the first stage.

Disorders of the Latent Phase

Latent phase arrest implies simply that labor has not truly begun. *Prolonged latent phase* refers to a latent phase of 20 hours or longer in the nulliparous patient or 14 hours or longer in the multiparous patient.[53] Although the duration of the latent phase of labor is highly variable and prolongation of the latent phase does not correlate with adverse perinatal outcome, this situation can be taxing to both the mother and the practitioner. Unless there is a maternal or fetal indication for expediting delivery, expectant management is usually recommended. Administration of an analgesic agent such as 15 to 20 mg of morphine may allow the patient to rest for a few hours or days (so-called therapeutic rest). If the decision is made to proceed with augmentation of labor, oxytocin infusion is the technique of choice. Amniotomy in such patients should be deferred because of the association between prolonged rupture of the membranes and intra-amniotic infection. Prolonged latent phase is not an indication for cesarean delivery.

Disorders of the Active Phase

Disorders of the active phase of the first stage of labor are classified into three broad categories.

A diagnosis of *primary dysfunctional labor* implies that the gravida has entered the active phase of labor but that the rate of active phase cervical dilatation is less than the fifth percentile, defined as less than 1.2 cm/h in nulliparas and less than 1.5 cm/h in multiparas[35,36,52] (Table 8–1 and Fig. 8–5). Although such pregnancies are at risk for secondary arrest primary dysfunctional labor is not itself an indication for cesarean delivery. In the nulliparous patient, inadequate uterine activity is the most common cause of primary dysfunctional labor. Once diagnosed, augmentation with amniotomy and/or oxytocin infusion should be attempted. In the multiparous patient, CPD due to malposition is the most common cause.

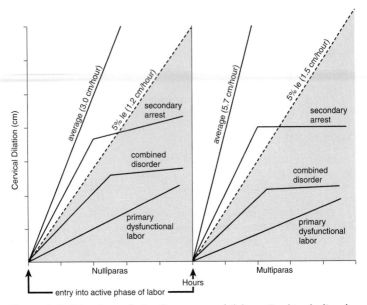

Figure 8–5. Disorders of the first stage of labor. Combined disorder implies an arrest in a gravida previously exhibiting primary dysfunctional labor.

Secondary arrest is defined as cessation of previously normal active phase cervical dilatation for a period of 2 hours or more.[56] Intrapartum management should include confirmation of adequate uterine contractions and exclusion of CPD. Vaginal examination should be performed to verify cervical dilatation as well as fetal presentation, position, and station. If uterine activity is suboptimal, amniotomy and/or oxytocin infusion should be initiated. The majority of gravidas with secondary arrest (70 to 80 percent) will respond to such maneuvers and resume progression of cervical dilatation, although such pregnancies remain at increased risk of second-stage abnormalities and operative deliveries. Continued arrest over 2 to 4 hours with adequate uterine contractions is an indication for cesarean delivery.

A *combined disorder* of active phase dilatation is defined as arrest of dilatation occurring when the patient has previously exhibited primary dysfunctional labor. This pattern is associated with a less favorable outcome with regard to vaginal delivery than in gravidas with secondary arrest alone.[56]

Abnormalities of the Second Stage

The second stage of labor is the interval between full cervical dilatation and delivery of the infant. Abnormalities of the second stage can be classified into two broad categories:

Protraction of Descent

Protraction of descent is defined as descent of the presenting part during the second stage of labor occurring at less than 1 cm/h in nulliparas and less than 2 cm/h in multiparas.[58] Review of electronic fetal heart rate tracings obtained during prolonged second stage labors has documented a high incidence of variable decelerations and prolonged decelerations[59] (see Chapter 9). The gradual fall in fetal scalp capillary pH that occurs throughout labor is accelerated during the second stage.[60] Deliveries complicated by prolonged second stage therefore place the fetus at increased risk of acidosis. Expectant management is reasonable provided that electronic fetal monitoring is reassuring, descent is progressive, and vaginal delivery is imminent.[61-64]

Arrest of Descent

Arrest (failure) of descent requires prompt reevaluation of uterine contractions, maternal and fetal well-being, and cephalopelvic relationships. Obvious problems such as inadequate uterine contractions, overdistended bladder, ineffectual maternal expulsive efforts, dense conduction anesthesia, or strong perineal resistance (soft-tissue dystocia) should be managed appropriately and are associated with a high expectation of success. The decision to continue oxytocin infusion or to proceed with operative intervention (assisted vaginal delivery or cesarean) should be individualized.

Abnormalities of the Third Stage

Separation of the placenta is a consequence of continued uterine contractions following expulsion of the fetus, which also control blood loss through compression of the spiral arterioles. The interval between delivery of the infant and delivery of the placenta and fetal membranes usually lasts less than 10 minutes and is complete within 15 minutes in 95 percent of all deliveries. After 30 minutes, intervention is indicated to expedite delivery of the placenta. Dilute intravenous oxytocin is superior to intravenous or intramuscular ergometrine in this regard.[65] If bleeding is excessive or if there is no response to uterotonic agents, manual removal of the placenta may be required. Prophylactic antibiotics should be administered to such patients to prevent postpartum endomyometritis.

INDUCTION OF LABOR

Induction of Labor

Induction of labor refers to the initiation of uterine contractions before the spontaneous onset of labor by medical and/or surgical means for the purpose of delivery. The patient and her family should be informed of the risks, benefits, and potential complications, including the possibility of cesarean delivery.

Indicated Induction of Labor

In general, induction of labor is indicated when the benefits of delivery to the mother and/or fetus outweigh the potential risks of continuing the pregnancy.

With recent technologic advances, the therapeutic armamentarium available to the obstetrician has increased, as has the temptation to intervene. A firm indication for delivery is a prerequisite for induction.

Elective Induction of Labor

Elective induction of labor is defined as termination of pregnancy without an acceptable medical indication. Such a strategy may be appropriate in select patients such as patients who live a great distance from the hospital or who have a history of rapid labors. The major potential complication of elective induction is iatrogenic prematurity, which can be minimized by using strict criteria for gestational age.

Cervical Ripening

The success of a labor induction is determined, in large part, by the initial state of the cervix. When induction of labor is attempted against an unfavorable cervix, the likelihood of a successful outcome is reduced.[71-74] In 1964, Bishop[75] developed a scoring system to evaluate multiparous patients for elective induction of labor at term. The scoring system is based on the properties of the cervix that can be assessed clinically; namely, dilatation, effacement, consistency; and position and station of the head. (Table 8–2). When the cervical score exceeds 8, the incidence of vaginal delivery subsequent to induction is similar to that for spontaneous labor. Enhancement of cervical maturation is an appropriate first step toward induction of labor when the cervix is unfavorable. Preinduction cervical maturation is associated with fewer failed inductions. A number of agents are available to facilitate cervical maturation (Table 8–3).

Table 8–2. ASSESSMENT OF ANTEPARTUM CERVICAL STATUS BY MODIFIED BISHOP SCORE

Parameter	Score			
	0	1	2	3
Dilatation (cm)	Closed	1–2	3–4	5 or more
Effacement (%)	0–30	40–50	60–70	80 or more
Station	−3	−2	−1 or 0	+1 or +2
Consistency	Firm	Medium	Soft	
Cervical position	Posterior	Midposition	Anterior	

Adapted from Bishop EH: Pelvic scoring for elective induction. Obstet Gynecol 24:266, 1964; American College of Obstetricians and Gynecologists, with permission.

Methods of Cervical Maturation and Labor Induction

A single technique is rarely effective on its own, and a combination of maneuvers may be required.

Nonpharmacologic Methods

Nonpharmacologic methods for cervical maturation and/or labor induction include stripping of the membranes, amniotomy and mechanical dilatation.

Table 8–3. METHODS OF CERVICAL RIPENING

Pharmacologic Methods	Nonpharmacologic Methods
Hormonal techniques Prostaglandins	Membrane stripping
Prostaglandin E_2 (dinoprostone [Prepidil], Cervidil)	Mechanical dilators
Prostaglandin E_1 (misoprostol [Cytotec])	Hygroscopic dilators (laminaria, lamicel, Dilapan)
Oxytocin	Balloon catheter (alone, with traction, with infusion)

Steroid receptor antagonists (?)
  RU-486 (Mifepristone)
  ZK98299 (Onapristone)
	Amniotomy

STRIPPING OF THE MEMBRANES. Stripping or sweeping of the fetal membranes refers to digital separation of the chorioamniotic membrane from the wall of the cervix and lower uterine segment. The vertex should be well applied to the cervix and the cervix must be dilated sufficiently to admit the practitioner's finger. Stripping of the membranes is believed to work by release of endogenous prostaglandins from the membranes and adjacent decidua.[82] Sweeping of the membranes is able to reduce the interval to spontaneous onset of labor, but there is no evidence of a reduction in operative vaginal delivery, cesarean section rates, or maternal or neonatal morbidity.[89]

AMNIOTOMY. The technique of amniotomy, artificial rupture of the membranes, involves perforation of the chorioamniotic membranes using either a toothed clamp or a plastic hook. Before amniotomy is performed, the vertex should be seen to be engaged in the pelvis and well applied to the cervix to prevent prolapse of the umbilical cord. The opening in the membranes should be widened by blunt dissection using the examining finger to retract the membranes over the vertex without dislodging the vertex. The amount and character of released amniotic fluid should be noted. In patients with a favorable cervical examination at term, amniotomy alone has been reported to be effective in inducing labor in 88 percent of cases[91] and to shorten the interval to delivery by 0.8 to 2.3 hours.[92,93] Whether this reduction in time to delivery translates into an improvement in clinical outcome is not clear.[96]

Advantages of amniotomy include (1) a high success rate for induction of labor; (2) observation of the amniotic fluid for blood or meconium; and (3) ready access to the intrauterine cavity and to the fetus for placement of an intrauterine pressure catheter, or a fetal scalp electrode. Although early amniotomy has been shown to reduce the length of labor, it does not appear to lower the rate of cesarean delivery.[92,93,97] Complications of amniotomy include (1) umbilical cord prolapse, (2) fetal injury, (3) prolonged rupture of the membranes, (4) adverse change in fetal position as amniotomy is associated with a greater frequency of malposition and asynclitism,[93] and (5) rupture of vasa previa and subsequent fetal hemorrhage. The fetal heart rate should be monitored during and immediately after amniotomy. A transient fetal tachycardia is common after amniotomy, but decelerations or bradycardia are rare in the absence of overt or occult cord prolapse.

MECHANICAL DILATORS. Mechanical dilators all rely on release of endogenous prostaglandins from the membranes and maternal decidua to promote cervical maturation. When compared with no preinduction cervical ripening, an intracervical balloon catheter has been shown to significantly shorten the induction to delivery interval and to increase the rate of vaginal delivery.[98] A randomized comparison between intracervical PGE_2 gel and intracervical Foley catheter for cervical ripening at term showed them to be equally effective, with no difference in side-effect profile, intrapartum complications, or mode of delivery.[99] Hygroscopic dilators — including laminaria Dilapan and lamicel rely on absorption of water to swell and forcibly dilate the cervix, and have been found to be at least as effective in promoting cervical maturation as PGE_2 gel.[100-102] A significant disadvantage of mechanical dilators, however, is patient discomfort both at the time of insertion and with progressive cervical dilatation. In specific clinical circumstances where prostaglandins should be avoided such as glaucoma or pulmonary disease mechanical dilators can be used both safely and effectively.

Pharmacologic Methods

Pharmacologic methods available for cervial maturation and/or induction of labor is summarized in Table 8–3.

PROSTAGLANDINS. Prostaglandins act locally at their site of production on contiguous cells. $PGF_{2\alpha}$ acts primarily to promote myometrial contractility, whereas PGE_2 appears to be important for cervical maturation. Exogenous PGE_2 preparations have been shown to be more potent at promoting cervical maturation than $PGF_{2\alpha}$.[104,109] Unlike oxytocin, the response of the uterus to prostaglandins does not change significantly throughout gestation. Thus prostaglandins are used to effect midtrimester pregnancy termination or induction of labor following intrauterine death remote from term. PGE_2 administered by any route improves the rate of spontaneous vaginal delivery and decreases the rate of both cesarean and operative vaginal delivery. Gastrointestinal side effects from PGE_2 are reported with all routes of administration, but appear to be minimized with vaginal administration. The most commonly used transvaginal PGE_2 preparation is dinoprostone gel (Prepidil). Placement of PGE_2 within the cervical canal will have a more marked effect on cervical maturation than placement in the posterior fornix of the vagina, but with no significant difference in labor or delivery outcomes.[115,116] A sustained release preparation of PGE_2 (Cervidil) unlike the gel can be easily removed if clinical complications such as tachysystole or uterine hypertonus ensue.

The PGE_1 analogues such as misoprostol (Cytotec) have been used for cervical ripening and induction of labor, although they are not FDA approved for this indication. They can be administered either transvaginally (25 μg every 3 hours to a maximum of eight doses[119]) or orally (50 μg every 4 hours[120]). Misoprostol is as effective as PGE_2 for cervical ripening and labor induction,[118] and the cost of misoprostol is a fraction that of any of the PGE_2 preparations. The optimal dosage regimen for PGE_1 preparations has yet to be determined. A higher prevalence of tachysystole, meconium passage, and possibly uterine rupture has been reported with its use,[118] and so misoprostol is not recommended for patients with a previous cesarean birth due to the possibility of uterine rupture.

Oxytocin

Oxytocin is a potent endogenous uterotonic agent that is capable of stimulating uterine contractions at intravenous infusion rates of 1 to 2 mIU/min at term.[125]

Only intravenous preparations are approved by the FDA for induction and augmentation of labor. Continuous low-dose (1 to 4 mIU/min) oxytocin infusion has been shown to be effective in promoting cervical maturation,[134] and appears to be as effective as PGE_2 gel preparations in this regard.[135] High-dose oxytocin significantly shortens labor without any adverse fetal effect.[136]

Overall, PGE_2 gel is probably a better agent for preinduction cervical ripening than oxytocin, being equally effective and easier to administer.

MANAGEMENT OF ABNORMAL LABOR AND DELIVERY

Augmentation of Labor at Term

Abnormalities of the first stage of labor may be either protraction or arrest disorders (Fig. 8–5). When such an abnormality is noted and uterine activity is suboptimal, administration of oxytocin is recommended. Variability in patient sensitivity and response to intravenous oxytocin is the rule. As such, the recommended rate of oxytocin administration is that which produces contractions every 2 to 3 minutes, lasting 60 to 90 seconds with a peak intrauterine pressure of 50 to 60 mm Hg and a resting uterine tone of 10 to 15 mm Hg. Dosage may vary from 0.5 to 30 to 40 mIU/min of oxytocin. Control of the intravenous dose is best achieved by using a constant-infusion pump. Augmentation is usually started at 0.5 mIU/min, and the rate is doubled every 15 to 20 minutes until adequate uterine contractions are observed. Approximately 30 to 40 minutes are needed for the full effect of an increase in dosage to be reflected in the contraction pattern. A slow rate of increase in oxytocin administration is as effective for inducing labor as a fast rate of increase, while at the same time minimizing oxytocin requirements.[146] When used in patients demonstrating a protraction disorder, oxytocin infusion rates greater than 6 mIU/min are rarely required.[148] It is unusual for a patient to require more than 30 to

40 mIU/min. As labor progresses, the frequency and intensity of contractions may increase, and the oxytocin infusion may need to be reduced.

Monitoring of uterine contractions and fetal heart rate is recommended throughout the induction and is best accomplished with continuous electronic monitoring. A number of complications of intravenously administered oxytocin are described.

Uterine Hyperstimulation

Uterine hyperstimulation refers to excessive frequency of contractions (polysystole) or increased uterine tone (hypertonia). Uterine hyperstimulation may produce a nonreassuring fetal heart rate tracing, placental abruption, or uterine rupture. The use of electronic fetal monitoring has increased the early detection of these potentially damaging maternal or fetal complications. The detection of fetal heart rate abnormalities secondary to uterine hyperstimulation should prompt discontinuation of the oxytocin infusion, positioning of the patient on her left side, and oxygen administration.

Water Intoxication

Oxytocin is structurally and functionally related to vasopressin (antidiuretic hormone). High-dose oxytocin infusions (30 to 40 mIU/min) have been associated with excessive fluid retention caused by binding of oxytocin to vasopressin and oxytocin receptors in the kidney leading to *water intoxication,* characterized by hyponatremia, confusion, convulsions, and coma. Fluid overload and hyponatremia can be prevented by strict recordings of fluid intake and output, use of balanced salt solutions, and by avoiding prolonged administration of high-dose oxytocin infusion.

Hypotension

Bolus injections of oxytocin may cause *hypotension.* Oxytocin should be administered intravenously as dilute solutions at recommended rates.

Uterine Rupture

Uterine rupture has been associated with excessive oxytocin administration. Other risk factors for uterine rupture include prior uterine surgery, fetal malpresentation, grandmultiparity, and a markedly overdistended uterus. After uterine rupture, contractions may cease even if the oxytocin infusion is continued.

Prostaglandins have been compared with oxytocin infusion for augmentation of labor at term. Since prostaglandins have more side effects and are more difficult to titrate, it is unlikely that prostaglandins will replace oxytocin for augmentation of labor.

Episiotomy

Episiotomy is an incision into the perineal body made during the second stage of labor to facilitate delivery. Although there is general agreement that episiotomy is indicated in association with an instrumental delivery or to expedite delivery in the setting of fetal heart rate abnormalities, the use of prophylactic episiotomy is widely debated. Cited advantages of prophylactic episiotomy include substitution of a straight surgical incision for a ragged spontaneous laceration, and reduction in the duration of the second stage.

Median (midline) episiotomy refers to a vertical midline incision from the posterior forchette towards the rectum. The incision should be performed when the fetal head has distended the vulva to 2 to 3 cm, and once adequate analgesia has been achieved. The size of the incision will depend on the length of the perineum but is generally around one half of the length of the perineum, and should be extended vertically up the vaginal mucosa for a distance of 2 to 3 cm. Complications of median episiotomy include increased blood loss, especially if the incision is made too early, and localized pain. Median episiotomies are associated with an increased incidence of third- and fourth-degree lacerations.[153,156] Such injuries are associated with a high incidence of long-term incontinence and pelvic prolapse. *Mediolateral episiotomy* is performed by incision at a 45 degree angle from the inferior portion of the hymeneal ring. The length of the incision is less critical than with median episiotomy, but longer incisions require more lengthy repair. Such incisions are less likely to be associated with damage to the anal sphincter and the rectal mucosa. They are the procedure of choice for women with inflammatory bowel disease because of the critical need to prevent rectal injury. Chronic complications such as unsatisfactory cosmetic results and inclusions within the scar may be more common with mediolateral episiotomies, and blood loss is greater.

Assisted Vaginal Delivery

Assisted vaginal delivery refers to any operative procedure designed to effect vaginal delivery, and includes forceps delivery and vacuum extraction. Randomized studies comparing forceps with vacuum have not shown a significant difference in success rate.[159–161]

Forceps-Assisted Vaginal Delivery

Obstetric forceps consist of two separate blades that are inserted into the vagina sequentially. Each half consists of the blade proper, which has a cephalic curvature designed to be applied to the fetal head, a shank, and a handle. The halves are joined by a lock usually located at the junction of the shanks and the handle. (Fig. 8–6)

"Classical" forceps have a cephalic curvature, a pelvic curve and an "English" lock in which the articulation is fixed. Examples include (1) Simpson forceps, which have fenestrated blades and separated (nonoverlapping) shanks; (2) Tucker-McLane forceps, which have solid (nonfenestrated) blades and overlapping shanks; and (3) Elliot forceps, which have fenestrated blades, overlapping shanks, and a greater cephalic curvature.

Rotational forceps such as Kielland forceps have a cephalic curvature to grasp the fetal head, but no pelvic curvature and a "sliding" lock, which permits movement between the forceps halves along the longitudinal axis of the shanks to correct for asynclitism of the fetal head. Once the fetal head has been rotated into the anteroposterior position, it is recommended that the rotational forceps be replaced by classical forceps, as the pelvic curvature of the classical forceps will minimize perineal trauma. *Forceps designed to assist vaginal breech deliveries* such as Piper forceps lack a pelvic curve and have blades below the plane of the shanks. Forceps deliveries are classified according to the station of the fetal head at the time of application (Table 8–4).

Forceps deliveries should be performed only after careful consideration of alternative approaches such as oxytocin administration, cesarean delivery, or simply expectant management. Once the decision has been made to proceed with forceps delivery, several criteria (summarized in Table 8–5) must be met before application of the forceps. A "phantom application" should be performed by the operator by positioning the forceps in front of the perineum in the correct position of the final application. A proper application is shown in Figure 8–7.

Vacuum-Assisted Vaginal Delivery

Vacuum suction induces an artificial caput succedaneum or chignon within the cup to which a traction force is applied in concert with uterine contractions. Current instruments are disposable and made of plastic, polyethylene, or silicone. There are two general types: those with a firm, mushroom-shaped rigid cup or with a pliable, funnel-shaped soft cup. Manual or electronically operated vacuum sources are available.

The suction cup should be placed on the fetal scalp symmetrically astride the sagittal suture with the posterior margin of the cup around 1 to 3 cm anterior to the posterior fontanelle. It should not be placed over the fontanelle. This placement will promote flexion of the fetal head with traction. After application, a low suction is applied to establish a vacuum as the cup is held in place. After

TYPES OF FORCEPS

① Classical forceps

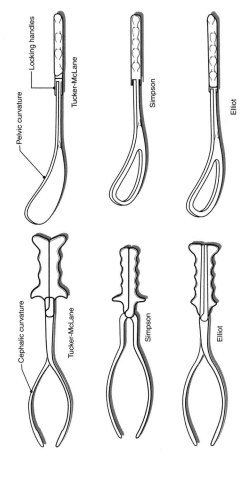

Cephalic curvature

Tucker-McLane

Simpson

Elliot

Locking handles

Pelvic curvature

Tucker-McLane

Simpson

Elliot

② Rotational forceps

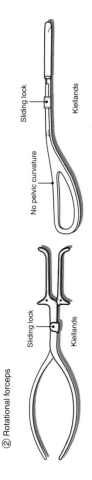

Sliding lock

Kiellands

No pelvic curvature

Sliding lock

Kiellands

③ Forceps for delivery of aftercoming head of the breech

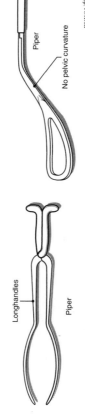

Longhandles

Piper

Piper

No pelvic curvature

JWKOJ Morley

Figure 8–6. Classification of forceps.

Table 8-4. CLASSIFICATION OF OPERATIVE VAGINAL DELIVERIES

Type of Procedure	Criteria
Outlet forceps	Scalp is visible at the introitus without separating the labia
	Fetal skull has reached the level of the pelvic floor
	Sagittal suture is in the direct anteroposterior diameter or in the right or left occiput anterior or posterior position
	Fetal head is at or on the perineum
	Rotation is ≤ 45 degrees
Low forceps	Leading point of the fetal skull (station) is $+ 2$ or more but has not as yet reached the pelvic floor
	1. Rotation is ≤ 45 degrees
	2. Rotation is > 45 degrees
Midforceps	The head is engaged in the pelvis but the presenting part is above $+ 2$ station
High forceps	(Not included in this classification)

Adapted from American College of Obstetricians and Gynecologists: Operative vaginal delivery, ACOG Technical Bulletin No. 196. Washington, DC, American College of Obstetricians and Gynecologists, 1994.

ensuring that no maternal soft tissue is trapped between the cup and the fetal head, suction is increased slowly to allow for the proper development of the chignon. Once a proper vacuum has been reached, sustained downward traction is applied along the pelvic curve using a two-handed technique in concert with uterine contractions and maternal expulsive efforts. Suction is released between contractions. Ideally, an episiotomy should be avoided, as pressure of the perineum on the vacuum cup will help to keep it applied to the fetal head and assist in flexion and rotation. It is suggested that the procedure be abandoned if the cup detaches three times, if no descent of the head is achieved, or if delivery is not effected within 30 minutes.

Indications for vacuum extraction-assisted delivery are similar to those for forceps delivery. One potential advantage of vacuum extraction is that delivery can be accomplished with minimal maternal analgesia. Relative contraindications include extreme prematurity (<34 weeks' gestation) and suspected fetal coagulation disorder. Although the overall rate of complications is similar between forceps and vacuum deliveries, the complication profile is

Table 8–5. PREREQUISITES FOR OPERATIVE VAGINAL DELIVERY: A NUMBER OF CRITERIA NEED TO BE FULFILLED PRIOR TO ATTEMPTING OPERATIVE VAGINAL DELIVERY

Maternal Criteria	Fetal Criteria	Uteroplacental Criteria	Other Criteria
Adequate analgesia Lithotomy position Bladder empty Clinical pelvimetry must be adequate in dimension and size to facilitate an atraumatic delivery Verbal or written consent	Vertex presentation The fetal head must be engaged in the pelvis The position of the fetal head must be known with certainty The station of the fetal head must be ≥ + 2 The attitude of the fetal head and the presence of caput succedaneum and/or moulding should be noted	Cervix fully dilated Membranes ruptured No placenta previa	Experienced operator who is fully acquainted with the use of the instrument The capability to perform an emergency cesarean delivery if required

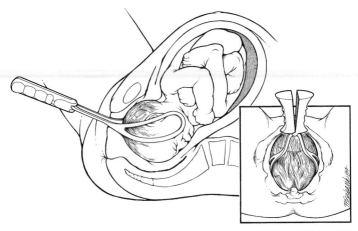

Figure 8–7. Proper application of obstetric forceps. (From O'Brien WF, Cefalo RC: Labor and delivery. *In* Gabbe SG, Niebyl JR, Simpson JL [eds]: Obstetrics: Normal and Problem Pregnancies, 3rd ed. New York, Churchill Livingstone, 1996 p 377, with permission.)

different. Failed delivery is commonly encountered using the vacuum extractor. Maternal perineal injuries are less common than with forceps deliveries. However, there is an increased incidence of fetal cephalohematoma or bleeding into the scalp which, if large, may be associated with neonatal jaundice, scalp lacerations and bruising.[160,169,170] Whether the incidence of fetal intracerebral hemorrhage is increased with vacuum extraction is not clear. In response to reports of 12 fetal deaths and 9 serious injuries over a 4-year period, the FDA issued a Public Health Advisory on May 21, 1998,[171] delineating the fetal risks associated with vacuum extraction and urging physicians to use caution when employing these devices. A follow-up statement by the ACOG[172] argued that "while no medical procedure is risk-free, vacuum extraction has an extraordinary low risk for adverse outcomes" (i.e., 5 adverse events per 228,354 vacuum deliveries per year).

INTRAPARTUM COMPLICATIONS

Cord Prolapse

Cord prolapse refers to passage of the umbilical cord into the vagina ahead of the presenting part following rupture of the fetal membranes. It is a true obstetric emergency, as fetal perfusion is rapidly diminished either by mechanical distortion in the vagina and/or by vasospasm triggered by the precipitous drop in temperature outside the uterus. Cord prolapse is a rare event in term cephalic pregnancies (0.4 percent), but is more common with malpresentations, especially footling breech presentations and transverse lies.[176,178] Diagnosis is made by palpation of the cord on vaginal examination with or without fetal bradycardia. Management involves pushing the presenting part up away from the cord, and immediate delivery, usually by emergent cesarean section. Prevention of iatrogenic cord prolapse can be achieved by performing amniotomy with fundal pressure and only when the vertex is well applied to the cervix.[179]

CONTROVERSIAL ISSUES IN LABOR MANAGEMENT

Active Management of Labor

There are two established methods of managing labor at term, traditional management and active management. The major difference between these two approaches is in the definition of failure to progress and in the oxytocin protocol chosen for labor augmentation.

Traditional Management

Traditional management uses a low dose oxytocin regimen with longer intervals between dose increments. Low-dose oxytocin infusion, starting at an infusion rate of 1 mIU/min and increasing by 1 to 2 mIU/min at intervals of not less than 30 minutes, significantly shortens the interval from initiation of oxytocin augmentation to full dilation as compared with physician-directed regimens.[77,148] High-dose oxytocin (starting at an infusion rate of 4 mIU/min and increasing by 4 mIU/min every 15 minutes "until adequate uterine contractility was obtained") may shorten the length of labor in both nulliparous and multiparous patients as compared with low-dose protocols.[136,182] It remains unclear, however, whether high-dose oxytocin actually improves obstetric outcome or whether it merely produces the same outcome in a shorter period of time.

Active Management of Labor

Active management of labor refers to a philosophy of labor management based on the premise that optimizing uterine contractions will improve the progress of labor and subsequent outcome.[24,54] An extension of this philosophy is the belief that fetal and maternal injuries are less with propulsion than with traction. It applies specifically to nulliparous patients in spontaneous labor with a cephalic presentation, and is not applicable to the multiparous patient or to patients undergoing induction of labor.

There are many other important components to this approach of management. The basic principles of active management include the following:

Strict criteria for admission to labor and delivery. In active management of labor protocols, labor is defined strictly as the presence of regular, painful contractions in conjunction with at least one further finding (complete cervical effacement, bloody show, or rupture of the fetal membranes).

Early amniotomy.

Hourly cervical examinations.

Early diagnosis of inefficient uterine activity. If the patient does not achieve and maintain a cervical dilatation rate of greater than or equal to 1.0 cm/h, a diagnosis of inefficient uterine activity is made and augmentation with intravenous oxytocin infusion is initiated immediately.

High-dose oxytocin infusion. In patients requiring oxytocin augmentation, a high-dose oxytocin infusion protocol is used. Oxytocin infusion is initiated at a rate of 6 mIU/min and increased by the same amount every 15 minutes until a uterine contraction frequency of seven contractions per 15 minutes is achieved or until the maximum oxytocin infusion rate of 36 mIU/min is reached.

Active intervention. Using this protocol, the expected duration of the first stage of labor is less than 12 hours and less than 2 hours for the second stage. If these expectations are not met, active intervention, operative vaginal or cesarean delivery, is recommended.

Patient education. Emphasis has been placed on antenatal education with a view to realistic expectations for the patient, close supervision by a senior obstetrician, and one-on-one nursing care.

The initial objective of the active management protocol was to shorten the length of nulliparous labor, not to lower the cesarean section rate. Since the rate of cesarean deliveries is dependent on a number of demographic factors, including maternal age and race, extrapolation from one population to another is difficult. Trials of active management have been carried out in several institutions around the world, some of whom have reported a decrease in cesarean deliveries as compared with historic controls.[184-185]

Active management is associated with a shortening in the duration of labor. It has been suggested that the aggressive introduction of high-dose oxytocin may overcome early, subclinical labor dystocia before uterine infection and fatigue make the uterus less responsive to augmentation.[192]

Premature Rupture of the Membranes at Term

Premature rupture of the membranes is defined as rupture of the fetal membranes prior to the onset of labor, and occurs in 8 percent of term pregnancies.[2] The management of this condition is controversial. Immediate delivery is indicated if there is evidence of chorioamnionitis, vaginal bleeding, and/or fetal compromise. It may also be prudent to expedite delivery in women colonized with group B streptococci, because of the increased risk of neonatal sepsis.[193] Premature rupture of the membranes is not a contraindication to cervical ripening using transvaginal prostaglandin preparations.[194,195] Immediate induction of labor with intravenous oxytocin, induction of labor with vaginal PGE_2 gel, and expectant management are all reasonable options for women and their babies if membranes rupture before the start of labor at term, since they result in similar rates of neonatal infection and cesarean delivery.[199,200] However, these is an increase in maternal chorioamnionitis and endometritis with expectant management.

Key Points

> ➤ The classical diagnosis of labor includes regular painful uterine contractions, progressive cervical effacement and dilatation, and a show (bloody discharge).

> ➤ The ability of the fetus to successfully negotiate the pelvis during labor and delivery is dependent on the complex interaction of three variables: the powers, the passenger, and the passage.

> ➤ The two major potential complications of elective induction of labor are iatrogenic prematurity and increased cesarean delivery resulting from failed induction. Routine induction of labor at 41 weeks' gestation is not associated with an increased risk of cesarean section regardless of parity, state of the cervix, or method of induction.

> ➤ When induction of labor is attempted against an unfavorable cervix, the likelihood of a successful outcome is reduced.

Box continued on following page

Key Points *Continued*

➤ In view of the lack of objective evidence of benefit of prophylactic episiotomy and the data suggesting that median episiotomy is associated with an increased incidence of severe perineal trauma, prophylactic median episiotomy should be discouraged.

➤ Abnormal labor itself, not the mode of delivery, may be the most important risk factor for intracranial hemorrhage in the neonate.

➤ Active management of labor refers to a philosophy of labor management based on the premise that optimizing uterine contractions will improve the progress of labor and subsequent outcome.

Chapter 9

Intrapartum Fetal Evaluation

THOMAS J. GARITE

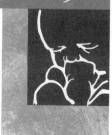

The question being asked by the clinician evaluating the fetus in labor is quite simple: What is the status of fetal oxygenation? If hypoxia is severe enough and lasts long enough, fetal tissue and organ damage will result, which may result in long-term injuries and/or death. Hypoxia severe enough to cause tissue damage virtually always occurs only in the face of a significant metabolic acidosis, and the term "asphyxia" is used in this situation (Fig. 9–1). To clarify the terminology used in these situations, a Glossary is provided.

Although there are other less frequent causes of fetal injury and/or death in labor hypoxia is by far the most common etiology and the one for which medical and surgical interventions have the potential for preventing injury and death. Prior to intensive intrapartum fetal heart rate (FHR) monitoring, relatively uniform intrapartum fetal death rates of 3 to 4 per 1,000 were reported.[1] Fetal hypoxia that is severe and associated with metabolic acidosis, but not sufficient to result in death, may alternatively cause asphyxial injury to the fetus and newborn. While the fetal central nervous system (CNS) is the organ system most vulnerable to long-term injury, the fetus destined to have permanent neurologic damage will virtually always have multiorgan dysfunction in the newborn period. Usually, complications such as seizures, respiratory distress, pulmonary hypertension with persistent fetal circulation, renal failure, bowel dysfunction, and pulmonary hemorrhage are seen in the baby who will ultimately have permanent neurologic injury.[2] Babies who recover from these complications and survive may be normal or may develop cerebral palsy, defined as a movement disorder, usually spastic in nature, that is present at birth, nonprogressive and often, but not always, associated with varying degrees of mental retardation.[3] Seizures are often seen in children with cerebral palsy. Mental retardation or seizures, in the absence of spasticity, are rarely the result of peripartum asphyxia. Cerebral palsy will develop in 0.5 percent of all births and is prevalent in about 0.1 percent of all school-age children.[3,4] Prematurity remains the leading cause of cerebral palsy. It is estimated that peripartum

215

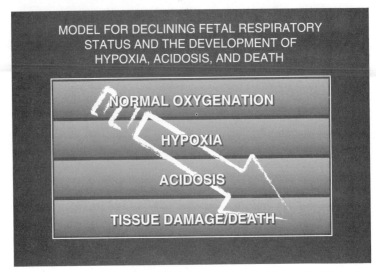

Figure 9–1. The purpose of FHR monitoring is to detect fetal hypoxia and metabolic acidosis. Many fetuses develop hypoxia intermittently but never progress to metabolic acidosis. The ideal is to avoid intervention for hypoxia, but to intervene in the presence of early metabolic acidosis before it can result in tissue damage or fetal death.

events contribute to no more than 25 percent of the overall rate of this disease.[5]

The goal of intrapartum monitoring is to detect hypoxia in labor and allow the clinician to implement nonoperative interventions such as positioning and oxygen (O_2) administration to correct or ameliorate the oxygen deficiency. If this is unsuccessful, the monitor should help the clinician to determine the severity and duration of the hypoxia and whether there is a metabolic acidosis. Finally, if there is sufficient hypoxia and metabolic acidosis present, the monitor should give adequate warning and time to permit the clinician to deliver the baby expeditiously, whether by operative vaginal means or cesarean section, to prevent damage or death from occurring.

INSTRUMENTATION FOR EFM

Today, Doppler devices coupled with autocorrelation formulas for signal processing have resulted in excellent external FHR recordings. External monitoring is necessary when the membranes are intact and cannot or should not be ruptured (Fig. 9–2). Certain

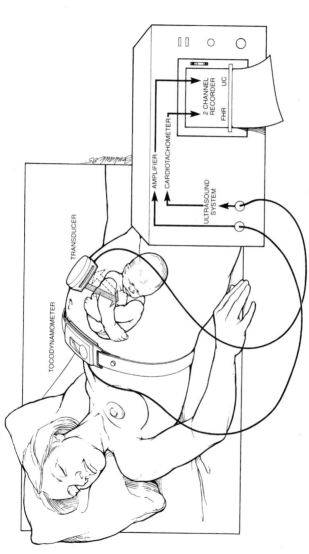

Figure 9–2. Instrumentation for external monitoring. Contractions are detected by the pressure-sensitive tocodynamometer, amplified, and then recorded. Fetal heart rate is monitored using the Doppler ultrasound transducer, which both emits and receives the reflected ultrasound signal that is then counted and recorded.

217

clinical situations such as maternal infection with human immun-odeficiency virus (HIV), hepatitis C, and herpes simplex, make it unwise to puncture the skin with a fetal electrode for fear of vertical transmission of infection to the fetus.

It is often necessary to apply an internal electrode to obtain a high-quality, accurate, continuous FHR tracing, especially in patients who are obese, those with a premature fetus, or when the mother or fetus is moving too much to obtain an adequate signal (Fig. 9–3). This is applied to the fetal scalp manually without additional instruments and without the requirement for a speculum to visualize the scalp. The FHR tracing results from the signal processor, which counts every R-R interval of the ECG from the scalp electrode, converts this interval to rate, and displays every interval (in rate as beats per minute) on the top channel of the two-channel fetal monitor recording paper. The signal is amplified by an automatic gain amplifier, which increases the amplitude (gain) until an adequate signal is available to count (Fig. 9–4).

Contractions can be monitored externally or internally. The external monitoring device, or tocodynamometer, is basically a ring-style pressure transducer attached to the maternal abdomen via a belt that maintains tight continuous contact. The tocodynamometer depicts the frequency of the contractions accurately, but the strength of the contractions only relatively, since it cannot measure actual intrauterine pressure. In addition, the apparent duration of the contraction varies with the sensitivity of the monitor, which is negatively affected by variables such as maternal obesity and premature gestational age. Contractions can be more accurately monitored via an intrauterine pressure catheter. The catheters require that the membranes be ruptured and are inserted transcervically beyond and above the fetal presenting part to rest within the uterine cavity. Once the catheter is electronically "zeroed" (calibrated), the contractions are accurately recorded in terms of frequency, duration, and intensity on the lower channel of the two-channel recording paper or television monitor. This channel is conveniently calibrated at 0 to 100 mm Hg on its vertical scale, from which contraction amplitude can be read.

The goal of monitoring is to maintain adequate, high-quality, continuous FHR and contraction tracings while maintaining maximum maternal comfort and avoiding the risk of trauma and/or infection to the fetus and mother. External devices minimize risk but often give less accurate information and are more uncomfortable for the mother. In general, when the FHR is reassuring and there is an adequate tracing and when the progress of labor is adequate, the external devices are fine. When better quality FHR monitoring is required or it becomes important to accurately assess uterine contraction duration and intensity, then internal device(s) may be necessary.

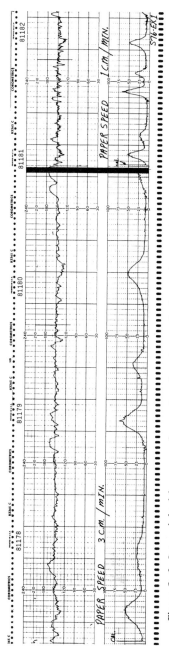

Figure 9–3. Internal fetal heart rate data gathered at the standard recording speed of 3 cm/min for the first portion. The same data are being recorded at a speed of 1 cm/min in the last segment. Normal long-term and short-term variabilities are present. Note that the uterine activity channel has been calibrated so that the intrauterine pressure readings can be measured correctly.

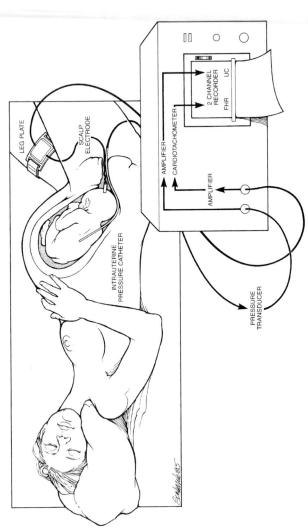

Figure 9–4. Techniques used for direct monitoring of fetal heart rate and uterine contractions. Uterine contractions are assessed with an intrauterine pressure catheter connected to a pressure transducer. This signal is then amplified and recorded. The fetal electrocardiogram is obtained by direct application of the scalp electrode, which is then attached to a leg plate on the mother's thigh. The signal is transmitted to the monitor, where it is amplified, counted by the cardiotachometer, and then recorded.

THE PHYSIOLOGIC BASIS OF FHR MONITORING

The basis of FHR monitoring is, in a real sense, fetal brain monitoring. The fetal brain is constantly responding to stimuli, both peripheral and central, with signals to the fetal heart that alter the heart rate on a moment-to-moment basis. Such stimuli to which the brain responds include chemoreceptors, baroreceptors, and direct effects of metabolic changes within the brain itself. The use of FHR to monitor fetal oxygenation is inherently crude and nonspecific, as many stimuli other than oxygen will either cause the brain to alter the fetal heart rate or may have a direct effect on the fetal heart itself. This really explains the most important basic premise of EFM: when the FHR is normal in appearance, one can be assured with high reliability that the fetus is well oxygenated, but when the FHR is not entirely normal, it may be the result of hypoxia or of other variables that may also affect fetal heart rate. In the past when the FHR became abnormal and the clinician decided intervention was necessary because of concern over fetal hypoxia, the term "fetal distress" was used. More often than not, however, such intervention results in the delivery of a well-oxygenated, nonacidotic, vigorous newborn. Thus, more recently, on the basis of recommendations of the American College of Obstetricians and Gynecologists (ACOG), the term "fetal distress" has been abandoned in favor of the term, "nonreassuring fetal status" (NRFS).[13]

Under normal circumstances during labor, the only variable that alters fetal oxygenation is the temporary interruption in blood flow to the placenta that occurs as a result of the compression of the spiral arteries by the wall of the uterus at the peak of the contraction. The duration that the spiral arteries will be compressed will thus depend on the duration and strength of the contraction. In most cases, the fetus tolerates these periods of stasis well without a significant change in its oxygen content. Contractions that are unusually long or unusually strong may, however, result in transient periods of fetal hypoxemia.

Other variables that have the potential for altering fetal oxygenation most commonly include those that affect uterine perfusion. A laboring woman in the supine position can develop supine hypotension as a result of vena caval compression from the uterus. Maternal hypotension with redistribution of blood flow away from the placenta occurs not infrequently with regional anesthesia. Maternal hemorrhage, such as in placenta previa or abruptio placentae, may have similar effects. Several forms of microvascular disease can impair fetal oxygenation from poor perfusion within the uteroplacental vascular bed including hypertension, preeclampsia/eclampsia, collagen vascular disease, diabetic vasculopathy, and postmaturity. Abruptio placentae may compromise fetal oxygenation due to maternal hypotension, a decrease in the surface area of the placenta, and uterine hyperactivity.

While the placenta functions as the fetal lung, the umbilical cord functions as its trachea, leading oxygen to the baby and carbon dioxide (CO_2) away. Alteration in umbilical cord blood flow is a very common occurrence during labor, either from direct compression or from stretch. Direct compression may occur when the cord becomes impinged between any part of the fetal body and the uterine wall, either with contractions or with fetal movement. This is especially more common when there is oligohydramnios, as there is less amniotic fluid to provide a cushion for the cord.[14] Alternatively, cord stretch may occur as the fetus descends into the pelvis.

It becomes important, therefore, to understand the physiologic mechanisms that control the fetal heart rate. This is so not only because the FHR may be used to determine the severity of the hypoxia and whether a metabolic acidosis is ensuing, but also because the FHR pattern can elucidate the mechanism of the reduction in fetal oxygenation. Thus, by knowing the cause of any hypoxia, the treatment, when possible, can be more specifically directed at the cause. Finally, an understanding of the mechanism and progression of the FHR pattern can often also provide an opportunity to predict how fetal oxygenation will progress over time.

The FHR has many characteristics that we are able to use to accomplish this interpretation. These include the *baseline rate*; the *variability* of the FHR from beat to beat; transient alterations below the baseline, termed *decelerations*; and transient alterations above the baseline, termed *accelerations*. Rate and variability are generally included as *characteristics of the baseline* FHR, and decelerations and accelerations as *periodic changes*.*

Tachycardia

The baseline FHR is typically between 120 and 160 bpm. Rates above 160 bpm are called *tachycardia*. The two most common causes of tachycardia are maternal fever and drugs that directly

---

*The terminology used in this chapter is fairly standard and is consistent with the most recent ACOG Technical Bulletin (Number 207–July, 1995)[16]; however, a recent publication from the National Institute of Child Health and Human Development Research Planning Workshop has some notable differences, and these are discussed.[17]

raise the fetal heart rate. Drugs that elevate the fetal heart rate fall into one of two categories: vagolytic such as atropine and β-sympathomimetic such as terbutaline.

Bradycardia

An FHR less than 120 bpm is termed a *bradycardia*. One must distinguish between a baseline FHR less than 120 bpm and a deceleration from a previous normal baseline. This is an important issue, since a baseline bradycardia is usually innocuous whereas a prolonged deceleration to less than 120 bpm lasting more than 60 to 90 seconds may often indicate significant fetal hypoxia. True fetal bradycardias are due to several possible causes. In the range of 90 to 120 bpm, a bradycardia may often be a normal variant, and these fetuses are usually bradycardic after birth, but are otherwise well oxygenated and normal. A fetal baseline heart rate in the range of 80 bpm or less, especially with reduced variability, may be caused by a complete heart block. Complete heart block may be caused by antibodies associated with maternal lupus erythematosus, may be seen with congenital cardiac anomalies, or is idiopathic.[22]

Variability

Differences in heart rate from beat to beat are recorded as "variability" reflected visually as a line that fluctuates above and below the baseline. This variability is a reflection of neuromodulation of the FHR by an intact and active CNS and also reflects normal cardiac responsiveness. Generally, the variability of the FHR is described as having two components: *short-term* and *long-term variability*. Short-term variability is the beat-to-beat irregularity in the FHR and is caused by the difference in rates between successive beats of the FHR. It is caused by the push–pull effect of sympathetic and parasympathetic nerve input, but the vagus nerve has the dominant role in affecting variability. Long-term variability is the waviness of the FHR tracing, and is generally seen in three to five cycles per minute. The National Institute of Child Health and Human Development (NICHD) Research Planning Workshop concluded that no distinction should be made between short- and long-term variability.[17]

FHR variability reflects the activity of the fetal brain. When the fetus is alert and active, the FHR variability is normal or increased. When the fetus is obtunded, due to whatever cause, the variability is reduced. Since severe hypoxia, especially when it reaches the level of metabolic acidosis, will always depress the CNS, normal variability reliably indicates the absence of severe hypoxia and acidosis. Reduced variability is a very nonspecific finding and must be interpreted in the context of other indicators of hypoxia, and other causes of reduced variability must be considered. In general, anything that is associated with depressed or reduced brain function will diminish variability including fetal sleep cycles; drugs, especially CNS depressants; fetal anomalies, especially of the CNS; and previous insults that have damaged the fetal brain. FHR variability is also affected by gestational age, and very immature fetuses of less than 26 weeks' gestation often have reduced variability.

Variability is usually described quantitatively, as normal, increased, reduced, or absent. The NICHD Research Planning Workshop suggested that FHR variability be defined as follows:

Absent: amplitude undetectable
Minimal: amplitude > undetectable and ≤5 bpm
Moderate: amplitude 6 to 25 bpm
Marked: > 25 bpm.[17]

PERIODIC CHANGES

Variability, tachycardia, and bradycardia are characteristic alterations of the baseline heart rate. Periodic changes of the FHR include decelerations and accelerations. These are transient changes in the fetal heart rate of relatively brief duration with return to the original baseline FHR. In labor, these usually occur in response to uterine contractions, but may also occur with fetal movement.

Decelerations

There are four principal types of decelerations: *early, late, variable,* and *prolonged.* These are named for their timing, relationship to contractions, duration, and shape, but are important distinctions more because they describe the cause of the decelerations.

Early Decelerations

Early decelerations are shallow, symmetric, uniform decelerations with onset and return that are gradual, resulting in a U-shaped deceleration (Fig. 9–5). They begin early in the contraction, have their nadir coincident with the peak of the contraction, and return to the baseline by the time the contraction is over. These decelerations rarely descend more than 30 to 40 bpm below the baseline rate. They are thought to be caused by compression of the fetal head by the uterine cervix as it overrides the anterior fontanel of

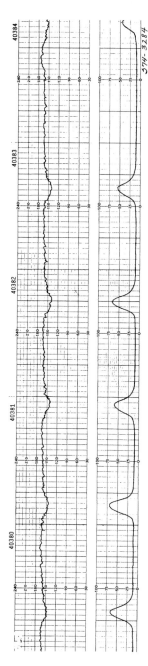

Figure 9-5. Early decelerations.

the cranium.[24] They do not indicate fetal hypoxia and are only significant in that they may be easily confused with late decelerations because of their similar shape and depth. They are the most infrequent of decelerations, occurring in about 5 to 10 percent of all fetuses in labor.

Late Decelerations

Late decelerations are similar in appearance to early decelerations. They too are of gradual onset and return, U-shaped, and generally descend below the baseline no more than 30 to 40 bpm, although there are exceptions. However, in contrast to early decelerations, late decelerations are delayed in timing relative to the contraction. They begin usually about 30 seconds after the onset of the contraction or even at or after its peak. Their nadir is after the peak of the contraction. FHR variability may be unchanged or even increased during the decelerations. These decelerations are not associated with accelerations immediately preceding or following their onset and return (Fig. 9–6).

Late decelerations are generally said to be caused by "uteroplacental insufficiency." This implies that uteroplacental perfusion is temporarily interrupted during the peak of strong contractions. The fetus that normally will not become hypoxic with this temporary halt in blood flow may do so if there is insufficient perfusion and/or oxygen exchange at other times. Physiologically, oxygen sensors within the fetal brain detect a relative drop in fetal oxygen tension in association with the uterine contraction. This change initially results in an increase in sympathetic neuronal response, causing an elevation in fetal blood pressure which, when detected by baroreceptors, produces a protective slowing in the FHR in response to the increase in peripheral vascular resistance. This has been referred to as the "reflex" type of late deceleration. This complex double reflex is probably the reason the deceleration is delayed.[25] There is also a second type of late deceleration, caused by "myocardial depression." As the hypoxia continues and becomes more severe, late decelerations are no longer vagally mediated and are seen even with interruption of the vagus nerve; thus, they are directly myocardial in origin. These decelerations are *not* proportional in their depth to the severity of the hypoxia, and actually may become more shallow as the hypoxia becomes quite severe. Because of this latter type of deceleration, it is generally agreed that the depth of the late deceleration *cannot* be used to judge the severity of the hypoxia. *Late decelerations always indicate fetal hypoxia.* Only the severity of the hypoxia and the overall duration of the late decelerations will determine whether a metabolic acidosis will occur, and this is highly unpredictable.

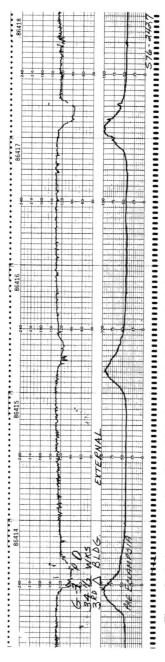

Figure 9–6. A case complicated by third-trimester bleeding in which the external heart rate and uterine activity data are collected. Note the presence of persistent late decelerations with only three contractions in 20 minutes as well as the apparent loss of variability of the fetal heart rate. The rise in baseline tone of the uterine activity channel cannot be evaluated with the external system.

Causes of late decelerations include any factor that can alter delivery, exchange, or uptake of oxygen at the fetal–maternal interface within the placenta. Excessive uterine contractions, usually seen with oxytocin, are the single most common cause of late decelerations.

Variable Decelerations

The most common type of decelerations seen in the laboring patient are variable decelerations. Variable decelerations are, in general, synonymous with umbilical cord compression, and anything that results in the interruption of blood flow within the umbilical cord will result in a variable deceleration. The term "variable" is by far the best single word to describe this type of deceleration. They are variable in all ways: size, shape, depth, duration, and timing relative to the contraction. The onset is usually abrupt and sharp. The return is similarly abrupt in most situations (Fig. 9–7).

When the umbilical cord is gradually compressed, the thinner walled umbilical vein collapses first and blood flow returning to the fetus is interrupted. This results in decreased cardiac return, fetal hypotension, and a baroreceptor reflex that leads the brain to accelerate the heart rate in order to maintain cardiac output. This increase in heart rate is the acceleration that precedes the variable deceleration. With continuing compression, the umbilical artery is compressed, and the fetus detects an increase in systemic vascular resistance as the previously low-resistance placental bed, to which 50 percent of fetal cardiac output normally flows, is occluded. The baroreceptors detect the increase in resistance and the heart slows as a protective mechanism.

It is most important to realize that variable decelerations are initially caused by a reflex in response to changes in pressure and not hypoxia. Thus, variable decelerations (even deep and prolonged) can be seen in fetuses with no change in oxygen saturation (Fig. 9–8).

Variable decelerations are seen in the vast majority of all labors, and most often these decelerations occur without fetal hypoxemia. It is apparent that additional criteria are needed to separate those benign variable decelerations not likely to be associated with hypoxia. A category of mild, moderate, and severe variable decelerations based on depth and duration is widely used (see box, Classifications of the Severity of Variable Decelerations).[30] While there is indeed a correlation between the severity of these decelerations and the likelihood of hypoxia, additional, characteristics of the fetal baseline are also used, including the development of tachycardia and loss of variability. Hypoxia is more likely to be associated with

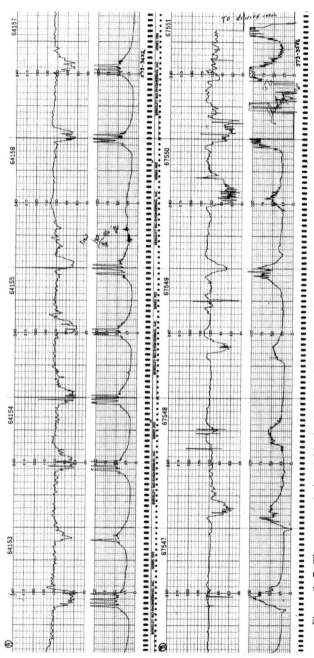

Figure 9-7. These are typical variable decelerations. Note that such decelerations are often recognized by the accelerations that precede and follow the decelerations.

229

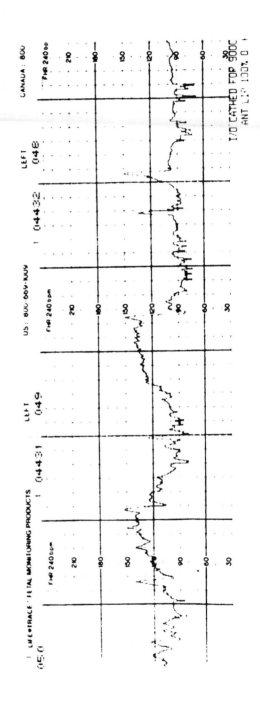

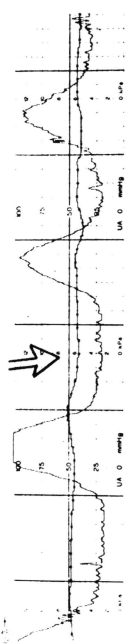

Figure 9–8. Superimposed on the contraction monitor tracing is a continuous tracing using a newly approved fetal pulse oximeter. The tracing shows an fetal oxygen saturation value ranging from 50 to 40 percent (normal = 35 to 60 percent). Note the consistently normal saturation values despite the prolonged FHR decelerations to 80 bpm.

231

Classifications of the Severity of Variable Decelerations

Mild
  Deceleration of a duration of <30 seconds, regardless of
    depth
  Decelerations not below 80 bpm, regardless of duration
Moderate
  Deceleration with a level < 80 bpm
Severe
  Deceleration to a level <70 bpm for >60 seconds

Data from Kubli et al.[30]

variable decelerations if they are severe, prolonged, and are associated with decreased variability, tachycardia; and a slow recovery.

Prolonged Decelerations

Prolonged decelerations are isolated decelerations lasting 90 to 120 seconds or more. Prolonged umbilical cord compression, profound placental insufficiency, or possibly even sustained head compression may lead to prolonged decelerations.

Accelerations

Accelerations are periodic changes of the FHR above the baseline (Fig. 9–9). Virtually all accelerations are a physiologic response to fetal movement.[32] Accelerations are usually short in duration, lasting no more than 30 to 90 seconds, but in an unusually active fetus they can be sustained as long as 30 minutes or more.

The presence of accelerations has virtually the same meaning as normal FHR variability, but the absence of accelerations means only that the baby is not moving. The 15 bpm above the baseline lasting for more than 15 seconds definition of an acceleration, first described with the nonstress test, is the definition usually used for defining accelerations in labor. Earlier in gestation, accelerations are less frequent and of lower amplitude. Fetuses of less than 32 weeks have been defined as having accelerations if they exceed 10 bpm for more than 10 seconds.[17] In fetuses having otherwise nonreassuring FHR patterns, the presence of accelerations, virtually always rules out a pH less than 7.20 on scalp sampling.[33] The presence of spontaneous accelerations or accelerations induced by stimulation of the fetal scalp or acoustic stimulation with a vibroacoustic stimulator has the same reliability.[34,35]

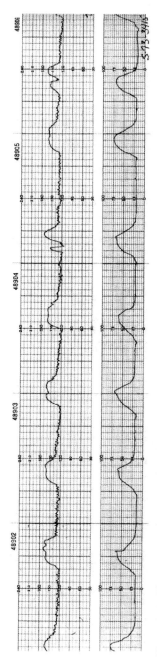

Figure 9–9. These are accelerations of the fetal heart. They are usually seen with fetal movement, and are often coincident with uterine contractions as well, as in this patient.

233

Sinusoidal Patterns

This pattern is rare, but significant. This pattern is strongly associated with fetal hypoxia, most often seen in the presence of severe fetal anemia. The criteria for identifying a sinusoidal FHR include (1) a stable baseline FHR of 120 to 160 bpm with regular sine wave–like oscillations, (2) an amplitude of 5 to 15 bpm, (3) a frequency of 2 to 5 cycles/min, (4) fixed or absent short-term variability, (5) oscillation of the sine wave above and below the baseline, and (6) absence of accelerations (Fig. 9–10).

Evolution of FHR Patterns

One of the sources of greatest confusion regarding FHR pattern interpretation and management is that the patterns have very poor specificity in terms of predicting fetal hypoxia and acidosis, newborn depression, or need for resuscitation. When patterns are normal or "reassuring," there is almost always normal oxygenation and the baby is born vigorous, with normal pH and Apgar scores. However, when the pattern is nonreassuring, the baby is more often normal than depressed or acidotic. In the fetus with persistent late decelerations who then loses FHR variability, the correlation with acidosis and depression should improve substantially because there was evidence that *hypoxia led to the acidosis*.

MANAGEMENT OF NONREASSURING FETAL HEART RATE PATTERNS

Interventions for Nonreassuring Fetal Status

The ideal intervention for fetal hypoxia is a cause-specific, noninvasive one that permanently reverses the problem. While not always possible, this should certainly be the goal. Obviously, the first step in achieving this goal is to recognize the cause of the abnormal FHR pattern. A thorough knowledge of the pathophysiology of FHR changes coupled with a careful clinical patient evaluation and a knowledge of common causes of specific FHR changes will maximize the opportunity for this goal to succeed. In addition to cause-specific types of interventions, virtually all cases of hypoxia should theoretically benefit by more generic interventions that have the potential to maximize oxygen delivery and placental exchange.

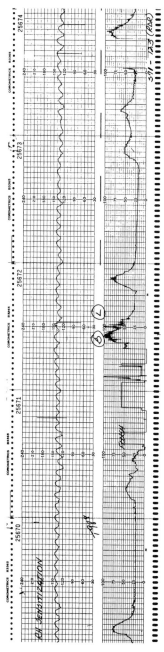

Figure 9–10. The sinusoidal heart rate pattern with its even undulations is demonstrated. Internal monitoring shows the absence of beat-to-beat variability characteristic of true sinusoidal patterns.

Nonsurgical Interventions

OXYGEN ADMINISTRATION. One of the most obvious ways to maximize oxygen delivery to the fetus is to give additional oxygen to the mother by face mask.

LATERAL POSITIONING. Ideally, all patients should labor in the lateral recumbent position, at least from the standpoint of maximizing uterine perfusion. The reasons for this are, at least theoretically, twofold: (1) in being inactive and recumbent, the body is required to deliver the least amount of blood flow to other muscles; and (2) in the lateral position, there is no compression by the uterus on the vena cava or aorta, thus maximizing cardiac return and cardiac output.

HYDRATION. By increasing fluid administration, there is the potential to maximize intravascular volume and thus uterine perfusion.

OXYTOCIN. In a patient with a nonreassuring pattern, the more time there is between contractions, the more time to maximally perfuse the placenta and deliver oxygen. In patients receiving oxytocin, there is potential to improve oxygenation by decreasing or discontinuing oxytocin.

TOCOLYTICS. Tocolytics are appropriate in at least two situations: (1) When patients are having spontaneous excessive contractions leading to nonreassuring FHR patterns, especially prolonged decelerations. The most commonly used agent is subcutaneous terbutaline, 0.25 mg and (2) intrauterine resuscitation after the decision is made to perform an operative delivery while waiting for preparations to be made.

AMNIOINFUSION. In situations where variable decelerations appear to be caused by oligohydramnios, reestablishing intrauterine fluid volume via a process called "amnioinfusion" has been demonstrated in numerous randomized studies to ameliorate the variable decelerations, improve Apgar scores and cord pH values, and even reduce the need for cesarean section for NRFS.[51–53] Intrauterine pressure catheters are now made with a port that allows the simultaneous administration of saline to accomplish this goal. Thus, in the patient with variable decelerations that suggest progression to more nonreassuring types, and where the cause is likely to be caused by oligohydramnios, the implementation of amnioinfusion is warranted.

Amnioinfusion also has been proposed, to avoid the fetal/neonatal pulmonary problems in the presence of meconium.[56] The evidence for efficacy in this setting is good. However, clear evidence that this modality avoids the meconium aspiration syndrome is lacking, since this complication is relatively infrequent. Some of these problems will be avoided with good oropharyngeal suctioning on the perineum and neonatal suctioning below the vocal cords when necessary.

MECONIUM. Meconium is not only a potential sign of fetal hypoxia but is also a potential toxin if the fetus aspirates this particulate matter with a gasping breath in utero or when it takes its first breaths following birth. The thickness of the meconium is also a reflection of the amount of amniotic fluid, and thick meconium virtually always reflects some degree of oligohydramnios. In general, meconium should alert the clinician to the potential for oligohydramnios, umbilical cord compression, placental insufficiency, and meconium aspiration. Fortunately, a reassuring FHR tracing is generally reliable, and patients with meconium can be managed expectantly.

Alternatives for Evaluating the Fetus with a Nonreassuring FHR Pattern

In the fetus with a persistently nonreassuring FHR pattern, where nonsurgical efforts at reversing or improving the pattern fail, the next step is to attempt to find out whether the hypoxia has progressed to metabolic acidosis.

FETAL SCALP PH. Determination of fetal scalp pH is historically the oldest and most well-tested method for determining if the fetus is acidotic. Technically, a plastic cone is inserted transvaginally against the fetal vertex. The cervix needs to be at least 4 to 5 cm dilated and the vertex at a −1 station or below to accomplish this. Mineral oil or another lubricant is applied to the scalp so blood will bead, and then using a lancet, the scalp is pricked and blood is then collected in a long capillary tube. A scalp pH less than 7.20 is consistent with fetal acidosis and a pH of 7.20 to 7.25 is borderline and should be repeated immediately. A reassuring value over 7.25 must be repeated every 20 to 30 minutes as long as the pattern persists and the fetus is not acidotic. In practice, because this technique is cumbersome, fraught with technical inaccuracy, uncomfortable for the patient, and with the requirement to perform repeated samples, it is used very infrequently.[58]

ACCELERATIONS. In the fetus with a nonreassuring pattern, spontaneous accelerations have the same significance as those elicited by scalp or acoustic stimulation. Thus, any acceleration—spontaneous or induced—indicates the absence of acidosis.

FETAL PULSE OXIMETRY. One of the most exciting recent developments in obstetrics is the introduction of fetal pulse oximetry. Since FHR monitoring is specifically intended to monitor fetal oxygenation and since this modality is so nonspecific, it stands to reason that what we should be using ideally is a device that directly monitors fetal oxygenation and/or pH. Fetal hemoglobin will alter absorption curves of the normally used red and infrared wavelengths. It was not until a special sensor was developed that is placed transcervically to lie against the fetal cheek that many of these problems were overcome (Fig. 9–11). This device accurately determines fetal oxygen saturation and continually records the value on the lower (contraction) channel of the electronic FHR monitor.

The second hurdle to overcome was to determine if there was a reliable "critical threshold" that could be determined. There is an extremely high correlation between the cutoff value of a saturation 30 percent and a scalp pH value of 7.20.[62] The saturation must remain below 30 percent for a substantial period of time (about 10 minutes or more) before a metabolic acidosis develops in most situations in labor.

Fetal pulse oximetry was approved by the Food and Drug Administration (FDA) for use in fetuses with nonreassuring FHR patterns in May 2000. The approval was based, in part, on the results of a large multicenter trial of over 1,000 patients comparing FHR monitoring alone versus FHR monitoring backed up by pulse oximetry in fetuses already having nonreassuring FHR patterns.[65] Whereas the trial did not demonstrate an overall reduction in cesarean section, there was a reduction in cesarean section for NRFS and an improved specificity and sensitivity of operative intervention for the fetus with depression, acidosis, and in need of resuscitation. Most importantly, in following the fetus with a nonreassuring FHR tracing but a reassuring oxygen saturation value (>30 percent), there was no increase in babies with adverse outcomes.

Therefore, fetal pulse oximetry may prove to be an excellent alternative to fetal scalp pH monitoring in patients with nonreassuring FHR patterns and may allow continued monitoring and avoid intervention of fetuses with apparently nonreassuring FHR patterns but with normal oxygenation. It is unlikely this modality will replace EFM for many years to come for several reasons. It cannot be used until the membranes are ruptured, and the cervix is at least 2 to 3 cm dilated. FHR monitoring is highly reliable when reassuring, and in the current format the monitor is needed to correlate and prognosticate changes in fetal oxygen saturation. Fetal pulse oximetry in its current form only gives an adequate signal about 70 percent of the time, although this will improve as the technology continues to be perfected.[65] Finally, the FHR pattern gives some clues as to the mechanism of hypoxia, allowing specific therapy to be provided, and the pulse oximeter only quantifies the degree of hypoxia. These modalities are complementary, and the potential for improving intrapartum assessment of the hypoxic fetus is vast.

Operative Intervention for Nonreassuring Fetal Status

When the fetus is determined to have a persistently nonreassuring FHR pattern and backup methods (scalp pH, accelerations, pulse oximetry) cannot provide reassurance that the fetus is not acidotic,

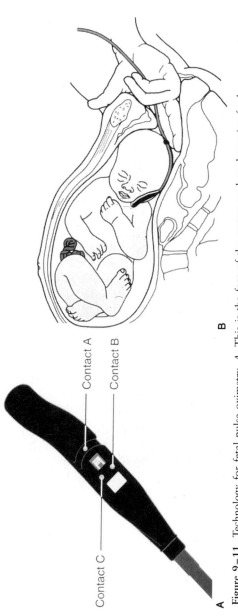

A

Contact C

Contact A

Contact B

B

Figure 9–11. Technology for fetal pulse oximetry. *A,* This is the face of the sensor used to determine fetal oxygen saturation. On its surface are three gold-plated electrodes (contacts A, B, and C), which determine adequate electrical contact, and a photoemittor and photodetector. *B,* This figure shows the technique for insertion of the sensor. The device is inserted transcervically, as with an intrauterine pressure catheter, to lie against the fetal face, where it is held in place simply by the pressure of the uterine cervix or pelvic sidewall. (see Fig. 9–8).

operative intervention is indicated to expeditiously deliver the baby to avoid further deterioration. Several questions arise when the decision has been made for intervention for NRFS. What is the best choice, operative vaginal delivery or cesarean section? How much time do we have to perform the delivery? What anesthetic should be used? What is the prognosis of the baby? And, finally, are there situations where the baby is already damaged or otherwise not likely to benefit from this intervention?

Choosing operative vaginal delivery or cesarean section is not difficult if the patient is in early labor. Except for the situation of a prolonged deceleration to less than 70 bpm with loss of variability that will not recover and requires the most rapid intervention safely possible, most other situations require judgment and integration of the entire clinical picture of mother and baby.

The question of how much time is available to perform an operative intervention in the face of a nonreassuring FHR pattern is a complex one. This judgment must be made on the basis of the severity of the FHR pattern and the overall clinical status of mother and baby must be integrated into this difficult decision.

MANAGEMENT OF NONREASSURING FHR PATTERNS—A PROPOSED PROTOCOL

The following algorithm for management of nonreassuring patterns is proposed.

1. When the pattern suggests the beginning development of hypoxia or is already nonreassuring:
   a. Identify when possible the cause of the problem (e.g., hypotension from an epidural).
   b. Correct the cause (e.g., fluids and ephedrine to correct the hypotension).
   c. Give measures to maximize placental oxygen delivery and exchange: oxygen by face mask, lateral positioning, hydration, consider decreasing or discontinuing oxytocin.

2. If the pattern becomes or remains nonreassuring and the above measures have been completed:
   a. Attempt to provide other measures of reassurance to rule out metabolic acidosis.
      • Accelerations—spontaneous or elicited
      • Scalp pH
      • Fetal pulse oximetry
   b. If reassurance using one of the above methods can be provided, and the pattern persists, continuous or intermittent

(every 30 minutes) evidence of absence of acidosis must be ascertained.
  c. If reassurance of the absence of acidosis cannot be provided, deliver expeditiously by the safest and most reasonable means (operative vaginal or cesarean section).

Patterns that qualify as nonreassuring and cannot be corrected and therefore warrant evidence of the absence of metabolic acidosis include:

1. Persistent late decelerations (>50 percent of contractions).
2. Nonreassuring variable decelerations.
   a. Progressively severe.
   b. With developing tachycardia and loss of variability.
   c. With developing slow return to baseline.
3. Sinusoidal tracing.
4. Recurrent prolonged decelerations.
5. The confusing pattern.
   a. The patient presents with a pattern of absent variability but without explanatory decelerations.
   b. An unusual pattern that does not fit into one of the categories defined above but does not have elements of a reassuring pattern.

Auscultation as an Alternative

Auscultation is an acceptable option for monitoring the fetus in labor when certain conditions are in place. The fetus should have a reassuring FHR on admission monitored electronically. The patient should have one-on-one nursing. The standards for frequency from the ACOG for auscultation are at least every 30 minutes in the first stage and every 15 minutes in the second stage for the low- risk patient and every 15 minutes in the first stage and every 5 minutes in the second stage for the high-risk patient.[16] Fetuses with abnormal FHR patterns on auscultation should have electronic monitoring to define the pattern and monitor for progression to worsening or nonreassuring patterns.

ASSESSMENT OF FETAL CONDITION AT BIRTH

The Apgar score was originally introduced as a tool to be used in guiding the need for neonatal resuscitation. Subsequently, this means of fetal assessment became used routinely for all births.

However, the Apgar score has been expected to predict far more than was originally intended. Such expectations have included evaluating acid–base status at birth (i.e., the presence or absence of perinatal asphyxia) and even predicting long-term prognosis. Unfortunately, the Apgar is a nonspecific measure of these parameters, as many other causes of fetal depression may mimic that seen with asphyxia, such as drugs, anomalies, prematurity, suctioning for meconium, and so forth. In situations where FHR patterns have been concerning and other back-up methods for evaluating fetal oxygenation or fetal acid–base status have been utilized, or in cases where the baby is unexpectedly depressed, it is important to specifically evaluate these parameters at birth, using umbilical cord blood gases. To accomplish this, a doubly clamped 10- to 30-cm section of umbilical cord is taken after the orginal cord clamping and separation of the baby from the cord. Using heparinized syringes, samples of umbilical artery and vein are separately obtained. These samples are evaluated for respiratory gases. Normal ranges for umbilical cord gases are shown in Table 9–1. Cord blood PO_2 or O_2 saturation is not useful, as many normal newborns are initially hypoxemic until normal extrauterine respiration is established. While cord pH, especially arterial, is the essential value, Pco_2 is also very important, as if the pH is low, the Pco is used to determine whether the acidosis is respiratory or metabolic. Respiratory acidosis is not predictive of newborn or long-term injury and should correlate with little or no need for resuscitation. In addition, the cord gases should be used to correlate

Table 9–1. NORMAL BLOOD GAS VALUES OF UMBILICAL ARTERY AND VEIN

	Mean Value	Normal Range*
Artery		
pH	7.27	7.15 to 7.38
Pco_2	50	35 to 70
Bicarbonate	23	17 to 28
Base excess	−3.6	−2.0 to − 9.0
Vein		
pH	7.34	7.20 to 7.41
Pco_2	40	33 to 50
Bicarbonate	21	15 to 26
Base excess	−2.6	−1.0 to −8.0

*Values are ± 2 SD and represent a composite of multiple studies. Data derived from Thorp and Rushing.[69]

interpretation of the FHR patterns, as previously described in the sections on their pathophysiology and to determine the appropriateness of operative intervention or lack of it. These gases can help the pediatrician in determining the etiology of immediate complications and the need for more intense observation of the baby. In addition, these values are often useful if the baby develops any long-term neurologic injury in determining whether any such injury may have been related to peripartum asphyxia. Studies have shown that if such asphyxia is present, in order for it to result in long-term injury it must have been severe (metabolic acidosis with a pH <7.0 to 7.05) and be associated with multiple organ dysfunction in the newborn period.[2]

RISKS AND BENEFITS OF EFM

Electronic FHR monitoring was introduced with the hope that this modality would reduce or eliminate the devastating consequences of asphyxia. Enthusiasm for this new technology established the role of continuous FHR monitoring in labor before studies demonstrated its accuracy. Initial retrospective studies evaluated more that 135,000 patients and showed more than a three-fold improvement in the intrapartum fetal death rate for patients monitored electronically.[1] However, the majority of subsequent prospective, randomized, controlled trials have failed to demonstrate an improvement in the intrapartum fetal death rate using EFM.[70-76] EFM has other potential benefits. These include an ability to understand the mechanism of developing hypoxia and treat it more specifically. It provides the ability to accurately monitor uterine contractions so we can better understand progress or lack of progress in labor as well as monitor the effects of oxytocin- stimulated contractions on fetal oxygenation. The monitor is ultimately, like all other monitors in intensive care situations, a labor-saving device allowing nurses to perform other tasks simultaneously.

EFM has several disadvantages, however. During the period in which FHR monitoring has risen in popularity, there was a parallel increase in the cesarean section rate. Certainly, this was not all caused by EFM, as there were many other changes in obstetric practice during this time period. In virtually all of the randomized controlled trials, EFM resulted in an increase in the cesarean section rate over intermittent auscultation without a concomitant improvement in outcome.[70-74]

The second major problem associated with EFM is the fear of a lawsuit should the child be compromised in any way. The monitor has created an expectation of perfect outcome. The interpretation of abnormal FHR tracings is highly subjective and variable, and "experts" often give diametrically opposite interpretations of the same tracing. The modality itself is nonspecific, and babies with anomalies or preexisting brain damage will often have abnormal FHR tracings easily confused with ongoing hypoxia. Finally, a jury cannot help but be sympathetic to a family and baby with debilitating cerebral palsy. However, these outcomes are not consistent with what we know about asphyxia. More than 75 percent of brain-damaged children have causes that are *not* related to perinatal asphyxia. Many cases of asphyxia occur *prior to* labor or early in labor before the patient arrives in the hospital. Very few of these cases are truly preventable.

SUMMARY

Electronic FHR monitoring has become the standard means for evaluating fetal oxygenation in labor. Because of fetal inaccessibility and the lack of alternatives to more specifically evaluate fetal oxygenation, this modality has been the only alternative. FHR monitoring is reliable when it tells us the fetus is well oxygenated, but more often unreliable when it suggests the fetus is "in distress." The recent change in terminology describing the abnormal FHR pattern as "nonreassuring" is a more accurate and honest depiction of the limitations of EFM in this situation. Despite or even because of these limitations, it is imperative that the clinician understand as much as possible about the underlying physiologic explanations of normal and abnormal FHR patterns, as this allows the only reasonable opportunity to appropriately evaluate and manage these changes. The goal of FHR monitoring should be to carefully and thoroughly monitor all patients in active labor; avoid unnecessary operative and nonoperative intervention for benign and innocuous FHR patterns; correct nonreassuring FHR patterns with noninvasive, etiology specific therapies when possible; or if not possible use appropriate means such as scalp pH, accelerations, or fetal pulse oximetry to rule out acidosis; and finally, if acidosis cannot be ruled out, operatively intervene in an expeditious manner appropriate for the entire clinical situation.

Key Points

➤ The goals of intrapartum fetal evaluation by electronic fetal heart rate monitoring and available back-up methods are to detect fetal hypoxia, reverse the hypoxia with nonsurgical means, or if unsuccessful, determine if the hypoxia has progressed to metabolic acidosis, and if so deliver the baby expeditiously to avoid the hypoxia and acidosis from resulting in any damage to the baby.

➤ EFM is an inherently suboptimal method of determining fetal hypoxia and acidosis, because many factors besides these variables may alter the FHR and mimic changes caused by hypoxia and acidosis. When the FHR is normal, its reliability in predicting the absence of fetal compromise is high, but when the FHR is abnormal, its reliability in predicting the presence of asphyxia is poor.

➤ The term "fetal distress" should be abandoned in favor of "nonreassuring fetal status," because when the fetal monitor suggests there may be a problem, in most circumstances we can only say that we are no longer reassured with a high degree of certainty that the fetus is well oxygenated.

➤ Late decelerations are always indicative of relative fetal hypoxia, and are caused by inadequate oxygen delivery, exchange, or uptake that is aggravated by the additional hypoperfusion of the placenta caused by contractions. Variable decelerations are caused by a decrease in umbilical cord flow resulting from cord compression or cord stretch. Prolonged decelerations may be caused by any mechanism that decreases fetal oxygenation.

➤ In labor, loss of variability, loss of accelerations, and tachycardia should only be interpreted as indicative of fetal compromise in the presence of nonreassuring decelerations (late, nonreassuring variable or prolonged decelerations), as signs of hypoxia should always precede signs of neurologic depression secondary to hypoxia.

➤ In the presence of oligohydramnios and variable decelerations, or with meconium, intrapartum amnioinfusion has been shown to decrease rates of cesarean delivery for NRFS and to decrease neonatal respiratory complications caused by meconium aspiration.

Box continued on following page

Key Points *Continued*

➤ In the presence of an otherwise nonreassuring FHR pattern, the presence of accelerations of the FHR, either spontaneous or elicited by scalp stimulation or vibroacoustic stimulation, indicate the absence of fetal acidosis. Their absence is associated with a 50 percent chance of fetal acidosis, but only in the setting of a nonreassuring FHR.

➤ Umbilical cord blood gases should be obtained and documented in situations where there is a nonreassuring or confusing FHR pattern during labor, where there is neonatal depression following birth, with premature babies, and when suctioning for meconium is performed. These values will help clarify the reasons for abnormal FHR patterns or for neonatal depression.

➤ Fetal pulse oximetry was approved in May 2000 by the FDA for use in term ≥ 36 weeks) patients with nonreassuring FHR patterns. This technology may improve our ability to more accurately interpret nonreassuring FHR patterns and may have the potential to decrease cesarean sections for NRFS.

➤ Although there is correlation between a nonreassuring FHR pattern and neonatal depression, the FHR is a poor predictor of long-term neurologic sequelae. Furthermore, fetuses with previous neurologic insults may have significantly abnormal FHR patterns even when they are well oxygenated in labor.

GLOSSARY

Acidemia – increased hydrogen ion concentration in blood.
Acidosis – increased hydrogen ion concentration in tissue.
Asphyxia – hypoxia with metabolic acidosis.
Base deficit – buffer base content below normal (this is calculated from a normogram using pH and Pco_2).
Base excess – buffer base content above normal.
Hypoxemia – decreased oxygen concentration in blood.
Hypoxia – decreased oxygen concentration in tissue.
pH – the negative log of hydrogen ion concentration ($7.0 = 1 \times 10^{-7}$

Chapter 10

Obstetric Anesthesia

JOY L. HAWKINS, DAVID H. CHESTNUT,
AND CHARLES P. GIBBS

The word "anesthesia" encompasses all techniques used by anesthesiologists: general anesthesia, regional anesthesia, local anesthesia, and analgesia.

Balanced general anesthesia is the type of general anesthesia used for cesarion sections; it usually refers to various combinations of barbiturates, inhalation agents, opioids, and muscle relaxants as opposed to high concentrations of potent inhalation agents alone.

In obstetrics, regional techniques include major blocks, such as spinal and lumbar epidural, as well as minor blocks, such as paracervical, pudendal, and local infiltration.

Psychoprophylaxis

Psychoprophylaxis is a nonpharmacologic method of minimizing the perception of painful uterine contractions. Relaxation, concentration on breathing, gentle massage (effleurage), and partner participation contribute to its effectiveness.

Although psychoprophylactic techniques may discourage the use of drugs, not all patients are alike and not all will be satisfied with psychoprophylaxis.[28] The greatest disadvantage is the potential for believing the use of drug-induced pain relief is a sign of failure and will harm the child. There are times when anesthesia will be *required* for vaginal or cesarean delivery, and no one would suggest that these patients avoid anesthesia.

Systemic Opioid Analgesia

All opioids provide pain relief, but can also produce respiratory depression in the mother and newborn.[32,33] Smaller doses of short-acting opioids are used and are administered via the more predictable intravenous route. Therefore, recent reports detail little neonatal depression.[35,36]

The reader is referred to the Appendix in *Obstetrics; Normal and Problem Pregnancies*, fourth edition for illustrations of anatomy relevant to this discussion.

The immediate treatment for respiratory depression caused by opioids is ventilation. Infants depressed by opioids may be sleepy and may not breathe adequately. Initially, they typically are not hypoxic, hypercarbic, or acidotic; however, if they are not ventilated, then these will result. If properly cared for, infants with opioid-induced depression will suffer no ill effects. Proper care includes ventilation, oxygenation, gentle stimulation, and the judicious use of the opioid antagonist naloxone. Positive-pressure ventilation is the single most effective measure and can be provided via face mask or intubation. Without ventilation, other measures are fruitless.

Naloxone, 0.1 mg/kg, should be given intravenously if possible, but it can be given intramuscularly or subcutaneously. This dose is higher than that previously recommended and should ensure an increased likelihood of effectiveness.[37] It may be repeated in 3 to 5 minutes if there is no immediate response. If there is no response after two or three doses, the depression is most likely *not* due to opioid effect.[38] Nursery personnel should be advised when naloxone has been given because it has a short duration of action, and therefore repeat administration may be necessary in the nursery. It should not be given routinely to all opioid-exposed newborns.[48]

An important and significant disadvantage of opioid analgesia is the prolonged effect of these agents on gastric emptying. If general anesthesia becomes necessary, the risk of aspiration is increased.[42–44]

Patient-Controlled Opioid Analgesia

In some centers, opioids are administered by patient-controlled intravenous infusion. The infusion pump is programmed to give a predetermined dose of drug upon patient demand. The physician may program the pump to include a lock-out interval (i.e., there is a minimum interval between doses of drug). Thus, the physician may limit the total dose administered per hour.

Sedatives

Sedatives do not possess analgesic qualities and are most often used early in labor to relieve anxiety or to augment the analgesic qualities and reduce the nausea associated with opioids. All sedatives and hypnotics cross the placenta freely. Except for the benzodiazepines, they have no known antagonists.

Because barbiturates and other sedatives are not analgesic, patients may be less able to cope with pain than if they had received no pharmacologic assistance at all; that is, normal coping mechanisms may be blunted.[58,59] The combination of barbiturate (100 mg secobarbital) with opioid (50 to 100 mg meperidine) increases the degree of neonatal depression.[32] Thus, these drugs should rarely be used during labor.

Phenothiazines

Promethazine chlorpromazine, and hydroxyzine are commonly administered. When given in small doses in combination with an opioid, these drugs do not seem to produce additional neonatal depression.[61,62] However, like the barbiturates, these agents rapidly cross the placenta and, in large doses, can depress the fetus, and have no known antagonist.

Benzodiazepines

A major disadvantage of diazepam is that it renders newborns less able to maintain body temperature.[63] The drug may persist in the fetal circulation for as long as 1 week.[64] Sodium benzoate, a buffer in the injectable form of diazepam, competes with bilirubin binding to albumin and could be a threat to infants susceptible to kernicterus.[66] Midazolam is water soluble, and is shorter acting than diazepam.[67]

A disadvantage of all the benzodiazepines is their tendency to cause maternal amnesia, a significant disadvantage if the drug is given near the time of delivery.[70] Flumazenil, a specific benzodiazepine antagonist, can reliably reverse benzodiazepine-induced sedation and ventilatory depression.[71]

Lumbar Epidural Analgesia/Anesthesia

Epidural blockade is a major regional anesthetic technique in which local anesthetic is injected into the epidural space. Epidural blockade may be used to provide *analgesia* during labor, or surgical *anesthesia* for vaginal or cesarean delivery. A large-bore needle is used to locate the epidural space. Next, a catheter is inserted through the needle, and the needle is removed over the catheter. Local anesthetic is injected through the catheter, which remains taped in place to the mother's back to enable subsequent injections throughout labor. Thus, it is often called continuous epidural analgesia. A test dose of local anesthetic is given first to be certain the catheter has not been unintentionally placed in the subarachnoid (spinal) space or in a blood vessel.

Two forms of epidural analgesia are used for labor: lumbar and caudal. The catheter is placed via a lumbar interspace in the former and via the sacral hiatus in the latter. More local anesthetic is necessary for the caudal technique, because the local anesthetic must fill the entire sacral canal before filling the epidural space up to T10.

Most anesthesiologists now prefer the lumbar approach and use a technique described as segmental epidural analgesia. Only the smallest amount and the weakest effective concentration of local anesthetic is injected via the L2-3, L3-4, or L4-5 interspace. Thus, both sensation and motor function of the perineum and lower extremities remain mostly intact. The patient can move about and perceive the impact of the presenting part on the perineum. If perineal anesthesia is needed for delivery, a larger concentration and dose of local anesthetic can be administered at that time through the catheter.

A new technique of labor analgesia involves passing a small-gauge spinal needle through the epidural needle prior to catheter placement. This combined spinal-epidural provides rapid onset of analgesia using a very small dose of opioid or a local anesthetic and opioid combination.[79,80] Because the dose of drug used in the subarachnoid space is much smaller than that used for epidural analgesia, the risks of local anesthetic toxicity or high spinal block are avoided. Side effects are usually mild, and include pruritus and nausea. Some practitioners have used this technique to allow parturients to ambulate during labor since there is little or no interference with motor function.[79]

Disadvantages of epidural analgesia include hypotension, local anesthetic toxicity, allergic reaction, high or total spinal anesthesia, neurologic injury, and spinal headache.

Spinal Headache

Spinal headache may follow uncomplicated spinal anesthesia. This complication can also occur when, during the process of administering an epidural block, the dura is punctured and spinal fluid leaks out (i.e., "wet tap"). Once a wet tap occurs, a spinal headache results in as many as 70 percent of patients. The incidence is much less following spinal anesthesia, because smaller needles are used. Characteristically the headache is more severe in the upright position and is relieved by the prone position.

Treatment of the headache may be initiated with oral analgesics, caffeine,[124] and continued hydration. If these simple measures do not prove immediately effective, an epidural blood patch is placed. Approximately 15 ml of the patient's own blood is placed aseptically into the epidural space; the blood coagulates over the hole in the dura and prevents further leakage.[125] The epidural blood patch has been found to be remarkably effective and nearly complication free.[127–129]

Whether there is an effect on the first stage of labor with epidural anesthesia is controversial. There is evidence that effective epidural analgesia may slightly prolong the second stage of labor.[141,142] However, a delay in the second stage is not necessarily harmful to infant or to mother, provided there is reassuring electronic fetal heart rate monitoring.[141,143-145] Indeed, the ACOG has defined a prolonged second stage as more than 3 hours in nulliparous patients *with* regional anesthesia as compared with more than 2 hours in nulliparous patients without regional anesthesia.[146]

MANAGEMENT OF EPIDURAL ANESTHESIA. *First,* it is preferable to avoid institution of epidural analgesia during early, latent-phase labor in most patients.

Second, a brief period of decreased uterine activity often follows the institution of epidural analgesia. In some patients, analgesia may seem to slow or to stop labor for longer, and the obstetrician should be willing to augment labor by giving oxytocin intravenously.

Third, analgesia should not be withheld routinely during the second stage. A dense epidural block may decrease the ability of some patients to push effectively. On the other hand, other patients will push more effectively in the presence of analgesia. If the block is too dense and the patient cannot push effectively, then there should be diminution of the level and/or intensity of analgesia.

Fourth, one should avoid arbitrary termination of the second stage. In some patients with effective epidural analgesia, it may be appropriate to allow a second stage of more than 3 hours, provided that there is continued progress in descent of the vertex and reassuring fetal monitoring.

Paracervical Block

Paracervical block analgesia is a simple, effective procedure. Usually, 5 to 6 ml of a dilute solution of local anesthetic without epinephrine is injected into the mucosa of the cervix at either the 4- and 8- or 3- and 9-o'clock positions; an Iowa trumpet prevents deep penetration of the needle (Fig. 10–1). The block can only be applied during the first stage of labor and it must be reapplied frequently during the course of a long labor. Furthermore, it has the major disadvantage of fetal bradycardia, which occurs in 2 to 70 percent of applications. It occurs within 2 to 10 minutes and lasts from 3 to 30 minutes. Although usually benign, it can be associated with fetal acidosis and occasionally with fetal death.[201-203]

There is no consensus regarding the mechanism of postparacervical block bradycardia. The theories include (1) high blood concentrations of local anesthetic in the fetus, (2) uterine artery vasoconstriction, and (3) postparacervical block increase in uterine activity.

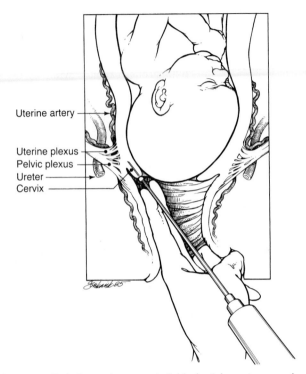

Figure 10–1. Technique of paracervical block. Schematic coronal section (enlarged) of lower portion of cervix and upper portion of vagina shows relation of needle to paracervical region. (Modified from Bonica JJ: Principles and Practice of Obstetric Analgesia and Anesthesia. Philadelphia, FA Davis, 1967, p 234.)

Regardless of etiology, the severity and duration of the bradycardia correlate with the incidence of fetal acidosis and subsequent neonatal depression. Freeman and colleagues[206] reported a significant fall in pH and a rise in base deficit only in those fetuses with bradycardia persisting more than 10 minutes. Paracervical block should not be used in mothers with fetuses in either acute or chronic distress.

Local Anesthesia

In the form of perineal infiltration, local anesthesia is widely used and very safe. Spontaneous vaginal deliveries, episiotomies, and outlet forceps can be accomplished with this simple technique.

Local anesthetic toxicity may occur if large amounts of local anesthetic are used or in the unlikely event that an intravascular injection occurs. Usually, 5 to 15 ml of 1 percent lidocaine suffices.

Pudendal Nerve Block

Pudendal nerve block is a minor regional block that is effective and safe. Using an Iowa trumpet and a 20-gauge needle, 5 to 10 ml of local anesthetic is injected just below the ischial spine. Because the hemorrhoidal nerve may be aberrant in 50 percent of patients,[210] some physicians prefer to inject a portion of the local anesthetic somewhat posterior to the spine.

The technique is satisfactory for all spontaneous vaginal deliveries and episiotomies and for some outlet or low-forceps deliveries, but may not be sufficient for deliveries requiring additional manipulation.

More than with perineal infiltration, the potential for local anesthetic toxicity exists with pudendal block because of the proximity of large vessels to the site of injection. Therefore, aspiration before injection is particularly important. Furthermore, the potential for large amounts of local anesthetic to be used increases when perineal and labial infiltration are required in addition to the pudendal block. In these instances, it is important to monitor closely the amount of local anesthetic given.

Spinal (Subarachnoid) Block

A saddle block is a spinal block in which the level of anesthesia is limited to little more than the perineum, that is, the saddle area. Spinal anesthesia is reasonably easy to perform and usually provides total pain relief in the blocked area. Therefore, spontaneous deliveries, forceps deliveries, and episiotomies can be accomplished without pain for the mother. The ability to push may be compromised.

ANESTHESIA FOR CESAREAN DELIVERY

Either spinal anesthesia or lumbar epidural anesthesia is preferred and is safer for the mother than general anesthesia.

Either general or regional anesthesia is safe for the infant; studies have reported Apgar scores and blood gas measurements as essentially the same for infants of mothers choosing either technique.

General Anesthesia

Failure to intubate and aspiration continue to be major causes of maternal mortality.[219-223] Maternal mortality rates are higher during general anesthesia than during regional anesthesia, perhaps as much as 17 times higher.

Antacids

Use of a clear antacid is considered routine for all parturients prior to surgery. Additional aspiration prophylaxis using an H_2-receptor blocking agent and/or metoclopramide may be given to parturients with risk factors such as morbid obesity, diabetes mellitus, a difficult airway, or those who have previously received narcotics. As soon as it is known that the patient requires cesarean delivery, be it with regional or general anesthesia, 30 ml of a clear, nonparticulate antacid, such as 0.3 M sodium citrate,[224] Bicitra,[225] or Alka Seltzer, 2 tablets in 30 ml water,[226] are administered to decrease gastric acidity and ameliorate the consequences of aspiration, should it occur.

Left Uterine Displacement

The uterus may compress the inferior vena cava and the aorta during cesarean delivery and so left uterine displacement is practiced. The induction-to-delivery time is not the crucial time, rather, it is the uterine incision-to-delivery interval that is predictive of neonatal status.[229] A uterine-incision interval of less than 90 seconds is optimal. Uterine manipulation and difficulty of the delivery are significant factors for the fetus during cesarean section.

Preoxygenation

Before patients become unconscious and paralyzed, it is best to wash all nitrogen from the lungs and replace it with oxygen. This is especially important in pregnant patients, because functional residual capacity is decreased and pregnant patients become hypoxemic more quickly than nonpregnant patients during periods of apnea.[230] Therefore, before starting induction, 100 percent oxygen is administered via face mask for 2 to 3 minutes. In situations of dire emergency, four vital capacity breaths of 100 percent oxygen via a tight circle system will provide similar benefit.[231]

Intubation

The patient at risk for a difficult or impossible intubation can often be identified prior to surgery. Examination of the airway is a critical part of the preanesthetic evaluation. When airway abnormalities are recognized by the obstetrician, patients should be referred for an early preoperative evaluation by the anesthesiologist.

Aspiration

The consequences of aspiration depend in part on the volume and nature of the aspirate. The conventional wisdom is that patients are at risk when their stomach contents are greater than 25 ml and when the pH of those contents is less than 2.5.[251] The pregnant patient is particularly at risk, as the enlarged uterus increases intra-abdominal pressure and thus intragastric pressure.[252] Gastric emptying is delayed primarily when patients have received opioids.[258] The type of aspiration that produces the most severe physiologic and histologic alterations is partially digested food. PaO_2 decreases more than with any other type of aspiration, and lung damage is considerably more destructive[259]. Because the necessity of a cesarean delivery cannot always be predicted, oral intake of anything but small sips of clear liquids or ice chips should be prohibited during labor.[241]

Key Points

➤ Analgesia during labor can reduce or prevent adverse hormonal and metabolic stress responses to the pain of labor.

➤ Use of parenteral opioids for labor analgesia can produce respiratory depression in the mother and newborn and delayed gastric emptying in the mother. However, when used appropriately, opioids are safe and effective.

➤ Regional analgesia is the most effective form of intrapartum pain relief currently available, and has the flexibility to provide additional anesthesia for spontaneous or instrumental delivery, cesarean delivery, and postoperative pain control.

➤ Spinal opioids provide excellent analgesia during much of the first stage of labor, while decreasing or avoiding the risks of local anesthetic toxicity, high spinal anesthesia, and motor block. Patients can often ambulate, although most will need additional analgesia later in labor and during the second stage.

➤ Side effects and complications of regional anesthesia include hypotension, local anesthetic toxicity, total spinal anesthesia, neurologic injury, and spinal headache.

➤ Epidural analgesia during labor is *associated* with an increased risk of prolonged labor and operative delivery, but whether there is a *cause-and-effect* relationship is controversial.

Box continued on following page

Key Points *Continued*

➤ General anesthesia can be associated with failed intubation and aspiration, the leading causes of anesthesia-related maternal mortality.

➤ Aspiration of gastric contents causes the worst physiologic consequences when there are food particles present and/or pH is less than 2.5; therefore, patients should be encouraged not to eat during labor.

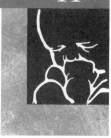

Chapter 11

Malpresentations

SUSAN M. LANNI AND JOHN W. SEEDS

Near term or during labor, the fetus normally assumes a vertical orientation or lie and a cephalic presentation with the fetal vertex flexed on the neck (Fig. 11–1). In about 5 percent of cases, however, deviation occurs from this normal lie, presentation, and flexion attitude, and such deviation constitutes a fetal malpresentation. Malpresentation are associated with increased risk to both the mother and the fetus.

This chapter examines malpresentations, possible etiologies, and the mechanics of labor and vaginal delivery unique to each situation.

CLINICAL CIRCUMSTANCES ASSOCIATED WITH MALPRESENTATION

Factors associated with malpresentation include (1) diminished vertical polarity of the uterine cavity, (2) increased or decreased fetal mobility, or (3) obstructed pelvic inlet. The association of great parity with malpresentation is presumably related to laxity of maternal abdominal muscular support and therefore loss of the normal vertical orientation of the uterine cavity. Placentation either high in the fundus or low in the pelvis is another factor that diminishes the likelihood of a fetus comfortably assuming a longitudinal axis. Uterine myomata, intrauterine synechiae, and müllerian duct abnormalities such as septate uterus or uterus didelphys are likewise associated with a higher than expected rate of malpresentation. Because both prematurity and hydramnios permit increased fetal mobility, there is an increased probability of a noncephalic presentation. Conditions such as autosomal trisomies, myotonic dystrophy, joint contractures from various etiologies, arthrogryposis or oligohydramnios, and fetal neurologic dysfunction result in decreased fetal muscle tone, strength, or activity and are also associated with an increased incidence of fetal malpresentation.

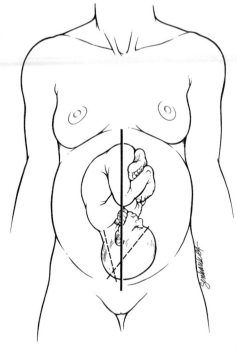

Figure 11-1. Frontal view of a fetus in a longitudinal lie with fetal vertex flexed on the neck.

Furthermore, preterm birth involves a fetus that is small relative to the maternal pelvis and results in increased fetal mobility. In these cases, pelvic engagement and descent with labor or rupture of membranes can occur despite malpresentation. Finally, the cephalopelvic disproportion associated with severe fetal hydrocephalus or with a frankly contracted pelvis is frequently implicated as an etiology of malpresentation because normal engagement of the fetal head is prevented.

ABNORMAL AXIAL LIE

The fetal "lie" indicates the orientation of the fetal spine relative to the spine of the mother. The normal fetal lie is longitudinal and by itself does not indicate whether the presentation is cephalic or breech. If the fetal spine or long axis crosses that of the mother, the fetus may be said to occupy a transverse or oblique lie (Fig. 11–2), resulting in a shoulder or arm presentation. The lie may be termed unstable if the fetal membranes are intact and there is great fetal mobility resulting in frequent changes of lie or presentation.[1]

Prematurity is often associated with abnormal lie, occuring in about 2 percent of pregnancies at 32 weeks, or six times the rate found at term.[9] Persistence of a transverse, oblique, or unstable lie beyond 37 weeks requires a systematic clinical assessment and plan for management, because rupture of membranes without a fetal part filling the inlet of the pelvis imposes a high risk of cord prolapse, fetal compromise, and maternal morbidity if neglected.

Great parity, prematurity, contraction or deformity of the maternal pelvis, and abnormal placentation are the most commonly reported clinical factors associated with abnormal lie,[2,5,9] although many cases manifest none of these.

The normally grown infant at term cannot undergo a safe vaginal delivery from an axial malpresentation.[4,7] Furthermore, a careful

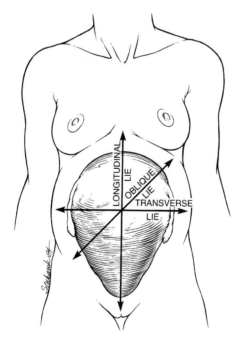

Figure 11–2. A fetus may occupy a longitudinal, oblique, or transverse axis, as illustrated by these vectors. The lie does not indicate whether the vertex or the breech is closest to the cervix.

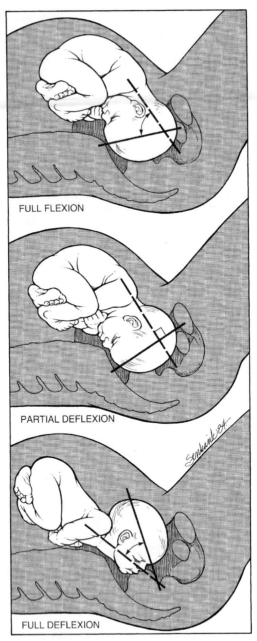

FULL FLEXION

PARTIAL DEFLEXION

FULL DEFLEXION

Figure 11–3. *See legend on opposite page.*

search for a potentially dangerous or compromising etiology of the malpresentation is indicated. A transverse/oblique or unstable lie late in the third trimester necessitates ultrasound examination to exclude a major fetal malformation and abnormal placentation.

External cephalic version followed by induction of labor after 37 weeks in the case of abnormal lie is a reasonable alternative to both expectant management and elective cesarean delivery. Although disputed by some,[3,14] external cephalic version has been found to be safe, with close monitoring, and effective in the majority of cases.[15]

If external version is unsuccessful or not attempted, if spontaneous rupture of membranes occurs, or if active labor has begun with an abnormal lie, cesarean delivery is the treatment of choice for the potentially viable infant.[1,3,14] There is no place for internal podalic version and breech extraction in the management of transverse or oblique lie or unstable presentation in singleton pregnancies because of the unacceptably high rate of fetal and maternal complications.[2]

A persistent abnormal axial lie, particularly if accompanied by ruptured membranes, also alters the choice of uterine incision at

---

Etiologic Factors in Malpresentation

Maternal
  Great parity
  Pelvic tumors
  Pelvic contracture
  Uterine malformation

Fetal
  Prematurity
  Multiple gestation
  Hydramnios
  Macrosomia
  Hydrocephaly
  Trisomies
  Anencephaly
  Myotonic dystrophy
  Placenta previa

Figure 11–3. The normal "attitude" *(top view)* shows the fetal vertex flexed on the neck. Partial deflexion *(middle view)* shows the fetal vertex intermediate between flexion and extension. Full deflexion *(lower view)* shows the fetal vertex completely extended, with the face presenting.

cesarean delivery. Although a low transverse cervical incision has many surgical advantages, up to 25 percent of transverse incisions require vertical extension for delivery of an infant from an abnormal lie to allow access to and atraumatic delivery of the vertex entrapped in the muscular fundus.[3,14] Furthermore, the lower uterine segment is often poorly developed. It makes no sense to perform a cesarean section to minimize birth trauma, then choose a transverse uterine incision if that incision makes fetal extraction more difficult. Therefore, when managing a transverse or oblique lie with ruptured membranes or a poorly developed lower segment, a vertical incision is more prudent.

DEFLECTION ATTITUDES

"Attitude" refers to the position of the fetal head with relation to the neck. The normal attitude of the fetal vertex during labor is one of full flexion on the neck, with the fetal chin against the upper chest. Deflexed attitudes include various degrees of deflection or even extension of the fetal head on the neck (Fig. 11–3). Spontaneous conversion to a more normal flexed attitude or further extension of an intermediate deflection to a fully extended position will commonly occur as labor progresses against resistance exerted by the pelvic bony and soft tissues. Although safe vaginal delivery is possible in most cases, experience indicates that cesarean delivery is the only appropriate alternative when arrest of progress is observed.

FACE PRESENTATION

A face presentation is characterized by a longitudinal lie and full extension of the fetal head on the neck, with the occiput against the upper back (Fig. 11–4). The fetal chin is chosen as the point of designation at vaginal examination. For example, a fetus presenting by the face whose chin is in the right posterior quadrant of the maternal pelvis would be called a *right mentum posterior* (RMP).

All clinical factors known to increase the general rate of malpresentation (see box, Etiologic Factors in Malpresentation, above) have been implicated in face presentation, but as many as 60 percent of infants with a face presentation are malformed. Anencephaly, for instance, is found in about one third of cases of face presentation.[5,25,26] Frequently observed maternal factors include a contracted pelvis or cephalopelvic disproportion in 10 to 40 percent of cases.[17,20,23]

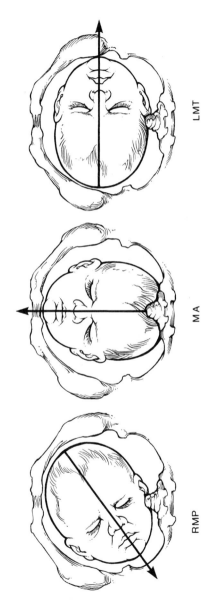

RMP   MA   LMT

Figure 11–4. The point of designation from digital examination in the case of a face presentation is the fetal chin relative to the maternal pelvis. *Left,* Right mentum posterior (RMP). *Middle,* Mentum anterior (MA). *Right,* Left mentum transverse (LMT).

Mechanism of Labor

Knowledge of the early mechanism of labor for face presentation is incomplete. Many infants with a face presentation probably begin labor in the less extended brow position. With descent into the pelvis, the forces of labor press the fetus against maternal tissues; either flexion or full extension of the head on the spine then occurs. The labor of a face presentation must include engagement, descent, internal rotation generally to a mentum anterior position, and delivery by flexion as the chin passes under the symphysis (Fig. 11–5). However, flexion of the occiput may not always occur. Delivery in the fully extended attitude is not uncommon.

Prognosis for labor with a face presentation depends on the orientation of the fetal chin. At diagnosis, 60 to 80 percent of infants with a face presentation are mentum anterior,[5,20,22,29] 10 to 12 percent are mentum transverse,[5,22,29] and 20 to 25 percent are mentum posterior.[5,20,22,29] Almost all average-sized infants presenting mentum anterior with adequate pelvic dimensions will achieve spontaneous or easily assisted vaginal delivery.[5,22,30,31] Furthermore, most mentum transverse infants will rotate to the mentum anterior position and deliver vaginally, and even 25 to 33 percent of mentum posterior infants will rotate and deliver vaginally in the mentum anterior position.[5,16,20] Persistence of mentum posterior with an infant of normal size, however, makes safe vaginal delivery less likely. Manual attempts to convert the face to a flexed attitude or to rotate a posterior position to a more favorable mentum anterior are rarely successful and increase both maternal and fetal risks.[16,22,26,32] Spontaneous delivery or cesarean delivery are the preferred routes for both fetal maternal safety.

Prolonged labor is a common feature of face presentation[5,8] and has been associated with an increased number of intrapartum deaths.[17] Therefore, prompt attention to an arrested labor pattern is recommended. The choice between augmentation of a dysfunctional labor or primary cesarean delivery rests on an assessment of uterine activity, pelvic adequacy, and fetal condition. In the case of an average or small fetus, adequate pelvis, and hypotonic labor, oxytocin may be considered. However, worsening of fetal condition during labor is common. Continuous intrapartum electronic fetal heart rate monitoring of a fetus with face presentation is considered mandatory, but extreme care must be exercised in the placement of an electrode, as ocular and cosmetic damage might result from this device. If external Doppler heart rate monitoring is inadequate and an internal electrode is considered necessary, placement of the electrode on the fetal chin is recommended.

No absolute contraindication to oxytocin augmentation of hypotonic labor in the case of a face presentation exists, but an arrest

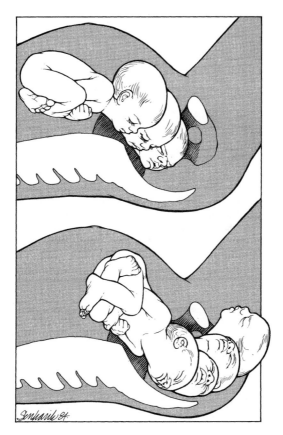

Figure 11–5. Engagement, descent, and internal rotation remain cardinal elements of vaginal delivery in the case of a face presentation, but successful vaginal delivery of a term size fetus presenting a face generally requires delivery by flexion under the symphysis from a mentum anterior position as illustrated here.

of progress despite adequate labor or nonreassuring fetal heart rate pattern should call for cesarean delivery.[8] Although cesarean delivery has been reported in up to 60 percent of cases of face presentation,[18,27] safe vaginal delivery may be accomplished in many, and a trial of labor with careful monitoring of fetal condition and progress is not contraindicated unless macrosomia or a small pelvis is identified. If cesarean delivery is warranted, care should be taken to flex the head gently both to accomplish elevation of the head through the hysterotomy incision as well as to avoid potential nerve damage to the neonate. However, forced flexion may also result in damage, especially with fetal goiter, or neck tumors.

Laryngeal and tracheal edema resulting from pressures of the birth process might require immediate nasotracheal intubation.[33]

BROW PRESENTATION

An infant in a brow presentation occupies a longitudinal axis, with a partially deflexed cephalic attitude, midway between full flexion and full extension (Fig. 11–6).[24] The frontal bones are the point of designation. If the anterior fontanel is on the mother's left side, with the sagittal suture in the transverse pelvic axis, the fetus would be in a left frontum transverse (LFT) position. Brow presentation will be detected more often in early labor before flexion occurs to a normal attitude. Less frequently, further extension results in a face presentation.

Factors that delay engagement are associated with persistent brow presentation. Cephalopelvic disproportion, prematurity, and great parity are often found and have been implicated in more than 60 percent of cases of persistent brow presentation.[5,35,38,39]

A persistent brow presentation requires engagement and descent of the largest (mento-occipital) diameter or profile of the fetal

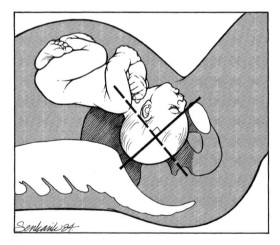

Figure 11–6. This fetus is a brow presentation in a frontum anterior position. The head is in an intermediate deflexion attitude.

head.[40] This process is possible only with a large pelvis or a small infant or both. However, brow presentations convert spontaneously by flexion or further extension to either a vertex or a face presentation and are then managed accordingly.[34,35] The earlier the diagnosis is made, the more likely conversion will occur spontaneously. Fewer than half of infants with persistent brow presentations undergo spontaneous vaginal delivery, but in most cases a trial of labor is not contraindicated.[5,36]

Prolonged labors have been observed in brow presentations,[5,20,35,38,39] and secondary arrest is not uncommon.[34] Forced conversion of the brow to a more favorable position with forceps is contraindicated,[34,35,38] as are attempts at manual conversion. One unexpected cause of persistent brow presentation may be an open fetal mouth pressed against the vaginal wall, splinting the head and preventing either flexion or extension[28,35]

In most brow presentations, as with face presentations, minimal manipulation yields the best results[35,41] if the fetal heart rate pattern remains reassuring. Expectancy is justified with a large pelvis, a small fetus, and adequate progress. If a brow presentation persists with a large baby, successful vaginal delivery is unlikely, and cesarean delivery may be most prudent.[20]

COMPOUND PRESENTATION

Whenever an extremity is found prolapsed beside the major presenting fetal part, the situation is referred to as a compound presentation[42] (Fig. 11–7). The combination of an upper extremity and the vertex is the most common.

This diagnosis should be suspected with any arrest of labor in the active phase or failure to engage during active labor.[44] Diagnosis is made by vaginal examination that discovers an irregular mobile tissue mass adjacent to the larger presenting part. Recognition late in labor is common, and as many as 50 percent of persisting compound presentations are not detected until the second stage.[42] Delay in diagnosis may not be detrimental because it is likely that only the persistent cases require significant intervention.

Maternal age, race, parity, and pelvic size have all been associated with compound presentation,[43,44] but prematurity is the most consistent clinical finding.[5,42] It is primarily the very small fetus that is at great risk of persistent compound presentation. In late pregnancy, external cephalic version of a fetus in breech position may increase the risk of a compound presentation.[46]

Fetal risk in compound presentation is specifically associated with birth trauma and cord prolapse. Maternal risks include soft tissue damage and obstetric laceration.

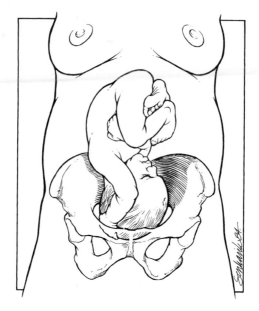

Figure 11–7. The compound presentation of an upper extremity and the vertex illustrated here most often spontaneously resolves with further labor and descent.

Labor is not necessarily contraindicated with a compound presentation; however, the prolapsed extremity should not be manipulated.[42–44,47] The accompanying extremity may retract as the major presenting part descends. Cruikshank and White[5] found that 75 percent of vertex/upper extremity combinations deliver spontaneously. Occult or undetected cord prolapse is possible, and therefore continuous electronic fetal heart rate monitoring is recommended.

The primary indications for surgical intervention are cord prolapse, nonreassuring fetal heart rate patterns, and failure to progress.[5] Cesarean delivery is the only appropriate clinical intervention.[42] Protraction of the second stage of labor has been noted to occur more frequently with persistent compound presentation, and dysfunctional labor patterns are said to be common.[42] As in other malpresentations, spontaneous resolution occurs more often and surgical intervention is less frequently necessary in those cases diagnosed early in labor. Persistent compound presentation is more likely with a small infant, as is the prognosis for successful vaginal delivery. Persistent compound presentation with a term-sized infant has a poor prognosis for safe vaginal delivery, and cesarean delivery is usually necessary.

BREECH PRESENTATION

The infant presenting as a breech occupies a longitudinal axis with the cephalic pole in the uterine fundus. This presentation occurs in 3 to 4 percent of labors overall, although it is found in 7 percent of pregnancies at 32 weeks and in 25 percent of pregnancies of less than 28 weeks' duration.[48] The three types of breech are noted in Table 11–1. The infant in the frank breech position is flexed at the hips with extended knees. The complete breech is flexed at both joints, and the footling breech has one or both hips partially or fully extended (Fig. 11–8).

The diagnosis of breech presentation may be made by abdominal palpation or vaginal examination and confirmed by ultrasound. Prematurity, fetal malformation, müullerian anomalies, and polar placentation are commonly observed causative factors. High rates of breech presentation are noted in certain fetal genetic disorders, including trisomies 13, 18, and 21; Potter's syndrome; and myotonic dystrophy.[49] Thus, conditions that alter fetal muscular tone and mobility also increase the frequency of breech presentation.

Mechanism and Conduct of Labor and Vaginal Delivery

The two most important elements for the safe conduct of vaginal breech delivery are continuous electronic fetal heart rate monitoring and noninterference until spontaneous delivery of the breech to the umbilicus has occurred. Early in labor, the capability for immediate cesarean delivery should be established. Anesthesia should be available, the operating room readied, and appropriate informed consent obtained. Two obstetricians should be in attendance as well as a pediatric team. Appropriate training and experience with vaginal breech delivery are fundamental to success. The instrument table should be prepared in the customary manner,

Table 11–1. BREECH CATEGORIES

Type	Overall Percent of Breeches	Risk (%)	
		Prolapse	Premature
Frank breech	48–73[31,46,48,54,70]	0.5[68]	38[48]
Complete	4.6–11.5[31,48,54,70]	4–6[68]	12[48]
Footling	12–38[31,48,54]	15–18[68]	50[48]

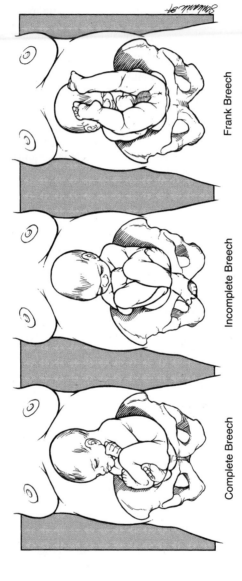

Complete Breech   Incomplete Breech   Frank Breech

Figure 11–8. The complete breech is flexed at the hips and flexed at the knees. The incomplete breech shows incomplete deflexion of one or both knees or hips. The frank breech is flexed at the hips and extended at the knees.

with the addition of Piper forceps and extra towels. There is no contraindication to epidural analgesia once labor is well established; many view epidural anesthesia as an asset in the control of the second stage.

The infant presenting in the frank breech position usually enters the pelvic inlet in one of the diagonal pelvic diameters (Fig. 11–9). Engagement has occurred when the bitrochanteric diameter of the fetus has passed the plane of the pelvic inlet, although by vaginal examination the presenting part may only be palpated at −2 to −4 station (out of 5) relative to the ischial spines. As the breech descends and encounters the levator ani muscular sling, internal rotation usually occurs to bring the bitrochanteric diameter into the anteroposterior (AP) axis of the pelvis. The point of designation in a breech labor is the fetal sacrum and, therefore, when the bitrochanteric diameter is in the AP axis of the pelvis, the fetal sacrum will lie in the transverse pelvic diameter.

If normal descent occurs, the breech will present at the outlet and begin to emerge, first as a sacrum transverse, then rotate to a sacrum anterior. Crowning occurs when the bitrochanteric diameter passes under the pubic symphysis. An episiotomy in the midline to but not through the anal sphincter may facilitate delivery but should be delayed until crowning begins. Some argue that a mediolateral episiotomy offers more room and less risk of extension through the anal sphincter, but considerable skill and experience are required to repair a mediolateral episiotomy properly, and this incision is associated with greater blood loss and pain. Premature

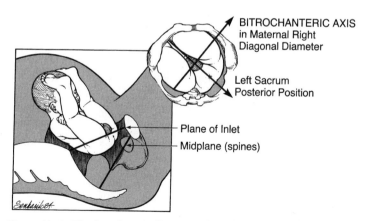

Figure 11–9. The breech typically enters the inlet with the bitrochanteric diameter aligned with one of the diagonal diameters, with the sacrum as the point of designation in the other diagonal diameter. This is a case of left sacrum posterior (LSP).

episiotomy will contribute to unnecessary blood loss and to the level of anxiety and perhaps a tendency to rush the delivery. As the infant emerges, rotation begins, usually toward a sacrum anterior position. This direction of rotation may reflect the greater capacity of the hollow of the posterior pelvis to accept the fetal chest and small parts. It is important to emphasize that operator intervention is not yet needed or helpful other than possibly to perform the episiotomy and encourage maternal expulsive efforts.

Premature or aggressive assistance may adversely affect the breech birth in at least two ways. First, cervical dilatation must be maximized and complete dilatation sustained for sufficient duration to retard retraction of the cervix and entrapment of the aftercoming fetal head. Rushing the delivery of the trunk may significantly diminish the effectiveness of this process. Second, the safe descent and delivery of the breech infant must be the result of expulsive forces from above to maintain flexion of the fetal vertex. Any traction from below in an effort to speed delivery would encourage deflexion of the vertex and result in the presentation of the larger occipitofrontal fetal cranial profile to the pelvic inlet. Such an event could be catastrophic. Rushed delivery also increases the risk of a nuchal arm, with one or both arms trapped behind the head above the pelvic inlet. Entrapment of a nuchal arm makes safe vaginal delivery much more difficult, as it dramatically increases the size of the aggregate object that must pass through the birth canal. Safe breech delivery of an average-sized infant, therefore, depends predominantly on maternal expulsive forces, and patience, not traction from below.

As the frank breech emerges farther, the fetal thighs are typically pressed firmly against the fetal abdomen, often splinting and protecting the umbilicus and cord. After the umbilicus appears over the maternal perineum, the operator may align his or her fingers medial to one thigh, then the other, pressing laterally as the fetal pelvis is rotated away from that side (Fig. 11–10). This results in external rotation of the thigh at the hip, flexion of the knee, and delivery of one and then the other leg. The dual movement of counterclockwise rotation of the fetal pelvis as the operator externally rotates the right thigh and clockwise rotation of the fetal pelvis as the operator externally rotates the fetal left thigh is most effective in facilitating delivery. The fetal trunk is then wrapped with a towel to provide secure support of the body while further descent results from expulsive forces from the mother. The operator primarily facilitates the delivery of the fetus by guiding the body through the introitus. The operator is not applying outward traction on the fetus that might result in deflexion of the fetal head or nuchal arm.

When the scapulae appear at the outlet, the operator may slip a hand over the fetal shoulder from the back (Fig. 11–11), follow the humerus and, with a lateral movement, sweep first one and then the other arm across the chest and out over the perineum.

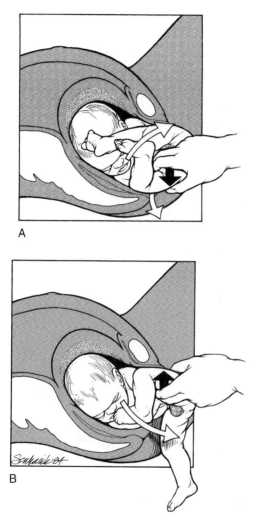

Figure 11–10. After spontaneous expulsion to the umbilicus, external rotation of each thigh *(A)* combined with opposite rotation of the fetal pelvis results in flexion of the knee and delivery of each leg *(B)*.

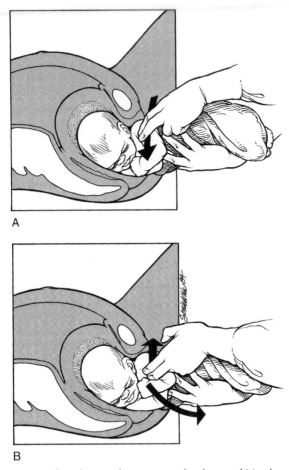

A

B

Figure 11-11. When the scapulae appear under the symphisis, the operator reaches over the left shoulder, sweeps the arm across the chest *(A)*, and delivers the arm *(B)*.

Gentle rotation of the fetal trunk counterclockwise assists delivery of the right arm, and clockwise rotation assists delivery of the left arm (turning the body "into" the arm). This accomplishes delivery of the arms by drawing them across the fetal chest in a fashion similar to that used for delivery of the legs (Fig. 11–12). Once both arms have been delivered, if the vertex has remained flexed on the neck, the chin and face will appear at the outlet, and the airway may be cleared and suctioned (Fig. 11–13).

With further maternal expulsive forces alone, spontaneous controlled delivery of the fetal head will often occur. If not, delivery may be accomplished with a simple manual effort to maximize flexion of the vertex using pressure on the fetal maxilla (not mandible; the Mauriceau-Smellie-Veit maneuver) along with suprapubic pressure (Credé's maneuver) and gentle downward traction (Fig. 11–14). Although maxillary pressure will maximize cephalic flexion, the main force effecting delivery remains the mother.

Alternatively, the operator may apply Piper forceps to the aftercoming head to facilitate delivery. The application requires very slight elevation of the fetal trunk by the assistant, while the operator kneels and applies the Piper forceps directly to the fetal head in the pelvis. In applying Piper forceps avoid *excessive* elevation by the assistant which may potentially harm to the neonate. Hyperextension of the fetal neck from excessive elevation of the fetal trunk should be avoided.

Piper forceps are characterized by absence of pelvic curvature. This modification allows *direct* application to the fetal head and avoids conflict with the fetal body that would occur with the application of standard instruments from below. The forceps are

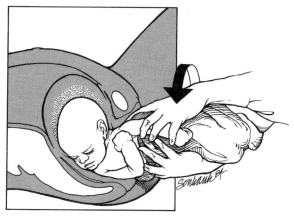

Figure 11–12. Gentle rotation of the shoulder girdle facilitates delivery of the right arm.

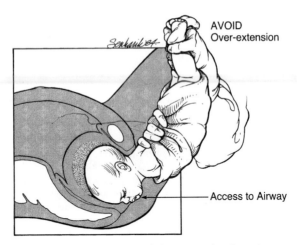

AVOID
Over-extension

Access to Airway

Figure 11–13. Following delivery of the arms, the fetus is wrapped in a towel for control and slightly elevated. The fetal face and airway may be visible over the perineum. Excessive elevation of the trunk is avoided.

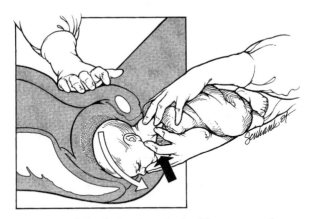

Figure 11–14. Cephalic flexion is maintained by pressure *(heavy arrow)* on the fetal maxilla (not mandible!). Often, delivery of the head is easily accomplished with continued expulsive forces from above and gentle downward traction.

inserted into the vagina from beneath the fetus. The blade to be placed on the maternal right is held by the handle in the operator's right hand and the blade inserted with the operator's left hand in the vagina along the right maternal sidewall and placed against the left fetal parietal bone. The handle of the left blade is then held in the operator's left hand and inserted by right hand along the left maternal sidewall and placed against the right fetal parietal bone. Forceps application controls the fetal head and prevents extension of the head on the neck. Gentle downward traction on the forceps with the fetal trunk supported on the forceps shanks results in controlled delivery of the vertex. Routine use of Piper forceps to the aftercoming head may be advisable both to ensure control of the delivery and to maintain optimal operator proficiency in anticipation of deliveries that may require their use.

Arrest of spontaneous progress in labor with adequate uterine contractions necessitates cesarean delivery. Vaginal interventions directed at facilitating delivery of the breech that is complicated by an arrest of spontaneous progress are discouraged, because fetal and maternal morbidity and mortality are both greatly increased. However, if labor is deemed to be hypotonic by internally monitored uterine pressures, oxytocin is not contraindicated.[50–52]

Mechanisms of descent and delivery of the footling and the complete breech are not unlike those of the frank breech described above, except one or both legs might already be extended and thus not require attention. The risk of cord prolapse or entanglement is greater and, hence, the possibility of emergency cesarean delivery increased. Furthermore, footling and complete breeches are not as effective a cervical dilator as either the vertex or the larger aggregate profile of the thighs and buttocks of the frank breech. Thus, the risk of entrapment of the aftercoming head is perhaps increased, and as a result primary cesarean delivery is often advocated for nonfrank breech presentations.

Management of the Term Breech

The reported perinatal mortality associated with breech presentation has varied from 9 to 25 percent,[54,55] three to five times that of the nonbreech infant at term.[56–58] The excess deaths associated with breech presentation are largely due to lethal anomalies and complications of prematurity, both of which are found more frequently among breech infants. Excluding anomalies and extreme prematurity, the corrected perinatal mortality reported by some investigators approaches zero regardless of the method of delivery, whereas others find that even with exclusion of these factors the term breech infant has been found to be at higher risk for birth trauma and asphyxia.[59–61] In order to assess the safety of breech delivery, an appropriately controlled randomized trial with sufficient number of study patients must be conducted. To date, only two randomized trials have been reported.[50,53] The remainder of reports surrounding the issue of safety of breech delivery is confined to cohort and observational types of studies, usually retrospective, and subject to significant risk of bias. Conclusions regarding safety of breech from a fetal standpoint will vary, but are summarized in Table 11–2. A well-publicized North American study coordinated from Canada has turned the tide toward routine cesarean delivery. Neonatal complications were unequivocally higher in the breech group randomized to vaginal delivery. However, this advice is not inviolate, and patients should be offered an option. A cooperative, compliant well informed patient is the most appropriate candidate for breech vaginal delivery. There remain many who believe that complete abandonment of vaginal delivery for the breech is not yet justified.[70,71] Moreover, sometimes time may preclude cesarean delivery; thus, the well-trained obstetrician must be familar with vaginal delivery of breech presentation.

Of special note is hyperextension of the fetal head, which is consistently associated with a high (21 percent) risk of spinal cord injury if the breech is delivered vaginally.[30,97,98] It is important to differentiate simple deflexion of the head from clear hyperextension, given that simple deflexion carries no excess risk.

Finally, footling breech carries a prohibitively high (16 to 19 percent) risk of cord prolapse during labor. In many cases, cord prolapse is manifest only late in labor, after commitment to vaginal delivery has been made.[60,85] Cord prolapse necessitates prompt cesarean delivery. Furthermore, the footling breech is a poor cervical dilator, and cephalic entrapment becomes more likely.

Table 11–2. INCIDENCE OF COMPLICATIONS SEEN WITH BREECH PRESENTATION

Complication	Incidence
Intrapartum fetal death	Increased 16–fold[65,67]
Intrapartum asphyxia	Increased 3.8–fold[65,67]
Cord prolapse	Increased 5– to 20–fold[48,55,68]
Birth trauma	Increased 13–fold[48]
Arrest of aftercoming head	8.8%[48]
Spinal cord injuries with extended head	21%[30,98]
Major anomalies	6–18%[55,65,67]
Prematurity	16–33%[31,54,60,63,69,82,83]
Hyperextension of head	5%[97]

External Cephalic Version

External cephalic version is an alternative to vaginal delivery or cesarean delivery for the breech infant.[15,54,56,117-120] External cephalic version significantly reduces the incidence of breech presentation in labor and is associated with few complications such as cord compression or placental abruption.[15,120] Reported success with external version varies from 60 to 75 percent, with a similar percentage of these remaining vertex at the time of labor.[15,121-124] Many infants in breech presentation before 34 weeks will convert spontaneously to a cephalic presentation, but few will do so afterward. Repetitive external version attempted weekly after 34 weeks is successful in converting over two thirds of cases and in reducing their breech presentation rate by 50 percent.[120]

Gentle constant pressure applied in a relaxed patient with frequent fetal heart rate assessments are key elements underlying success.[54,56,117] Methodology varies, although the "forward roll" is more widely supported than the "back flip" (Fig. 11-15).[117] The mechanical goal is to squeeze the fetal vertex gently out of the fundal area to the transverse and finally into the lower segment of the uterus.

Tocolysis and epidural anesthesia during the procedure may also be helpful.

In the case of the gravida with a previous cesarean delivery, external cephalic version is controversial.

SHOULDER DYSTOCIA

Shoulder dystocia is diagnosed when, after delivery of the fetal head, further expulsion of the infant is prevented by impaction of the fetal shoulders within the maternal pelvis. Specific efforts are necessary to facilitate delivery (Fig. 11-16).

Although a difficult shoulder dystocia occurs infrequently, one does not soon forget the experience. Often, but not always, at the end of a difficult labor, the fetal head may be delivered spontaneously or by forceps, but the neck then retracts. The fetal head appears to be drawn back with the chin close to the maternal perineum or thigh, creating difficulty suctioning the infant's mouth. As maternal expulsive efforts are encouraged, the fetal head becomes plethoric, and the danger to the infant is apparent if delivery cannot be promptly accomplished.

The neonatal morbidity of greatest concern is brachial plexus injury, resulting from trauma to cervical nerve root V and VI.

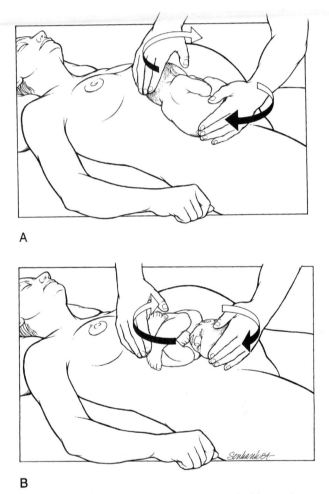

A

B

Figure 11–15. External cephalic version is accomplished by gently "squeezing" the fetus out of one area of the uterus and into another. Here, the "forward roll," often the most popular, is illustrated.

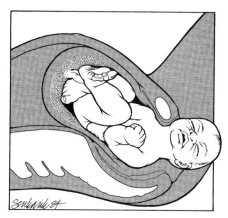

Figure 11–16. When delivery of the fetal head is not followed by delivery of the shoulders, the anterior shoulder has often become caught behind the symphysis as illustrated here. The head may retract toward the perineum. Desperate traction on the fetal head is not likely to facilitate delivery and may lead to trauma.

Fortunately, most cases are transient, with full recovery observed in 90 to 95 percent of infants.[139]

Etiology

Although shoulder dystocia has traditionally been strongly associated with macrosomia, up to one half of cases of shoulder dystocia occur in neonates under 4,000 g.[140,141] With macrosomia or continued fetal growth beyond term, the trunk and particularly the chest grow larger relative to the head. Chest circumference exceeds the head circumference in 80 percent of cases.[140] Arms also contribute to the greater dimensions of the upper body. Macrosomia shows the strongest correlation with shoulder dystocia of any clinical factor and occurs more often with gestational diabetes and twice as often in postdate pregnancies. Other clinical factors associated with shoulder dystocia appear to be related to macrosomia as well and include maternal obesity,[137,142] previous birth of an infant weighing over 4,000 g,[137,140,142,143] diabetes mellitus,[142,143] prolonged second stage of labor,[141–143] prolonged deceleration phase (8 to 10 cm),[127] instrumental midpelvic delivery,[144] and previous shoulder dystocia,[143] which has been found to have a recurrence risk of almost 14 percent. Increased maternal age and excess maternal weight gain have been found by some but not all investigators[137,142–144] to increase the risk of macrosomia and shoulder dystocia.[143]

Clinical efforts to detect macrosomia prenatally could be helpful in anticipating problems with delivery of the shoulders. Such efforts, however, have been disappointing. Numerous sonographic markers have been assessed to determine their usefulness in predicting macrosomia. These include the estimation of fetal weight using a variety of fetal dimensions and the comparison of chest to head circumference. Numerous efforts in the literature repeatedly demonstrate the shortcomings of both clinical and ultrasonographic estimations of fetal weight, and have concluded that the best estimation is a combination of the two.

There is a growing trend to consider cesarean delivery of any infant with an estimated weight over 4,500 g or of any infant of a diabetic mother with an estimated weight over 4,000 g[141,144] to avoid birth trauma, particularly brachial plexus injury. Any consideration of elective abdominal delivery on the basis of estimated fetal weight alone, however, must consider the technical error of the method. If 90 percent confidence is desired that the actual fetal weight is at least 4,000 g, the sonographic estimate by most current methods must exceed 4,600 g. This is a result of the expected methodologic error of ± 10 percent (± 1 SD). Furthermore, the fetal vertex is often too deeply engaged in the pelvis to allow accurate measurement of head circumference. Estimated fetal weight should be only one of several factors considered in the management of the laboring patient. In the obsese diabetic patient with an estimated fetal weight over 4,500 g and showing poor progress in labor, cesarean delivery may be the most prudent course. However, in most other cases, the risks of cesarean to the mother, the accuracy of prediction of macrosomia, and the alternative of a carefully monitored trial of labor should be discussed.

The occurrence of brachial plexus injury in the absence of shoulder dystocia has been described and attributed to in utero forces, such as the posterior shoulder impacting on the sacral promontory (although anterior injuries have been described as well),[157] malpresentations,[158] and dysfunctional labor, mostly precipitate labor.[141,159] Interestingly, in neonates with brachial plexus injury without shoulder dystocia, there was a trend toward lower birth weight, more clavicular fractures, injuries to the brachial plexus of the posterior arm, and longer persistence of the condition than their counterparts in the shoulder dystocia-present group.[157]

Management during Vaginal Delivery

Successful management follows anticipation and preparation. Anticipation involves the prenatal suspicion of macrosomia by clinical and/or sonographic means. One must be aware of the clinical features that have been cited and consider a pregnancy at high risk for macrosomia and therefore for shoulder dystocia. Strong consideration for cesarean delivery is recommended when a prolonged second stage occurs in association with macrosomia.

Deliveries are best managed in a delivery room. Deliveries in bed increase the difficulty of reducing a shoulder dystocia because the bedding precludes fullest use of the posterior pelvis and outlet.

Once a vaginal delivery has begun, the obstetrician must resist the temptation to rotate the head forcibly to a transverse axis. Maternal expulsive efforts should be used rather than traction. Gentle manual pressure on the fetal head inferiorly and posteriorly will push the posterior shoulder into the hollow of the sacrum, increasing the room for the anterior shoulder to pass under the pubis (Fig. 11–17). This pressure is not outward traction and must be symmetric. If the head is pressed asymmetrically, as if to "pry" the anterior shoulder out, brachial plexus injury is more likely.

If delivery is not accomplished, a deliberate, planned sequence of efforts should then be initiated. One must not pull desperately on the fetal head. Fundal expulsive efforts, including maternal pushing and any fundal pressure, should be temporarily stopped. Aggressive fundal pressure prior to disimpaction or rotation of the shoulders will not facilitate delivery and may work against rotation and disimpaction.

The McRoberts maneuver[160] is a simple, logical, and usually successful measure to promote delivery of the shoulders. The McRoberts maneuver involves hyperflexion of maternal legs on the

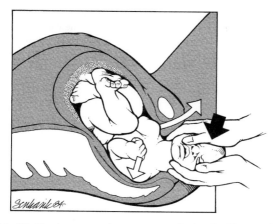

Figure 11–17. Gentle, symmetric pressure on the head will move the posterior shoulder into the hollow of the sacrum and encourage delivery of the anterior shoulder. Care should be taken not to "pry" the anterior shoulder out asymmetrically, as this might lead to trauma to the anterior brachial plexus.

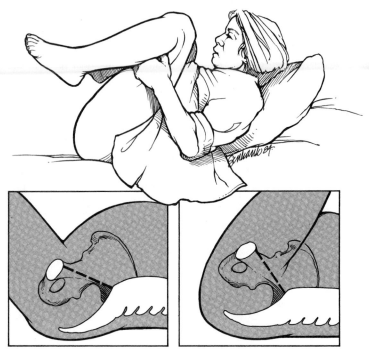

Figure 11–18. The least invasive maneuver to disimpact the shoulders is the McRoberts maneuver. Sharp ventral flexion of the maternal hips results in ventral rotation of the maternal pelvis and an increase in the useful size of the outlet.

maternal abdomen that results in flattening of the lumbar spine and ventral rotation of the maternal pelvis and symphysis (Fig. 11–18). This maneuver may increase the useful size of the posterior outlet, resulting in easier disimpaction of the anterior shoulder. The McRoberts maneuver significantly reduces shoulder extraction forces, brachial plexus stretching, and likelihood of clavicular fracture. In a retrospective review of shoulder dystocia, one study found that the McRoberts maneuver was the only step required in 42 percent of 236 cases.[162] When shoulder dystocia occurs because of failure of the bisacromial diameter to engage, the Walcher position, which entails dropping the maternal legs down toward the floor with concurrent suprapubic pressure in a dorsal-caudal direction, has been advocated. Only then, while constant suprapubic pressure is being maintained, should the parturient be placed in the McRoberts position; this may allow for the disimpaction of the fetal shoulder from the symphysis by increasing the AP diameter of the inlet prior to increasing the outlet.[163] Additionally, the "all fours," or Gaskin maneuver, which differs from the knee-chest position, may relieve the dystocia.[164] Use of this maneuver is reasonable only in the setting of a mobile parturient with no significant motor blockade from regional anesthetic, and a stable and wide surface on which to assume this position in order to avoid the potential for injury during transition to this position.

If the shoulders remain undelivered, often only moderate suprapubic pressure is required to disimpact the anterior shoulder and allow delivery. If this is not effective, the operator's hand may be passed behind the occiput into the vagina, and the anterior shoulder may be pushed forward to the oblique, after which, with maternal efforts and gentle posterior pressure, delivery should occur (Fig. 11–19).[131] Alternatively, the posterior shoulder may be rotated forward, through a 180-degree arc, and passed under the pubic ramus as in turning a screw (Wood's screw maneuver). As the posterior shoulder rotates anteriorly, delivery will often occur.[165]

Many authorities have advocated delivery of the posterior arm and shoulder should the above methods fail. The operator's hand is passed into the vagina, following the posterior arm of the fetus to the elbow. The arm is flexed and swept out over the chest and the perineum (Fig. 11–20). In some cases, delivery will now occur without further manipulation. In others, rotation of the trunk, bringing the freed posterior arm anteriorly, is required.[131,140] These maneuvers are highly likely to fracture the clavicle (up to 25 percent), humerus (up to 15 percent), or both or result in transient or permanent nerve injury (up to approximately 9 percent).[165] Overall, similar rates of bone fracture were noted when any type of manipulation was performed to accomplish delivery of an impacted fetal shoulder.[166] Deliberate fracture of the clavicle is possible and will facilitate delivery by diminishing the rigidity and size of the shoulder girdle. It is best if the pressure is exerted in a direction away from the lung to avoid puncture. Sharp instrumental transection of the clavicle is not recommended, since lung puncture is common with such a method, and infection of the bone through the open wound is a serious possible complication.

Two techniques rarely used in the United States for the management of shoulder dystocia include vaginal replacement of the fetal head with cesarean delivery (Zavanelli maneuver) and subcutaneous symphysiotomy. O'Leary and Cuva[168] described 35 cases of the Zavanelli manueuver, 31 of which were considered successful. One needed a hysterotomy incision to disimpact the fetal shoulders and facilitate vaginal delivery when the fetal head could not be replaced into the vagina from below.

Subcutaneous symphysiotomy has been practiced in some countries such as South Africa for many years as an expedient alternative

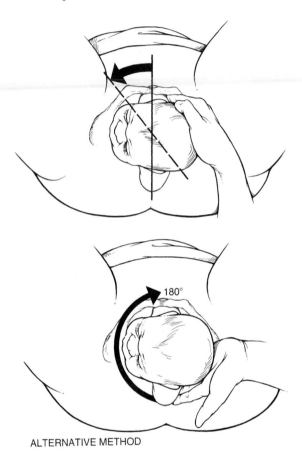

ALTERNATIVE METHOD

Figure 11-19. Rotation of the anterior shoulder forward through a small arc or the posterior shoulder forward through a larger one will often lead to descent and delivery of the shoulders. Forward rotation is preferred, as it tends to compress and diminish the size of the shoulder girdle, while backward rotation would open the shoulder girdle and increase the size.

to cesarean delivery with very good results.[169] The procedure can be safe and effective as long as attention is paid to the three main points in the procedure: lateral support of the legs, partial sharp dissection of the symphysis, and displacement of the urethra to the side with an indwelling urinary catheter.[170] However, symphysiotomy has

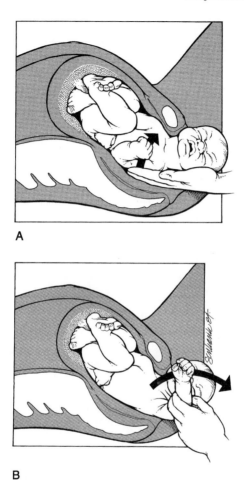

A

B

Figure 11–20. The operator here inserts a hand and sweeps the posterior arm across the chest and over the perineum. Care should be taken to distribute the pressure evenly across the humerus to avoid unnecessary fracture.

been widely or often used in obstetric practice in the United States. Attempted implementation of either method by the inexperienced practitioner before the trial of more conventional remedies may increase risk to the child, the mother, and the clinician.

> **Key Points**

➤ The "fetal lie" indicates the orientation of the fetal spine relative to that of the mother. Normal fetal lie is longitudinal and by itself does not connote whether the presentation is cephalic or breech.

➤ Cord prolapse occurs far more often with an abnormal axial lie than it does with a cephalic presentation.

➤ Fetal malformations are observed in more than half of infants with a face presentation.

➤ Face presentation must deliver mentum, anterior, often after awaiting spontaneous rotation from mentum posterior.

➤ External cephalic version of the infant in breech presentation near term is a safe and often successful management option. Use of tocolytics and/or epidural anesthesia may improve success. A recent randomized trial has led to recommendations that cesarean delivery be offered in all breech presentation, because of increased fetal safety. However, not all patients will accept and sometimes delivery occurs too rapidly to allow cesarean delivery.

➤ Appropriate training and experience is a prerequisite to the safe vaginal delivery of selected infants in breech presentation.

➤ Shoulder dystocia cannot be precisely predicted or prevented but is often associated with macrosomia, maternal obesity, gestational diabetes, and a postdate pregnancy.

➤ The clinician must be prepared to deal with shoulder dystocia at every vaginal delivery with a deliberate, controlled sequence of interventions that emphasize suprapubic pressure and maternal hip flexion.

Chapter 12

Obstetric Hemorrhage

THOMAS J. BENEDETTI

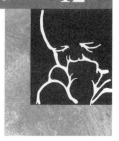

The normal pregnant patient frequently loses 500 ml of blood at the time of vaginal delivery and 1,000 ml at the time of cesarean delivery. Appreciably more blood can be lost without clinical evidence of a volume deficit as a result of the 40 percent expansion in blood volume that occurs by the 30th week of pregnancy.

The pregnant patient does not exhibit early signs of volume loss. When 1,000 ml is rapidly removed from the circulatory blood volume, vasoconstriction occurs in both the arterial and venous compartments in order to preserve essential body organ flow (Fig. 12–1). Blood pressure is initially maintained by increases in systemic vascular resistance. As volume loss exceeds 20 percent, the fall in cardiac output accelerates and blood pressure can no longer be maintained by increases in resistance. Thereafter blood pressure and cardiac output fall in parallel. In addition, if the volume loss has occurred more than 4 hours earlier, significant fluid shifts from the interstitial space into the intravascular space will partially correct the volume deficit. This movement of fluid, termed *transcapillary refill*, can replace as much as 30 percent of lost volume. With more chronic bleeding, the final blood volume deficit may amount to as little as 70 percent of the actual blood lost.

CLASSIFICATION OF HEMORRHAGE

A standard classification for volume loss secondary to hemorrhage is illustrated in Table 12–1. Hemorrhage can be classified as one of four groups, depending on the volume lost. The determination of the class of hemorrhage reflects the volume deficit, which may not be the same as the volume loss. The average 60-kg pregnant woman has a blood volume of 6,000 ml at 30 weeks, and an unreplaced volume loss of less than 900 ml falls into class 1. Such patients rarely exhibit signs or symptoms of volume deficit.

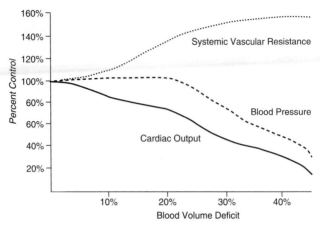

Figure 12–1. Relationships among systemic vascular pressure, cardiac output, and blood pressure in the face of progressive blood volume deficit.

A blood loss of 1,200 to 1,500 ml is characterized as class 2 hemorrhage. These individuals will begin to show expected physical signs, the first being a rise in pulse rate and/or a rise in respiratory rate. Tachypnea is a nonspecific response to volume loss and, although a relatively early sign of mild volume deficit, is frequently overlooked. Doubling of the respiratory rate may be observed in this circumstance. If the patient appears to be breathing rapidly, the minute ventilation is usually twice its normal value. This finding should not be interpreted as an encouraging sign, but rather one of impending problems.

Table 12–1. CLASSIFICATION OF HEMORRHAGE IN THE PREGNANT PATIENT*

Hemorrhage Class	Acute Blood Loss†	Percentage Lost
1	900	15
2	1,200–1,500	20–25
3	1,800–2,100	30–35
4	2,400	40

*Total blood volume = 6,000 ml.
†In the usual clinical setting, very few episodes of volume loss occur without some infusion of intravenous fluids, usually crystalloid-containing solutions such as lactated Ringer's solution, or normal saline. Therefore, the amount of blood loss preceding physical signs and symptoms will usually exceed the values listed. Adapted from Baker R: Hemorrhage in obstetrics. Obstet Gynecol Annu 6:295, 1997.

Patients with class 2 hemorrhage will frequently have orthostatic blood pressure changes and may have decreased perfusion of the extremities. However, this amount of blood loss will not usually result in the classic cold, clammy extremities. However, a more subtle test may document blood loss. One can squeeze the hypothenar area of the hand for 1 to 2 seconds and then release the pressure. A patient with normal volume status will have an initial blanching of the skin, followed within 1 to 2 seconds by a return to the normal pink coloration. A patient who has a volume deficit of 15 to 25 percent will have delayed refilling of the blanched area of the hand.

Narrowing of the pulse pressure is another sign of class 2 hemorrhage. When a patient loses blood, compensatory mechanisms are activated that help ensure perfusion to vital body organs (brain, heart). The initial response, vasoconstriction, diverts blood away from nonvital body organs (skin, muscle, kidney). Blood loss results in sympathoadrenal stimulation, which causes a rise in diastolic pressure. Because the systolic pressure is usually maintained with small volume deficits (15 to 25 percent), the first blood pressure response seen with volume loss is narrowing of the pulse pressure (120/70 to 120/90 mm Hg). That is, pulse pressure changes from 50 mm Hg to 30 mm Hg. When pulse pressure drops to 30 mm Hg or less, the patient should be carefully evaluated for other signs of volume loss.

Class 3 hemorrhage is defined as blood loss sufficient to cause overt hypotension. In the pregnant patient, this usually requires a blood loss of 1,800 to 2,100 ml. These patients exhibit marked tachycardia (120 to 160 beats/min) and may have cold, clammy skin and tachypnea (respiratory rate of 30 to 50 breaths/min).

In class 4 patients, the volume deficit exceeds 40 percent. These patients are in profound shock and frequently have no discernible blood pressure. They may have absent pulses in their extremities and are oliguric or anuric. If volume therapy is not quickly begun, circulatory collapse and cardiac arrest will soon result.

After acute blood loss, the hematocrit will not change significantly for at least 4 hours, and complete compensation requires 48 hours. Infusion of intravenous fluids can alter this relationship, resulting in earlier lowering of measured hematocrit. When significant hemorrhage is thought to have occurred, a hematocrit should always be obtained. If this result shows a significant fall from a previous baseline value, a large amount of blood has been lost. Measures should immediately be taken to evaluate the source of the loss and whether the hemorrhage is ongoing but unrecognized.

Narcotics, which are frequently used for pain relief in the immediate postoperative period, can significantly reduce the ability of the sympathetic nervous system to effect vasoconstriction of the arterial and venous compartments. If these medications are given to a hypovolemic patient, serious hypotension can result. Signs and symptoms of hypovolemia should always be sought before the postoperative patient is given narcotic analgesics on the first post-partum day.

URINE OUTPUT—"THE WINDOW OF BODY PERFUSION"

In hypovolemic patients, urine output must be carefully monitored. In many cases, the urine output will fall before other signs of impaired perfusion are manifest. In contrast, adequate urine volume in patients who have not received diuretics strongly suggests perfusion to vital body organs is adequate.

Reasonable correlation exists between renal blood flow and urine output. If the urine output is low, renal blood flow is often low as well. When there is a rapid decrease in renal blood flow, there is usually a reduction in urine output. Urine will become more concentrated and will have a lower concentration of sodium and a higher osmolarity. With a gradual fall in renal blood flow, the urine sodium and osmolarity will often be affected before any significant fall in urine output. A urine sodium concentration of less than 10 to 20 mEq/L or a urine/serum osmolar ratio of greater than 2 usually indicates reduced renal perfusion.

BLOOD LOSS IN SEVERE PREECLAMPSIA

Major blood loss in a patient with severe preeclampsia may present a confusing picture. One must be aware of the altered hemo-dynamic status of these patients to appreciate the extent of the volume loss and to ensure appropriate fluid replacement. In severe preeclampsia, the blood volume has frequently failed to expand and is similar to that in a nonpregnant woman. These patients will not have the protective effect of the usual volume expansion of pregnancy and will show signs of blood loss earlier. In these cases, however, blood pressure can be a misleading indicator of volume. A blood pressure appropriate for a previously normotensive patient could indicate serious volume depletion in the preeclamptic woman. It is especially important to record serial pressures. If the blood pressure shows a significant drop during the immediate postoperative or postpartum period, a volume deficit should be suspected because hypertension usually persists for days to weeks in patients with severe preeclampsia.

When significant hemorrhage occurs in the woman with hypertension, it may be important to supplement the crystalloid fluid resuscitation with colloidal fluids pending the availability of the best colloid, whole blood. Albumin (5 percent) may be given in the ratio of 500 ml of albumin for every 4 L of crystalloid. This form of therapy will help compensate for the low albumin and total protein concentrations present in the patient with severe preeclampsia. It is not uncommon for these women to have total protein levels less than 5.0 g/dl with an albumin concentration below 2.5 g/dl. If crystalloid fluids are given alone, massive fluid accumulation in the already overexpanded extravascular space can occur and may result in cerebral as well as pulmonary edema.[1]

TREATMENT

Patients showing signs of class 2 or greater volume loss should receive crystalloid intravenous fluids pending the arrival of blood and blood products. The infusion rate should be rapid, between 1,000 and 2,000 ml in 30 to 45 minutes, or faster if the patient is obviously hypotensive. This infusion may serve as a therapeutic trial to help determine the amount of blood loss. If the physical signs and symptoms return to normal and remain stable after this challenge, no further therapy may be needed. If blood loss has been severe and the patient continues to bleed, however, this favorable response may be only transient. In this situation, typed and cross-matched blood should be given. The initial administration of a balanced salt solution will reduce the amount of whole blood needed to restore an adequate blood volume.[2]

Blood and Blood Products

Whole Blood

The use of whole blood has been discouraged and in many instances discontinued by blood banking centers around the United States. In obstetrics, the main indication for whole blood rather than component therapy is massive blood loss requiring more than a 4,000-ml replacement (Table 12–2).

For many years, the anticoagulant cpda-1 has been used to preserve whole blood. With cpda-1 the useful life of a unit of whole blood is 35 days. Recently, a new system for red cell preservation has been developed using the red cell preservative Optisol. This extends the shelf life of red cells from 35 days to 42 days, and the ability to extract larger volumes of fresh frozen plasma (FFP) from each unit of whole blood. The expansion of the shelf life is a

Table 12-2. BLOOD REPLACEMENT

Product	Cost/Unit	Contents	Volume (ml)	Effect
Whole blood (WB)	$97	Red blood cells (2,3—DPG) White blood cells (not functional after 24 hours) Coagulation factors (50%—V, VIII after 7 days) Plasma proteins	500	Increase volume (ml/ml) Increase hematocrit 3%/unit
Packed red cells	$97	Red blood cells—same as whole blood White blood cells—less than whole blood Plasma proteins—few	240	Same red blood cells as whole blood Less risk febrile, or WBC transfusion reaction Increase hematocrit 3%/unit
Platelets	$47	55×10^6 platelets/units, few white blood cells	50	Increase platelet count 5,000–10,000 µl/unit Give 6 packs minimum
Fresh frozen plasma	$50	Clotting factors V and VIII, fibrinogen	250	Only source of factors V, XI, XII Increase fibrinogen 10 mg/dl/unit
Cryoprecipitate	$30	Factor VIII 25% Fibrinogen von Willebrand factor	40	Increase fibrinogen 10 mg/dl/unit
Albumin 5%	$54	Albumin	500	
Albumin 2.5%	$54	Albumin	50	

particular advantage and should make the autologous blood donation available to more patients. The main disadvantage is that its
adoption by the blood bank eliminates the availability of whole
blood for transfusion. The other consideration is for neonates in
whom large volumes of adenine and mannitol contained in Optisol
may be toxic.

Massive Blood Transfusion

Massive transfusion is an ill-defined term but can generally be
thought of as the need to replace a patient's entire blood volume in
24 hours or less.[3] In a pregnant patient, this is usually 10 or more
units of blood. Essentials of management of the patient requiring
massive transfusion include maintenance of circulation, blood volume, oxygen-carrying capacity, hemostasis, colloid osmotic pressure, and biochemical balance. If massive obstetric bleeding exists,
two units of O-negative packed cells are immediately sent to the
delivery suite from the hospital emergency supply and an order is
also sent to the blood center for immediate release of 4 units of
uncross-matched packed red cells, 6 units of platelets, and 10 bags
of cryoprecipitate. Emergency blood studies include coagulation
studies, arterial blood gas, and an additional tube for cross-match.
(If platelets are $<100,000$, 6 units of platelets are transfused; if
fibrinogen is <125 mg/dl, 10 bags of cryoprecipitate are transfused;
if international normalized ratio [INR] is >1.5 or massive bleeding
is encountered, then 4 units of AB plasma are thawed and transfused.) A flow sheet is useful to keep track of products used, medications given, laboratory results, and intravenous fluids.

Metabolic derangements are less common than once encountered
with massive transfusion. Hypocalcemia is a theoretical problem,
but clinical syndromes from this problem are infrequently described
and the possible complications of prophylactic calcium infusion
may be more harmful than hypocalcemia. Hypocalcemia can be
clinically important if combined with hyperkalemia and hypothermia, a triad that can lead to cardiac arrhythmias. Hypothermia can
be a problem if the recently refrigerated blood is administered at
a rate of 1 unit every 5 to 10 minutes. If this rate of administration
is required, attempts should be made to warm the blood above
4 °C before transfusion. Close attention should also be paid to the
electrocardiogram. If arrhythmias are noted, supplemental calcium
should be considered.

Acid–base problems, namely citrate toxicity are rarely a problem
because the healthy liver can metabolize the citrate in a unit of
blood in 5 minutes. Unless transfusion rates exceed 1 unit per
5 minutes or the liver is previously diseased, citrate toxicity should
not be a problem. Stored blood has an acid pH, but acidosis is

uncommon because metabolism of citrate produces alkalosis. Prolonged acidosis is more often the result of hypoperfusion and shock rather than blood replacement. Blood gas measurement should guide the therapy with bicarbonate in this instance.

Packed Red Blood Cells

Packed red blood cells (PRBCs) are the most effective and efficient way to provide increased oxygen-carrying capacity to the anemic patient. Unless a patient has suffered massive blood loss, PRBCs and crystalloid will satisfy most clinical needs. Oxygen-carrying capacity may become impaired in the euvolemic patient when the hemoglobin level drops below 7 g/dl. If adequate volume replacement has not been accomplished, patients may exhibit orthostatic blood pressure changes or other signs of impaired oxygen-carrying capacity at hemoglobin levels above 7 g/dl. Because a unit of PRBCs has small amounts of white blood cells (WBCs) and iso-hemagglutinins (anti-A and anti-B), its use reduces the incidence of nonhemolytic transfusion reactions compared with that of 1 unit of whole blood. However, care should be taken to administer PRBCs with normal saline rather than lactated Ringer's or dextrose solutions. These solutions can cause the blood to clot or the red cells to lyse.

Platelets

A unit of platelets derived from a single unit of whole blood has a shelf life of 72 hours. Transfusion of a single unit of platelets can raise the platelet count between 5,000 and 10,000/µl in a patient who has no antiplatelet antibodies and a normal sized spleen. The survival of transfused platelets can be as long at 3 to 5 days but will be shorter if disseminated intravascular coagulation (DIC) is present. Platelets should be administered rapidly, over 10 minutes, with repeat laboratory evaluation performed 2 hours after infusion. For the obstetric patient, platelets should be ABO and Rh specific. Sensitization can be prevented by concomitant administration of Rh-immune globulin. One 300-µg dose will prevent sensitization for 30 platelet packs. Each unit of random donor platelets carries the transfusion risk of a single unit of blood.

In general, platelet counts below 50,000/µl will require transfusion prior to or during surgery. However, when the need for a cesarean delivery arises in patients with platelet counts ranging from 20,000 to 50,000 platelets, transfusion may be avoided or the amount reduced if the transfusion is delayed until the need becomes apparent. This is usually evident from bleeding from skin edges, as hemostasis in the uterus is primarily a function of uterine muscle contraction, not platelet function.

Cryoprecipitate

Prepared by warming fresh frozen plasma and collecting the precipitate, cryoprecipitate contains significant amounts of factor VIII, factor XIII, fibrinogen, and von Willebrands' factor. ABO compatibility is necessary only in infants, given their small size. In pregnant patients, Rh-compatible cryoprecipitate should be used whenever possible. If not possible, Rh-immune globulin should be administered within 72 hours of transfusion. One 20-ml unit of cryoprecipitate will contain 200 mg of fibrinogen, but results in only a 5 mg/dl rise in fibrinogen per bag of cryoprecipitate transfused because only 75 percent of the fibrinogen remains in the intravascular space after transfusion.

Fresh Frozen Plasma

Fresh frozen plasma is the plasma harvested from a unit of whole blood. FFP contains all coagulation factors in normal concentrations without platelets, leukocytes, or red blood cells. Transfusion of FFP need not be Rh compatible but should be ABO compatible. Fresh frozen plasma should be administered when both volume replacement and coagulation factors are needed. The main clinical indication for this therapy is the massively hemorrhaging patient. If the prothrombin time (PT) or partial thromboplastin time (PTT) are at least 50 percent prolonged or the international normalized ratio (INR) is greater than 1.5, there is usually a 70 percent reduction in factor levels present. A 10 percent increase in factor levels will usually be required for significant change in coagulation status. The required dose of FFP in this instance will be 4,250-ml units.

Recently introduced to the market is a second type of FFP, manufactured by the Vitex Corporation, solvent/detergent-treated plasma and produced by pooling approximately 2,500 units of donor plasma. The product is treated with a solvent and a detergent, which together are very effective in destroying the lipid envelope viruses. Coagulation factors are equivalent to FFP, with elimination of the risk of viruses. Disadvantages include exposure of many donors because of the pooled nature of the preparation, and cost, approximately three times that of FFP.

Autologous Transfusion

Primarily as the result of fear of acquiring the acquired immunodeficiency syndrome (AIDS) virus from blood transfusion, interest in autologous blood transfusion for pregnant patients was heightened in past years. Autologous transfusion can be accomplished in two ways. In the most common approach, blood is collected and stored during the weeks before delivery. In the past this presented some logistic problems for the pregnant patient, since 3 weeks was the longest time that blood can be stored. Currently, blood storage has been extended to 35 days and, with the advent of a new solution for blood storage, another week can be added to the shelf life of donated blood (see prior section). Although predelivery autologous blood donation is generally safe for both mother and fetus, the low incidence of blood transfusion in patients at the time of childbirth and the safety of allogeneic transfusion has limited enthusiasm on the part of health care professionals. Studies have questioned the cost effectiveness of autologous transfusion in general.[4] Since the incidence of transfusion in pregnant patients is significantly lower than the incidence of transfusion in operative patients, predelivery autologous blood donation in pregnant patients is probably not cost effective.

The chance of acquiring HIV from a unit of donated and screened blood is now approximately 1 in 700,000. Antepartum patients inquiring about antalogous transfusion should be counseled that the chance of needing a blood transfusion is about 1 in 80 overall. Risk exceeds 1 percent when emergency cesarean delivery becomes necessary or if placenta previa exists.[5-7] Coupled with the low risk of acquiring HIV from a donated unit of blood, the a priori risk of a low-risk patient needing a blood transfusion and subsequently acquiring HIV is less than 1 in 20 million.

A second type of autologous donation involves intraoperative blood salvage, which can occur at the time of excessive blood loss. This technique has limitations in the obstetric setting. Heavy bacterial contamination is one contraindication, and the use during cesarean delivery had been questioned because of the possibility of amniotic fluid, fetal debris, and bacterial contamination. Recently, a clinical report of 139 patients who were transfused with autologous blood using Cell Saver technology (Haemonetics, Braintree, MA) has been published.[8] There were no differences in infections, respiratory, or coagulation abnormalities when the autologous transfused patients were compared to patients with similar conditions transfused with donor blood products. This technique may be useful in patients in whom anticipated blood loss is high. It may be acceptable to Jehovah's Witness patients and has the potential to add a significant margin of safety for these patients.

Transfusion Risks

PRBCs, fresh frozen plasma, cryoprecipitate, and platelets have the same risk of transmitting infectious diseases as a unit of whole blood. See the box "Risks of Blood Transfusion" for common risks of blood transfusion when blood is procured from volunteer donors. The risks of serious complications from blood transfusion have fallen to very low rates, although blood obtained from paid sources can be expected to have higher rates of many of the complications listed in the box.

Risks of Blood Transfusion: Transfusion Risks Table[9-11]

A. Viral infection
   HIV-1, HIV-2   1/700,000
   Hepatitis B   1/140,000
   Hepatitis C*   1/90,000
   HTLV I and II   1/641,000

B. Bacterial contamination
   Red cells   1/500,000
   Platelets   1/12,000

C. Reactions
   Acute hemolytic reaction   1/600,000
   Delayed hemolytic reaction   1/1,000
   Acute lung injury   1/5,000

---

*In 1999, trials were begun to screen blood with a PCR test for HCV RNA. It is anticipated that there will be a significant reduction in the transmission of hepatitis C but reliable data are not currently available.

Transfusion of an incompatible blood component results in a hemolytic transfusion reaction. They are usually due to clerical errors or to misidentification of the patient or unit of blood. Naturally occurring antibodies in the ABO system are the usual causes. Hemolytic transfusion reactions may result in DIC or acute renal failure. The clinical signs of acute hemolytic transfusion reaction may include some or all of the following: severe anxiety, flushing, chest or back pain, fever, hypotension, tachycardia, or dyspnea. In an anesthetized patient, hemoglobinuria may be the first noticeable sign. A rapid diagnostic test is the discovery of reddish plasma after centrifugation of a red-top tube of blood. Upon recognition, the transfusion should be stopped, and the blood returned to the blood center along with a tube of the patient's blood. Treatment with fluids, diuretics, and transfusion support for bleeding are the cornerstone of therapy.

Fever after or during transfusion is usually, but not always, related to sensitization of antigens on cell components, usually leukocytes. However, fever can also be the first sign of sepsis related to bacterial contamination of red cells or platelets.

Transfusion-related acute lung injury is an acute respiratory distress syndrome occurring within 4 hours of transfusion. It is characterized by dyspnea and hypoxemia secondary to noncardiogenic pulmonary edema and is estimated to occur with a frequency of greater than 1 in 5,000 transfusions.

ANTEPARTUM HEMORRHAGE

Abruptio Placenta

The premature separation of the normally implanted placenta from the uterus is called *abruptio placenta* or *placental abruption*. Diagnosis of placental abruption is certain when inspection of the placenta shows an adherent retroplacental clot with depression or disruption of the underlying placental tissue; however, this frequently is not found if the abruption is of recent onset. Clinical findings indicating placental abruption include the triad of external or occult uterine bleeding, uterine hypertonus and/or hyperactivity, and fetal distress and/or fetal death. Placental abruption can be broadly classified into three grades that correlate with clinical and laboratory findings.

Grade 1: Slight vaginal bleeding and some uterine irritability are usually present. Maternal blood pressure is unaffected, and the maternal fibrinogen level is normal. The fetal heart rate pattern is normal.

Grade 2: External uterine bleeding is mild to moderate. The uterus is irritable, and tetanic or very frequent contractions may be present. Maternal blood pressure is maintained, but the pulse rate may be elevated and postural blood volume deficits may be present. The fibrinogen level may be decreased. The fetal heart rate often shows signs of fetal compromise.

Grade 3: Bleeding is moderate to severe but may be concealed. The uterus is tetanic and painful. Maternal hypotension is frequently present and fetal death has occurred. Fibrinogen levels are often reduced to less than 150 mg/dl; other coagulation abnormalities (thrombocytopenia, factor depletion) are present.

Etiology

Studies have suggested an increased incidence of abruption in patients with advanced parity or age, maternal smoking, poor nutrition, cocaine use, and chorioamnionitis.[15–19]

Maternal hypertension (>140/90 mm Hg) seems to be the most consistently identified factor.[22] This relationship is true for all grades of placental abruption but is most strongly associated with grade 3 abruption, in which 40 to 50 percent of cases are found to have hypertensive disease of pregnancy.[20,22]

Blunt external maternal trauma is an increasingly important cause of placental abruption. Two conditions account for the majority of blunt abdominal trauma leading to placental abruption: motor vehicle collision and maternal battering. Historically, 1 to 2 percent of grade 3 abruptions have been attributed to maternal trauma.[22,23] However, recent epidemiologic studies show an alarmingly high incidence of maternal battering in some populations.[24] These data make it incumbent on the obstetrician to consider placental abruption when a history of trauma is elicited and vice versa.

Rapid decompression of the overdistended uterus is an uncommon cause of placental abruption. This may occur in patients with multiple gestations and those with polyhydramnios. When rapid decompression of the uterus is apparent, abruption is usually observed after the delivery of the first fetus. To avoid rapid decompression of the uterus in polyhydramnios, amniotic fluid should be slowly released by amniocentesis before induction of labor or once spontaneous labor has been established.

Acquired or inherited thrombophilias are also significant factors in the etiology of placental abruption.[25] In one study of Jewish women, mutations of one or more of three thrombolphilic mutations (e.g. factor V Leiden mutation) were present in 60 percent of women who had suffered placental abruption. However the presence of factor V Leiden mutation in the control population was much higher (17 percent) than in the comparable white United States population (5 percent).

There exists a significant recurrence rate for placental abruption. This figure has been reported to vary from 5 percent to 17 percent.[13,17,22] If a patient has suffered an abruption in two pregnancies, the chance for recurrence is 25 percent. The recurrence rate of severe placental abruption again resulting in fetal demise is 11 percent.

Diagnosis and Management

Ultrasound can identify three predominant locations for placental abruption. These are subchorionic (between the placenta and the membranes), retroplacental (between the placenta and the myometrium), and preplacental (between the placenta and the amniotic fluid). Hematomas identified by ultrasound during the early phases of vaginal bleeding and pain are most likely to be hyperechoic or isoechoic compared with the placenta. As the hematoma resolves, it will become hypoechoic within a week and sonolucent within 2 weeks.[29] Because of the changing character of the hematoma, misinterpretation of a hematoma as uterine myoma, succenturiate placental lobe, chorioangioma, or molar pregnancy may occur.

Nearly 80 percent of patients who eventually prove to have a placental abruption will present with vaginal bleeding, but 20 percent fail to exhibit external signs of bleeding. These patients have a concealed abruption and are commonly given the diagnosis of premature labor. On some occasions, the abruption may progress despite successful tocolysis, and fetal death may result. Other signs of placental abruption include increased uterine tenderness and tone.

Once the diagnosis of placental abruption has been made, precautions should be taken to deal with the possible life-threatening consequences for both mother and fetus. At least 4 units of blood should be available for maternal transfusions. A large-bore (16-gauge) intravenous line must be secured and the infusion of a crystalloid solution begun. Blood should be drawn for hemoglobin and hematocrit determinations and coagulation studies (fibrinogen, platelet count, fibrin degradation products, PT, PTT). A red-topped tube should also be obtained and used to perform a clot test. If a clot does not form within 6 minutes or forms and lyses within 30 minutes, a coagulation defect is probably present and the fibrinogen level is less than 150 mg/dl. Continuous fetal monitoring should be used to record fetal heart rate and document uterine activity.

In many cases of placental abruption, delivery will be the treatment of choice. During labor, careful attention must be paid to several maternal and fetal parameters. Because 60 percent of fetuses may exhibit signs of intrapartum fetal distress, continuous fetal heart rate monitoring is essential. In a similar manner, continuous monitoring of maternal volume status is important. Serial maternal hematocrit determinations should be made regularly at intervals of 2 to 3 hours. The goal of therapy should be to maintain a maternal urine output of 1 ml/min and a hematocrit of at least 30 percent.

Placental abruption frequently stimulates the clotting cascade, resulting in DIC. Intravascular fibrinogen is converted to fibrin by activation of the extrinsic clotting cascade. In the usual clinical setting, platelets and clotting factors V and VIII are also depleted. Serial measurements of plasma fibrinogen provide valuable information regarding the coagulation status of the patient and will help estimate the volume of blood loss that has occurred.

The normal maternal fibrinogen concentration in the third trimester is 450 mg/dl. When the fibrinogen value drops below 300 mg/dl, significant coagulation abnormalities are usually present. Most women with significant falls in fibrinogen will require blood transfusion to maintain a normal circulating volume. If fibrinogen is less than 150 mg/dl, most patients will have already lost 2,000 ml of blood. The signs and symptoms of such blood loss may not be obvious because, as noted earlier, the normal hypervolemia of pregnancy protects the mother from a volume loss that a nonpregnant individual could not tolerate. Rapid crystalloid infusion of at least 1,000 ml pending the availability of whole blood should be done to maintain euvolemia. Two to 3 ml of crystalloid should be given for each 1 ml of blood lost.

If urine output fails to reach 30 ml/h despite adequate volume replacement, consideration should be given to inserting a central venous pressure (CVP) catheter to determine the adequacy of intravascular volume. The absolute level of CVP is less important than the response of the CVP to volume infusion, so long as the CVP is less than 7 cm H_2O in response to the preceding 250-ml aliquot. If this response has been achieved but the urine output is still inadequate, consideration should be given to replacing the CVP catheter with a pulmonary artery catheter.

Considerable controversy remains regarding the appropriate method of delivery in patients with placental abruption. A number of patients present with a live fetus, only to have that fetus die undelivered while awaiting vaginal delivery.[12,15] Retrospective reviews show increased fetal survival in patients who have undergone cesarean delivery once the maternal condition has been stabilized. However, these reports surveyed a period in which intrapartum fetal monitoring was routine. Currently, the use of continuous electronic fetal monitoring in this situation is associated with excellent fetal survival, and cesarean delivery can be reserved for cases with fetal distress or other traditional obstetric indications.[13] The cesarean section rate associated with placental abruption is 50 to 75 percent, depending on the clinical aggressiveness of the physicians managing the patient.[35]

Restoration of a normal blood volume and coagulation status is the sine qua non of treatment. Patients with severe placental abruption often have a blood pressure that appears quite normal. However, this is a false interpretation because 50 percent of patients will exhibit hypertension once adequate volume replacement has been accomplished. Adequate volume status in this situation is best achieved by ensuring a urine output of at least 30 ml/h.

Some clinicians believe that if placental abruption has progressed to fetal death and severe coagulopathy, cesarean delivery will result in the quickest resolution of maternal problems. However, operating in the presence of a coagulopathy can result in prolonged operative times secondary to surgically uncontrollable bleeding. Bleeding from all cut surfaces at the time of cesarean delivery usually occur with fibrinogen levels of less than 150 mg/dl. Hemorrhage after vaginal delivery is not correlated with fibrinogen levels unless there were extensive vaginal lacerations or uterine atony. In current obstetric practice, administration of coagulation factor replacement along with PRBCs is the treatment of choice in patients with DIC. Even in the face of a severe coagulopathy, induction to delivery times exceeding 18 hours may result in equal or better maternal outcome as long as maternal volume status and coagulation status can be maintained.[14]

Irrespective, induction of labor should be initiated soon as adequate volume status is accomplished and blood products are available. This can usually be accomplished with oxytocin. Many patients are already experiencing some uterine activity, oftentimes hypertonic in nature.

When cesarean delivery is necessary, extravasation of blood into the uterine muscle to produce red to purple discoloration of the serosal surface will be found in 8 percent of patients. This finding, known as a Couvelaire uterus, has been feared to result in a high incidence of uterine hemorrhage secondary to atony. However, atony is the exception and most patients with a Couvelaire uterus demonstrate an appropriate response to the infusion of oxytocin. Hysterectomy should be reserved for cases of atony and hemorrhage unresponsive to conventional uterotonics.

Placenta Previa

In placenta previa implantation of the placenta occurs over the cervical os. There are three recognized variations of placenta previa: total, partial, and marginal (Fig. 12–2). In total placenta previa, the cervical os is completely covered by the placenta. This type presents the most serious maternal risk, as it is associated with greater blood loss than either marginal or partial placenta previa. Partial placenta previa is defined as the partial occlusion of the cervical os by the placenta. A marginal placenta previa is characterized by the encroachment of the placenta to the margin of the cervical os. It does not cover the os. The differentiation of the latter two degrees of placenta previa is dependent on the dilatation of the cervix and the method of diagnosis (ultrasound or direct examination).

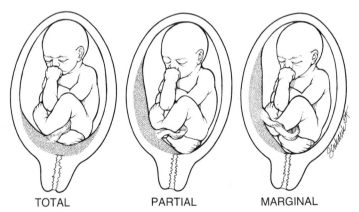

TOTAL   PARTIAL   MARGINAL

Figure 12–2. Three variations of placenta previa.

A leading cause of third-trimester hemorrhage, placenta previa presents classically as painless bleeding. Bleeding is thought to occur in association with the development of the lower uterine segment in the third trimester. Placental attachment is disrupted as this area gradually thins in preparation for the onset of labor. When this occurs, bleeding occurs at the implantation site, as the uterus is unable to contract adequately and stop the flow of blood from the open vessels.

Significant epidemiologic risk factors are maternal age above 35 years and black or other minority races and previous cesarean delivery. The risk for placenta previa occurring in the pregnancy following a cesarean delivery has been reported to be between 1 and 4 percent.[41,44–47] There is a linear increase in placenta previa risk with the number of prior cesarean deliveries, such that patients with four or more cesarean deliveries the risk of placenta previa approaches 10 percent.[44]

Whereas third-trimester bleeding was once a common presentation for placenta previa, most cases of placenta previa are now detected antenatelly prior to the onset of significant bleeding. The common practice of second-trimester ultrasound for detection of fetal anomalies has led to this change. However, because most cases of placenta previa diagnosed in the second trimester will resolve, management of placenta previa diagnosed in the second trimester will differ from the same diagnosis in the third trimester. At 17 weeks' gestation, evidence of placental tissue covering the cervical os will be found in 5 to 15 percent of all patients.[42] More than 90 percent of these patients will have a normal ultrasound by 37 weeks' gestation.[48] This phenomenon has been termed *placental migration*. Changes in architecture secondary to differential growth of the lower uterine segment during the second and third trimesters probably account for this observation. Total placenta previa diagnosed in the second trimester will persist into the third trimester in 26 percent of cases, whereas marginal or partial placenta previa will persist in only 2.5 percent of cases.[49]

In patients diagnosed prior to 24 weeks' gestation, a repeat ultrasound should be scheduled between 24 and 28 weeks' gestation to confirm the resolution of the radiographic diagnosis of placenta previa. However, if patients have vaginal bleeding during this time period, they should be assumed to have placenta previa. Similarly, placenta previa should be suspected in all patients presenting with bleeding after 24 weeks' gestation.

For the patient who is remote from term (24 to 36 weeks' gestation), expectant management is the treatment of choice. The essence of this approach is maintenance of the fetus in a healthy intrauterine environment without jeopardizing maternal condition. Maternal blood loss should be replaced in order to maintain the maternal hematocrit between 30 and 35 percent. Even an initial blood loss in excess of 500 ml can be expectantly managed with adequate volume replacement.

Patients with third-trimester bleeding though due to placenta previa should be treated similar to that outlined in the section on abruptio placenta (e.g., maternal stabilization, fetal monitoring). However, blood studies do not need to be as extensive as those ordered for patients with placental abruption because DIC is rare in cases of placenta previa.

In the patient who is unequivocally at 37 weeks' gestation with evidence of uterine activity or with persistent bleeding, delivery is the treatment of choice. In previous years, a double setup examination was the initial step in this process. With the early diagnosis of placenta previa and rapid and reliable ultrasound availability and interpretation, this technique is now unnecessary in the most cases.

Rarely, vaginal delivery may still be considered with marginal or partial placenta previa in women who present in labor with minimal bleeding.

Although obstetricians are most concerned about maternal hemorrhage, they must remember that fetal blood can also be lost during the process of placental separation. Rh-immune globulin should be given to all at-risk patients with third-trimester bleeding who are Rh-negative and unsensitized.

Because of the reduced risk of cardiovascular complications, magnesium sulfate has become the agent of choice for the treatment of patients in preterm labor with placenta previa at many institutions. Infusion of a 6-g loading dose followed by 3 g/h or more are often necessary to control uterine irritability because of the increased maternal glomerular filtration rate. Once the patient has been stabilized on magnesium sulfate, the use of oral tocolytics has been advocated by some, although no conclusive studies demonstrate improved outcome with oral tocolytic therapy for any indication. Patients may occasionally require more than 1 week of continuous intravenous tocolytic therapy. The use of antenatal corticosteroids to accelerate fetal pulmonary maturity is effective in reducing the incidence of neonatal respiratory distress syndrome, intracranial hemorrhage, and neonatal death.[57,58] Given a high incidence of respiratory distress syndrome in the infants of mothers requiring delivery after failed expectant management (24 to 41 percent),[42,59] antenatal steroids should be given in patients presenting between 25 and 33 weeks. Data on safety of repeated weekly doses of steroids are concerning enough that this practice is currently not recommended outside of investigational protocols.

If the mother responds to conservative management, she should be treated with bed rest, preferably in the hospital setting. Blood should always be available for maternal transfusion in the event of sudden hemorrhage.

Approximately 25 to 30 percent of patients can be expected to complete 36 weeks' gestation without labor or repetitive bleeding forcing earlier delivery. In these patients, amniocentesis should be performed and, if the analysis of amniotic fluid documents pulmonary maturity, a cesarean delivery planned.

When encountering a patient with placenta previa, the possibility of a placenta accreta or one of its variations, placenta percreta or placenta increta, should be considered (Fig. 12–3).[62] In this condition, the placenta forms an abnormally firm attachment to the uterine wall. There is absence of the decidua basalis and incomplete development of the fibrinoid layer. The placenta can be attached directly to the myometrium (accreta), invade the myometrium (increta), or penetrate the myometrium (percreta). Antenatal diagnosis with ultrasound or MRI is possible.[63,64] Ultrasound findings most predictive of placenta accreta are thinning and distortion of the uterine serosa–bladder interface. Color Doppler imaging can also be useful.

Prior cesarean delivery and other uterine surgery are the factors most often associated with placenta accreta. In patients with previous cesarean delivery who have placenta previa, the incidence of placenta accreta is approximately 10 to 35 percent.[44,47] In patients with multiple cesarean deliveries and placenta previa the risk of accreta is 60 to 65 percent. At least two thirds of the patients with placenta previa/placenta accreta will require cesarean hysterectomy.[42,65,66] However, in cases where uterine preservation is highly desired and no bladder invasion has occurred, bleeding after pla-

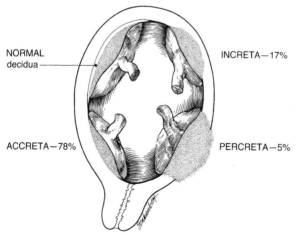

Figure 12–3. Uteroplacental relationships found in abnormal placentation.

cental removal has been successfully controlled with a variety of surgical techniques.

If uterine preservation is not important, or if maternal blood loss is excessive, hysterectomy offers the best chance for survival and will minimize morbidity.[70] If uterine preservation is important, four treatment options are available:

1. *Placental removal and oversewing the uterine defects.* After removing as much of the placenta as possible, the bleeding defects are oversewed and the patient treated with oxytocics and antibiotics (this option is probably most useful when there is significant bleeding from a partially separated placenta with only a focal accreta).

2. *Localized resection and uterine repair.*

3. *Curettage of the uterine cavity, and leaving the placenta in situ.* For the patient who wishes to maximize her chances for uterine preservation and who is not actively bleeding, the placenta may be left in situ. The umbilical cord should be ligated and cut as close to its base as possible. The patient should then be treated with antibiotics. This approach has been successful when bleeding has not necessitated more aggressive surgical procedures.[71] Some authors have advocated treatment with methotrexate in this instance, but there is presently no consensus on whether this therapy is any more effective than observation.

4. In rare cases, placenta accreta invades the maternal bladder. In this instance, it is probably best to treat in a manner similar to abdominal pregnancy and avoid placental removal. However, this may not obviate the need for eventual hysterectomy and partial cystectomy.[72,73]

Vasa Previa and Succenturiate Placenta

A rare but important cause of third-trimester bleeding is rupture of a fetal vessel. Vasa previa is a condition in which the fetal vessels traverse the membranes in the lower uterine segment and cover the cervical os and occurs in approximately 1 in 1,000 to 1 in 5,000 pregnancies. With velamentous insertion of the umbilical cord, vessels often run between the chorion and amnion without the protection of Wharton's jelly. In other instances, a succenturiate placenta will have vascular communications between placental cotyledons. The classic presentation is spontaneous rupture of membranes, laceration of a fetal vessel, and rapid fetal death.

Ultrasound imaging now makes it possible to diagnose this condition in some instances, prior to the onset of fetal bleeding. Diagnosis of a succenturiate placental cotyledon or the discovery of an anomaly of the umbilical cord insertion should prompt the use of color Doppler examination of the membranes over the cervix. Both transabdominal and transcervical imaging have been used for this purpose. When umbilical arterial waveforms are documented at the same rate as the fetal heart rate, diagnosis is confirmed. When this occurs, careful observation and timing of elective cesarean section upon documentation of fetal pulmonary maturity should be considered.

When the fetal vessel ruptures, often acute vaginal bleeding is associated with an abrupt change in the fetal heart rate. The fetal heart rate pattern often shows an initial fetal tachycardia followed by bradycardia with intermittent accelerations. Short-term variability may be maintained.

One must make the diagnosis rapidly and institute definitive therapy and delivery to optimize fetal outcome. The fetal mortality in this condition has been reported to be greater than 50 percent.[74,75]

On occasion when the fetal heart rate is not abnormal and the source of the bleeding is in question, an examination of the blood passed vaginally can be performed. Adult oxyhemoglobin is less resistant to alkali than fetal oxyhemoglobin, permitting tests for fetal hemoglobin using alkaline denaturation: Apt, Ogita, and Loendersloot.[76] All take from 5 to 10 minutes to perform and have good sensitivity for detection of pure fetal blood. However, the Ogita test is most reliable.

However, usually there is no time to perform this test. The diagnosis must be based on clinical findings unless there has been prior ultrasound suspicion of vasa previa.

POSTPARTUM HEMORRHAGE

Acute blood loss is the most common cause of hypotension in obstetrics. Hemorrhage usually occurs immediately preceding or after delivery of the placenta. Excessive blood loss most commonly results when the uterus fails to contract after the delivery of its contents. The prospect for dire problems becomes clear when one realizes that approximately 600 ml/min of blood flows through the placental site. Effective hemostasis after separation of the placenta is dependent on contraction of the myometrium to compress severed vessels. Failure of the uterus to contract can usually be attributed to myometrial dysfunction and retained placental fragments. Factors predisposing to myometrial dysfunction include overdistention of the uterus as in multiple pregnancy, fetal macrosomia, hydramnios, oxytocin-stimulated labor, uterine relaxants, and amnionitis.

Prevention

Reduction of excessive blood loss after vaginal birth or cesarean delivery can be aided by recognizing high-risk factors for postpartum hemorrhage (Table 12–3) and by applying proven methods to limit bleeding. Dilute solutions of oxytocin in addition to gentle cord traction reduces cesarean delivery associated blood loss by 31 percent compared with manual removal of the placenta.[77] Umbilical cord clamping within 30 seconds of delivery and gentle cord traction followed by administration of intramuscular or dilute solutions of intravenous oxytocin before delivery of the placenta reduce postpartum blood loss and postpartum transfusion requirements.[78] Administration of oxytocin before delivery of the placenta is associated with a reduction in the length of the third stage of labor (mean 5 minutes) and a low incidence of manual removal of the placenta (2 percent) compared with physiologic management of the third stage of labor (15 minutes and 2.5 percent, respectively).[78] In the absence of significant maternal hemorrhage, 30 minutes or more of expectant management can be allowed because half of the retained placentas will deliver spontaneously during this time, avoiding the need for manual removal, anesthesia, and excessive blood loss.

Upon encountering postpartum hemorrhage, manual digital exploration of the uterus should be quickly accomplished to rule out the possibility of retained placental fragments (Fig. 12–4). If retained tissue is not detected, manual massage of the uterus should be started (Fig. 12–5). Simultaneously, pharmacologic methods should be employed to control uterine bleeding. Initial therapy includes the administration of a dilute solution of oxytocin, usually 10 to 20 units of oxytocin in 1,000 ml of physiologic saline solu-

Table 12–3. RISK FACTORS FOR OBSTETRIC HEMORRHAGE OF >1,000 ML

Factor	Risk Increase
Placental abruption	12.6
Placenta previa	13.1
Multiple pregnancy	4.5
Obesity	1.6
Retained placenta	5.2
Induced labor	2.2
Episiotomy	2.1
Birth weight >4 kg	1.9

From Stones RW, Paterson CM, Saunders NJ: Risk factors for major obstetric hemorrhage. Eur J Obstet Gynecol Reprod Biol 48:15, 1993, with permission.

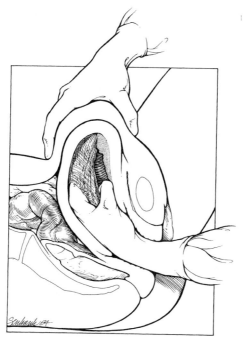

Figure 12–4. Digital exploration of the uterus and removal of retained membranes. A sponge has been wrapped around the examiner's fingers.

tion. The solution can be administered in rates as high as 500 ml in 10 minutes without cardiovascular complications. However, an intravenous bolus injection of as little as 5 units of oxytocin may be associated with maternal hypotension, further stressing an already compromised maternal cardiovascular system.

When oxytocin fails to produce adequate uterine contraction, most clinicians now administer synthetic 15-methyl-$F_{2\alpha}$ prostaglandin (Prostin, Upjohn). The efficacy and safety of prostaglandin medications in this instance have obviated the need to use ergonovine (0.2 mg intramuscularly) in most instances. Initial studies with prostaglandin medications for postpartum hemorrhage were performed with the naturally occurring $F_{2\alpha}$-prostaglandin compound, which required direct intrauterine injection. The total dose used was 1 to 2 mg diluted in 10 to 20 ml of saline.[80] Subsequently, clinical trials of the synthetic 15-methyl-$F_{2\alpha}$-prostaglandin produced promising results.[82] This compound should be given in 0.25-mg doses in the deltoid muscle every 1 to 2 hours. As many as five doses may be administered without adverse effect.

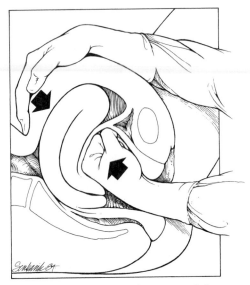

Figure 12–5. Manual compression and massage of the uterus to control bleeding from uterine atony.

Misoprostol, may represent a promising new medical option. O'Brien et al. recommend 1,000 μg of misoprostol per rectum in patients with refractory uterine bleeding prior to the administration of 15-methyl-$F_{2\alpha}$-prostaglandin.[81]

When pharmacologic methods fail to control hemorrhage from atony, surgical measures should be undertaken to arrest the bleeding before it becomes life threatening. However, before a laparotomy, a careful inspection of the vagina and cervix should be made to confirm that the uterus is the source of the bleeding.

A laceration of maternal soft tissues is the likely cause of continued vaginal bleeding. Careful inspection of the cervix and vagina will often indicate the source of the bleeding. Lacerations of the perineum must be recognized and repaired. Adequate exposure for the repair of such lacerations is critical and, if needed, assistance should be summoned to aid in retraction.

In cervical laceration, it is important to secure the base of the laceration, which is often a major source of bleeding. This area is frequently difficult to suture. Valuable time can be lost trying to expose the angle of such a laceration. A helpful technique especially when help is limited or slow in responding, is to start to suture the laceration at its proximal end, using the suture for traction to expose the more distal portion of the cervix until the apex is in view (Fig. 12–6). This technique has the added advantage of arresting significant bleeding from the edges of laceration.

When uterine bleeding is not responsive to pharmacologic methods and no vaginal or cervical lacerations are present, surgical exploration may be necessary. Laceration of uterine vessels during the birth process will occasionally be found. On occasion, bleeding will be similar to that from uterine atony, but the uterus will appear contracted. On other occasions, substantial episodic hemorrhage followed by periods of relatively little blood flow will occur. Longitudinal lacerations of the inner myometrium may be the cause of bleeding refractory to the usual techniques.[83]

If hemorrhage is secondary to atony, vascular ligation will often be necessary to control bleeding. Hypogastric artery ligation, a technique recommended for many decades to control postpartum hemorrhage, has fallen out of favor because of the prolonged operating time, technical difficulties and inconsistent clinical response.

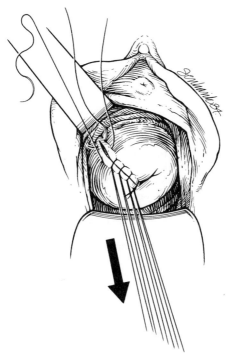

Figure 12–6. Repair of a cervical laceration, which begins at the proximal part of the laceration, using traction on the previous sutures to aid in exposing the distal portion of the defect.

Instead, a stepwise progression of uterine vessel ligation should be rapidly accomplished. Ligation of the ascending branch of the uterine arteries should be attempted as a first step if hemorrhage is unresponsive to oxytocin or prostaglandin[84,85] (Fig. 12–7A and B). The uterine artery should be located at the border between the upper and lower uterine segment and suture ligated with 0 or No. 1 chromic suture. The suture should be placed 2 cm medial to the uterine artery and the needle driven from the anterior surface of the uterus posteriorly and tied. Because the suture is placed high in the lower uterine segment, the ureter is not in jeopardy and the bladder usually does not need to be mobilized. In approximately 10 to 15 percent of cases of atony, unilateral ligation of the uterine artery is sufficient to control hemorrhage. Bilateral ligation will control an additional 75 percent.[85]

If bleeding continues, attention should next be paid to interrupting the blood flow to the uterus from the infundibulopelvic ligament (Fig. 12–7C). The easiest method involves ligation of the anastomosis of the ovarian and uterine artery, high on the fundus, just below the uterovarian ligament. A large suture on an atraumatic needle can be passed from the uterus, around the vessel, and tied. If bilateral uterovarian vessel ligation does not stop the bleeding, temporary occlusion of the infundibulopelvic ligament vessels may be attempted. This can be accomplished with digital pressure or with rubber-sleeved clamps. It may be an especially useful technique if the patient is of low parity and future childbearing is of great importance. If this appears to control hemorrhage, ligation of the infundibulopelvic ligament can be performed by passing an absorbable suture from anterior to posterior through the avascular area inferior to and including the ovarian vessels. Although the ovarian blood supply may be decreased, successful pregnancy has been reported after all major pelvic vessels were ligated to arrest postpartum hemorrhage.[72,73]

Two other surgical techniques can control of hemorrhage secondary to uterine atony: hemostatic suturing and the B-Lynch surgical technique.[87,88] Both of these techniques use surgical tamponade of the uterus to control bleeding. These techniques may be considered prior to hysterectomy in women of low parity in whom preservation of childbearing is desired.

A prerequisite to successful use of the B-Lynch or brace suture technique is the control of uterine bleeding with manual compression of the uterus. Assessment of bleeding should be done by direct visualization through the vagina by placing the patient in a supine frogleg position during the operation.

A final hemostatic suturing technique recently described involves placing multiple 2- to 3-cm^2 sutures in the myometrium using a through-and-through suture of No. 1 chromic. With this procedure, segments of the anterior and posterior uterine wall are sewn together and tied tightly, compressing the intervening myometrium.

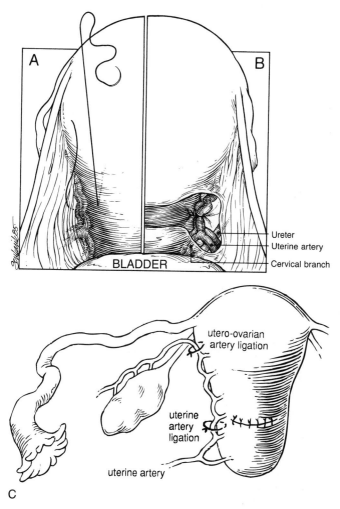

Figure 12–7. Ligation of the uterine artery. *A* and *B*, This anterior view of the uterus demonstrates the placement of a suture around the ascending branch of the uterine artery and vein as described by O'Leary and O'Leary. Note that 2 to 3 cm of myometrium medial to the vessels has been included in the ligature. The vessels are not divided. *C*, View of sutured uterus: ligated uterine artery, and ligated utero-ovarian artery.

Selective Arterial Embolization

Arterial embolization is currently an increasingly common therapeutic option for various types of obstetric hemorrhage. In the absence of coagulopathy, the success rate of arterial embolization has been reported to be greater than 90 percent.

Procedure-specific complications occur in less than 10 percent of cases. Postprocedure fever and pelvic infection are most commonly reported. Much less common, but potentially more serious, is reflux of embolic material to nontargeted pelvic structures. Premature ovarian failure may occur in older patients. Currently, there are no procedure-related deaths described in obstetric patients.

Pelvic Hematoma

Blood loss leading to cardiovascular instability is not always visible. In some instances, traumatic laceration of blood vessels may lead to the formation of a pelvic hematoma. Pelvic hematomas may be divided into three main types: vulvar, vaginal, or retroperitoneal.

Vulvar Hematoma

This type of hematoma results from laceration of vessels in the superficial fascia of either the anterior or posterior pelvic triangle. The usual physical signs are subacute volume loss and vulvar pain. The blood loss in this case is limited by Colle's fascia and the urogenital diaphragm. In the posterior area, the limitations are the anal fascia. Because of these fascial boundaries, the mass will extend to the skin and a visible hematoma will result.

Surgical management calls for wide linear incision of the mass through the skin and evacuation of blood and clots. As this condition is often the result of bleeding from small vessels, the lacerated vessel will not usually be identified. Once the clot has been evacuated, the dead space can be closed with sutures. The area should then be compressed by a large sterile dressing and pressure applied. An indwelling catheter should be placed in the bladder at the start of the surgical evacuation and left in place for 24 to 36 hours. Compression can be removed after 12 hours.

Vaginal Hematoma

Vaginal hematomas may result from trauma to maternal soft tissues during delivery. These hematomas are frequently associated with a forceps delivery but may occur spontaneously. They are less common than vulvar hematomas. In this instance, blood accumulates in the plane above the level of the pelvic diaphragm. It is unusual for large amounts of blood to collect in this space. The most frequent complaint in such cases is severe rectal pressure. Examination will reveal a large mass protruding into the vagina.

Vaginal hematomas should be treated by incision of the vagina and evacuation. As with vulvar hematomas, it is uncommon to find a single bleeding vessel as the source of bleeding. The incision need not be closed, as the edges of the vagina will fall back together after the clot has been removed. A vaginal pack should be inserted to tamponade the raw edges. The pack is then removed in 12 to 18 hours.

Retroperitoneal Hematoma

Retroperitoneal hematomas are the least common of the pelvic hematomas but are the most dangerous to the mother. Symptoms from a retroperitoneal hematoma may not be impressive until the sudden onset of hypotension or shock. A retroperitoneal hematoma occurs after laceration of one of the vessels originating from the hypogastric artery. Such lacerations may result from inadequate hemostasis of the uterine arteries at the time of cesarean delivery or after rupture of a low transverse cesarean delivery scar during a trial of labor. In these patients, blood may dissect up to the renal vasculature.

Treatment of this life-threatening condition involves surgical exploration and ligation of the hypogastric vessels on both the lacerated side and on the contralateral side if unilateral ligation does not arrest the bleeding. On occasion, it may be possible to open the hematomas and identify the bleeding vessel.

Inversion of the Uterus

Occasionally, the third stage of labor is complicated by partial delivery of the placenta followed by rapid onset of shock in the mother. These events characterize uterine inversion. Uterine inversion is an uncommon but life-threatening event. Hypotension usually results before significant blood loss has occurred. The inexperienced obstetrician may mistake an inversion of the uterus for a partially separated placenta or aborted myoma.

Treatment of uterine inversion should include fluid therapy for the mother and restoration of the uterus to its normal position. This latter is best accomplished using the technique illustrated in Figure 12–8 and should be attempted immediately upon recognition of the inversion. Separation of the placenta before replacement of the uterus will only increase maternal blood loss.[98] If possible, the uterus should be replaced without removing the placenta. Initial efforts to replace the uterus should be made without the use of uterine-relaxing agents. If initial efforts fail, the use of either β-mimetic agents or magnesium sulfate should be tried. In the case

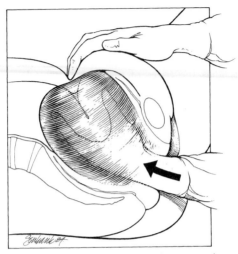

Figure 12–8. Manual replacement of an inverted uterus.

of severe maternal hypotension, magnesium sulfate is probably the best choice.

Occasionally, it is impossible to reposition the subacutely inverted uterus vaginally and laparotomy is necessary.

Once the uterine inversion has been corrected, the anesthetic agents used for uterine relaxation should be discontinued and oxytocic agents given to produce uterine contraction. If oxytocin fails to contract the uterus, prostaglandin $F_2\alpha$ should be used. The same dosage and intervals used to arrest postpartum hemorrhage with uterine atony are appropriate in this circumstance.

Coagulation Disorders

Continued bleeding in the third stage of labor that is unresponsive to usual treatment should cause the clinician to consider uncommon but serious maternal coagulation disorders.

The most frequent disorder, von Willebrand disease (VWD), is a hemorrhagic disorder that affects both men and women. This coagulopathy is inherited in an autosomal dominant pattern and is characterized by the following laboratory abnormalities: prolonged bleeding time, decreased factor VIII activity, decreased factor VIII–related antigen, and decreased von Willebrand factor. The latter is a plasma factor that is essential for proper platelet function and aggregation.

VWD is variable in its clinical course, severity, and laboratory abnormalities, even in the same patient. It is therefore possible for a patient with this disorder to go undetected throughout pregnancy until bleeding problems develop postpartum. The usual increase in factor VIII coagulant activity associated with pregnancy may also mask VWD. Only those patients with very low levels (<5 percent) before gestation fail to exhibit this rise.

When VWD is diagnosed before parturition, factor VIII activity should be monitored serially and transfusion with cryoprecipitate given to keep the factor VIII activity near term at 40 percent. If factor VIII levels are inadequate, the patient should be given one bag of cryoprecipitate per 10 kg body weight 24 hours before the planned induction of labor or cesarean delivery. This infusion will immediately restore the factor VIII activity level, but it will take 24 hours for the associated platelet defect to be corrected. If one suspects this disorder in a patient with unexplained postpartum hemorrhage, coagulation studies should be ordered and a hematologist consulted. However, since time is often limited, it would be prudent to notify the blood bank that cryoprecipitate may be needed emergently. In this situation, at least 6 units of cryoprecipitate are required, to be given every 12 hours for the next 3 to 5 days.[100]

Amniotic Fluid Embolism/Anaphylactoid Syndrome of Pregnancy

Amniotic fluid embolism (AFE) is a rare but frequently fatal obstetric emergency.

The classic clinical presentation of the syndrome has been described by five signs that often occur in the following sequence: (1) respiratory distress, (2) cyanosis, (3) cardiovascular collapse, (4) hemorrhage, and (5) coma.

Important new findings are the certainty of fetal distress accompanying this syndrome and the high incidence of maternal coagulopathy. In many cases, fetal distress is the initial presenting symptom, rapidly followed by maternal distress.

Only scanty information is available on which to base the treatment of the initial syndrome. Early airway control usually necessitating endotracheal intubation has been stressed in the few patients surviving the full-blown syndrome.[106,107] Once maximal ventilation and oxygenation have been achieved, attention should be paid to restoration of cardiovascular equilibrium. Central monitoring of fluid therapy with a pulmonary artery catheter is very helpful if the patient can be stabilized long enough to allow time for its placement. Hypotension results from myocardial failure; thus, efforts should be used to provide myocardial support.[104] These would include inotropic agents such as dopamine, as well as volume therapy.[108] If the patient survives the initial cardiorespiratory collapse, there is a high likelihood that coagulopathy will develop if it has not been previously clinically apparent. DIC results in the depletion of fibrinogen, platelets, and coagulation factors, especially factors V, VIII, and XIII. The fibrinolytic system is activated as well.[109] Most patients will have profound hypofibrinogenemia, with values less than 200 mg/dl being the rule. PT and PTT will also be abnormal in nearly all patients. Platelet counts are more variable, with 60 percent having values less than $100,000/\mu l$. Supportive coagulation and volume therapy (blood, fresh frozen plasma, or cryoprecipitate) should be administered as soon as they are available.

The neonatal outcome in patients suffering this catastrophe is better than the maternal outcome. If the fetus is alive at the time of the event, nearly 80 percent will survive the delivery. Unfortunately, 50 percent of the survivors will incur neurologic damage.[103] The two main factors influencing neonatal outcome are the presence or absence of maternal cardiac arrest and the time from arrest to delivery.

Disseminated Intravascular Coagulation

DIC results from the loss of local control of the body's clotting mechanisms. Normally, there are four essential elements in the maintenance of local control of the hemostatic system: vascular integrity, platelet function, the coagulation system, and clot lysis.[110] The body must maintain vascular integrity for the survival of the organism. To minimize blood loss, any break in this system initiates the entire hemostatic cascade.

During DIC, the body is forming and lysing fibrin clots throughout the circulation rather than in the localized physiologic process. Therefore, the loss of localization of the clotting process is the main defect in DIC. The lyric process may be activated as well but occurs only in response to the activation of the clotting system.

In obstetrics, DIC causing hemorrhage may involve any of the four mechanisms involved in the localization process. Activation of the coagulation cascade by the presence of large amounts of tissue phospholipid is the most common stimulus for DIC in obstetrics. Such conditions include abruptio placenta, retained dead fetus, and amniotic fluid embolism. These tissue phospholipids contribute to the utilization of large amounts of clotting factors and lead to a consumption coagulopathy. Once this widespread coagulation has taken place, the lytic process is called into action. The degradation of large amounts of fibrin produces fibrin split products, or fibrin degradation products (FDPs). These factors have their own physiologic activity and, when present in large amounts, contribute to bleeding by inhibiting fibrin cross-linking and producing platelet dysfunction.

The platelet count and fibrinogen level are the most clinically useful tests in evaluating the patient with DIC. Because platelets and fibrinogen have a half-life of 4 to 5 days, they are not immediately replaced by the body's own mechanisms and will give an accurate reflection of ongoing consumption as well as the effectiveness of factor replacement.

The sine qua non of successful management of DIC is treatment of the initiating event. Once the cause has been located and treated, the process should resolve. However, depleted factors must be restored to permit orderly repair of injured tissues. Successful therapy involves the replacement of essential factors faster than the body is consuming them. These factors are platelets, coagulation factors derived from fresh frozen plasma or cryoprecipitate, and fibrinogen supplied by cryoprecipitate of fresh frozen plasma. The obstetrician should attempt to achieve a platelet count of more than $100,000/\mu dl$ and a fibrinogen level of greater than 100 mg/dl. Heparin has no use and will only cause the bleeding to worsen.

Key Points

➤ Considerable blood loss can occur in the pregnant patient prior to occurrence of signs that would be readily evident in the non-pregnant patient

➤ Blood loss up to 1500 ml (20–25%) volume may be characterized only by narrowed pulse pressure and hypothenar blanchris following pressure.

➤ Tachycardia and tachypnea usually require loss of 1800–2100 ml, whereas profound shock indicates loss of 40% of blood volume (2400 ml).

➤ In patients with abruptio placentae, cesarean delivery usually should be performed for obstetric or fetal indications, not maternal coagulopathy.

➤ Expectant management of patients with abruptio placentae or placenta previa can be safely accomplished in many patients.

➤ In patients with postpartum hemorrhage secondary to uterine atony, dilute solutions of oxytocin (intravenous) and 15-methyl-F-2α prostaglandin (intramuscular) should be the first two drugs administered. Misoprostal may also be helpful.

Box continued on following page

Key Points *Continued*

➤ The maternal risks from heterologous blood transfusion have decreased significantly in the last 5 years.

➤ The clinical presentation of amniotic fluid embolism is more heterogenous than previously described. Treatment focuses on ventilation and providing myocardial support.

➤ When uterine inversion is encountered, the uterus should be replaced and reinverted before placental removal is attempted.

➤ Oxytocin given before placental expulsion and separation can minimize postpartum blood loss.

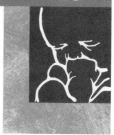

Chapter 13

Cesarean Delivery

RICHARD DEPP

Cesarean birth has become the most common hospital-based operative procedure in the United States, accounting for more than 22 percent of all live births in 1999.[1-3] The increase has been attributed to the liberalization of indications for "fetal distress," cephalopelvic disproportion/failure to progress, breech presentations, as well as elective repeat cesarean delivery.[4] In many medical centers, the present overall rate would be significantly higher were it not for a recent change in attitude facilitating acceptance of vaginal birth after cesarean birth.[5]

As the percentage of laboring patients presenting with a prior cesarean birth has increased, there has been an associated increase in more difficult repeat cesarean deliveries and complications, including a higher incidence of placenta previa, placenta accreta, symptomatic uterine rupture, hemorrhage, requirement for transfusion, and need for unplanned hysterectomy.

CESAREAN BIRTH RATES

The early onset of a change in the overall cesarean delivery rate is dramatically demonstrated by data from the Chicago Lying-In Hospital, which had a fivefold increase in the cesarean rate from 0.6 percent in 1910 to 3 percent in 1928.[20] The rate of cesarean delivery in the United States increased dramatically from 4.5 percent in 1965 to 16.5 percent in 1980, finally peaking at 24.7 percent in 1988.[21] At least 90 percent of the increase between 1980 and 1985 was attributable to three factors: repeat cesarean deliveries (48 percent), dystocia (29 percent), and "fetal distress" (16 percent).

In 1979, the National Institute of Child Health and Human Development (NICHD) established a task force on cesarean childbirth and in 1980 sponsored a consensus development conference to consider the issue of cesarean delivery in the United States.[25] The task force recommended that efforts be made to diminish the impact of elective repeat cesarean delivery and the diagnosis of "dystocia" because these indications were the two major causes of the increase in cesarean birth rates that were likely to be susceptible to reduction.

Recently, the U.S. Department of Health and Human Services, as part of its Healthy People 2000 program, identified a number of health-related objectives, including (1) reduction of the primary cesarean delivery rate to 12 percent and (2) increase of the number of vaginal births after cesarean (VBACs) to greater than or equal to 35 per 100 women who have had a prior cesarean section.[2,29]

In 1997, the American College of Obstetricians and Gynecologists (ACOG) appointed a task force on cesarean delivery rates to determine the factors that contribute to the cesarean delivery rates in the United States.[28] The task force noted that the highest variation in primary cesarean delivery rates occurred among nulliparous women with a singleton fetus in a cephalic presentation without other complications. The task force also observed that patients with a prior cesarean varied in the frequency with which they were offered a trial of labor and how often the trial of labor was successful. Using data from the National Center for Health Statistics, the task force established two benchmark rates based on the 25th to 75th percentiles of state rankings for these two patient groups. The task force advised that the targets for these two categories be set at the 25th percentile for primary cesarean delivery rates and the 75th percentile for VBAC rates. For nulliparous women at 37 weeks with a singleton fetus and a cephalic presentation, the national 1996 cesarean delivery rate was 17.9 percent. The group recommended a benchmark rate of 15.5 percent, at the 25th percentile. For multiparous women with one prior low transverse cesarean delivery at 37 weeks' gestation or greater with a singleton fetus and a cephalic presentation, the national 1996 VBAC rate was 30.3 percent. The task force recommended a benchmark rate of 37 percent, at the 75th percentile. The task force emphasized that in examining the cesarean rate of obstetricians or the institutions in which they practice it is essential that the rate be adjusted for the risk factors in the patient population. The task force proposed that using case-mix adjusted cesarean delivery rates and these benchmarks would be helpful in evaluating practice patterns and developing strategies to lower the rate of cesarean sections.[28]

Vaginal breech deliveries have been abandoned by many clinicians in favor of cesarean delivery. Most breech presentations are now delivered by cesarean birth, with rates in some medical centers as high as 79 and 92 percent.[21,35] A recently published large prospective randomized trial comparing planned cesarean delivery with planned vaginal birth for term frank or complete breech presentations demonstrated that perinatal mortality, neonatal mortality, and serious neonatal morbidity were all significantly lower in the planned cesarean group.[36]

BENEFITS AND RISKS OF CESAREAN BIRTH

Maternal Mortality

Maternal mortality as a result of cesarean delivery fortunately is an infrequent occurrence, but the overall rate is estimated to be several-fold higher than that following vaginal delivery. Approximately 300 maternal deaths occur annually in the United States in just over 4 million deliveries of all types per year, an overall rate less than 10 per 100,000 live births. Maternal mortality following cesarean birth has been assessed in two publications[6,47] with a sufficient number of cesarean deliveries (400,000 and 121,000) to provide meaningful. The cesarean delivery-associated maternal mortality can be estimated to range from 6.1 to 22 per 100,000 live births. Approximately one third to one half of maternal deaths of these patients can be attributed directly to the cesarean procedure itself.

Perinatal Morbidity and Mortality

The hypothesis that cesarean birth offers a major opportunity to improve perinatal outcome has, with few exceptions, not been proven.

INDICATIONS FOR CESAREAN DELIVERY

Fetal Indications

Fetal indications for cesarean birth are in large part designed to minimize neonatal morbidity and possibly long-term consequences of profound intrapartum metabolic or mixed metabolic acidemia and/or deliveryrelated trauma or transmission of infection.[55] Accepted indications, often used selectively, include the following: "significant" nonremediable and nonreassuring FHR patterns, especially when associated with progressive loss of variability; various categories of breech presentation at risk for head entrapment and/or cord prolapse; the VLBW fetus; and active genital herpes. The decision to use cesarean delivery may be selective, based on the results of ultrasound or cordocentesis studies (i.e., major fetal congenital anomalies). In such cases, a planned, controlled delivery with predictable access to pediatric surgical support may be desirable.

Maternal–Fetal Indications

Placental abnormalities such as placenta previa or placental abruption in which hemorrhage poses a significant risk to both mother and fetus as well as labor "dystocia," are indications for which cesarean delivery offers a potential benefit to both mother and fetus.

Dystocia is a term used to describe indications for cesarean birth arising from one or more of the "three Ps": relatively large fetus (passenger), relatively small "passage" (pelvis), or relatively insufficient or inefficient uterine contractions (power). Included in dystocia are failure to progress (FTP), relative cephalopelvic disproportion (CPD), and absolute CPD on the rare occasion when the latter can be diagnosed. Some include failed inductions under this designation. CPD is almost always a relative term; the CPD diagnosis is made only after application of a number of diagnostic and therapeutic measures including oxytocin. In most instances it involves a normal-sized fetus.[58]

Maternal Indications

There are only a few indications for cesarean delivery that are solely maternal. They include mechanical obstructions of the vagina from large vulvovaginal condylomata, advanced lower genital tract malignancy, and placement of a permanent abdominal cerclage with a desire for future pregnancies.

HOSPITAL REQUIREMENTS FOR CESAREAN DELIVERY

Facility and Personnel Requirements

Any hospital that provides labor and delivery services should be equipped to perform an "emergency" cesarean delivery. In the past, it was recommended that a hospital offering obstetric services should provide the professional and institutional resources to respond to "acute obstetric emergencies" (i.e., a cesarean delivery) within 30 minutes, when indicated, from the time a decision is made until the procedure is begun.[60] The nursing, anesthesia, neonatal resuscitation, and obstetric personnel required must be either in the hospital or readily available. In its 1999 Practice Bulletin, the ACOG recommended that, if a VBAC-TOL is considered, a physician capable of monitoring the labor and performing an emergency cesarean delivery should be "immediately" available.[3]

At this time, there is no consensus standard that defines an acceptable time interval for performance of a cesarean delivery. Under most circumstances (i.e., protraction and arrest disorders of labor) cesarean delivery is not necessary within a 30-minute time frame.

ABDOMINAL INCISIONS

Selection of Incision Type

The surgeon may choose either a vertical or a transverse skin incision (Fig. 13–1) when performing a cesarean delivery. The ultimate choice hinges on factors such as the urgency of the procedure, the presence of prior abdominal scars, and associated nonobstetric pathology, if any. The midline vertical, transverse Maylard, and transverse Pfannenstiel incisions are the three most commonly used types.

In general, vertical incisions allow more rapid access to the lower uterine segment, have less blood loss, provide greater feasibility for incisional extension around the umbilicus, and allow easier examination of the upper abdomen. In pregnancy, speed of entry through a midline vertical incision is facilitated by the common occurrence of diastasis of the rectus muscles.

Transverse incisions are somewhat more time consuming; the difference in time of entry between the two incision types is approximately 30 to 60 seconds in the hands of an experienced clinician. Transverse incisions are preferred cosmetically, are generally less painful, have been associated with a lower risk of subsequent herniation, and yet provide equal, if not better, visualization of the pelvis.

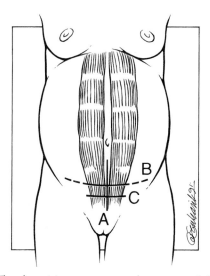

Figure 13–1. The obstetrician most commonly uses one of three abdominal incisions: (A) midline, (B) Maylard, and (C) Pfannenstiel. *Hatched lines* indicate possible extension. (Modified from Baker C, Shingleton HM: Incisions. Clin Obstet Gynecol 31:701, 1988.)

The Maylard incision (Fig. 13–1) differs from the Pfannenstiel incision in that it involves transverse incision of the anterior rectus sheath and the rectus muscles bilaterally.[86] The Pfannenstiel incision (Fig. 13–1) is a curvilinear incision that is best suited for the nonobese patient. The incision is generally made approximately 3 cm above the symphysis pubis within the pubic hair line at its midpoint. The determination of its lateral extension should, to some extent, be a function of the estimated fetal size.

Skin Incision in the Obese Patient

The obese patient is at significant additional risk for wound complications. Should the patient be massively obese, it may be better to use an incision that does not involve the underside of the panniculus, an area that is more heavily colonized with bacteria and is difficult to prepare surgically, to keep dry, and to inspect in the postoperative period. The objective is to enter the abdomen directly over the lower uterine segment. The surgeon may choose either a vertical midline incision, which is developed periumbilically both above and below the umbilicus or, alternatively, a transverse incision closer to the umbilicus. The actual selection of the site of incision, whether it be vertical or transverse, can be made by retracting the panniculus in a caudad direction so as to place the incision directly overlying the uterine segment.

In closing the fascia of an obese patient, placement of the sutures in the fascia should be at least 1.5 to 2 cm lateral to the cut margin of the fascia, with successive bites approximately 1.5 cm apart along the longitudinal axis of the incision. Subcutaneous sutures may be used and the skin closed with suture staples, left in place for 7 to 10 days. Subcutaneous closure will reduce the risk of wound disruption in women with 2 cm or more of subcutaneous fat.[90]

Figure 13–2. Uterine incisions for cesarean delivery. *A,* Low transverse incision. The bladder is retracted downward, and the incision is made in the lower uterine segment, curving gently upward. If the lower segment is poorly developed, the incision can also curve sharply upward at each end to avoid extending into the ascending branches of the uterine arteries. *B,* Low vertical incision. The incision is made vertically in the lower uterine segment after reflecting the bladder, avoiding extension into the bladder below. If more room is needed, the incision can be extended upward into the upper uterine segment. *C,* Classic incision. The incision is entirely within the upper uterine segment and can be at the level shown or in the fundus. *D,* J incision. If more room is needed when an initial transverse incision has been made, either end of the incision can be extended upward into the upper uterine segment and parallel to the ascending branch of the uterine artery. *E,* T incision. More room can be obtained in a transverse incision by an upward midline extension into the upper uterine segment.

Selection of Lower Uterine Incision

The most commonly used uterine incisions (Fig. 13–2) are the low transverse incision and the low vertical incision.[16] A low transverse (Kerr) incision is used in more than 90 percent of all cesarean births. The low transverse incision has the following advantages over a

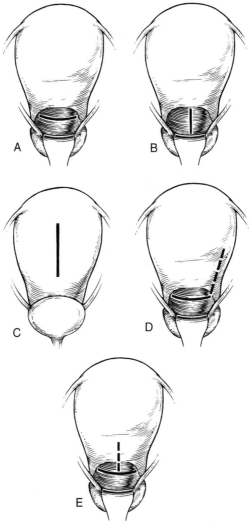

Figure 13–2. *See legend on opposite page*

vertical incision: less risk of entry into the upper uterine segment, greater ease of entry, less bladder dissection, less operative blood loss, less repair, easier reperitonealization, and less likelihood of adhesion formation to bowel or omentum. Importantly, in subsequent pregnancies the obstetrician can feel more comfortable offering a VBAC trial because there is less likelihood of uterine rupture.[93]

A vertical incision (classic or low vertical) may be advantageous if the patient has not been in labor and the lower uterus is narrow and poorly developed or if the fetus is not in a cephalic presentation, particularly a back-down transverse lie or preterm breech. Should a transverse incision be performed under such circumstances, there is a greater likelihood of lateral extension of the incision into the vessels of the broad ligament. However, individualization is reasonable. Other possible indications for a vertical incision include leiomyomata obstructing exposure to the lower segment and structural uterine anomalies.

The classic uterine incision involves the upper active uterine segment. Its primary advantage is the rapidity of entry into the uterus. More commonly encountered complications associated with classic incisions include subsequent adhesion formation and greater risk of uterine rupture with later pregnancies.[95] Patients who have had a prior classic incision should consider an appropriately timed elective repeat cesarean birth because of the risk of uterine rupture even before labor has started.

PERFORMING THE CESAREAN DELIVERY

Development of Bladder Flap

After placement of a bladder catheter and entry into the peritoneal cavity, the obstetrician should palpate the uterus to determine the degree and direction of uterine rotation. In most instances, the uterus is dextrorotated such that the left round ligament may be visualized more anteriorly and closer to the midline than is the right. The uterovesical peritoneum (serosa) is grasped in the midline and undermined with Metzenbaum scissors inserted between the peritoneum and underlying myometrium to develop bluntly a retroperitoneal space bilaterally to the lateral margins of the lower uterine segment. The peritoneal reflection is then incised bilaterally in an upward direction and the vesicouterine fold is grasped with forceps and the bladder lifted anteriorly, allowing blunt separation of the bladder from the underlying lower uterine segment. Once the dissection is complete in the midline, the fingers may be carefully swept laterally in each direction to free the bladder more completely. After the bladder flap is adequately developed, a universal retractor or bladder blade is used to retract the bladder anteriorly and inferiorly to facilitate exposure of the intended incision site.

Low Transverse Cesarean Incision

The lower uterine segment incision (Fig. 13–2A) is begun 1 to 2 cm above the site of the original upper margin of the bladder. A small midline incision is first made with a scalpel through the lower uterine segment to the fetal membranes. Continuous suction should be available to facilitate visualization of the operative field and to evacuate amniotic fluid should the incision perforate through the fetal membranes. Care should be taken to avoid laceration of the fetus.

After suctioning, the incision may be extended laterally and slightly upward (cephalad) to the lateral margin of the lower uterine segment so as to maximize incisional length and avoid extension into the uterine vessels. Extension of the incision may be accomplished by either of two methods: (1) sharp dissection, taking care to avoid fetal fingers and toes; or (2) blunt dissection by spreading the incision with each index finger.

Low Vertical Incision

Should the fetus present as a breech or transverse lie, particularly back-down, there is often advantage to a low vertical (Figs. 13–2B) uterine incision, particularly if the lower uterine segment is not well developed. The bladder is displaced downward to expose the lower uterine segment more inferiorly so that the low vertical incision will be less likely to extend into the upper segment. Once the anticipated site is exposed, an incision is made at the inferior margin of the lower segment and extended cephalad with either bandage scissors or knife.

Although vertical cesarean incisions are traditionally categorized into low vertical and classic types, the performance of a true low vertical incision that does not enter the upper contractile portion of the uterus is actually uncommon. The clinical implication is that the low vertical incision poses considerably less risk in a subsequent VBAC trial than would be the case with a classic incision; nonetheless, the risk of rupture is probably somewhat greater than that of a low transverse incision.

Classic Cesarean Incision

The initial incision (Fig. 13–2C) is made with a scalpel 1 to 2 cm above the bladder reflection. Once the fetus or membranes are visualized, the incision is extended cephalad with bandage scissors, the size of the incision varying with the estimated size of the fetus. The patient should also be advised of this occurrence and its importance to future pregnancies should a VBAC trial be considered.

Delivery of the Fetus

Upon completion of the incision, the retractors are removed and a hand is inserted into the uterine cavity to elevate and flex the fetal head through the uterine incision. Should the head be deeply wedged within the pelvis, it can be dislodged by an assistant applying upward pressure vaginally. Once the occiput presents into the incision, moderate fundal pressure may facilitate expulsion. On occasion the head may be delivered with shorthandled Simpson forceps or vacuum. Once delivery of the fetal head is completed, the nose and oropharynx are suctioned with a bulb syringe. If meconium is present, suction can be accomplished with continuous wall suction. When suctioning is complete, expulsion of the remainder of the newborn is facilitated by moderate uterine fundal pressure. The cord is then doubly clamped and cut, and the infant is transferred to the resuscitation team.

Operative Techniques for the Preterm Fetus

The uterine incision to be used for the delivery of the preterm fetus is best selected after entry into the maternal abdomen. At least 50 percent of cases will require a low vertical or classic incision for indications such as malpresentation or a poorly developed lower uterine segment. Low transverse cesarean incisions may require a T or J extension (Fig. 13–2D and E) for malpresentation, usually of a preterm fetus, for a poorly developed lower uterine segment, or when the fetal head was deeply arrested in the midpelvis.

Manual Versus "Spontaneous" Placental Expulsion

Following delivery of the fetus, 20 to 40 units of oxytocin can be administered in an isotonic crystalloid solution. While subsequent removal of the placenta is commonly done manually, several studies have demonstrated that spontaneous delivery of the placenta is associated with significantly less blood loss and a lower incidence of endometritis. Following its removal, the placenta should be inspected for possible missing cotyledons.

Repair of the Uterine Incision

Closure of the uterine incision may be aided by manual delivery of the uterine fundus through the abdominal incision.[103] Delivery of the uterine fundus through the abdominal incision facilitates uterine massage and observation of uterine tone, as well as routine examination of the adnexa and tubal ligation. The fundus may be covered with a moistened laparotomy pad and the uterine incision inspected for obvious bleeding points, which are controlled with either Ring forceps or Allis clamps until suture closure can be accomplished. The uterine cavity may then be inspected and wiped clean with a dry laparotomy sponge to remove fetal membranes and placental fragments.

Midline placement of a ring forceps or Allis clamp may be used to elevate the lower portion of the low transverse uterine incision, facilitating visualization of the field and approximation of the incision. Allis clamps can be routinely placed at the angles of the incision to control bleeding and to identify the end of the incision.

Reapproximation of the lower uterine incision may be performed in either one or two layers (Fig. 13–3) using 0 or double 0 chromic suture or similar absorbable synthetic suture such as Vicryl, the second layer inverting the first. The initial suture should be placed lateral to the angle of a transverse incision or inferior to the lower margin of a vertical incision. Subsequent stitches may be run in a continuous or continuous-locking manner to the opposite end

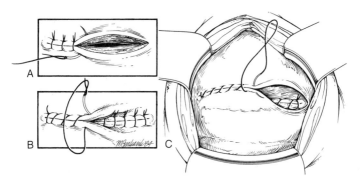

Figure 13–3. Closure of low transverse incision. *A,* The first layer can be either interrupted or continuous. A continuous locking suture is less desirable, despite its reputed hemostatic abilities, because it may interfere with incision vasculature and, hence, with healing and scar formation. *B,* A second inverted layer created by using a continuous Lembert's or Cushing's stitch is customary but is really needed only when apposition is unsatisfactory after application of the first layer. Inclusion of too much tissue produces a bulky mass that may delay involution and interfere with healing. *C,* The bladder peritoneum is reattached to the uterine peritoneum with fine suture.

of the incision. The sutures may be placed through the entire myometrium. Reapproximation of the visceral (vesicouterine) and parietal peritoneum is not necessary.

Closure of a classic cesarean incision involving the more thickened upper segment most often will require a two-layer closure. Should the uterine wall be unusually thick, it may be necessary to use a third layer.

Abdominal Closure

Once the uterine incisional reapproximation is completed, the incision should once again be inspected for bleeding points, which can be individually ligated, coagulated, or controlled with figure-of-eight sutures. Before closing the abdomen, the uterus, fallopian tubes, and ovaries should be examined for unsuspected pathology. Some routinely examine the appendix. The pelvis and lower abdomen may be irrigated, especially if there is coexistent chorioamnionitis or if there has been heavy spillage of meconium outside the operative field. The operating team should confirm that the needle and sponge counts are correct.

There is no need to reapproximate the parietal peritoneum or rectus muscles. The rectus fascia may be closed with either interrupted or continuous (nonlocking) sutures. Suture choice is important in fascial healing. If the suture is absorbed too rapidly, tensile strength may be reduced, thus increasing the likelihood of wound breakdown. Chromic suture should be avoided when possible. Selection of a suture for its duration of strength is particularly important for patients at risk for wound dehiscence. Unlike their chromic counterparts, synthetic braided sutures maintain tensile strength throughout fascial healing. They are predictably broken down by hydrolysis. If the surgeon is dealing with a patient at risk for wound breakdown from chronic corticosteroid therapy, for example, delayed absorbable material such as PDS or polyglyconate (Maxon) or permanent material such as nylon or polypropylene (Prolene) may have merit.

Large bites using larger gauge suture material are less likely to transect tissue than are small bites with narrow-gauge suture material. Suture entry and exit sites should be well beyond the 1-cm inner zone of collagenolysis at the margin of the wound. Sutures should be placed at approximately 1-cm intervals approximately 1.5 cm from the incision line.

It is acceptable to use a running suture in closing the fascia in patients with a clean incision. Approximation of fascia should allow maintenance of adequate blood flow; unnecessarily tight sutures will cause hypoxia and potentially interfere with predictable wound healing.[116,117] Should a patient be at high risk for wound

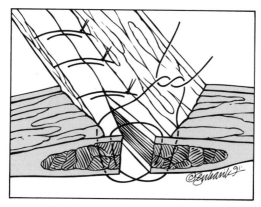

Figure 13–4. Modification of far-near, near-far Smead-Jones suture. Suture passes deeply through lateral side of anterior rectus fascia and adjacent fat, crosses the midline of the incision to pick up the medial edge of the rectus fascia, then catches the near side of the opposite rectus sheath, and, finally, returns to the far margin of the opposite rectus sheath and subcutaneous fat. (Modified from American College of Obstetricians and Gynecologists: Prolog. *In* Gynecologic Oncology and Surgery. Washington, DC, ACOG, 1991, p 187.)

dehiscence, it is preferable that the fascia not be closed with continuous suturing, particularly on a vertical incision. If the patient is at high risk for abdominal distention and wound breakdown, a mass or Smead-Jones (Fig. 13–4) closure is preferable.

It is generally not necessary to reapproximate the subcutaneous tissue unless the patient is markedly obese, in which case subcutaneous closure may reduce wound disruption. Skin may be closed with staples or a subcuticular stitch. If staples are used, they may be replaced with Steristrips 3 or 4 days after surgery to decrease scarring.

INTRAOPERATIVE COMPLICATIONS

Uterine Lacerations

Lacerations of the lower uterine incision are more common when a low transverse incision is used in the presence of a macrosomic fetus or a noncephalic presentation. Fortunately, these lacerations are usually easily sutured as long as they only extend laterally to the margin of the myometrium or inferiorly into the vagina. Care must be taken to avoid ligation of the ureters.

Bladder Injuries

Although the risk of bladder injury can be minimized by preoperative catheterization of the bladder and careful entry into the peritoneal cavity, it is not always possible to avoid injury during a repeat procedure. When the bladder is more adherent than usual, sharp dissection of the "webbing" between the bladder base and the lower uterine segment and vagina, as opposed to blunt dissection with a sponge stick or gauze-covered finger, will reduce, but not eliminate, the incidence of unplanned cystotomy.

Should a bladder laceration be encountered, the bladder may be repaired with a two-layer closure with 2-0 or 3-0 chromic. After the bladder has been repaired, a catheter can be left in place for 7 to 10 days.[120,123]

Uterine Atony

Initial efforts to control uterine atony include uterine massage and medical therapy with (1) intravenous oxytocin, 20 to 40 units/L; (2) methergotamine, 0.2 mg, or ergonovine administered intramuscularly; or (3) 15 methylprostaglandin $F_{2\alpha}$ (Hemabate), which can be administered either intramuscularly or directly into the myometrium. Should the initial dose of prostaglandin be insufficient, successive dosages of 250 µg, up to a total dose of 1.0 to 1.5 mg, can be used. Should medical treatment fail, the surgeon must decide between ligation of the uterine arteries, hypogastric artery ligation, and hysterectomy. Uterine or hypogastric artery ligation may be the desirable approach should the patient be stable cardiovascularly and desirous of future pregnancy. Hypogastric artery ligation can be accomplished by ligation of the ascending branch, which can usually be found at the inferior and lateral extreme of the low transverse incision ascending retroperitoneally within the broad ligament (Fig. 13–5). Should uterine or hypogastric artery ligation also fail to control the hemorrhage, it may be necessary to proceed to hysterectomy.

Placenta Accreta

Placenta accreta is now the most common indication for postcesarean hysterectomy. Approximately 25 percent of patients having a cesarean delivery for placenta previa in the presence of a prior uterine incision subsequently require cesarean hysterectomy for placenta accreta. The risk of placenta accreta appears to increase with the number of prior incisions. This obstetric complication may be rising because of the growing number of previous cesarean sections.[128,129]

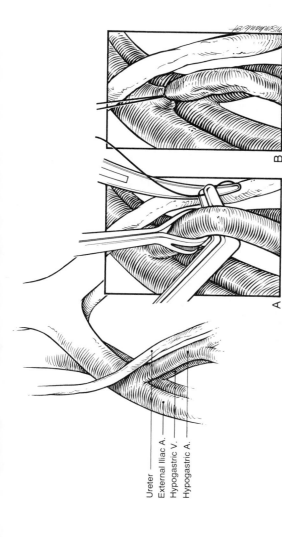

Ureter
External Iliac A.
Hypogastric V.
Hypogastric A.

Figure 13–5. Hypogastric artery ligation. Approach to the hypogastric artery via the peritoneum, parallel and just lateral to the ovarian vessels, exposing the interior surface of the posterior layer of the broad ligament. The ureter will be found attached to the medial leaf of the broad ligament. The bifurcation of the common iliac artery into its external and internal (hypogastric) branches is exposed by blunt dissection of the loose overlying areolar tissues. Identification of these structures is essential. A and B, To avoid traumatizing the underlying hypogastric vein, the hypogastric artery is elevated by means of a Babcock clamp before passing an angled clamp to catch a free tie. (Adapted from Breen J, Gregori CA, Kindzierski JA: Hemorrhage in Gynecologic Surgery. Hagerstown, MD, Harper & Row, 1981, p 438.)

If the accreta is focal and the patient desires future pregnancies, it may be possible to excise the site of trophoblastic invasion, oversewing bleeding areas with several figure-of-eight sutures. If that is not possible, hysterectomy should be initiated. A complete hysterectomy will usually be required because a placenta accreta commonly involves the lower uterine segment and, in such cases, a supracervical hysterectomy will not be effective in controlling the bleeding.

PREOPERATIVE AND INTRAOPERATIVE FLUID GUIDELINES

Extracellular (interstitial and intravascular) water constitutes approximately one third of total body water and 20 percent of total body weight. Ordinary daily physiologic fluid needs are approximately 2,000 to 2,500 ml.[134] In the pregnant patient, daily physiologic fluid losses are estimated to be 1,000 ml in excess of urinary output and include urinary output (800 to 1,500 ml), insensible loss (800 ml) from both skin and lungs, and stool loss (200 ml). Insensible loss in the laboring patient can be considerably greater.

There will be little problem with dehydration if intravenous fluid intake has been maintained at 100 to 125 ml/h during labor. Should this not be the case, fluid losses can be estimated based on the average hourly need (100 to 125 ml) times the cumulative number of hours since the time of last fluid intake.

Should the patient be only mildly hypovolemic in the first 24 hours, normal isotonic saline or Ringer's lactate solution in 5 percent dextrose is preferable to more hypotonic solutions because there is greater retention of fluids in the intravascular space providing volume expansion. In contrast, infusion of a 5 percent dextrose in water solution (D_5 W) will result in distribution of fluid evenly throughout all water spaces, two thirds being in the intracellular space.

Intraoperative fluid requirements, apart from blood replacement, range from 500 to 1,000 ml/h, up to a maximum of 3 L in a 4-hour interval under ordinary surgical conditions.

POSTOPERATIVE COMPLICATIONS

Maternal Morbidity and Mortality

Major sources of morbidity and associated mortality relate to complications of maternal sepsis, anesthesia, and thromboembolic disease and its complications.

Endomyometritis and Wound Infection

For a discussion of endomyometritis and wound infection, see Chapter 25.

Fascial Dehiscence

Dehiscence of a wound through the fascia is infrequent, occurring in approximately 5 percent of wound infections.[150] Dehiscence is suggested by the presence of a large amount of discharge from the wound. If loops of small bowel protrude through the incision, the small bowel should be immediately covered with wet sterile dressings. The wound should be opened and inspected and emergency closure performed in the operating room under sterile conditions. If a dehiscence is confirmed, the wound should be cleansed, debrided, and closed with either Smead-Jones or retention sutures (Fig. 13–4).

Urinary Complications

Urinary tract infections rank second to endomyometritis as a cause of postcesarean febrile morbidity. The reported incidence varies from as low as 2 percent to as high as 16 percent.[165,166] Urethral catheterization contributes to 80 percent of nosocomial urinary tract infections in hospitalized patients, particularly when indwelling catheters are used. The incidence is increased with longer duration of catheter use, in diabetic patients, and in patients who are critically ill.[164] Attention to detail in terms of proper preparation and insertion of the catheter and the use of a closed drainage system have decreased this risk.

Gastrointestinal Complications

Most patients undergoing cesarean delivery have little if any gastrointestinal problems postoperatively. However, anesthesia and narcotics employed to treat postoperative pain may contribute to bowel dysfunction. As a result, an occasional patient may have postoperative nausea or mild transient abdominal distention in the first 24 hours.

Ileus should be suspected if prolonged nausea or vomiting together with signs such as abdominal distention, absence of bowel sounds, and failure to pass flatus are persistent. Distended loops of bowel with or without air–fluid levels on radiography will provide confirmatory evidence. In most instances, simply withholding oral intake, providing adequate fluid replacement, and being observant are sufficient. If the ileus is persistent, nasogastric suction may be required.

Thromboembolic Disorders

The risk of deep venous thrombophlebitis (DVT) after cesarean delivery is approximately three to five times greater than after vaginal delivery.[170] Compounding risk factors include obesity, inability to ambulate, advanced maternal age, and higher parity. Should the DVT go untreated, approximately 15 to 25 percent of patients will develop pulmonary emboli, and 15 percent will sustain a fatal pulmonary embolus (PE). However, if recognized early and treated appropriately, the risks of PE and death are reduced to 4.5 and 0.7 percent, respectively.[169,171]

Classic symptoms for DVT include unilateral leg pain, tenderness, and swelling. A 2-cm difference in leg circumference between the affected and normal limb is generally required for diagnosis. Other clinical signs include edema, a palpable cord, and a change in limb color. A positive Homan's sign (calf pain on passive dorsiflexion of the foot) suggests DVT.

Unfortunately, the first sign of DVT may be the occurrence of a PE, which can present with symptoms of tachypnea (90 percent), dyspnea (80 percent), pleuritic chest pain with or without splinting (>70 percent), apprehension (~60 percent), tachycardia (40 percent), and cough (>50 percent).[172,173] Other findings include atelectatic rales, a friction rub, accentuated second heart sound, and a gallop. Patient evaluation is complicated in the postcesarean delivery patient, since splinting from incisional pain and tachypnea are not unusual findings. Doppler studies have a sensitivity of 90 percent for popliteal, femoral, or iliac thromboses, but only 50 percent for calf involvement because of abundant collateral vessels. Impedance plethysmography (IPG) is sensitive in approximately 95 percent of proximal thromboses, but is not as effective as Doppler for pelvic vessel thrombosis and will generally identify most cases, especially above the calves. Should Doppler and IPG be inconclusive, ascending venography, the most accurate of the three tests, should be performed. IPG can be used as a first-line test postpartum in the nonlactating mother. Should PE be suspected, a baseline arterial blood gas, chest radiograph, and electrocardiogram, as well as prothrombin time and partial thromboplastin time, should be obtained. Oxygen therapy should also be administered. Once the diagnosis has been established, heparin therapy should be started. The diagnosis and treatment of a PE are discussed in the section on Pulmonary Disease in Chapter 24.

Septic Pelvic Thrombophlebitis

For a discussion of septic pelvic thrombophlebitis, see Chapter 25.

POSTOPERATIVE MANAGEMENT

Postoperative Analgesia

Analgesia should be provided in a dose and at a frequency that will neither obtund nor cause respiratory depression and yet allow the patient (1) to avoid the consequences of extremes in analgesic blood levels resulting in unnecessary pain and (2) to cooperate with normal postoperative management. The patient receiving inadequate analgesia may, in an effort to protect her wound, maintain a shallow breathing pattern without deep breaths and, hence, develop atelectasis.[175]

Commonly used analgesics include meperidine (50 to 75 mg) or morphine (10 mg, depending on maternal size), administered intravenously or intramuscularly every 3 to 4 hours. Intrathecal or epidural narcotic administration used with agents such as morphine can also be used for postoperative anesthesia, which may last as long as 30 hours following delivery, providing an advantage to a patient who has undergone a regional block (see Chapter 10).[176]

Ambulation

Early ambulation is important in reinstitution of inflation of the most dependent alveoli and the prevention of pulmonary complications, particularly in the patient who has had general anesthesia. Early ambulation also promotes the return of normal urinary and bowel activity. Under most circumstances, the uncomplicated patient can be allowed to sit up within 8 to 12 hours following the procedure, even after epidural anesthesia. The patient generally can ambulate within the first day after surgery, and by the second day can shower without fear of injury to the incision.

Oral Intake

Active bowel sounds are commonly not observed until the second postoperative day. Nonetheless, in most instances the patient will easily tolerate oral fluids the day after surgery. Only rarely, when the patient has been septic or there has been extensive intra-abdominal manipulation, will there be a need to withhold oral fluids, even though the patient may have diminished bowel sounds and not pass gas. Most clinicians feel comfortable in providing clear liquids and ice chips with only a small amount of liquid as soon as nausea subsides to relieve complaints of a dry mouth. The progression of the diet also varies according to clinician. Some advance the patient rapidly to a regular diet, whereas others await the return of normal bowel sounds and passage of flatus to indicate return of colonic function before a regular diet is begun.

Bladder Management

The urinary catheter is ordinarily removed within 12 to 24 hours following surgery unless there have been intraoperative complications.

Postoperative Wound Care

The incision is generally covered for the first day with a light dressing, until the wound is sealed. The dressing is removed after the first postoperative day.

Laboratory Studies

Blood loss arising from an uncomplicated cesarean delivery is approximately 1,000 ml.[177] As a consequence of blood loss as well as intra- and postoperative hydration, the postoperative hematocrit may be expected to drop by approximately 2 to 3 percentage points during the initial 2 days following surgery, independent of hydration status.

Postoperative Fluids

The normal postpartum period is generally characterized by mobilization of the physiologic accumulation of fluid during pregnancy. As a consequence, large volumes of intravenous fluids are seldom required after cesarean delivery. In the low-risk patient, fluid replacement needs during a 24-hour interval are generally only 1,000 ml above urinary output. Three liters of a salt-containing solution will thus generally suffice during the first 24 hours unless urinary output falls below 30 ml/h. Under certain circumstances there may be increased requirements for fluids: following prolonged labor, febrile illness, vomiting and diarrhea, or even prior use of diuretics or salt restriction. More complex patients may have additional needs. Potassium is ordinarily not required during the first 24 hours by uncomplicated patients because of intracellular potassium release from cell destruction. After the first 24 hours, intravenous fluid replacement with 5 percent dextrose in 0.45 percent sodium chloride is commonly used, unless volume expansion is an issue. If it is anticipated that the patient will require prolonged intravenous fluids, potassium may be administered as 60 to 80 mEq/day. Should the patient be oliguric, potassium is generally not given until the patient has a normal urinary output.

Average Length of Stay

Depending on postoperative morbidity/complications and availability of care at home, hospital discharge may occur as early as the second to as late as the fifth postoperative day. The average length of stay is approximately 3 days. The length of hospitalization associated with cesarean birth, like those associated with vaginal delivery, has declined dramatically.[1,2,26]

Discharge Management

The mother's activities at home for the first week should be limited to personal care and to care of the newborn. By the third to fourth week, the patient can generally resume most activities at home.

REDUCING THE CURRENT CESAREAN BIRTH RATE

Table 13–1 summarizes potential clinical strategies to reduce the current cesarean rate. The strategy most likely to have a significant impact is one that strongly encourages vaginal birth after cesarean-trial of labor (VBAC-TOL).

The cesarean birth rate rose 44 percent between 1978 and 1984, and 47 percent of the rise was attributable to the performance of elective repeat cesarean deliveries.[1,2,4] The total cesarean rate in the United States peaked in 1988 at 24.7 percent; of these, 36.3

Table 13–1. POTENTIAL APPROACHES TO REDUCE CESAREAN BIRTHS

Vaginal birth after cesarean trial of labor (VBAC-TOL)
Dystocia/CPD/FTP
   Disciplined approach to labor management
   Active management of labor
Breech presentation/transverse lie
   External version
   Selective vaginal delivery of breech
Fetal hypoxia/acidosis
   Develop more predictive markers for acidosis
   Fetal capillary blood gases for reassurance
   Fetal stimulation for reassurance

Data from Taffel et al.[26]

percent (351,000) were repeat cesarean deliveries. In the 1989 to 1991 interval, the cesarean rate appeared to reduce or plateau. Changing VBAC-TOL rates appear to be largely responsible, increasing 47 percent from 1988 (12.6 percent) to 1989 (18.5 percent). The VBAC rate peaked in 1996 at 28.3 percent.

VAGINAL BIRTH AFTER CESAREAN BIRTH

Benefits and Risks of VBAC-TOL

VBAC-TOL is successful in 60 to 80 percent of acceptable candidates.[194-197] If applied to all patients presenting with a prior cesarean procedure (8.2 to 8.5 percent), there is a potential to increase the rate of overall vaginal delivery by approximately 5 percent. Furthermore, there is evidence from a large multicenter trial that VBAC-TOL reduces the incidence of postpartum infection, the need for postpartum transfusion, and maternal length of stay; as a result, there is significant cost savings.[197,198,199] Data compiled for 1996 by the Health Insurance Association of America on 40,967 vaginal deliveries and 10,305 cesarean sections across the country reveal average charges of $11,450 for a cesarean delivery and $7,090 for a normal vaginal delivery, including both the hospital and physician components.[198]

In 1988, the ACOG published *Guidelines for Vaginal Delivery After a Previous Cesarean Birth*, recommending VBAC- TOL as an option that should be selected based on available evidence available at that time.[61] Suggested 1988 guidelines include the following:

1. Repeat cesarean birth should be by specific indication.
2. Women with two or more prior cesarean deliveries should not be discouraged from attempting a VBAC-TOL.
3. Normal patient activity should be encouraged during the latent phase of labor. There is no need for restriction prior to the onset of the active phase of labor.
4. Professional and institutional resources should be available to respond to "intrapartum obstetric emergencies" such as performing a cesarean delivery within 30 minutes from the time the decision is made until the "surgical procedure is begun."
5. A physician capable of evaluating labor and performing a cesarean delivery should be "readily available."

ACOG has recently modified its recommendations. VBAC after one prior low transverse cesarean delivery is encouraged, and after two it may be allowed recognizing the increased risk of uterine rupture.[213] The ACOG advises that the use of prostaglandin gel or oxytocin require close monitoring. Patients with a true low vertical incision are candidates for VBAC. The major change has been the recommendation that the obstetrician be "immediately available" to provide emergency care.[3]

One of the first questions to be raised by a patient when considering a VBAC-TOL is, what is the likelihood for a successful vaginal birth according to the indication for the prior cesarean birth? Obstetric history regarding preexisting conditions is helpful in the prediction of VBAC success. Women who have previously given birth vaginally or women whose prior cesarean delivery was for nonrecurring conditions are more likely to succeed.

The likely success of a VBAC trial will depend to some degree on whether the indication for the prior cesarean is a recurring or nonrecurring one. Patients with a nonrecurring indication (breech presentation, so-called fetal distress–nonreassuring FHR pattern, and conditions such as placenta previa, abruption, or maternal hemorrhage) are more likely (82 to 86 percent) to achieve success than is the patient who has undergone a prior cesarean for a potentially recurring condition (70 percent) such as dystocia (failure to progress and/or CPD), approximating the success rate for the so-called low-risk nulliparous patient.[208,218,225]

Considerations in Management of VBAC-TOL

Management of the patient undergoing a VBAC-TOL is similar to that of patients attempting to achieve a vaginal delivery.[3,233] As a consequence, it is appropriate to use oxytocin and epidural anesthesia as one would in other labors. Potential problems such as suspected fetal macrosomia will be encountered and management will be no different from that in normal labor. The major difference will arise from some heightening of concern for uterine dehiscence and/or rupture. *Uterine incisional dehiscence* is commonly used to describe the occult or asymptomatic scar separation or thinning that is occasionally observed at surgery in patients with a prior low transverse incision. A useful operational definition of *dehiscence* is a uterine scar separation that does not penetrate the uterine serosa, does not produce hemorrhage, and does not cause major clinical problems.[5]

Uterine rupture is symptomatic and may have presenting signs that require acute intervention. With uterine rupture, the intrauterine and peritoneal cavities communicate. Dehiscence is uncommon (≤2 percent) and rupture is relatively rare (<1 percent). Routine uterine exploration to detect uterine dehiscence after a sucessful VBAC is not necessary.

Prior Low Vertical Incision

A prior low vertical uterine incision, limited to the lower, more passive, noncontractile portion of the uterine segment, is not a contraindication for a VBAC-TOL.[60,212]

Prior Classic Incision

It is likely that we will continue on occasion to be confronted with patients who have had a prior classic incision. A TOL should be strongly discouraged in such cases.[60] Patients with prior classic incision have an associated 12 percent risk of symptomatic uterine rupture during labor.[212,236] Since approximately one third of ruptures occur prior to labor, it is currently recommended that women who have a prior classic cesarean delivery be delivered by repeat cesarean procedure upon achieving fetal pulmonary maturity prior to the onset of labor. Such patients should be warned of the hazards of an unintended labor and the signs of possible uterine rupture.[237]

Known Versus Unknown Incision Type

In an era when prior medical records are not always readily available, it is reassuring that the overall risk of dehiscence or rupture is low even among women undergoing a TOL with an unknown prior cesarean incision type. Overall, 90 to 95 percent of women with unknown scars will have had a low transverse incision.[202]

Prostaglandin Gel and Misoprostol Usage

Although the use of prostaglandin E_2 gel for cervical ripening is extensive and is likely to have been employed in many prior VBAC candidates, reported data are limited. A recent population-based, retrospective cohort analysis of women whose first child was delivered by cesarean section in Washington State reported a .5% risk for uterine rupture in women who entered spontaneous labor. This risk increased to .8% in women induced without prostaglandins and 2.4% when prostaglandins were administered for induction. These data, collected before the widespread use of misoprostol, suggest that caution should be exercised when utilizing prostaglandins for a VBAC-TOL. Misoprostol has been associated with an increased risk of uterine rupture and should *not* be used in VBAC-TOL patients.[246]

Fetal Monitoring

In most cases, a significant alteration in FHR pattern is the presenting sign (Fig. 13–6); on occasion, an alteration (increased frequency and/or intensity) in uterine contraction pattern (if monitored externally) or a loss of intrauterine pressure (if monitored

Text continued on page 350

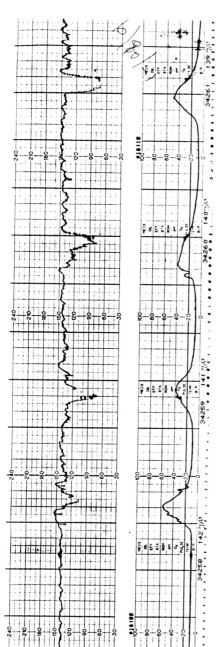

Figure 13–6. The patient is a 37-year-old gravida 7 para 3 AB3 woman at 41 weeks' gestation who presented for induction of labor. She had had two prior vaginal deliveries but her last baby was born at 33 weeks by low transverse cesarean section for nonimmune hydrops caused by a cardiac malformation. The patient's induction was begun with prostaglandin gel. Her cervix changed from fingertip dilated, 50 percent effaced, to 1 cm dilated, 70 percent effaced with a cephalic presentation at −2 station. Oxytocin was then begun at 1 milliunit/min. The patient progressed well, and epidural anesthesia was administered at 4 to 5 cm dilatation, 90 percent effaced, and 0 station. The patient was at 6 cm dilatation with a tracing demonstrating normal heart rate variability and variable decelerations.

Illustration continued on following page

347

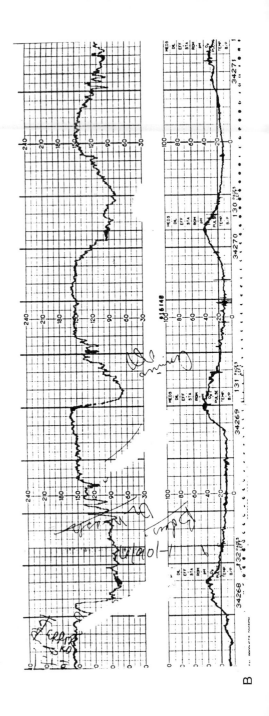

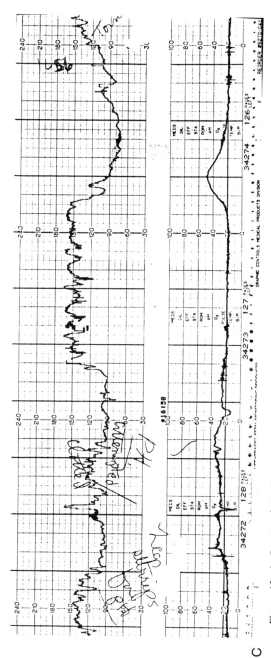

Figure 13–6. *Continued B,* 30 minutes after the above tracing was recorded, the fetal heart rate pattern changed to severe variable decelerations. *C,* The tracing then demonstrated prolonged decelerations at 90 bpm. The patient was taken to the operating room for an emergency cesarean delivery. Uterine rupture had occurred along the site of the previous uterine incision. A female fetus weighing 3,200 g with Apgar scores of 7 and 8 was delivered. The umbilical arterial pH was 7.17 and the venous pH 7.22. The uterine incision had not extended and was easily closed. The baby did well.

with an internal pressure catheter) is the presenting sign.[199] The clinical detection and management of a possible uterine rupture will involve interpretation and reaction to a nonreassuring FHR observation (i.e., a sudden prolonged deceleration, late decelerations, or repetitive "significant" variable deceleration of a degree requiring intervention under the circumstances of the case). It would appear prudent to proceed more rapidly to cesarean delivery under such circumstances than would be the case in the absence of a prior uterine incision. Unfortunately, use of intrauterine pressure catheters does not reliably assist in the diagnosis of rupture.[248,249]

Two series, one involving more than 11,000 and one more than 17,000 women with prior cesarean births, provide data specific for risk of rupture.[195,197,211] In one series, the overall risk of rupture (117 cases) was 0.7 percent (0.5 percent for those not undergoing a trial and 0.7 percent for those attempting a trial) in all women presenting with a prior cesarean.[211] In the two other reports summarizing experience from Kaiser-Permanente Hospitals in California, the overall incidence of rupture during the past decade was 0.5 percent ([10 of 5,733] in the interval between 1984 and 1988 and 0.8 percent [39 of 5,022] during the 1990 to 1992 interval).[195,197]

Perinatal Morbidity and Mortality

The perinatal mortality rate for VBAC-TOL is slightly higher than that for women having an elective repeat cesarean section, 5.8 per 1,000 versus 3.4 per 1,000. However, should uterine rupture occur the perinatal mortality rate is increased 10 fold.

Two reports have summarized the outcomes of 20 uterine ruptures. There were no maternal deaths in either study, but only 14 of 20 (70 percent) had good perinatal outcomes. There were four perinatal deaths and four cases with newborn neurologic sequelae. Unfortunately, three of the four perinatal deaths involved women who were laboring at home without fetal monitoring.[248,260]

Timing of Elective Repeat Cesarean Delivery

Should the patient refuse a VBAC-TOL or have a recurring indication for cesarean delivery, the clinician has four possible options to determine when elective cesarean delivery should occur. According to the ACOG, fetal maturity may be assumed and amniocentesis need not be performed if the criteria of one of the four options in Table 13–2 are met.[237,264] The criteria do not preclude use of menstrual dating, particularly if one of the four confirm menstrual dates in a patient with normal menstrual cycles and no immediately recent use of oral contraceptives. Ultrasound is considered confirmatory if there is agreement between menstrual-gestational age and

Table 13–2. FETAL MATURITY ASSESSMENT PRIOR TO ELECTIVE REPEAT CESAREAN DELIVERY

Option 1 (FHR)	One or more of the following is present for the stated duration: For 20 weeks: FHR by nonelectronic fetoscope For 30 weeks: FHR by Doppler
Option 2 (hCG)	For 36 weeks: positive serum or urine pregnancy test
Option 3* (Ultrasound)	At 6–12 weeks' gestation: Ultrasound crown-rump length supports gestational age of ≥ 39 weeks
Option 4* (Ultrasound)	At 12–20 weeks, multiple ultrasound measures confirm gestational age of ≥ 39 weeks as determined by clinical history and physical examination
Option 5	Await spontaneous onset of labor
Option 6	Fetal pulmonary maturity documented by amniotic fluid surfactant assessment

*Does not preclude use of menstrual age with agreement within 7 days (option 3) or 10 days (option 4).
Data from ACOG.[264]
Adapted from American College of Obstetricians and Gynecologists, Committee Opinion: Fetal Maturity Assessment Prior to Elective Repeat Cesarean Delivery. No. 98. September 1991.

crown–rump age at 6 to 11 weeks or by the average gestational age determined by multiple measurements at 12 to 20 weeks within 1 week and within 10 days, respectively.

INFORMED CONSENT

Informed Consent Is a Process

Informed consent should be considered a process that includes sharing of information and discussion of the choices reflected in the informed consent document.[266] Ordinarily, effective informed consent requires active participation by both the physician and the patient. It is the physician's responsibility to make sure that the patient is well informed; has under ordinary circumstances reasonable time to contemplate the information provided; and is encouraged to ask questions when necessary. It is the patient's responsibility to provide accurate and complete information and, if matters are unclear, to pose questions.[267]

Because likelihood of a successful VBAC is only minimally dependent on the indication for the prior cesarean delivery, the physician should present the chances of success in a positive manner. An increasing number of clinicians do obtain written consent. ACOG has recently stated that "the ultimate decision to attempt this procedure (VBAC) or undergo a repeat cesarean delivery should be made by the patient and her physician. . . . Global mandates for a trial of labor after a previous cesarean delivery are inappropriate because individual risk factors are not considered. . . ."[3]

PERIPARTUM HYSTERECTOMY

Peripartum or obstetric hysterectomy is the surgical removal of the uterus at the time of a planned or unplanned cesarean delivery or in the immediate postpartum period.

Unplanned Emergency Indications

Most peripartum hysterectomies are unplanned and follow cesarean delivery.[125] The most common indications are uterine atony, placenta accreta, uterine rupture, uterine myomata, and extension of the uterine scar. Most are performed after more conservative efforts to control bleeding have been unsuccessful. Although hysterectomy may be the ultimate remedy for control of obstetric hemorrhage, conservative measures remain the primary approach; hysterectomy is reserved for circumstances in which these efforts either fail or are not applicable as would often be the case with abnormal placentation.[274]

Prior cesarean delivery heightens the risk for subsequent placenta previa, placenta accreta, and symptomatic uterine rupture, each of which increases the likelihood for an emergency hysterectomy.[272,275] The adverse impact of placenta previa as a risk factor for unplanned hysterectomy in patients with a prior cesarean is well established.[91,276] Placenta accreta has been reported in 25 percent of cases of placenta previa and a single prior cesarean delivery and 50 percent of cases with two prior cesarean deliveries.

Maternal morbidity and mortality associated with peripartum hysterectomy is not simply the product of the procedure itself. Maternal mortality and morbidity will in large part depend on whether (1) the procedure is a planned/scheduled or an unplanned/emergency procedure, (2) the patient was previously in labor and had significant risk factors for infection, or (3) the patient had coincidental pregnancy-related complications. Unplanned hysterectomies have a greater risk for maternal mortality than planned procedures, since they are commonly performed in response to life-threatening hemorrhage with independent morbidity and mortality consequences. Nonetheless, the risk is very low. The combined mortality rate from three series is 3.2 per 100,000 (1 in 310).

Key Points

> Even when morbidity and mortality arising from the indications leading to cesarean delivery are excluded, maternal morbidity and mortality remain many times higher for cesarean delivery than for vaginal delivery.

> As the percentage of laboring patients presenting with prior cesarean births has increased, there have been associated increases in more difficult repeat cesarean deliveries and complications, including a higher incidence of placenta previa, placenta accreta, symptomatic uterine rupture, hemorrhage, requirement for transfusion, and need for unplanned hysterectomy.

> The reported incidence of maternal mortality following cesarean delivery is estimated to range from 6.1 to 22 per 100,000 live births. Approximately one third to one half of maternal deaths can be attributed directly to the cesarean procedure itself.

> There are no well-documented prospective trials demonstrating benefit to the fetus or to the mother that would justify the extent of the increase in the primary cesarean delivery rate over the past two decades. Although perinatal mortality rates have decreased as cesarean birth rates have increased, the improvement is largely attributable to major advances in prenatal and intrapartum care, as well as dramatic improvements in neonatal intensive care implemented in the same time frame.

> If the patient is massively obese, it may be better to use an incision directly over the lower uterine segment that does not involve the underside of the panniculus, an area that is more heavily colonized with bacteria and that is difficult to prepare surgically, to keep dry, and to inspect in the postoperative period.

Box continued on following page

Key Points *Continued*

➤ The physician contemplating a cesarean delivery for placenta previa, particularly a repeat procedure, should consider the possibility of hysterectomy. The reported incidence of placenta accreta (1 in 2,500 deliveries) increases to approximately 4 percent in patients with a placenta previa and may approach 25 percent in patients with a prior cesarean birth.

➤ Although cesarean delivery is often elected to minimize trauma to the preterm breech fetus, the actual delivery mechanism via the cesarean incision is essentially identical to that of the vaginal route. Should head entrapment be encountered, the first action should be to extend the abdominal incision and to enlarge the uterine incision.

➤ Elective repeat cesarean delivery is estimated to be responsible for a significant proportion of the increase in the cesarean birth rate during the past two decades. VBAC-TOL lowers the self-perpetuating contribution of the indication of previous cesarean birth.

➤ Most patients with a prior cesarean birth are candidates for VBAC. The only established contraindication is a prior classical incision. VBAC reduces the incidence of postpartum infection, the need for postpartum transfusion, maternal length of stay and, as a result, offers the potential to generate significant cost savings.

➤ VBAC trial candidates are no more likely to require a cesarean delivery than a population of women with no prior cesarean deliveries. VBAC trial of labor is successful in 60 to 80 percent of acceptable candidates.

Chapter 14

Surgical Procedures in Pregnancy

JACK LUDMIR AND
PHILLIP G. STUBBLEFIELD

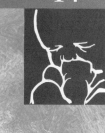

Approximately 0.2 to 2.2 percent of pregnant women require surgery in pregnancy.[1-3] Changes in the maternal cardiovascular system and increased uterine perfusion and size during gestation require special adaptation of anesthesia and surgical technique to the pregnant patient (see the box "Maternal Physiologic Changes Relevant to Surgery").[4-10] Advances in diagnostic modalities, including computed tomographic (CT) imaging, magnetic resonance imaging (MRI), high-resolution ultrasound, and Doppler studies have improved our ability to make the diagnosis of surgical conditions during gestation.[11-14] Furthermore, new surgical therapeutic modalities, including laparoscopy, are now being evaluated in the management of the pregnant patient with a surgical condition.[15-22] The patient and physician facing the possibility of surgery during pregnancy are concerned about the possible ill effects of anesthesia and surgery on the developing fetus versus the consequences of delaying such surgery. In the largest study to date of surgical procedures in pregnancy, surgery was performed in the first trimester in 41 percent, compared with 35 percent in the middle, and 24 percent in the third trimester. Abdominal surgery constituted one fourth of all operations, and almost 20 percent were gynecologic and urologic procedures. Although laparoscopy was the most commonly performed first-trimester operation to rule out ectopic gestation, appendectomy was the most common procedure in the second trimester. One half of the surgeries were performed using general anesthesia, and in 90 percent of the cases, nitrous oxide was given. The rate of congenital malformation and stillbirth were not significantly increased. However, the rate of low-birth-weight infants, as well as neonatal deaths during the first 7 days of life in patients undergoing surgery, was significantly increased. The authors concluded that surgery, in particular nonobstetric, during pregnancy could increase the rate of poor obstetric outcomes. This increase in perinatal morbidity was thought to be secondary to the surgical disease process affecting the pregnancy rather than to the adverse effects of anesthesia or

Maternal Physiologic Changes Relevant to Surgery

Cardiovascular changes
  Increased cardiac output
  Increased blood volume
  Decreased systematic vascular resistance
  Decreased venous return from the lower extremities

Respiratory changes
  Increased minute ventilation
  Decreased functional residual capacity

Gastrointestinal changes
  Decreased gastric motility
  Delayed gastric emptying

Coagulation changes
  Increased clotting factors II, V, VII, VIII, IX, X, and XII
  Increased fibrinogen
  Increased risk for thromboembolic disease

Renal changes
  Increased renal plasma flow and glomerular filtration rate
  Ureteral dilatation
  Increased bladder capacity

surgery. In approaching the pregnant patient requiring surgery, re-assurance can be given regarding the rate of birth defects and stillbirths, but prematurity and growth restriction may be significantly increased, secondary to the ill-effects of the underlying condition requiring surgery.

CERVICAL CERCLAGE

Cervical function in gestation is described by a bell-shaped curve that correlates to length.[25] Cervical function could change secondary to interaction with different variables, such as physical activity, infection, uterine distention, and uterine contractility.[30] This new concept of a continuum in cervical competence is helpful in explaining why a cervix that appears and feels long and closed could result in an early pregnancy loss, whereas a cervix that feels short and soft could carry a pregnancy to term. The traditional criteria used for performing a cervical cerclage are a classic history of painless dilatation with delivery of a premature infant, history of rapid labors, history of recurrent premature rupture of membranes (particularly in patients with prior history of cervical surgeries or trauma), or a history of diethylstilbestrol (DES)-exposure. These criteria are

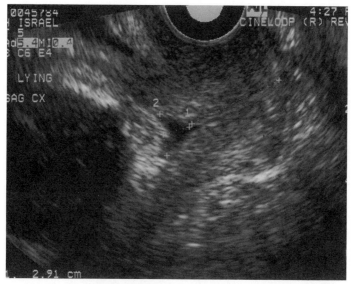

Figure 14-1. Transvaginal sonogram of the cervix at 22 weeks' gestation. Patient is at risk for cervical incompetence. Note minimal evidence of cervical funneling.

currently being challenged as the only criteria (see the box "Diagnostic Criteria for Cervical Incompetence").[31-37] The use of vaginal sonography in gestation to evaluate the cervix longitudinally may be a more objective way of screening patients at risk for cervical incompetence and of helping the clinician to decide which women would benefit from a cerclage. Sonographic parameters such as cervical shortening and/or funneling (Figs. 14-1 and 14-2)[38-43] may

---

Diagnostic Criteria for Cervical Incompetence

Historical factors
  History of painless cervical dilatation with preterm delivery
  History of forceful cervical dilatation and evacuation
  History of obstetric trauma: cervical lacerations, prolonged
    second stage followed by cesarean
  Prior cervical surgery: cone, loop
  DES exposure in utero
Cervical sonography
  Short cervical length
  Cervical funneling

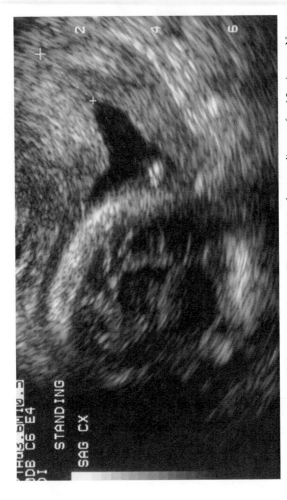

Figure 14–2. Transvaginal sonogram of the same patient as Figure 14–1 after standing up for 15 minutes. Note cervical funneling and decreased cervical length.

be particularly helpful in the patient in whom a classic history of painless dilatation cannot be elucidated and the benefit of placing a prophylactic cerclage remains unclear. The ideal cervical length at which to place a cerclage has not been determined. Studies have recommended cerclage for cervical lengths varying from as low as 1.5 to 2.5 cm in length.[43–45] It remains to be seen if cerclage, pessary, or bed rest are justifiable therapeutic interventions in patients demonstrating sonographic cervical change.

Cerclage Technique

Prophylactic Cerclage

In 1955, Shirodkar reported successful management of cervical incompetence with a submucosal band.[48] Initially, he used catgut suture, and later Mersilene placed at the level of the internal cervical os. The procedure required anterior displacement of the bladder in an attempt to place the suture as high as possible at the level of the cervical internal os. This type of procedure resulted in a greater number of patients being delivered via cesarean section because of the difficulty in removing the suture buried under the cervical surface and may require leaving the suture in place postpartum. Several years later, McDonald described a suture technique in the form of a purse string, not requiring cervical dissection, easily placed during pregnancy.[49] This technique involves taking four or five bites as high as possible in the cervix, trying to avoid injury to the bladder or the rectum, with placement of a knot anteriorly to facilitate removal (Fig. 14–3). Several types of suture material have been used.[50] We have been successful in using a Mersilene tape. However, the use of thinner suture material, such as Prolene or other synthetic nonabsorbable sutures like Ethibond is advocated by others, with the argument that the width of the Mersilene tape places the patient at greater risk for infection.[50,51] Currently, there is no evidence that placing two sutures results in better outcomes than placing one.[52–54] Preoperative patient preparations, including the use of prophylactic antibiotics or tocolytics, have not been proven to be of benefit. We perform a culture for group B streptococcus and give preoperative penicillin to the patient with a positive culture. Prophylactic cerclage placement is performed after the first trimester, to avoid the risk of spontaneous loss most likely attributable to chromosomal abnormalities.[52,53] The choice of anesthesia for cerclage varies.[55] Chen et al.[56] did not show difference. Both general and regional anesthesia may be used. In our experience, a short-acting regional anesthetic is sufficient. We advise patients to remain on bed rest for the first 48 hours after cerclage and to avoid intercourse until follow-up postoperative visit. Decisions regarding physical activity and intercourse are individualized and based on the status of the cervix as determined by

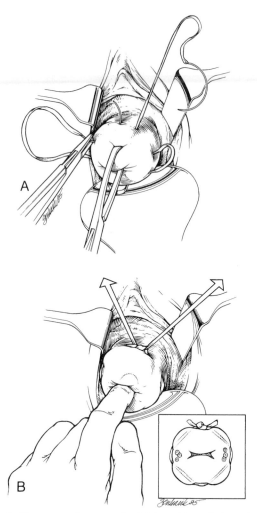

Figure 14–3. Placement of sutures for McDonald cervical cerclage. *A*, We use a double-headed Mersilene band with four "bites" in the cervix, avoiding the vessels. *B*, The suture is placed high upon the cervix close to the cervical-vaginal junction, approximately the level of the internal os.

outpatient digital evaluation or sonographic findings[39,40,57–59] The suture is usually removed at 37 weeks electively.[52,53]

In patients with a hypoplastic cervix, such as those exposed to DES in utero, history of large cervical conization, or prior history of failed vaginal cerclage, an abdominal cerclage has been recom-

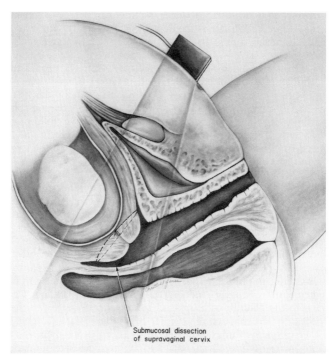

Submucosal dissection
of supravaginal cervix

Figure 14–4. Transvaginal cerclage under ultrasound guidance. (Modified from Ludmir J, Jackson GM, Samuels P: Transvaginal cerclage under ultrasound guidance in cases of severe cervical hypoplasia. Obstet Gynecol 78:1067, 1991.)

mended.[60] This procedure is usually done at 11 weeks and requires a laparotomy. A bladder flap is created and a Mersilene tape is placed at the level of the junction between the lower uterine segment and the cervix.[61] This procedure is associated with greater morbidity including injury to the uterine vessels and requires delivery by cesarean section. We have described the placement of a transvaginal cerclage when there is a hypoplastic cervix, or the cervix is flush against the vaginal wall.[62] Under ultrasound guidance, the supravaginal portion of the cervix is dissected away from the bladder and a suture is placed either in a purse-string fashion, or in cross fashion from 12 to 6 o'clock and 3 to 9 o'clock (Fig. 14–4).

Therapeutic and Emergent Cerclage

The gestational age limit for cerclage placement is ill defined. Although some clinicians will offer this therapeutic modality up to

28 weeks,[64] we do not advocate the use of therapeutic cerclage beyond 24 weeks' gestation, because of fetal viability concerns and potentially causing a preterm delivery while placing the cerclage. Some of these patients have been managed successfully with strict bed rest.[44] If the decision is made to place a cerclage, we treat preoperatively with antibiotics and nonsteroidal anti-inflammatory agents, such as indomethacin. The patient is placed on strict bed rest for the first 72 hours and is advised to refrain from intercourse and strenuous physical activity for the remainder of the pregnancy. We follow these patients with frequent sonographic assessment of the cervix and recommend strict bed rest if the membranes are prolapsing to the level of the suture.[58] Prophylactic tocolytics are not used after the procedure.

In situations in which the cervix has dilated enough to allow visualization of the membranes or the membranes have prolapsed into the vagina, placing an emergent cerclage constitutes a heroic maneuver.[64-68] These patients are at high risk of having a subclinical infection and subsequent poor outcome.[65,69] To rule out infection, some clinicians advocate amniocentesis prior to cerclage placement.[70] Several techniques have been described to reduce the prolapsing membranes, including the following: placing the patient in Trendelenburg position; the use of a pediatric Foley catheter to tease the membranes into the endocervical canal, and instilling 1 L of saline into the bladder with upper displacement of the lower uterine segment.[67,68,70,71] Although the efficacy of antibiotics or tocolytics has not been properly studied, some case series advocate their use. Although clinicians have been reluctant to offer cerclage in patients with protruding membranes, some reports have suggested salvage rate in excess of 70 percent despite advanced cervical dilatation.[72-74]

Risks of Cerclage

Cervical lacerations at the time of delivery are one of the most common complications from a cerclage, occurring in 1 to 13 percent of patients.[52] Three percent of patients require cesarean birth because of the inability of the cervix to dilate secondary to cervical scarring and dystocia.[52] Although the risk of infection is minimal with a prophylactic cerclage, the risk increases significantly in cases of advanced dilatation with exposure of membranes to the birth canal.[69] Cervical cerclage displacement occurs in a small number of patients. When the clinician is faced with premature rupture of membranes distant from term in a patient with cerclage, the decision to remove or leave the suture is controversial. Our own data suggests that with suture retention, there is an increased period of latency, at the expense of increased risk for neonatal sepsis and mortality.[75] These data have been recently challenged by reports suggesting increased latency period without increase in neonatal morbidity.[76,77] Decisions to remove the suture at time of ruptured membranes should be individualized until more information becomes available.

Efficacy of Cervical Cerclage

Most reports demonstrating improvement in pregnancy outcome with cerclage placement have done so by using each patient as her own historical control. Four prospective, randomized, controlled trials of cerclage, including one for multiple gestations, failed to demonstrate significant improvement in pregnancy outcome in patients receiving prophylactic cerclage.[79-82] Unfortunately, these trials did not involve patients with classic indications for cerclage, but used as criteria for randomization increased risk for preterm birth, or cases in which obstetricians were unsure as to whether a cerclage should be placed. The introduction of sonography in assessing the cervix during gestation will provide additional diagnostic criteria to help the clinician decide if therapeutic intervention with cerclage is indicated.[43-45] Initial information from ongoing randomized trials in patients at high risk for cervical incompetence do not demonstrate differences in preterm delivery between prophylactic cerclage versus sonographically indicated therapeutic cerclage.[43] Based on this new information, it seems prudent to incorporate cervical sonography in the management of patients at risk for cervical incompetence.

MYOMECTOMY

Uterine myomas (fibroids) are the most common pelvic masses found in gestation. Myomas can increase in size during gestation, and place the patient at risk for preterm birth, abruption, dystocia, and bleeding.[83] When myomas outgrow their blood supply, they can develop cystic areas of red degeneration resulting in severe pain requiring nonsteroidal agents or narcotic medication.[83] Small fibroids increase in size during the second trimester, but during the third trimester, most fibroids decrease in size, regardless of their initial size. Most of the complications in pregnant patients with myomas are secondary to myoma location in the uterus.[86-88] The removal of a fibroid in pregnancy is contraindicated unless there is the presence of a pedunculated myoma twisting its stalk and giving the patient severe discomfort. Laparoscopic removal of this type of fibroid could be considered, but lack of experience with this situation precludes its routine use. The finding of myomas at time of cesarean section constitutes a challenge to the obstetrician.[88,89] If the myomas are encountered on the uterine incision line, careful myomectomy may be performed,[89] but may cause profuse bleeding and even may require hysterectomy to control hemorrhage. To avoid massive hemorrhage, routine myomectomy at time of cesarean section should be avoided; most myomas will involute in size in the nonpregnant state.

OOPHORECTOMY

The frequent use of ultrasound in early gestation has resulted in a significant number of asymptomatic adnexal masses diagnosed early in pregnancy. This knowledge creates a dilemma for the clinician: the appropriate management of an asymptomatic adnexal mass on the pregnant patient.[90] Ovarian masses in pregnancy could undergo torsion, rupture, and cause obstruction of labor.[91] They also carry a small risk of malignancy.[92] If the clinical presentation is consistent with torsion, rupture, or hemorrhage, immediate surgical intervention is indicated. If an adnexal mass is identified coincidentally at the time of cesarean section, some advocate its removal including those masses smaller than 5 cm. In one study, only 2 of 41 masses smaller than 5 cm were functional cysts. While some authors have advocated aspiration and cytologic evaluation of cysts in selected cases, a malignancy could be missed even with simple smooth-walled cysts especially if it is greater than 5 cm. The patient with a simple sonographic cyst, smaller than 5 cm, has a very small risk for malignant change.[95] This patient can be followed during gestation without surgical intervention.[96,97] For those patients demonstrating masses greater than 5 cm, and with presence of solid elements, surgical intervention should be considered during the early second trimester, to minimize fetal risk. Surgery in the second trimester is felt to be safest. The risk of surgical intervention may favor a conservative approach on the basis of sonographic findings (Table 14–1). Laparoscopy offers a newer approach to the pregnant patient with an adnexal mass (see the boxes "Laparoscopy During Pregnancy Guidelines [SAGES]" and "Relative Contraindications to Laparoscopy in Pregnancy").

Table 14–1. RISK OF OVARIAN MALIGNANCY BASED ON SONOGRAPHIC FINDINGS

Low risk of malignancy	Simple smooth wall cyst
	Size <5 cm
Increased risk of malignancy	Solid mass
	Nodules
	Thick septations
	Size >5 cm

Laparoscopy During Pregnancy Guidelines (SAGES)

Pneumatic compression devices
Lead shield with selective fluoroscopy
Dependent position
Obstetric consultation
Intraoperative fetal monitoring
Minimal pneumoperitoneum (8–12 mm Hg)
Serial arterial blood gas analysis
Second-trimester deferment
Open technique

Modified from Guidelines for laparoscopic surgery during Pregnancy. Surg Endosc 4:100, 1998.

Relative Contraindications to Laparoscopy in Pregnancy

Access issues
    Late second or third trimester
    Multiple gestations
    Advanced disease process (e.g., walled-off abscess)
    Retrocecal location of appendix
Medical complications
    Intra-abdominal sepsis
    Bleeding disorders
    Ileus

TUBAL STERILIZATION

Advantages for postpartum tubal sterilization include the use of one anesthesia for labor, delivery, and sterilization, and only one hospitalization.[99] Tubal ligations after vaginal delivery are performed through a minilaparotomy incision at the level of the uterine fundus, usually subumbilically. The same surgical techniques are applied if tubal ligation is performed at time of cesarean section. The long-term failure rate is approximately 1 percent overall.

Modified Pomeroy

The Pomeroy technique includes grasping the fallopian tube at its midportion, creating a small knuckle, and then ligating the loop

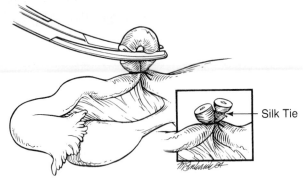

Silk Tie

Figure 14–5. Pomeroy sterilization. A knuckle of tube is ligated with absorbable suture, and a small segment is being excised. Note that the ligation is performed at a site that will favor reanastomosis, should that become desirable. Some surgeons place an extra tie of nonabsorbable suture around the proximal stump as added protection against recanalization.

of tube with a double strand of No. 1 catgut suture. It is critical that the fallopian tube be conclusively identified. Visualizing the fimbriated portion of the tube and identifying the round ligament as a separate structure can accomplish this. Absorbable sutures are used so that the tubal ends will separate quickly after surgery, leaving a gap between the proximal and distal ends. Modifications include placing nonabsorbable suture in the proximal ends of each resected tube. In performing the procedure, care should be taken to make the loop of fallopian tube sufficient in size to ensure that complete transection of the tubal lumen will occur. After the loop of fallopian tube is ligated, the mesosalpinx of the ligated loop should be perforated using scissors, and the knuckle of the tube is transected (Fig. 14–5). It is important not to resect the fallopian tube so close to the suture that the remaining portion of the fallopian tube slips out of the ligature and causes delayed bleeding.

The Uchida Procedure

In this sterilization procedure,[104] the fallopian tube muscular portion is separated from its serosal cover and grasped approximately 6 to 7 cm from the uterotubal junction, saline solution is injected subserosally, and the serosa is then incised. The muscular portion of the fallopian tube is grasped with a clamp and divided. The serosa over the proximal tubal segment is bluntly dissected toward the uterus, exposing approximately 5 cm of the proximal tubal segment. The tube is then ligated with chromic suture near the uterotubal junction, and

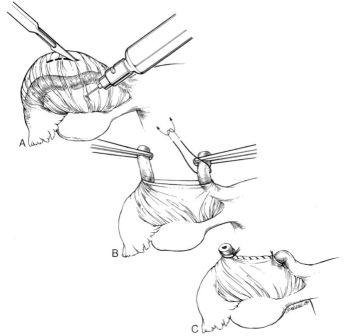

Figure 14-6. Uchida sterilization. The leaves of the broad ligament and peritubal peritoneum are infiltrated with saline so that the tube can be easily isolated from these structures, divided, and ligated. The broad ligament is then closed, burying the proximal stump between the leaves and including the distal stump in the line of closure.

approximately 5 cm of the tube is resected. The shortened proximal tubal stump is allowed to retract into the mesosalpinx. The serosa around the opening in the mesosalpinx is sutured in a purse-string with a fine absorbable stitch; when the suture is tied the mesosalpinx is gathered around the distal tubal segment (Fig. 14-6).

SPECIFIC SURGICAL PROBLEMS IN PREGNANCY

Appendicitis

Appendicitis is one of the most common surgical complications of pregnancy, with an incidence of 1 to 2 per 1,000 gestations.[105] This incidence is roughly similar to that in the nonpregnant population.

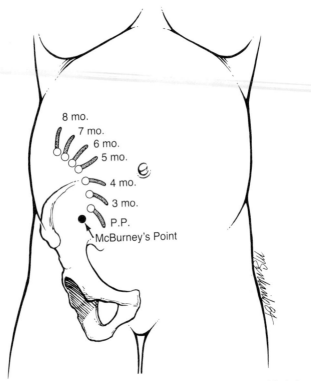

Figure 14-7. Locations of the appendix in pregnancy. As modified from Bauer et al., the approximate location of the appendix during succeeding months of pregnancy is diagrammed. In planning an operation, it is better to make the abdominal incision over the point of maximum tenderness unless there is a great disparity between that point and the theoretical location of the appendix. (Modified from Baer JL, Reis RA, Arens RA: Appendicitis in pregnancy with changes in position and axis of the normal appendix in pregnancy. JAMA 98:1359, 1932.)

Appendiceal location changes during pregnancy with upper displacement of the appendix with advancing gestation (Fig. 14-7). The change in appendiceal location with advancing gestation would change the location of perceived pain toward the patient's right upper quadrant or right flank. Nevertheless, pain in the right lower quadrant of the abdomen remains the most common symptom of appendicitis regardless of gestational age. The diagnosis of appendicitis in pregnancy is difficult secondary to a clinical picture mimicking common symptoms in gestation including nausea, vomiting, and abdominal discomfort.[109]

Early in the course of appendicitis, temperature and pulse rate may be normal; later, a low-grade temperature elevation or even a normal temperature may be present. Only 20 percent of patients exhibit rectal or vaginal tenderness. The normal leukocytosis of pregnancy (14,000/mm^3) might mask appendicitis. Radiographic studies are rarely helpful, but most recently ultrasound and CT scan of the abdomen have been advocated.[14,110] Even though the diagnosis is only found in 50 percent of patients undergoing surgery, it is better to operate unnecessarily rather than postpone surgery until generalized peritonitis has developed. Surgery can minimize maternal–fetal morbidity by preventing progression to appendiceal rupture and peritonitis.[105,106,109] Fetal mortality is low when acute appendicitis is diagnosed and treated, but may rise significantly in the presence of peritonitis. Maternal death may occur in the presence of peritonitis and overwhelming intra-abdominal sepsis. Cesarean section is rarely indicated at the time of appendectomy. A recent abdominal incision presents no problem during labor and vaginal delivery. Recently, several small case series of laparoscopic appendectomies in pregnancy have been reported demonstrating success during all trimesters, without complications.[15,18,19,111]

Acute Cholecystitis

After appendicitis, biliary tract disease is the second most common general surgical condition encountered in pregnant women. Its incidence varies from 1 in 2,000 to 1 in 4,000 pregnancies.[112] Pregnancy increases the risk of gallstones, probably secondary to high progesterone levels that inhibit smooth muscle contractility. This results in greater gallbladder volume with retention of cholesterol crystals prerequisite for gallstone formation.[113]

Cholecystitis during pregnancy usually develops when there is obstruction of the cystic duct. This clinical entity ranges from intermediate attacks of biliary colic to persistent pain radiating into the subcapsular area in cases where the common duct is obstructed by a stone. There is usually right subcostal tenderness along with a low-grade fever. Ultrasound is helpful in detecting the presence of stones as small as 2 mm, and confirms the diagnosis of gallstones in about 90 percent of patients.[11] The differential diagnoses for cholecystitis include conditions unique to pregnancy such as acute fatty liver of pregnancy and severe preeclampsia. Initial attacks of cholecystitis should be treated conservatively, with intravenous fluids, nasogastric suction, antibiotics, and antispasmodics. Without prompt resolution of symptoms, surgery should be considered. Eighty percent of patients with an initial attack will get relief with conservative medical treatment. In the presence of common duct obstruction or pancreatitis, cholecystectomy is necessary.[114] Delaying surgery for cholecystitis results in increased perinatal morbidity, with lower morbidity found in those patients managed surgically, particularly in cases of bile duct obstruction.[117]

Laparoscopic cholecystectomies have revolutionized the management of the pregnant patient with cholecystitis.[16,115,116] Small case series demonstrate the same good outcomes compared with open laparotomies.

Intestinal Obstruction

The incidence of bowel obstruction in pregnancy is similar to that of the general population, approximately 1 in 3,000 deliveries.[119] Intestinal obstruction usually involves the small bowel, and is commonly caused by an adhesive band or hernia (Table 14–2).[120] Prior abdominal and pelvic surgery are the most frequent causes for intestinal obstruction. Intestinal obstruction is a grave complication of pregnancy and results from pressure of the growing uterus on intestinal adhesions. Patients with bowel obstruction present with colicky midabdominal pain associated with hyperactive peristalsis. Nausea and vomiting is found in 80 percent of cases. As time passes, the intestinal peristalsis decreases and the abdomen finally becomes silent. Bowel distention may be marked, and difficult to access in pregnancy. Limited radiography studies are clearly indicated. In cases of small bowel obstruction, radiologic findings include dilatation of small bowel loops with air–fluid levels. Initial treatment of intestinal distention includes decompression with a nasogastric tube or long tube, adequate fluid resuscitation, and correction of electrolyte imbalance. If after 6 to 8 hours of treatment

Table 14–2. CAUSES OF INTESTINAL OBSTRUCTION IN PREGNANCY

Cause	%
Adhesions	60
Volvulus	25
Ileus	8
Intussusception	5
Hernia, appendicitis	6

From Perdue PW, Johnston HW Jr, Stafford PW: Intestinal obstruction complicating pregnancy. Am J Surg 164:384, 1992, with permission.

there is no satisfactory patient response, laparotomy should be performed before bowel necrosis and perforation occur. The uterus rarely interferes with the surgery, and if preterm labor follows the procedure, tocolytics can be used.

Trauma

Trauma from accidental injuries complicates 6 to 7 percent of all pregnancies.[124] The majority of these patients suffer only minor injuries and would not require hospital admission in the absence of pregnancy.[125] Unfortunately, trauma is the leading nonobstetric cause of maternal mortality, accounting for 20 percent of maternal deaths.[126] The risk of fetal demise from major blunt trauma increases from 8.7 percent in the first trimester, to 40 to 50 percent during the second and third trimesters.[127] Domestic violence during pregnancy is an increasingly common cause of maternal injury.

Automobile restraint systems with a shoulder harness prevent forward flexion of the maternal torso, and when used correctly reduce fetal death rates by preventing ejection of the mother from the vehicle. A waist-type seat belt can produce distortion of the uterus produced by the sudden compression of the belt resulting in placental abruption.[129,130] Blunt trauma may result in rupture of the membranes and preterm labor. Placental abruption is the most common cause of fetal demise when the maternal injuries are not lethal.[131] Placental separation may manifest at the time of injury or later, with the great majority of them in the first 24 hours. For this reason, even moderate blunt trauma should be an indication for fetal heart rate monitoring and close observation.[132-134]

Management of the pregnant trauma patient requires a team effort and complete understanding of the physiologic changes unique to gestation. Initially, the "ABCs" (airway, breathing, and circulation) should be assessed. If possible, the injured pregnant woman who is more than 20 weeks' gestation should be kept in the lateral decubitus position. Once the maternal vital signs have been stabilized, appropriate diagnostic studies to rule out internal injury, including CT scan and MRI are performed, if necessary. Fetal assessment with continuous electronic monitoring is advocated, as well as uterine contraction monitoring.[133,134] Possible placental abruption is predicted by using continuous electronic monitoring and findings of frequent uterine contractions.[124]

The American College of Obstetricians and Gynecologists (ACOG) recommends that any pregnant woman sustaining trauma beyond 22 to 24 weeks' gestation should undergo fetal monitoring for a minimum of 24 hours. In the presence of ruptured membranes, bleeding, fetal arrhythmia, fetal heart rate deceleration, or more than four contractions per hour, the patient should be admitted with continuous fetal monitoring for at least 24 hours.[136] Ultrasound is useful to determine gestational age, to determine fetal well-being if monitoring is equivocal, and to confirm fetal death.

Several studies have established that fetal maternal hemorrhage is increased in women who have suffered trauma in pregnancy.[124] The use of the Kleihauer-Betke test is advocated in RhD-negative women, so adequate anti-D immune globulin can be administered. A Kleihauer-Betke test is not helpful in RhD-positive women.

Key Points

➤ Surgery in pregnancy requires knowledge and understanding of the physiologic alterations in gestation.

➤ Symptoms of gastrointestinal disease during gestation can mimic pregnancy-related symptomatology. Careful evaluation of the patient with abdominal pain in pregnancy is mandatory.

➤ Delay in surgical intervention for patients with intra-abdominal surgical pathology results in increased maternal and fetal morbidity and mortality.

➤ Elective surgery early during the second trimester is associated with the most favorable outcome for both mother and fetus.

➤ Decisions regarding cervical cerclage placement require careful evaluation of the patient's history and cervical status.

➤ Evaluation of the cervix by ultrasound is helpful in the management of patients at risk for cervical incompetence.

➤ Surgery for asymptomatic adnexal masses in pregnancy should include sonographic evaluation of the mass.

➤ High index of suspicion for appendicitis is required for the pregnant patient presenting with right lower quadrant abdominal pain.

➤ Recent series of laparoscopic appendectomies and cholecystectomies during gestation demonstrate similar outcomes to an open approach.

➤ The performance of laparoscopic surgery in gestation should be subject to specific guidelines to ensure maternal and fetal well-being. Further studies are necessary before making absolute recommendations regarding the safety of this technique.

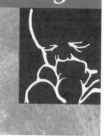

Postpartum Care

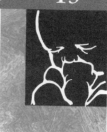

Chapter 15

Delivery Room Management of the Neonate

ADAM A. ROSENBERG

The first 4 weeks of an infant's life, the neonatal period, are marked by the highest mortality rate in all of childhood. The greatest risk occurs during the first several days after birth. Critical to survival during this period is the infant's ability to adapt successfully to extrauterine life. During the early hours after birth, the newborn must assume responsibility for thermoregulation, metabolic homeostasis, and respiratory gas exchange, as well as undergo the conversion from fetal to postnatal circulatory pathways. Successful accouplishment of this process begins with proper management in the delivery room, specifically resuscitation.

RESUSCITATION OF THE NEWBORN

When an asphyxiated infant is expected, a resuscitation team should be in the delivery room. The team should have at least two persons, one to manage the airway and one to monitor heart rate and provide whatever assistance is needed. The necessary equipment for an adequate resuscitation is listed in Table 15–1.

Steps in the resuscitation process[91,92] are as follows (Fig. 15–1):

1. Dry the infant well and place under the radiant heat source on the back or side with the neck slightly extended.
2. Gently suction the oropharynx and nose.
3. Assess the infant's condition (Table 15–2). The best criteria to assess are the infant's respiratory effort (apneic, gasping, regular) and heart rate (more or less than 100). A depressed heart rate indicative of hypoxic myocardial depression is the single most reliable indicator of the need for resuscitation.[90,93]
4. Generally, infants who are breathing with heart rates over 100 bpm will require no further intervention. If the infant is breathing with an adequate heart rate, but is cyanotic, provide supplemental oxygen. Infants with heart rates less than 100 bpm with

Table 15-1. EQUIPMENT FOR NEONATAL RESUSCITATION

Clinical Needs	Equipment
Thermoregulation	Radiant heat source with platform, mattress with warm sterile blankets, servo control heating, temperature probe
Airway management	*Suction:* bulb suction, meconium aspirator, wall vacuum suction with sterile catheters
	Ventilation: manual infant resuscitation bag connected to pressure manometer capable of delivering 100% oxygen, appropriate masks for term and preterm infants, oral airways, stethoscope, gloves
	Intubation: neonatal laryngoscope with #0 and #1 blades; extra bulbs and batteries; endotracheal tubes 2.5, 3.0, and 3.5 mm OD with stylet; scissors, adhesive tape
Gastric decompression	Nasogastric tube, 8.0 Fr
Administration of drugs/volume	Sterile umbilical catheterization tray, umbilical catheters (3.5 and 5.0 Fr), volume expanders (lactated Ringer's, normal saline), drug box with appropriate neonatal vials and dilutions, sterile syringes, and needles
Transport	Warmed transport isolette with oxygen source

apnea or irregular respiratory efforts should be vigorously stimulated by rubbing the baby's back with a towel while blowing oxygen over the face.

5. If the baby fails to respond rapidly to tactile stimulation, proceed to bag and face mask ventilation, using a soft mask that seals well around the mouth and nose. Choice of ventilation bags includes a flow-inflating bag (500 to 750 ml) with a pressure gauge and flow control valve or a self-inflating bag (240 to 750 ml) with an oxygen reservoir and pressure release valve. For the initial inflations, pressures of 30 to 40 cm H_2O may be necessary to overcome surface active forces in the lungs. Adequacy of ventilation is assessed by observing expansion of the infant's chest with bagging and a gradual improvement in color, perfusion, and heart rate. After the first few breaths, attempts should

Table 15–2. THE APGAR SCORING SYSTEM

Sign	0	1	2
Heart rate	Absent	<100 bpm	>100 bpm
Respiratory effort	Apneic	Weak, irregular, gasping	Regular
Reflex irritability*	No response	Some response	Facial grimace, sneeze, cough
Muscle tone	Flaccid	Some flexion	Good flexion of arms and legs
Color	Blue, pale	Body pink, hands and feet blue	Pink

*Elicited by suctioning the oropharynx and nose.
Modified from Apgar V: A proposal for a new method of evaluation of the newborn infant. Anesth Analg 32:260, 1953.

be made to lower the peak pressure to 15 to 20 cm H_2O. Rate of bagging should not exceed 40 to 60 bpm.

6. Most neonates can be effectively resuscitated with a bag and face mask. If the infant does not initially respond to bag and mask ventilation, try to reposition the head (slight extension), reapply the mask to achieve a good seal, consider suctioning the mouth and oropharynx, and try ventilating with the mouth open. It may be necessary to increase the pressure used. However, if there is not favorable response in 30 to 40 seconds, one must proceed to intubation:

   a. The head should be stable, with the nose in the sniffing position (pointing straight upward).
   b. Insert the laryngoscope blade, and sweep the tongue to the left.
   c. Advance the blade to the base of the tongue, and identify the epiglottis.
   d. Pick up the proper size endotracheal tube (2.5 mm OD for infants <1,000 g, 3.0 mm for infants 1,000 to 2,000 g, and 3.5 mm for larger infants) with the right hand.
   e. Slide the laryngoscope anterior to the epiglottis, and gently lift along the angle of the handle of the laryngoscope (Fig. 15–2).
   f. Identify the vocal cords.
   g. Insert the tube in the right side of the mouth, and visualize the tube passing through the vocal cords. The tube should be located 7 cm at the lip for a 1,000-g infant, 8 cm for a 2,000-g infant, and 9 cm for a 3,000-g infant.

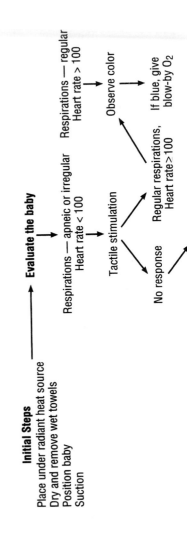

Initial Steps
Place under radiant heat source
Dry and remove wet towels
Position baby
Suction

↓

Evaluate the baby

Respirations — apneic or irregular   Respirations — regular
Heart rate < 100   Heart rate > 100

↓   ↓

Tactile stimulation   Observe color

No response   Regular respirations,   If blue, give
               Heart rate >100   blow-by O₂

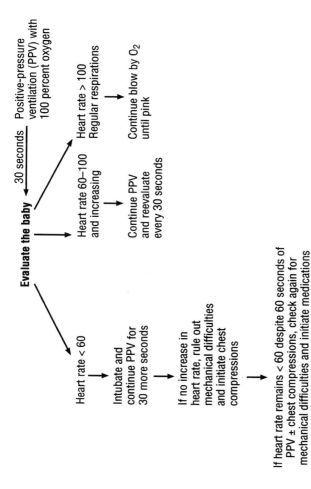

Evaluate the baby — 30 seconds — Positive-pressure ventilation (PPV) with 100 percent oxygen

Heart rate > 100
Regular respirations

Continue blow by O₂ until pink

Heart rate 60–100 and increasing

Continue PPV and reevaluate every 30 seconds

Heart rate < 60

Intubate and continue PPV for 30 more seconds

If no increase in heart rate, rule out mechanical difficulties and initiate chest compressions

If heart rate remains < 60 despite 60 seconds of PPV ± chest compressions, check again for mechanical difficulties and initiate medications

Figure 15–1. Delivery room management of the newborn. PPV, positive-pressure ventilation.

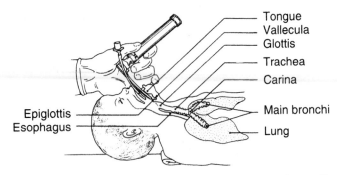

Tongue
Vallecula
Glottis
Trachea
Carina
Epiglottis
Esophagus
Main bronchi
Lung

Figure 15–2. Anatomy of laryngoscopy for endotracheal intubation. From the American Heart Association and American Academy of Pediatrics: Textbook of Neonatal Resuscitation. Washington, DC, American Heart Association, 1994, with permission (but the 1994 edition is out of print as of 2000).

   h. Ventilate as described above.
   i. Failure to respond to intubation and ventilation can result from (i) mechanical difficulties (Table 15–3), (ii) profound asphyxia with myocardial depression, and (iii) inadequate circulating blood volume.
   j. The mechanical causes listed in Table 15–3 should be quickly ruled out. Check to be sure the endotracheal tube passes through the vocal cords. Occlusion of the tube should be suspected when there is resistance to bagging and no chest wall movement. If the endotracheal tube is in place and not occluded, and the equip-

Table 15–3. MECHANICAL CAUSES OF FAILED RESUSCITATION

Category	Examples
Equipment failure	Malfunctioning bag, oxygen not connected or running
Endotracheal tube malposition	Esophagus, right mainstem bronchus
Occluded endotracheal tube	
Insufficient inflation pressure to expand lungs	
Space-occupying lesions in the thorax	Pneumothorax, pleural effusions, diaphragmatic hernia
Pulmonary hypoplasia	Extreme prematurity, oligohydramnios

ment is functioning, a trial of bagging with higher pressures is indicated. The other causes listed in Table 15–3 are rare compared with equipment failure or tube problems. A pneumothorax is characterized by asymmetric breath sounds not corrected by repositioning the tube above the carina. Pleural effusions usually occur with fetal hydrops, while a diaphragmatic hernia should be ruled out in the setting of asymmetric breath sounds and a scaphoid abdomen. Pulmonary hypoplasia should be considered if the pregnancy has been complicated by oligohydramnios. It is very unusual for a neonatal resuscitation to require either cardiac massage or drugs. Almost all newborns respond to ventilation with 100 percent oxygen.

7. If mechanical causes are ruled out, external cardiac massage should be performed for persistent heart rate at less than 60 bpm. Compression of $\frac{1}{3}$ the anterior-posterior diameter of the chest should be performed, interposed with ventilation at a 3:1 ratio (90 compressions, 30 breaths per minute).

8. If drugs are needed for a persistent heart rate less than 60 bpm after ventilation and chest compressions (Table 15–4), the drug of choice is 0.1 to 0.3 ml/kg of 1:10,000 epinephrine through the endotracheal tube or preferably an umbilical venous line. Sodium bicarbonate 1 to 2 mEq/kg of the neonatal dilution (0.5 mEq/ml) can be used in prolonged resuscitation efforts in which response to other measures is poor or with a documented metabolic acidosis. If volume loss is suspected (e.g., documented blood loss with clinical evidence of hypovolemia), 10 ml/kg of a volume expander (normal saline) should be administered through an umbilical venous line. The appropriateness of continued resuscitative efforts should always be reevaluated in an infant who fails to respond to all of the above efforts. Today, resuscitative efforts are made even in "apparent stillbirths," that is, infants whose 1-minute Apgar scores are 0 to 1. However, efforts should not be sustained in the face of little or no improvement over a reasonable period of time (i.e., 10 to 15 minutes).[94]

Infants in whom respiratory depression secondary to narcotic administration is suspected may be given naloxone (Narcan). However, this should not be done until the airway has been managed and the infant resuscitated in the usual fashion. In addition, naloxone should not be given to the infant of an addicted mother, as it will precipitate withdrawl. A second special group are preterm infants. Minimizing heat loss improves survival, so prewarmed towels should be available, and the environmental temperature of the delivery suite should be raised. In the extremely-low-birth-weight infant (<1,000 g), proceed quickly to intubation. Volume expanders and sodium bicarbonate should be infused slowly to avoid rapid swings in blood pressure.

Table 15-4. NEONATAL DRUG DOSES

Drug	Dose	Route	How Supplied
Epinephrine	0.1–0.3 ml/kg	IV or ET	1:10,000 dilution
Sodium bicarbonate*	1–2 mEq/kg	IV	0.5 mEq/ml (4.2% solution)
Volume†	10 ml/kg	IV	Whole blood, lactated Ringer's, normal saline
Naloxone (Narcan)‡	0.1 mg/kg	IV, ET, IM, or SC	1 mg/ml

*For correction of metabolic acidosis only after adequate ventilation has been achieved; give slowly over several minutes.
†Infuse slowly over several minutes.
‡After proceeding with proper airway management and other resuscitative techniques.
IV, intravenous; ET, endotracheal; IM, intramuscular; SC, subcutaneous.
Modified from American Heart Association and American Academy of Pediatrics: Neonatal Resuscitation Textbook. American Academy of Pediatrics and American Heart Association, 2000.

MECONIUM ASPIRATION SYNDROME

Meconium aspiration syndrome (MAS) is a form of aspiration pneumonia that occurs most often in term or postterm infants who have passed meconium in utero (10 to 15 percent of all deliveries[95]).

Current clinical and experimental data support that MAS is the result of intrauterine asphyxia. The best method of prevention is to identify the fetus at risk (postterm, oligohydramnios). Intrapartum management should emphasize treatments that enhance uteroplacental perfusion. Aminoinfusion in cases with oligohydramnios may reduce cord compression, gasping, and intrapartum aspiration.[107] The management of the infant's airway remains controversial, but a reasonable approach is as follows:

1. The obstetrician carefully suctions the oro- and nasopharynx after delivery of the head with a suction apparatus, hooked to wall suction.
2. The delivery is then completed and the baby given to the resuscitator.
3. If the baby is active and breathing and requires no resuscitation, the airway need not be inspected, thus avoiding the risk of inducing vagal bradycardia.
4. Any infant in need of resuscitation should have the airway inspected and suctioned before instituting positive-pressure ventilation.
5. Suction the stomach when airway management is complete and vital signs are stable.

Postpartum Care and Breast-Feeding

WATSON A. BOWES, JR., VERN L. KATZ,
AND EDWARD R. NEWTON

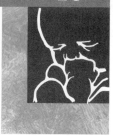

POSTPARTUM INVOLUTION

The Uterus

Hemostasis immediately after birth is accomplished by arterial smooth muscle contraction and compression of vessels by the involuting uterine muscle. Within 2 weeks after birth the uterus has usually returned to the pelvis, and by 6 weeks it is usually normal size, as estimated by palpation.

The postpartum uterine discharge or lochia begins as a flow of blood lasting several hours, rapidly diminishing to a reddish brown discharge through the third or fourth day postpartum. This is followed by a transition to a mucopurulent discharge, lochia serosa, for about 3 weeks. In the majority of patients, the lochia serosa is followed by a yellow-white discharge, lachia alba. Sometimes a sudden but transient increase in uterine bleeding occurs between 7 and 14 days postpartum. This corresponds to the slough of the eschar over the site of placental attachment. Although it can be profuse, this bleeding episode is usually self-limited, requiring nothing more than reassurance of the patient. If it does not subside within 1 or 2 hours, the patient should be evaluated for possible retained placental tissue with ultrasound. Ultrasound examination efficiently detects patients who have retained tissue and who will therefore benefit from uterine evacuation and curettage. Those who have an empty uterine cavity will respond to therapy with oxytocin or methylergonovine.[12]

Ovarian Function

It has long been recognized that women who breast-feed their infants will be amenorrheic for long periods of time, often until the infant is weaned. Several studies, using a variety of methods to indicate ovulation, have demonstrated that ovulation occurs as

385

early as 27 days after delivery, with the mean time being approximately 70 to 75 days in nonlactating women.[17,18] Among those women who are breast-feeding their infants, the mean time to ovulation is about 6 months.

Menstruation resumes by 12 weeks' postpartum in 70 percent of women who are not lactating, and the mean time to the first menstruation is 7 to 9 weeks. The duration of anovulation depends on the frequency of breast-feeding, the duration of each feed, and the proportion of supplementary feeds.[19] The risk of ovulation within the first 6 months' postpartum in a woman exclusively breast-feeding is 1 to 5 percent.

Weight Loss

By six weeks postpartum, 28 percent of women will have returned to their prepregnant weight. The remainder of the weight loss occurs from 6 weeks postpartum until 6 months after delivery. Women with weight gain in pregnancy of more than 35 lb are likely to have a net gain.[22]

Thyroid Function

The postpartum period is associated with an increased risk for the development of a transient autoimmune thyroiditis that may in some cases lead to permanent hypothyroidism.[27] Asymptomatic postpartum thyroid dysfunction may occur in as many as 10 percent of parturients.[28]

Cardiovascular System and Coagulation

By the third postpartum day, plasma volume has increased by 900 to 1,200 ml because of a shift of extracellular fluid into the vascular space.[32] Patients who deliver vaginally have a 5 percent increase in hematocrit, whereas those who have a cesarean delivery have on average a 6 percent decrease in hematocrit.[33]

The Urinary Tract and Renal Function

The urinary tract becomes dilated during pregnancy, especially the renal pelves and the ureters above the pelvic brim, the right kidney more than the left. These changes are caused by compression of the ureters by adjacent vasculature, by compression from the enlarged uterus, and by the effect of progesterone. Ureteral tone above the pelvic brim returns to nonpregnant levels immediately after delivery.[41]

Hair Loss

Hair growth slows in the puerperium. Often, women will experience hair loss, as temporarily more hair is lost than is regrown. This is a transient phenomenon, and the patient may be reassured that hair patterns return to normal within a few months.

Management of the Puerperium

If a patient has adequate support at home (i.e., help with housekeeping and meal preparation), there is little value in an extended hospital stay, provided the mother is adequately educated about infant care and feeding, family planning, and identification of danger signs in either the infant or herself. For mothers who are insecure about infant care and feeding, extending the hospital stay will provide time for them to gain adequate education and some measure of self-confidence.[59] Also, home nursing visits can be helpful in providing support, education, and advice to mothers.

Physical activity, including walking up and down stairs, lifting heavy objects, riding in or driving a car, and performing muscle-toning exercises, can be resumed without delay if the delivery has been uncomplicated. Mothers whose lethargy persists beyond several weeks must be evaluated, especially as regards thyroid dysfunction and depression.

Sexual activity may be resumed when the perineum is comfortable. The desire and willingness to resume sexual activity in the puerperium varies greatly among women, depending on the site and state of healing of perineal or vaginal incisions the amount of vaginal atrophy secondary to breast-feeding, and the return of libido.[65]

Six weeks is regarded as the normal period of "disability" following delivery[69] for employed mothers, and eight weeks after a cesarian delivery.

Perineal Care

Analgesia can be accomplished in most patients with nonsteroidal anti-inflammatory drugs such as ibuprofen. These drugs have been shown to be superior to acetaminophen or propoxyphene for episiotomy pain and uterine cramping[72] and are safe for nursing mothers.

When a patient complains of inordinate perineal pain, the first and most important step is to reexamine the perineum, vagina, and rectum to detect and drain a hematoma or to identify a perineal infection. Perineal pain may be the first symptom of the rare but potentially fatal complications of angioedema, necrotizing fasciitis, or perineal cellulitis.[73–75]

Sitz baths also provide pain relief. Although hot sitz baths have long been customary therapy for perineal pain, cold or "iced" sitz baths provide immediate pain relief as a result of decreased excitability of free nerve endings and decreased nerve conduction. Further pain relief comes from local vasoconstriction, which reduces edema, inhibits hematoma formation, and decreases muscle irritability and spasm.

The technique for administering a cold sitz bath is first to have the patient sit in a tub of water at room temperature to which ice cubes are then added. The patient remains in the ice water for 20 to 30 minutes.

Frequently, what appears to be severe perineal pain is, in fact, the pain of prolapsed hemorrhoids. Witch hazel compresses, suppositories containing corticosteroids, or local anesthetic sprays or emollients may be helpful. Occasionally, a thrombus will occur in a prolapsed hemorrhoid. It is a simple task to remove the thrombus through a small scalpel incision using local anesthesia. Dramatic relief of pain usually follows this procedure.

Postpartum Infection

The standard definition of postpartum febrile morbidity is a temperature of 38.0 °C (100.4 °F) or higher on any 2 of the first 10 days after delivery, exclusive of the first 24 hours.[82] The most common cause of postpartum fever is endometritis, but the differential diagnosis includes urinary tract infection, lower genital tract infection, wound infections, pulmonary infections, thrombophlebitis, and mastitis. (see Chapter 25.)

Maternal–Infant Attachment

It is now recognized that there should be opportunities for parents to be with their newborns even from the first few moments after birth and as frequently as possible during the first days thereafter. Separation of mother and infant in the first hours after birth has been shown to diminish or delay the development of characteristic mothering behaviors,[84] or "bonding."

The modern hospital maternity ward should enhance and encourage parent–infant attachment by such policies as flexible visiting hours for the father, encouragement of the infant rooming with the mother, and supportive attitudes about breast-feeding.

Lactation Suppression

For those patients who for personal or medical reasons will not breast-feed, breast support, ice packs, and analgesic medications are helpful in ameliorating the symptoms of breast engorgement, which will usually last for 24–48 hr.

Natural Methods

The natural family planning methods, which depend on predicting the time of ovulation by use of basal body temperature or assessment of cervical mucus, cannot be used until regular menstrual cycles have resumed.[128] In the first weeks or months following birth, provided there is little or no supplemental feeding for the infant, breast-feeding will provide 98 percent contraceptive protection for up to 6 months. At 6 months, or if menses return, or if breast-feeding ceases to be full or nearly full before the sixth month, the risk of pregnancy increases.[129]

Barrier Methods

The proper size of the diaphragm should be determined at the 6-week postpartum visit. The use of condoms alone or in combination with spermicides is often advised for women who are lactating.

Steroid Contraceptive Medications

In patients who are not breast-feeding, oral contraceptive agents can be taken as early as 3 weeks after delivery. Combined-type oral contraceptive agents have a suppressive effect on lactation. Progestin-only medications (e.g., norethindrone 0.35 mg every day or depot medroxyprogesterone acetate 150 mg IM every 3 months) do not diminish lactation performance and are recommended for nursing mothers. It is recommended that the use of these medications be delayed until lactation has been established.[138]

Pregnancy rates in women using the levonangestral subdermal implants are lower than with any other reversible contraception.[143] Implants inserted 4 weeks after delivery have no effect on lactation or growth of an infant who is nursing even though small amounts of levonorgestrel are excreted in the milk. Irregular uterine bleeding, expense, and the occasional difficulty in removing the implants are the major drawbacks.

Intrauterine Devices

The copper-containing T shaped device (copper-T IUD, ParaGard T380A) and the progesterone-releasing device (Progestasert) are highly effective in preventing pregnancy (2 to 3 pregnancies per 100 woman-years).[145,146] The advantage of the copper-containing

IUD is that it is effective for 10 years; its disadvantage is an increase in irregular uterine bleeding. The device that releases progesterone reduces uterine bleeding, but it must be replaced annually.

The major side effects and complications are uterine perforation, abnormal uterine bleeding, uterine and pelvic infection, and ectopic pregnancy.[110]

Sterilization

The 10-year failure rate of postpartum partial salpingectomy is 0.75 percent.[155] There are several modifications of this procedure: the Pomeroy, Parkland, Uchida, and Irving (see Chapter 14).[156,159] The Pomeroy or Parkland procedures are as effective as the more complicated procedures.

Perhaps more important than the type of procedure is the decision about the timing of the procedure or whether it should be performed at all. Puerperal sterilization compared with interval sterilization is associated with increased incidence of guilt and regret.[161] With increasing frequency, couples are postponing tubal ligation procedures until after delivery. This provides time to ensure that the infant is healthy and to review all the implications of the decision.

There has also been concern about poststerilization depression.[164] Because depression is common in women of childbearing age and is even more common in the puerperium, it is difficult to know whether sterilization procedures are independent risk factors for depression. It is obvious, however, that the loss of fertility associated with a sterilization procedure will have important conscious and subconscious implications for many women. It is therefore not surprising that some patients manifest transient grief reactions in response to tubal ligation. The loss of libido that may occur in such situations may be frightening to some women and equally disturbing to their partners. Reassurance that such reactions are temporary and are not necessarily symptoms of a seriously disturbed psyche is an important means of support during this crisis.

Obstetricians must remember that vasectomy is often a more advisable and desirable alternative for a couple considering sterilization.[165,166] It can be performed as an outpatient procedure under local anesthesia with insignificant loss of time from work or family. Furthermore, almost all the failures (about 3 to 4 per 1,000 procedures) can be detected by a postoperative semen analysis. This is a decided advantage over the tubal ligation, in which failures are discovered only when a pregnancy occurs. Furthermore, vasectomy is less expensive and overall is associated with fewer complications.

Tubal ligation can be reversed, but a patient should not undergo sterilization if she is contemplating reversal. Success as measured by the occurrence of pregnancy following tubal reanastamosis varies from 40 to 85 percent, depending on the type of tubal ligation performed and on the length of functioning tube that remains.

POSTPARTUM PSYCHOLOGICAL REACTIONS

A common psychological reaction experienced following childbirth is a relatively mild, physiologic, and transient "maternity blues" (50 to 70 percent of women). True depression occurs in 8 to 20 percent, and frank puerperal psychosis occurs in 0.14 to 0.26 percent.

Postpartum Blues

The most common psychological manifestation of the puerperium is a state of tearfulness, anxiety, irritation, and restlessness, described as "maternity blues" or "postpartum blues." As it occurs in up to 70 percent of parturients,[170] it might well be considered a normal involutional phenomenon. The symptoms may appear on any day within the first week after delivery and usually have resolved by postpartum day 10. The disruptive sleep patterns in the first weeks following delivery have been shown to contribute to an increase in dysphoric mood experienced by women during this time.[172]

Because the syndrome is transient and of short duration, no therapy is indicated. Some of the symptoms may be exacerbated by sleep deprivation, and increased rest may be helpful.

Postpartum Depression

The signs and symptoms of postpartum depression are not different from those in nonpregnant patients, but may be difficult to differentiate from normal involutional phenomena (e.g., weight loss, sleeplessness) or from the transient "maternity blues."[183] However, in addition to the more common symptoms of depression, the postpartum patient may manifest a sense of incapability of loving her family and manifest ambivalence toward her infant.

There is a high risk of recurrence (50 to 100 percent) of postpartum depression in subsequent pregnancies and a 20 to 30 percent risk of postpartum depression in women who have had a previous depressive reaction not associated with pregnancy.

Puerperal hypothyroidism often presents with symptoms including mild dysphoria; consequently, thyroid function studies may be useful in patients presenting with suspected postpartum depression.

Treatment for postpartum depression should be begun early. Optimal treatment includes both counseling and medications. In women with a previous episode of postpartum depression, it has been suggested that prophylactic serotonin selective reuptake inhibitor (SSRI) medications be started 2 to 3 weeks prior to delivery. This approach allows these drugs to achieve an effective level by the postpartum period.[193] If there is no prompt response to general supportive measures and initial use of medication, psychiatric consultation is advisable. The prognosis for treated postpartum depression is good, although symptoms may persist for up to a year. Unfortunately, untreated postpartum depression has significant consequences. Depression may progress to frank suicidal psychosis.

Postpartum Psychosis

Schizophrenia and bipolar disorders are seen with increased frequency in the puerperium, suggesting that there is a psychosis specific to the postpartum condition. During the immediate postpartum period, the early signs of depression may be difficult to distinguish from "maternity blues," but if suicidal thoughts or attempts occur, or if frankly delusional thoughts are expressed, the diagnosis of postpartum psychosis can be made.[195]

Clearly, all patients with puerperal psychosis require hospitalization for at least initial evaluation and institution of therapy. Antipsychotic agents, eletroconvulsive therapy, antidepressants, neuroleptics, and lithium carbonate have all been recommended for specific subgroups of puerperal psychosis. There is recent evidence, however, that sublingual estradiol (1 mg 3–6 times daily) results in substantial improvement in patients with postpartum psychosis.[199] Whatever therapy for these conditions is instituted, it should be conducted or supervised by a psychiatrist.

Women with postpartum psychosis should be supervised at all times. These patients have a 5 percent rate of suicide, and a 5 percent rate of infanticide!

MANAGING PERINATAL GRIEVING

When a patient and her family experience a loss associated with a pregnancy, special attention must be given to the grieving patient and her family. Grief will occur with any significant loss whether it is the actual death of an infant or the loss of an idealized child in the case of the birth of a handicapped infant.[200]

There are five manifestations of normal grieving. These include somatic symptoms of sleeplessness, fatigue, digestive symptoms, and sighing respirations; preoccupation with the image of the deceased; feelings of guilt; feelings of hostility and anger toward others; and disruption of the normal pattern of daily life. Pathologic grief may occur if acute mourning is suppressed or interrupted. Some of the manifestations of this so-called morbid grief reaction are overactivity without a sense of loss; appearance or exacerbations of psychosomatic illness; alterations in relationships with friends and relatives; furious hostility toward specific persons; lasting loss of patterns of social interaction; activities detrimental to personal, social, and economic existence; and agitated depression.

It is important that the characteristics of the grieving patient be recognized and understood by health professionals caring for such patients. What is actually beneficial at such a time is a sympathetic listener and an opportunity to express and discuss feelings of guilt, anger, and hopelessness and the other symptoms of mourning.

It is not surprising that postpartum depression is more common and more severe in families that have suffered a perinatal loss. In one study, the prolonged grief response occurred more often in those women who became pregnant within 5 months of the death of the infant.[207]

The regionalization of perinatal health care has resulted in a large proportion of the perinatal deaths occurring in tertiary centers. In some of these centers teams of physicians, nurses, social workers, and pastoral counselors have evolved to aid specifically in the management of families suffering a perinatal loss.[211-214] While this approach ensures an enlightened, understanding, and consistent approach to bereaved families, it suggests that the support of a grieving patient is a highly complex endeavor, to be accomplished only by a few specially trained individuals who care for postpartum patients. Enlightened and compassionate counseling of parents who have suffered a perinatal loss may be accomplished by any of the mother's health care professionals by using the guidelines listed in the box (Guidelines for Managing Perinatal Loss).[214] Clearly, management of grief is not solely a postpartum responsibility. This is particularly true when a prenatal diagnosis is made of fetal death or fetal abnormality. A continuum of support is essential as the patient moves from the prenatal setting, to labor and delivery, to the postpartum ward, and finally to her home. Relaxation of many of the traditional hospital routines may be necessary to provide the type of support these families need. For example, allowing a loved one to remain past visiting hours, providing a couple a private setting to be with their deceased infant, or allowing unusually early

Guidelines for Managing Perinatal Loss

Keep parents informed; be honest and forthright.

Recognize and facilitate anticipatory grieving.

Inform parents about the grieving process.

Encourage support person to remain with the mother throughout labor.

Encourage the mother to make as many choices about her care as possible.

Support parents in seeing, touching, or holding the infant.

Describe the infant in detail, especially for couples who choose not to see the infant.

Allow photographs of the infant.

Prepare the couple for hospital paperwork, such as autopsy requests.

Discuss funeral or memorial services.

Assist the couple in how to inform siblings, relatives, and friends.

Discuss subsequent pregnancy.

Liberal use of follow-up home or office visits.

Modified from Kowalski K: Managing perinatal loss. Clin Obstet Gynecol 23:1113, 1980.

discharge with provisions for frequent phone calls and follow-up visits will often facilitate the resolution of grief.

It is also important to realize that the fathers of infants who die have somewhat different grief responses than do the mothers. Their grief is characterized by the necessity to keep busy with increased work, feelings of diminished self-worth, self-blame, and limited ability to ask for help. Stoic responses are typical of men and may obstruct the normal resolution of grief.

Postpartum Posttraumatic Stress

Posttraumatic stress disorder may occur after any physical or psychological trauma. It may lead to behavioral sequelae including flashbacks, avoidance, and inability to function. Emergency operative deliveries, both vaginal and abdominal, and severe unexpected pain have been reported to have produced posttraumatic stress. The reaction may lead to fear of a subsequent delivery that may become incapacitating, as well as generalized symptoms of this disorder. Whenever an emergency procedure is indicated, debriefing afterwards, both early and a few weeks later, may help to decrease the incidence of this problem. Women with adverse outcomes frequently will experience transference of their previous experience as the next delivery approaches.[216–219]

BREAST-FEEDING

Breast-feeding is the global standard for infant feeding. The American Academy of Pediatrics has recently published an endorsement for breast-feeding at least through the first year of life and as an exclusive method for the first 6 months.[1] Unfortunately, the majority of American infants are not given this opportunity. The latest survey (1995)[2] reports that 59.7 percent of women initiate breast-feeding in the hospital and only 21.6 percent of those are still breast-feeding at 6 months. Less than 10 percent of American infants meet the standard of breast-feeding 1 year or more.

Fortunately, since 1989 more women at greatest risk for feeding their infants artificial breast milk are initiating breast-feeding in the hospital.[2]

Dysfunctional cultural and familial attitudes are outside the direct control of medicine, and may directly affect the care delivered by physicians. The normal function of the breasts, to produce breast milk, is muted by two cultural attitudes. One cultural attitude is the association of breasts with sexual attraction. The media is replete with examples that show beautiful, well-formed breasts as a sexual ideal. A corollary of this attitude is that breast-feeding will cause the breasts to sag and lose their sex appeal. The other opposing cultural attitude is that breast-feeding restricts self-fulfillment; mothers who stay at home to breast-feed and care for their babies are considered poor examples of the modern, independent professional woman. These attitudes are exacerbated by a lack of knowledge about breast-feeding and lactation. The lack of exposure to successful, experienced breast-feeding mothers seriously compromises the chances of success for the women who attempt to breast-feed.

A recent national survey of physician knowledge revealed that 20 to 40 percent of physicians (obstetricians, pediatricians, and family practitioners) did not know that breast-feeding is the "gold standard" for infant feeding, and similar percentages have serious and sometimes dangerous gaps in their knowledge in the management of breast-feeding problems.[3] A 1999 survey of fellows of the American Academy of Pediatricians revealed that only 65 percent recommended exclusive breast-feeding during the first month of life, and more than half agreed with or had a neutral opinion about the statement that breast-feeding and formula-feeding are equally acceptable methods for feeding infants.[4]

In order to support the breast-feeding mother, the obstetrician must be convinced of the biologic superiority of breast-feeding and human breast milk over artificial breast milk (formula).

In this chapter we review the morbidity and mortality associated with infant feeding using artificial breast milk, and describe the vast differences between breast milk and artificial breast milk, a difference directly related to unique needs of the human infant.

BENEFITS OF BREAST-FEEDING

Epidemiologic research shows that human milk and breast-feeding of infants provide significant advantages to general health, growth, and development. In contrast, infant feeding with artificial breast milk is associated with higher incidences of acute and chronic diseases than in infants who are fed human milk through breast-feeding. The studies of predominantly middle class populations in developed countries show that infant feeding with artificial breast milk is associated with higher incidences and greater severity of diarrhea,[8-12] lower respiratory infection,[13-15] otitis media,[9,16-18] bacteremia,[19,20] bacterial meningitis,[19,21] urinary tract infection,[22] and necrotizing enterocolitis[23,24] than similar populations who were breast-fed. Numerous studies show higher incidences of sudden infant death syndrome,[25-27] type I (insulin-dependent) diabetes,[28,29] adolescent obesity,[30] Crohn's disease,[31,32] ulcerative colitis,[32] lymphoma,[33] allergic diseases,[34-38] and other chronic digestive diseases among infants fed artificial breast milk.[36-38] In high-risk populations, preterm infants, and phenylketonurics, as well as healthy middle class populations of infants, breast-feeding has been associated with enhancement of cognitive development and intelligence quotients.[39-44]

Increase in acute medical diseases will manifest as increased costs of medical care for those families who choose to feed their infant artificial breast milk. The nonmedical costs of artificial breast milk feeding are considerably higher than breast-feeding. The direct costs of artificial breast milk feeding includes the cost of the artificial formula bottles, and supplies. A major indirect cost of artificial breast milk feeding is the environmental impact of large dairy herds to supply the milk substrate.

Breast-feeding provides the right amount of a superior product at precisely the right time and at the right temperature. The nonmedical costs of breast-feeding include the cost of increased calorie and protein needs, nursing bras and breast pads, and increased numbers of diapers in the first 2 to 3 months. If an electric breast pump is used when the woman returns to work, the cost of breast-feeding will increase.

Breast-feeding accrues multiple benefits to the mother that are not shared by women who feed their infants artificial breast milk. Breast-feeding through increased release of oxytocin results in faster uterine involution and less postpartum blood loss[49]; the incidence of postpartum anemia may be reduced. Breast-feeding is associated with 1 to 3 kg less retained postpartum weight.[49,50] Exclusive breast-feeding delays ovulation with increased child spacing.[51]

BREAST ANATOMY AND DEVELOPMENT

The breast is located in the superficial fascia between the second rib and sixth intercostal cartilage in the midclavicular line. There is usually a projection of the central disk into each axilla, the *tail of Spence*. The mature breast weighs about 200 g in the nonpregnant state; during pregnancy, 500 g; and during lactation, 600 to 800 g. As long as glandular tissue and the nipple are present, the size or shape of the breast has little to do with the functional success of the breast. The adequacy of glandular tissue for breast-feeding is ascertained by inquiring whether a woman's breasts have enlarged during pregnancy. If there is failure of the breast to enlarge as the result of pregnancy, especially if associated with minimal breast tissue on examination, the clinician should be wary of primary failure of lactation.

The nipple, or *papilla mammae,* is a conical elevation in the middle of the areola. The areola is a circular pigmented area, which darkens during pregnancy. The areola contains multiple small elevations, *Montgomery's tubercles,* which enlarge during pregnancy and lactation. Montgomery's tubercles contain multiple ductular openings of sebaceous and sweat glands. These glands secrete lubricating and anti-infective substances (IgA) that protect the nipples and areola during nursing. These substances are washed away when the breasts and nipples are washed with soap or alcohol-containing compounds, leaving the nipple prone to cracking and infection.

The areola and nipple contain smooth muscle and collagenous and elastic tissue. With light touch or anticipation, these muscles contract and the nipple erects to form a teat. The contraction pulls the lactiferous sinuses into the nipple–areola complex, which allows the infant to milk the breast milk from these reservoirs.

The tip of the nipple contains the openings (0.4 to 0.7 mm in diameter) of 15 to 20 milk ducts (2 to 4 mm in diameter). Each of the milk ducts empties one tubuloalveolar gland, which is embedded in the fat of the body of the breast. A sphincter mechanism at the opening of the duct limits the ejection of milk from the breast. The competency of this mechanism is variable. About 20 percent of women do not demonstrate milk ejection from the contralateral breast when milk ejection is stimulated. If milk leakage is demonstrated from the contralateral breast during nursing, there is supporting evidence of milk transfer to the infant.

Five to 10 mm from their exit, the milk ducts widen (5 to 8 mm) into the lactiferous sinuses (Fig. 16–1). When these sinuses are pulled into the teat during nursing, the infant's tongue, facial muscles, and mouth squeeze the milk from the sinuses into the infant's oropharynx.[56,57] The tubuloalveolar glands (15 to 20) form lobi, which are arranged in a radial fashion from the central nipple–areola complex. The lobi and lactiferous ducts extend into the tail of Spence. Ten to 40 lactiferous ducts connect to each lactiferous sinus, each forming a lobulus. Each lobulus arborizes into 10 to 100 alveoli for tubulosaccular secretory units. The alveoli are the critical units of the production and ejection of milk. A sac of alveolar cells is surrounded by a basket of myoepithelial cells. The alveolar cells are stimulated by prolactin to produce milk. The myoepithelial cells are stimulated by oxytocin to contract and eject the recently produced milk into the lactiferous ducts, lactiferous sinuses, and beyond.

The radial distribution of lactiferous ducts prompts important considerations relative to breast surgery on women who are breast-feeding or who will breast-feed. Surgical skin incisions parallel to the circumareolar line, especially at the circumareolar line, have better cosmetic healing and are often chosen by surgeons. However, if the incision is taken deep into the parenchyma, the lactiferous ducts may be compromised; a superficial, parallel skin incision and a radial deep incision are preferred. In women who intend to breast-feed, a circumareolar incision is to be avoided. The incision compromises breast-feeding in three ways: occlusion of lactiferous ducts, restriction of the formation of a teat during nursing, and injury to the lateral cutaneous branch of the fourth intercostal nerve.

Surgical disruption of the lateral cutaneous branch of the fourth intercostal nerve can have devastating effects on the success of breast-feeding.[58,59] This nerve is critical to the production and ejection of breast milk. Furthermore, the nerves provide organ-specific control of regional blood flow, and a tremendous increase in mammary blood flow occurs during a nursing episode.[60] Disruption of this autonomic control may severely compromise lactation performance. The rate of breast-feeding failure is two to three times higher when a circumareolar incision is performed.[58] The obstetrician needs to be alert to old surgical incisions when a pregnant patient expresses a desire to breast-feed or when a breast biopsy is anticipated in a reproductive-aged woman.

As a mammal, humans have the potential to develop mammary tissue, glandular or nipple tissue, anywhere along the milk line (*galactic band*). The milk line extends from the axilla and inner

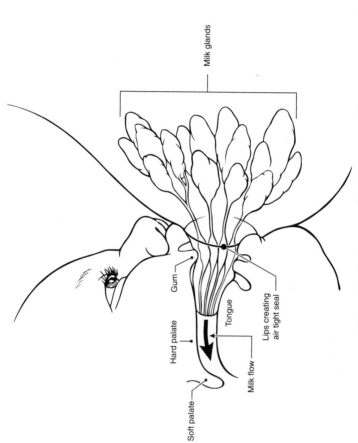

Hard palate

Soft palate

Gum

Tongue

Milk flow

Lips creating
air tight seal

Milk glands

Figure 16–1. Anatomy of the breast. *Illustration continued on following page*

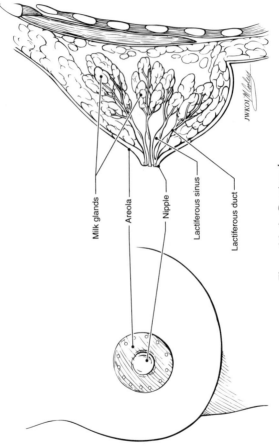

Milk glands

Areola

Nipple

Lactiferous sinus

Lactiferous duct

Figure 16–1. *Continued*

upper arm to its current position, down the abdomen along the midclavicular line to the upper lateral mons and upper inner thigh. When accessory glands occur, this is termed hypermastia. This may involve accessory glandular tissue, supernumerary nipples, or both. Two to 6 percent of women have hypermastia, and the response to pregnancy and lactation is variable. The most common site for accessory breast tissue is the axilla. These women may present at 2 to 5 days postpartum (galactogenesis) with painful enlargements in the axilla. Ice and symptomatic therapy for 24 to 48 hours is sufficient. Supernumerary nipples (*polythelia*) are associated with renal abnormalities (11 percent).

Full alveolar development and maturation of the breast must await the hormones of pregnancy (progesterone, prolactin, and human placental lactogen) for completion of the developmental process. By midpregnancy, the gland is competent to secrete milk (colostrum), although full function is not attained until the tissues are released from the inhibition of high levels of circulating progesterone. This is termed *lactogenesis stage 1*. Lactogenesis stage 2 occurs as the progesterone levels fall after delivery of the placenta, during the first 2 to 4 days after birth. Stage 2 includes dramatic increases in mammary blood flow and oxygen/glucose uptake by the breast. At 2 to 3 days postpartum, the secretion of milk is copious and "the milk comes in." This is the most common time for engorgement if the breasts are not drained by efficient, frequent nursing. Until lactogenesis stage 2 is developed, the breasts secrete colostrum. Colostrum is very different than mature milk in volume and constituents.[61,62] Colostrum has more protein, especially secretory immunoglobulins, lactose, and lower fat content than mature milk. Prolactin and glucocorticoids play important promoter roles in this stage of development.

After lactogenesis stage 2 (4 to 6 days postpartum) lactation enters an indefinite period of milk production formerly called galactopoiesis, now termed lactogenesis stage 3. The duration of this stage is dependent on the continued production of breast milk and the efficient transfer of the breast milk to the infant. Prolactin appears to be the single most important galactopoietic hormone, since selective inhibition of prolactin secretion by bromocriptine disrupts lactogenesis. Oxytocin appears to be the major galactokinetic hormone. Stimulation of the nipple and areola or behavioral cues cause a reflex contraction of the myoepithelial cells that surround the alveoli and ejection of milk from the breast.

During a feeding episode the lipid content of milk rises by more than two to threefold (1 to 5 percent) The rising lipid content during a feed has practical implications in breast-feeding management. If a woman limits her feeds to less than 4 minutes, but nurses more frequently, the calorie density of the milk is lower and the infant's hunger may not be satiated. The infant wishes to feed sooner and the frequency of nursing accelerates. This stimulates more milk production and creates a scenario of a hungry infant despite apparent good volume and milk transfer.[71] Lengthening the nursing episode or using one breast for each nursing episode often solves the problem.

The final stage of development is involution and cessation of breast-feeding. As the frequency of breast-feeding is reduced to less than six episodes in 24 hours and milk volume is less than 400 ml/24 h, prolactin levels fall and a cyclic pattern ends in the total cessation of milk production. After 24 to 48 hours of no transfer of breast milk to the infant, intraductal pressure[63] and lactation inhibitory factor[64] appear to initiate apoptosis of the secretory epithelial cells and proteolytic degradation of the basement membrane. Lactation inhibitory factor is a protein secreted in the milk, whose increasing concentration in the absence of drainage appears to decrease milk production by the alveolar cells.[64-66] It counterbalances pressures to increase milk supply (increased frequency of nursing) and allows for the day-to-day adjustment in infant demands.

Milk Production and Transfer

Does diet affect the volume and constitution of breast milk? For the average American woman with the range of diets from teenagers to mature, health-conscious adults, the answer is "no." There is no convincing evidence that the macronutrients in breast milk, protein, fats, and carbohydrates, vary across the usual range of American diets. Volume may vary in the extremes. In a controlled experiment,[73] well-nourished European women reduced their calorie intake by 33 percent for 1 week. Milk volume was not reduced when the diet was maintained at greater than 1,500 kcal/day. If the daily energy intake was less than 1,500 kcal/day, milk volume was reduced 15 percent. Moderate dieting and weight loss postpartum (4.5 lb/mo) are not associated with changes in milk volume,[50] nor does aerobic exercise have any adverse effect.[74]

In the first year of life, the infant undergoes tremendous growth; infants double their birth weight in 180 days. Infants fed artificial breast milk lose up to 5 percent of their birthweight during the first week of life, while breast-milk-fed infants lose about 7 percent of their birthweight. A maximum weight loss of 10 percent of birthweight is tolerated in the first week of life in breast-fed infants. If this threshold is exceeded, the breast-feeding dyad needs immediate intervention by a trained health care provider. While supplementation with donor breast milk or artificial breast milk may be a necessary part of the intervention, the key focus of intervention is establishing good breast milk transfer by ensuring adequate production, correct nursing behavior, and adequate frequency. Once stage 3 of lactogenesis occurs, "the milk has come in"; the term breast-fed infant will gain about 1 oz/day with adequate milk transfer. By 14 days, the breast-fed infant should have returned to birthweight.

As long as nursing frequency is maintained at greater than eight times for 10 to 20 minutes with each episode in 24 hours, the serum prolactin levels will suppress the LH surges and ovarian function.[75]

Serum oxytocin levels also rise with nipple stimulation. Positive sights, sounds, or smells related to nursing often stimulate the production of oxytocin, which, in turn, causes the myoepithelial cells to contract and milk to leak from the breasts. This observation is a good clinical clue indicating an uninhibited *let-down reflex*.

Pain, anxiety, and insecurity may be hidden reasons for breast-feeding failure through the inhibition of the let-down reflex. In contrast, the playing of a soothing motivational/educational audiotape to women who were pumping milk for their premature infants has improved milk yields.[77] These observations have been confirmed by measuring the inhibition of oxytocin release by psychological stress.[78]

Several trials with random assignment of subjects to early nursing (delivery room) or late nursing (2 hours after birth) demonstrated a 50 to 100 percent increase in the number of mothers who are breast-feeding at 2 to 4 months postpartum who nursed in the delivery room.[83] One of the keys to obstetric management is to have the mother nurse her newborn in the delivery room.

The initial step of milk transfer to the infant is good latch-on. With light tactile stimulation of the cheek and lateral angle of the mouth, the infant reflexively turns its head and opens its mouth, as in a yawn (Fig. 16–2). The nipple is tilted slightly downward using a "C-hold", or *palmar grasp*. In this hand position, the fingers support the breast from underneath and the thumb lightly grasps the upper surface 1 to 2 cm above the areola-breast line. The infant is brought firmly to the breast by the supporting arms while being careful to not push the back of the baby's head. The nipple and areola are drawn into the mouth as far as the areola-breast line (Figs. 16–3 and 16–4). The posterior areola may be less visible than the anterior areola, and the lower lip of the infant is often curled out. The infant's lower gum lightly fixes the teat over the lactiferous sinuses. A slight negative pressure exerted by the oropharynx and mouth holds the length of the teat and breast in place and reduces the "work" to refill the lactiferous sinuses after they are drained. The milk is extracted, not by negative pressure, but by a peristaltic action from the tip of the tongue to the base. There is no stroking, friction, or in-and-out motion of the teat; it is more of an undulating action. The buccal mucosa and tongue mold around the teat, leaving no space.

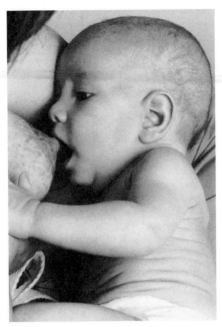

Figure 16–2. The latch-on reflex.

The peristaltic movement of the infant's tongue is most frequent in the first 3 minutes of a nursing episode; the mean latency from latch-on to milk ejection is 2.2 minutes. After milk flow is established, the frequency of sucking falls to a much slower rate.[84] The change in cadence is recognizable as "suck-suck-swallow-breath." Audible swallowing of milk is a good sign of milk transfer. At the start of a feed the infant obtains 0.10 to 0.20 ml per suck. As the infant learns how to suck and as he matures he becomes more efficient at obtaining more milk in a shorter period of time. Eighty to 90 percent of the milk is obtained in the first 5 minutes the infant nurses on each breast, but the fat-rich and calorie-dense hind milk is obtained in the remainder of the time sucking at each breast, usually less than 20 minutes total.[85,86] A bottle-feeding infant sucks steadily in a linear fashion, receiving about 80 percent of the artificial breast milk in the first 10 minutes.

Sucking on a bottle is mechanically very different than nursing on the human teat (Fig. 16–5). The relatively inflexible artificial nipple resists the milking motion of the infant's tongue and mouth. The diameter of the artificial nipple expands during a suck, whereas the human teat collapses during the milk flow. The infant who is sucking on a bottle learns to generate strong negative

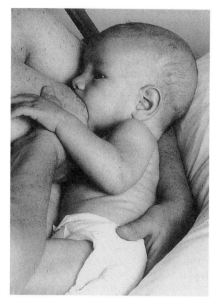

Figure 16–3. Appropriate latch-on.

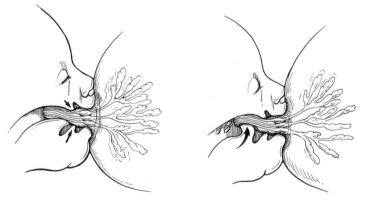

Figure 16–4. The mechanics of nursing.

pressures (>100 mm Hg) in order to suck the milk out of the bottle. Since rapid flow from the bottle can gag the infant, he or she quickly learns to use the tongue to regulate the flow. When the infant who has learned to bottle-feed is put to the breast, the stopper function of the tongue may abrade the tip of the nipple and force the nipple out of the infant's mouth. The efficiency of milk

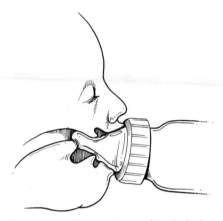

Figure 16–5. The mechanics of bottle-feeding.

transfer falls drastically and the hungry infant becomes frustrated and angry. A similar rejection may occur at 4 to 8 weeks when the exclusively breast-feeding infant is given a bottle in preparation for the mother's return to work.

Milk transfer is made more efficient by proper positioning of the infant to the breast. Rotating positions of nursing allows improved drainage of different lobules, an observation important in the management of a "plugged" duct. Maternal comfort and convenience are the major reasons for changing nursing positions; the football hold position and the side-lying position are more comfortable if there is an abdominal incision.

Baseline prolactin levels appear to be the major determinant of the hormonal state during lactation, a state of high-prolactin, low-estrogen, and low-progesterone levels. As the frequency of nursing decreases below eight in 24 hours, the baseline prolactin levels drop to below a level where ovulation is suppressed (35 to 50 ng/ml), LH levels rise, and menstrual cycling is initiated.[74,85,87] Serum prolactin levels in women who feed their infants artificial breast milk drop to prepregnant levels (8 to 14 ng/ml) within days. The total number of nursing episodes per day (more than eight per 24 hours) and night nursings are critical to the successful management of breast-feeding.

The most logical time to start solid food substitution is when the infant has reached the neurologic maturity to grasp and bring food to its mouth from his or her mother's plate. The required neurologic maturity to perform this behavior usually occurs at about 6 months. As the infant matures, his or her ability to feed improves and the proportion of the diet supplied by solid food gradually increases.

BREAST MILK: THE GOLD STANDARD

One of the most common misperceptions by physicians and the lay public is that modern formulas for artificial breast milk are equivalent to breast milk. Human breast milk is uniquely suited to our biologic needs and remains the best source of nutrition for the human infant. It has a composition very different than that of bovine milk or soybean plants from which artificial breast milk is produced.

In contrast with most other animals, the human secretory immune system is not completely functional at birth. While the passive transplacental transfer of maternal IgG starts at 20 weeks, fetal levels do not approach maternal levels until term. By 3 months of age, the infant must rely on its own secretory response. The newborn's IgM and IgA responses are naive and incomplete. For example, in the presence of active antigen-positive cytomegalovirus infection at birth, 20 percent of infants will be IgM negative. A newborn's cellular response is likewise immature; functional impairment is evident for months after birth. Breast milk provides necessary support for the developing immune system.[89,90] The powerful anti-infective qualities of breast milk are measured by decreased infant mortality in developing countries, where exclusive breast-feeding is the norm. In first-world countries, the anti-infective benefits of exclusive breast-feeding are measured by decreased morbidity[35] and fewer hospitalizations.[48]

Most artificial breast milk products use bovine milk as a substrate. Minerals, vitamins, protein, carbohydrates, and fats are added to pasteurized bovine milk for perceived nutritional needs as well as marketing needs in order to make a product that will successfully compete with human breast milk. Human breast milk appears "thinner" than bovine milk. Artificial breast milk manufacturers add constituents such as palm or coconut oil to make artificial breast milk appear rich and creamy. In 1980, the U.S. Congress passed the Infant Formula Act (with revisions in 1985) as the result of severe health consequences when artificial breast milk failed to include key vitamins and minerals in new formula compositions.[91] This law now requires that all formulas for artificial breast milk contain minimum amounts of essential nutriments, vitamins, and minerals. Although life-threatening omissions are unlikely, current formulas for artificial breast milk have major differences in the total quantities and qualities of proteins, carbohydrates, and fats when compared to human milk.[92-96]

The nutritional differences between artificial breast milk and human milk are reflected in differences in the growth patterns of infants who are exclusively breast-fed for 4 to 6 months and infants who are fed artificial breast milk.[97] In general, breast-fed infants have faster linear and head growth, whereas artificial breast milk–fed infants tend to have greater weight gain and fat deposition. The greater deposition in fat may relate in part to the earlier introduction of solid foods in the infant fed artificial breast milk, a factor that has not been adequately controlled in current studies. Regardless of the cause, greater fat deposition in infants fed artificial breast milk has important adverse effects on the child and the future health of the society. Infant feeding using artificial breast milk is associated with a higher incidence of adolescent obesity,[30,36] which predicts significant increases in adult morbidity such as obesity, type II (insulin-resistant) diabetes, coronary heart disease, and hypertension.[98]

At birth, the fetus enters an unsterile world with an immature immune system. Breast milk has a wide array of anti-infective properties that will support the developing immune system.[89,90] The major mechanisms for the protective properties of breast milk include active leukocytes, antibodies, antibacterial products, and competitive inhibition. Active leukocytes[99] are completely eliminated by pasteurization or freezing.

Immunoglobulins are a unique component to breast milk and absent in artificial breast milk.[89,90] Immunoglobulins constitute a sizable portion of protein content of early milk (colostrum) for the first 2 to 4 days. In serum, the concentration of monomeric IgA is one fifth the concentration of IgG. In breast milk, the ratio is reversed.

The binding of iron to lactoferrin also enhances iron absorption; less iron is required in breast milk in order to satisfy the iron needs of the infant.

THE ROLE OF THE OBSTETRICIAN

The obstetrician plays the primary role in the initiation of breast-feeding and is largely responsible for which women go home from their postpartum hospitalization breast-feeding. From then on, the obstetrician/gynecologist performs a critical supporting role to the pediatrician in the maintenance of breast-feeding. He or she provides the medical support for breast-specific problems or issues relative to maternal health, as pediatricians are uncomfortable with the examination of the adult breast and accepting the mother as their patient.

The obstetrician/gynecologist amplifies support for breast-feeding by community advocacy, office environment, and personal choices. The office environment needs to be "breast-feeding friendly." Visible, active support of breast-feeding includes the presence of breast-feeding mothers, patient educational programs on breast-feeding, a quiet area for nursing mothers, the absence of material supplied by formula companies, and visible support for office personnel who choose to breast-feed.

The support of the obstetrician starts at the first prenatal visit and continues through the mother's total breast-feeding experience. At the first prenatal visit, the method of infant feeding is identified, her choice to breast-feed is verbally reinforced, gaps in her knowledge are identified, and an educational plan is recommended. The educational plan may include reference reading, specific classes on breast-feeding, identification of a "breast-feeding–friendly pediatrician," and introduction to community resources, such as support groups (La Leche League International). At the initial physical examination the breasts are examined for anatomic abnormalities that might influence the success of breast-feeding, such as hypoplasia, nipple inversion and surgical scars.

At delivery and during the postpartum hospitalization, the obstetrician is the champion for the application of breast-feeding physiology; early to the breast (<1 hour) after birth, frequent feeds (>10 per day), appropriate nursing behavior (latch-on), continuous mother–infant contact (rooming-in), and no infant supplementation unless directed by the infant's physician. As an advocate for breast-feeding the obstetrician must be willing to confront administrative and nursing protocols that are designed for control and efficiency rather than optimal care for the breast-feeding dyad.

In 1989 the World Health Organization initiated the Baby Friendly Hospital initiative. The ten steps by which a hospital might be designated "baby friendly" are outlined in the highlighted box. As of the year 2000, less than 40 of the more than 1,500 hospitals worldwide who have been designated baby friendly are in the United States. The biggest challenge to hospitals in the United States in becoming baby friendly is the forebearance of artificial breast milk donations and direct in-hospital marketing by the artificial breast milk companies. The obstetrician has a role in supporting the baby-friendly initiative.

When the obstetrician remains a verbal participant in the mother's breast-feeding experience at the 4- to 6-week postpartum visit, the likelihood that the mother will continue to breast-feed at 16 weeks is almost doubled.[103]

The successful management of breast-feeding requires the active cooperation of the mother, her support group, the obstetric care provider, and infant care provider. In our current culture, a lactation consultant often becomes an active participant in the care of the breast-feeding dyad. There are numerous reliable reference texts for additional information. They include *Breast-feeding: a Guide For The Medical Profession*,[104] *The Breastfeeding Answer Book*,[105] *The Womanly Art of Breastfeeding*,[106] *Drugs In Pregnancy and Lactation*,[107] and *Medication and Mother's Milk*.[108]

Ten Steps to Successful Breast-Feeding

1. Have a written policy to support breast-feeding.
2. Train all health care providers.
3. Inform all pregnant women about the benefits of breast-feeding.
4. Initiate breast-feeding within 1-hour after birth.
5. Show mothers how to breast-feed and maintain lactation even if they are separated from their infants.
6. Give newborn infants no food or drink other than breast milk, unless medically indicated.
7. Allow mothers and infants to remain together 24 hours a day (i.e., rooming in).
8. Encourage breast-feeding on demand.
9. Give no artificial teats or pacifiers.
10. Foster the establishment of breast-feeding support groups and refer mothers to them on discharge from the hospital or clinic.

Adapted from WHO/UNICEF: Protesting, Promoting and Suporting Breastfeeding: The Special Role of Maternity Services, A Joint WHO/UNICEF Statement. Geneva, World Health Organization, 1989.

ANATOMIC ABNORMALITIES OF THE BREAST

Congenital abnormalities of the breasts (excluding inverted nipples) are rare, less than 1 in 1,000 women. The most significant defect is glandular hypoplasia. These women have no development or abnormal development of one or both breasts during sexual maturation. Women with no development of the breasts often have normally shaped and sized nipples and areolas, and they may have sought consultation from a plastic surgeon. One manifestation of abnormal development is referred to as the *tubular breast*. The nipple and areola, which are often normal in size, shape, and appearance, are attached to a tube of fibrous cords. Whatever the shape or size of the breasts in a nonpregnant woman, the final evaluation of adequate glandular tissue must await the expected growth during pregnancy. The size of the average breast will grow from 200 g to 600 g during pregnancy; most women will easily recognize this growth. A routine screening question at the 36-week prenatal visit should be, "Have your breasts grown during pregnancy?" If the response is negative in a woman with unusually small or abnormally shaped breasts, lactational failure is a possibility and prenatal consultation with a lactation expert is recommended. Unilateral abnormalities are usually not a problem except for increased asymmetry, as the normal breast can usually produce more than enough milk for the infant.

Congenital tethering of the nipple to underlying fascia is diagnosed by squeezing the outer edge of the areola as normally, the nipple will protrude. Severe tethering is manifested by an inverted nipple, which occurs in less than 1 percent of women. While successful breast-feeding is possible in these severe cases, prenatal consultation and close follow-up are very important to identify and treat poor milk transfers. Three prenatal methods of treating tethered nipples have been described: nipple pulling, Hoffman's exercises, and nipple cups (shells). A recent controlled trial failed to demonstrate efficacy[109] of either shells or Hoffman's exercises and recommended that these should be abandoned.

In the early neonatal period, a breast pump may be of help in women with flat or inverted nipples. The breast is gently pumped at low settings until the teat is drawn out. The infant is immediately offered that breast. Usually this is only required for a few days. If it is required for more than a few days, a relatively cheap alternative can be created from a 10- or 20-ml plastic syringe.

Washing the breast with harsh soaps, buffing the nipple with a towel and using alcohol, benzoin, or other drying agents are not helpful and may increase the incidence of cracking of nipples. Normally, the breast is washed with clean water and should be left to air-dry. Trials involving application of breast cream or expression of colostrum have not shown a reduction in nipple trauma or sensitivity, when compared to those with untreated nipples.

Previous breast surgery may have significant adverse effects on breast-feeding success. The major issues are loss of sensation in the nipple or areola by nerve injury or compromise of the lactiferous ducts. Women who have had breast surgery, breast biopsy, chest surgery, or augmentation, have a threefold higher incidence of unsuccessful breast-feeding.[58] Circumareolar skin incisions may compromise both the nerve and ducts. Breast augmentation has significant potential to disrupt breast-feeding.[111] In a carefully studied, prospective series, 27 of 42 (64 percent) of women who exclusively breast-fed after preconceptional breast augmentation had insufficient lactation. Circumareolar incision was the dominant predictor. One half of women with a submammary or axillary incision had insufficient lactation, whereas all 11 women after a circumareolar incision for breast augmentation had lactation failure. If the woman has had a silicone implant, she can be reassured that there is no evidence that breast-feeding places her infant at risk. Large epidemiologic studies of infants who have nursed from breasts with silicone implants have not shown excess adverse events.[113]

Reduction mammoplasty is always associated with lactation insufficiency. In any case of reconstructive surgery on the breast, augmentation or reduction, the breast-feeding dyad is considered at high risk for lactation failure. Prenatal referral to an expert on lactation is appropriate.

LABOR AND DELIVERY MANAGEMENT

Most obstetric interventions reduce the success of lactation by indirect interference with physiology. Induction of labor is not associated with lactation failure, but a long, tiring induction and labor will reduce the likelihood that the mother will get appropriate amounts of infant contact in the delivery room and in the first 24 hours after birth. Cesarean delivery reduces the incidence of breast-feeding by 10 to 20 percent in the first week after birth. After most cesarean sections, the infant is not put to the breast immediately after birth nor will the mother breast-feed her infant more than eight times in the first 24 hours. Well-meaning nurses become concerned for the baby's nutrition and artificial breast milk is given to the infant until the mother "recovers." Labor analgesia (i.e., meperidine and promethazine) has long been associated with poor breast-feeding success. Intrapartum narcotics appear to adversely affect the infant's ability to nurse effectively.[82,114–116] Epidural anesthesia with local anesthetic agents seems to be better for breast-feeding than parenteral narcotics.

In the recovery room and on the ward, the best place for the neonate is with the mother. This maximizes mother–infant bonding and allows "on-demand" feeding every 1 to 2 hours. Rooming-in allows the mother to participate in the care of her baby and gives her an opportunity to ask questions. The mother should be encouraged to sleep when the neonate sleeps. Since the hospital runs on an adult diurnal pattern, the patient should be discharged early in order to get her rest.

The frequency of early feeding is proportional to milk production and weight gain in neonates.[85,120–122] Therefore, supplementation with glucose or formula should be discouraged. Supplementation decreases milk production through a reduction in nursing frequency by satiation of the neonate and slower digestion of formula. Supplementation also undermines the mother's confidence about her lactational adequacy.[123–126] A randomized trial of giving or withholding free formula samples at the time of discharge demonstrated a significantly reduced incidence of breast-feeding at 1 month and an increased likelihood of solid food introduction by the mothers given the formula samples.[123]

BREAST MASSES DURING LACTATION

One to 3 percent of all breast cancers occur during pregnancy and lactation. Recently, researchers in Japan have analyzed breast cancer in age-matched control women (n = 192), women who were pregnant at diagnosis (n = 72), and women who were lactating at diagnosis (n = 120).[128] The prognosis for breast cancer that is diagnosed during pregnancy or lactation is poorer than for breast cancer diagnosed at other times. The 10-year survival for age-matched controls without lymph node metastasis was 93 percent; for women who were diagnosed during pregnancy or lactation the survival was 85 percent. When the lymph nodes are involved, the 10-year survival was 62 percent and 37 percent in controls and women who were diagnosed during pregnancy or lactation, respectively. The difference in survival is partially explained by a longer duration of symptoms prior to diagnosis (6.3 vs. 5.4 months), and tumor size on palpation (4.6 vs. 3.0 cm).

The lactating woman is most likely to recognize a breast mass through her daily manipulations of her breasts. In her framework of reference, she usually considers this mass a "plugged duct." She should be encouraged to report a plugged duct that persists more than 2 weeks despite efforts to initiate drainage of that lobule. Her provider faces an expanded differential diagnosis. Fibromas and fibroadenomas are more common in young women. These solid tumors are rubbery, nodular, and mobile, and they may grow rapidly with the hormonal stimulation of pregnancy. The most common diagnosis is a dilated milk duct, a completely benign diagnosis.

A needle aspiration of the mass is the mainstay of diagnosis. Percutaneous fine-needle aspiration is performed in the same manner as in nonpregnant women. If milk or greenish fluid (fibrocystic disease) is found and the lesion disappears, no further diagnostic procedures need to be performed. If the tumor is solid or fails to disappear completely after aspiration, the needle is passed several times through the lesion under strong negative pressure. The aspirated tissue fluid is air-dried on a slide and sent for cytologic evaluation. Fine-needle aspiration biopsy appears to have the same accuracy in pregnancy and lactation as in the nonpregnant, nonlactating woman. Gupta et al.[129] performed 214 fine-needle aspirations during pregnancy and lactation. Eight (13.7 percent) were cancer.

Ultrasound is an accurate method of determining the cystic nature of a breast mass in lactating women. Mammography is more difficult to interpret during lactation. Young breasts are generally more dense, and the massive increase in functioning glands may obscure small cancers. However, the accuracy is still good if the films are interpreted by experienced radiologists.

A core biopsy using ultrasound or radiographic guidance is a reasonable option to avoid a surgical procedure. If the mother nurses just before the procedure, she will empty the breast, which makes the surgery easier, and will allow 3 to 4 hours until the next feed. The mother should be allowed to nurse on schedule.

Surgical biopsy usually has little effect on breast-feeding performance unless the procedure is done in the periareolar area or the nerves supplying the nipple are compromised. Circumareolar incisions are to be avoided if possible. Milk fistulas are an uncommon risk (5 percent) of central biopsy. The fistulas are usually self-limited and will spontaneously heal over several weeks. Prohibiting breast-feeding does not change the likelihood of ultimate healing.

MATERNAL NUTRITION

The efficiency of conversion of maternal foodstuff to milk is about 80 to 90 percent. If the average milk volume per day is 900 ml, and milk has an average energy content of 75 kcal/dl, the mother must consume an extra 794 kcal/day, unless stored energy is used. During pregnancy, most women store an extra 2 to 5 kg (19,000 to 48,000 kcal) in tissue, mainly as fat, in physiologic preparation for lactation. These calories and nutrients supplement the maternal diet during lactation. As a result, the required dietary increases are easily attainable in healthy mothers and infants.

In lactation, most vitamins and minerals should be increased 20 to 30 percent over nonpregnant requirements. Folic acid should be doubled. Calcium, phosphorus, and magnesium should be increased by 40 to 50 percent, especially in the teenager who is lactating. The appropriate intake of vitamins can be ensured by continuing prenatal vitamins with folic acid through the lactation. The mother should drink at least 1 extra liter of fluid per day to make up for the fluid loss through milk.

Vegetarianism may cause dietary deficiencies of B vitamins (especially B_{12}), total protein, and the full complement of essential amino acids. The dietary history should focus on protein, iron, calcium, and vitamins D and B: Nursing mothers can supplement with soy flour, molasses, or nuts and use vegetable protein combinations.

BREAST AND NIPPLE PAIN

Breast or nipple pain is one of the most frequent complaints of lactating mothers. The frequency is related to failure in the initial management of lactation: late first feed, decreased frequency of feedings, poor nipple grasp, and/or poor positioning. The differential diagnosis of breast pain includes problems with latching-on, engorgement, nipple trauma, mastitis and, occasionally, the let-down reflex.

Symptoms assist with the differential diagnosis. One type of problem with latching-on is the anxious, vigorous infant who sucks strongly against empty ducts until the let-down occurs. The other is the nipple-confused infant who chews on the nipple and abrades the tip with his tongue. In these cases, the nipple and breast pain starts with latching-on and diminishes with let-down. Contact pain suggests nipple trauma and may persist as long as the nipple is manipulated. Engorgement causes a dull, generalized discomfort in the whole breast, worse just before a feed and relieved by it. Localized, unilateral, and continuous pain in the breast may be caused by mastitis. Occasionally, women describe the let-down reflex as painful; this occurs after the first minute of sucking and usually lasts only a minute or two as the ductal swelling is relieved by nursing.

Infection may be a co-factor associated with the pain of nipple injury. When the microbiology of the nipple/milk of 61 lactating women with nipple pain was compared to 64 lactating women without nipple pain and 31 nonlactating women, *Candida albicans* (19 percent) and *Staphylococcus aureus* (30 percent) were more common in women with pain and nipple fissures than in controls (3 to 5 percent).[132]

The management of breast pain consists of general as well as specific steps. Appropriate nursing technique and positioning will prevent, or significantly decrease, the incidence of nipple trauma, engorgement, and mastitis. Rotation of nursing position will reduce the suction pressure on the same part of the nipple, as well as ensuring complete emptying of all lobes of the breast. Frequent nursing will reduce engorgement and milk stasis. The use of soaps, alcohol, and other drying agents on the nipples tends to increase nipple trauma and pain. The nipples should be air-dried for a few minutes after each feed, and clean water is sufficient to cleanse the breast.

Stimulating a let-down and manual expression of milk can be useful in the management of many breast problems. The flow of milk can be improved by placing the mother in a quiet, relaxed environment.[77] The let-down produced by manual expression is never as complete as a normally elicited one. An effective let-down can be elicited by initiating nursing on the side without nipple trauma or mastitis. This will effectively reduce breast pain.

In the first 5 days after birth, about 35 percent of the nipples of breast-feeding mothers show damage, and 69 percent of mothers have nipple pain.[133,134] The management of painful, tender, or injured nipples includes prefeeding manual expression, correction of latching-on, rotation of positions, and initiation of nursing on the less painful side first, with the affected side exposed to air. Drying is facilitated by the application of dry heat (e.g., with a hair dryer on low setting) for 20 minutes four times per day. Analgesics given $1/2$ hour before nursing may be helpful in severe cases. Engorgement can be avoided, but if it occurs, feeding frequency should be maintained or increased. Lanolin can be applied to traumatized nipples, and soap and alcohol have been shown to injure nipples.[133,134] Nipple shields should be used only as a last resort because of a 20 to 60 percent reduction in milk consumption.

Engorgement of the breast occurs when there is inadequate drainage of milk.[136] Swollen, firm, and tender breasts are caused by distention of the ducts and increased extravascular fluid. Aside from the discomfort, engorgement leads to dysfunctional nursing behavior and nipple trauma. The firm breast tissue pushes the infant's face away from the nipple.

The best treatment is prevention, but when this has not occurred, management is centered on symptomatic support and relief of distention. Proper elevation of the breasts is important. The mother should wear a firm-fitting nursing brassiere, with neither thin straps nor plastic lining. A warm shower or bath, with prefeed manual expression, is effective. Frequent suckling (every 1 to 2 hours) is the most effective mechanism to relieve engorgement; postfeed electric pumping from each breast may be helpful. In selected cases, intranasal oxytocin may be given just prior to each feed if let-down seems to be inhibited.

GALACTOGOGUES: DRUGS TO IMPROVE MILK PRODUCTION

Numerous agents have been shown to increase prolactin production; and galactorrhea is a clinical issue for women on phenothiazines or metoclopramide. It is reasonable that these drugs might be used where milk supply seems insufficient.[137] The most understandable clinical scenarios include premature delivery requiring mechanical pumping, glandular hypoplasia, reduction mammoplasty, and relactation (nursing an adoptive child). Clinical trials with random assignment of subjects have demonstrated the effectiveness of metoclopramide,[138,139] sulpiride,[140,141] and nasal oxytocin[142] for increasing milk production.

Metoclopramide (Reglan) is used to promote gastrointestinal tone; however, a secondary effect is to increase prolactin levels.

Most studies demonstrate a multiplefold increase in basal prolactin levels[143] and a 60 to 100 percent increase in milk volume.[137] The effects of metoclopramide are very dose dependent; the usual dose is 10 to 15 mg three times a day. The side effects, gastric cramping, diarrhea, and depression may limit its use. The incidence of depression increases with long-term use; treatment should be tapered over time and limited to less than 4 weeks. There appears to be little effect on the infant.

Sulpiride is a selective dopamine antagonist used in Europe as an antidepressant and antipsychotic. Smaller doses (50 mg twice daily) do not produce neuroleptic effects in the mother, but prolactin and milk production are increased significantly.[144] Clinical studies suggest an increase in milk production (20 to 50 percent) less than that seen with metoclopramide. The transfer of sulpiride to the breast milk is minimal and no adverse effects are seen in the infants. Sulpiride is not available in the United States.

Intranasal oxytocin substitutes for endogenous oxytocin to contract the myoepithelial cells and cause milk let-down. Oxytocin is destroyed by gastrointestinal enzymes and is not given orally. Until recently, oxytocin intranasal spray was available commercially, but it has been taken off the market. A pharmacist can prepare an intranasal spray with a concentration of 2 IU per drop. The let-down dose is a spray (3 drops) to each nostril; the total let-down dose is approximately 12 IU. This is taken within 2 or 3 minutes of each nursing episode. In a double-blind trial, intranasal oxytocin alone was used to enhance milk production in women during the first 5 days after delivery of a premature infant. The cumulative volume of breast milk obtained between the second and fifth days was 3.5 times greater in primiparas given intranasal oxytocin than in primiparas given placebo.[142] Because of oxytocin's complementary mechanism to prolactin-stimulating medications, they are often used in combination.[145]

MASTITIS AND BREAST ABSCESS

Mastitis is an infectious process of the breast characterized by high fever (39° to 40 °C), localized erythema, tenderness, induration, and palpable heat over the area. Often these signs are associated with nausea, vomiting, malaise, and other flu-like symptoms. Mastitis occurs most frequently in the first 2 to 4 weeks postpartum and at times of marked reduction in nursing frequency. Risk factors include maternal fatigue, poor nursing technique, nipple trauma, and epidemic *Staphylococcus aureus*. The most common organisms associated with mastitis are *S. aureus, S. epidermidis,* streptococci and, occasionally, gram-negative rods. The incidence of sporadic mastitis is 2 to 5 percent in lactating and less than 1 percent in nonlactating mothers.

The management of mastitis includes the following: (1) breast support; (2) fluids; (3) assessment of nursing technique; (4) nursing initiated on the uninfected side first to establish let-down; (5) the infected side emptied by nursing with each feed (occasionally, a breast pump helps to ensure complete drainage); and (6) dicloxacillin, 250 mg every 6 hours for 7 days. Erythromycin may be used in patients allergic to penicillin. It is important to continue antibiotics for a full 7 days, since abscess formation is more likely with shorter courses. Hand washing before each feed and by nursing staff reduces nosocomial infection rates.

Breast abscess will occur in about 10 percent of women who are treated for mastitis. The signs include a high fever (39° to 40 °C), and a localized area of erythema, tenderness, and induration. In the center a fluctuant area may be difficult to palpate. *S. aureus* is usually cultured from the abscess cavity.

The management of breast abscess is similar to that for mastitis, except that (1) drainage of the abscess is indicated and (2) breast-feeding should be limited to the uninvolved side during the initial therapy. The infected breast should be mechanically pumped every 2 hours and with every let-down. The abscess can be drained by serial percutaneous needle aspiration under ultrasound guidance[150]; however, the most common method is surgical drainage. The skin incision should be made over the fluctuant area in a manner parallel to and as far as possible from the areolar edge. While the skin incision follows skin lines, the deeper extension should be made bluntly in a radial direction. Once the abscess cavity is entered, all loculations are bluntly reduced and the cavity irrigated with saline. American surgeons pack the wound open for drainage and secondary closure. British surgeons advocate removal of the abscess wall and primary closure.[151] In either case, wide closure sutures should be avoided, as they may compromise the ducts. Patients have a protracted recovery of 18 to 32 days and recurrent abscess formation in 9 to 15 percent of cases. Breast-feeding from the involved side may be resumed, if skin erythema and underlying cellulitis have resolved, which may occur in 4 to 7 days.

Candida albicans infection is considered a common cause of breast pain. Candida infection of the breast is a commonly diagnosed by clinical presentation. Women describe severe pain when the infant nurses. She will describe the pain as "like a red hot poker being driven through my chest." Often she has received antibiotics recently, she is a diabetic, or the infant has evidence of oral thrush or diaper rash *(Candida albicans)*. A potassium hydroxide (KOH) smear can confirm the diagnosis. The initial treatment is to massage nystatin cream or miconazole oral gel into both nipples after each feed and in the infant's mouth three times a day for 2 weeks. Recurrent or persistent candida mastitis can be treated by swabbing the infant's mouth with gentian violet liquid (0.5 percent) and immediately latching the baby to the breast, twice a day for 3 days. The major disadvantage of this therapy is the permanent staining associated with gentian violet. An alternative therapy in severe cases is oral fluconazole, 200-mg loading dose followed by 100 mg/day for 14 days.

DRUGS IN BREAST MILK

Most medications taken by the mother appear in the milk (see Chapter 3), but the calculated dose consumed by the nursing infant ranges from 0.001 to 5 percent of the standard therapeutic doses and are tolerated by infants without toxicity.[152,153] Two good references are *Drugs in Pregnancy and Lactation*[107] and *Medications in Mother's Milk*.[108] Very few drugs are absolutely contraindicated. These include anticancer agents, radioactive materials, lithium, chloramphenicol, phenylbutazone, atropine, and the ergot alkaloids.

The following guidelines are helpful:

1. Evaluate the therapeutic benefit of medication. Diuretics given for ankle swelling provide very different benefits from those for congestive heart failure. Are drugs really necessary, and are there safer alternatives?
2. Choose drugs most widely tested and with the lowest milk/plasma ratio.
3. Choose drugs with the lowest oral bioavailability.
4. Select the least toxic drug with the shortest half-life.
5. Avoid long-acting forms. Usually, these drugs are detoxified by the liver or bound to protein.
6. Schedule doses so that the least amount gets into the milk. The rate of maternal absorption and the peak maternal serum concentration are helpful in scheduling dosage. Usually, it is best for the mother to take the medication immediately after a feeding.
7. Monitor the infant during the course of therapy. Many pharmacologic agents for maternal use are also used for infants. This implies the availability of knowledge about therapeutic doses and the signs and symptoms of toxicity.

MATERNAL DISEASE

In the vast majority of cases of lactating mothers with intercurrent disease, there is no medical reason to stop breast-feeding. A hospitalized nursing mother should have her nursing baby with her in the hospital for on-demand feedings. This situation stretches the flexibility of hospital administrators and nursing services, but the problem can be overcome by education.

The first principle is to maintain lactation. An acute hospitalization for a surgical procedure is a common complication. If breast milk was the neonate's only source of nutrition, an acute reduction in nursing may lead to breast engorgement, confusing postoperative fever, and mastitis. The infant should be put to the breast just before premedication, and the breasts should be emptied in the recovery room. The most effective way is to have the mother nurse. Although some anesthetic may be present in the milk, most are compatible with lactation.[107,108,119,153] If there is legitimate concern or if the mother cannot communicate (on a ventilator), the breasts should be pumped mechanically and subsequently emptied every 2 to 3 hours by nursing or pumping.

The second principle is to adjust for the special nutritional requirements of nursing mothers. This principle is especially pertinent when intake is restricted postoperatively and when maternal diet must be manipulated, as in diabetes.[154] In the postoperative period, the surgeon must account for the calories and fluid required for lactation. Until oral intake is established, a lactating mother needs an additional 500 to 1,000 ml of fluid per day. Early return to a balanced diet is essential to offset the additional energy and protein requirements of lactation and wound healing.

Infection is the most common area where breast-feeding is questioned. In general, the necessary exposure of the infant to the mother in day-to-day care is such that breast-feeding does not add to the risk. This recommendation assumes that appropriate therapy is being given to both mother and infant. Isolation of infected areas should still be practiced, such as a mask in the case of respiratory infection and lesion isolation in herpes. The three acute infections in which breast-feeding is contraindicated are herpes simplex lesions of the breast, untreated active (not just purified protein derivative [PPD]-positive) tuberculosis, and human immunodeficiency viral (HIV) disease.

MILK TRANSFER AND INFANT GROWTH

When is an exclusive diet of breast milk insufficient to supply the nutritional needs of the growing infant? It is apparent that a healthy and successfully breast-feeding mother can supply enough nutrition through breast milk alone for 6 months. The clinical markers for adequate breast milk transfer include an alert, healthy appearance, good muscle tone, good skin turgor, six wet diapers per day, eight or more nursing episodes per day, three or four loose stools per day, consistent evidence of a let-down with operant conditioning, and consistent weight gain.

The infant should be evaluated for failure to thrive or slowed growth if (1) it continues to lose weight after 7 days of life (after "the milk has come in" the infant should gain 1 oz/day); (2) does not regain birth weight by 2 weeks; or (3) gains weight at a rate below the 10th percentile beyond the first months of age. If the infant is premature, ill, or small for gestational age, weight, height, and skin-fold thickness can be used to define adequate growth.

BACK-TO-WORK ISSUES

Breast-feeding during employment is both possible and fulfilling.[157] Preparation, milk storage, and choice of child-care are the cornerstones to easy adaptation to employment. Preparation involves preemployment change in lifestyle to accommodate the increased stresses. Lactation should be well established with frequent nursing (10 to 14 times per day) and no supplementation prior to return to work. Return to full-time work prior to 4 months has a greater negative impact than return to work after 4 months.[157,158] Part-time work lessens the impact. About 2 weeks prior to work, the mother should change her nursing schedule at home. During the workday, she should express or pump her breasts two or three times, while increasing her nursing with short, frequent feeds before and after work times. The infant is fed bottles of stored breast milk by a different person in a different place to allow it to adapt more easily.

During the 2 weeks prior to employment, the day-care arrangements should be carefully selected and observed. In addition to references, several questions are pertinent to the selection of the day-care setting. Is the sitter a mother herself, and does the sitter have experience with nursing babies? Is the mother welcome to use the child-care site for a midday nursing? Does the day-care center provide in-arm feeding, or does it use high chairs and propped bottle-feedings? Is the time and activity of the center highly structured and rigid, or is it flexible to mother or infant needs and requests? Does the staff treat the parents and children with respect? Many of these questions can answered by an extended (1 to 2 hours) observation of the center and its children.

Fatigue is the number one enemy of the working mother. Emotional and physical support of the mother is critical. Some helpful suggestions include (1) bringing the infant's bed into the parents' room, or the construction of a temporary extension to the parents' bed; (2) use of labor saving devices, division of domestic chores, and the elimination of less important household chores to reduce the workload; and (3) taking naps and frequent rest periods to conserve energy.

Continued stimulation of the breast during working hours is important. Pumping not only improves milk supply but it also supplies human milk for the infant. Manual expression and/or mechanical pumping should be performed more frequently (two to three times) in the first 6 months postpartum. After 6 months, the frequency can be reduced and eliminated as the infant is supplemented by fluids or solids during the day.

The collection of breast milk has become simple with the wide variety of mechanical pumps available in the market. Mechanical pumps that employ a bulb syringe produce the least amount of milk and have the highest rate of bacterial contamination. Cyclic electric pumps produce the most milk with the least amount of nipple trauma. The most efficient pumps are not as effective as the efficiently nursing boby in increasing milk volume and raising prolactin levels.[159]

Freshly refrigerated milk should be used within 2 days. Four to 6 oz of human milk can be frozen in partially filled resealable (Ziploc) plastic bags. When human milk is frozen, it should be cooled briefly prior to transfer to the freezer. The milk will keep for 2 to 4 weeks in the refrigerator freezer and up to 6 months in a freezer set at 0 °F. The milk should be stored in layers and thawed quickly in warm tap water. Frozen milk should not be thawed in the microwave, as the heating is uneven and severe oral burns have been reported. After it is thawed it should be used within 6 to 8 hours.

WEANING

The American Academy of Pediatrics recommends exclusive breast-feeding for the first 6 months of life and continuation at least through the first 12 months of life. Dettwyler[161] makes a very cogent argument for the "natural" age of weaning in the human to be 3 to 4 years. As the infant supplements an increasing proportion of its nutritional needs with solid or liquid food, the mother will begin to ovulate. Subsequent pregnancy is increasingly more likely. Breast-feeding, through its suppression of gonadal function, mantains a birth interval of 3 to 4 years. Clearly, breast-feeding into the third or fourth year is a cultural exception in the United States, but prolonged breast-feeding does not constitute abnormal behavior. As we learn more about the benefits of long-term lactation, our culture may return to more reasonable expectations for duration of breast-feeding.

Key Points

➤ By 6 weeks postpartum, 28 percent of women will have returned to their prepregnant weight.

➤ Approximately 50 percent of parturients experience diminished sexual desire during the 3 months following delivery.

➤ Postpartum uterine bleeding of sufficient quantity to require medical attention occurs in 1 to 2 percent of parturients. In patients requiring curettage, 40 percent will be found to have retained placental tissue.

➤ Late-onset endometritis (after 7 days) is frequently caused by *Chlamydia trachomatis.*

➤ *Candida* infection is a common cause of persistent nipple soreness in women who are breast-feeding.

➤ Most women with puerperal mastitis can be adequately treated with penicillin V, ampicillin, or dicloxacillin while they continue to breast-feed their infants.

➤ Progestin-only contraceptive medication (norethindrone 0.35 mg daily) does not diminish lactation performance.

➤ Postpartum, major depression occurs in 8 to 20 percent of parturients.

➤ Puerperal hypothyroidism often presents with symptoms that include mild dysphoria; consequently, thyroid function studies are suggested in the evaluation of patients with suspected postpartum depression that occurs 2 to 3 months after delivery.

➤ Breast-feeding will result in 98 percent contraceptive protection for up to 6 months following delivery, provided there is little or no supplemental feeding of the infant.

➤ The American Academy of Pediatrics and the American College of Obstetricians and Gynecologists endorse breast-feeding as the gold standard for infant feeding.

➤ Breast-feeding accrues many health benefits for the infant, including protection against infection, less allergy, better growth, better neurodevelopment, and lower rates of chronic disease such as insulin-dependent diabetes and childhood cancer.

Box continued on following page

Key Points *Continued*

➤ Breast-feeding accrues more health benefits for the mother, including faster postpartum involution, improved postpartum weight loss, less premenopausal breast cancer, better mother–infant bonding, and less economic burden.

➤ Artificial breast milk lacks key components including defenses against infection, hormones and enzymes to aid digestion, polyunsaturated fatty acids, which are necessary for optimal brain growth, and adequate composition for efficient digestion.

➤ Contact with the breast within one half hour after birth increases the duration of breast feeding. A frequency of nursing greater than eight per 24 hours, night nursing, and a duration of nursing longer than 15 minutes are needed to maintain adequate prolactin levels and milk supply.

➤ Prolactin is the major promoter of milk synthesis. Oxytocin is the major initiator of milk ejection. The release of prolactin and oxytocin results from the stimulation of the sensory nerves supplying the areola and nipple.

➤ Oxytocin released from the posterior pituitary can be operantly conditioned and is influenced negatively by pain, stress, or loss of self-esteem.

➤ The nursing actions on a human teat versus on an artificial teat are very different. Poor lactation is the major cause of nipple injury and poor milk transfer. Perceived or real lack of milk transfer is the major reason why lactation fails.

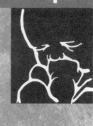

Complicated
Pregnancies

Chapter 17

Fetal Wastage

JOE LEIGH SIMPSON

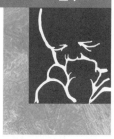

Not all conceptions result in a liveborn infant. Of clinically recognized pregnancies, 10 to 15 percent are lost. A subset of women (1–2 percent) manifest repetitive spontaneous abortions as opposed to merely representing random untoward events. This chapter considers the causes of fetal wastage, and the management of couples experiencing repetitive losses. Ectopic gestations are also discussed.

FREQUENCY AND TIMING OF PREGNANCY LOSSES

Pregnancy is not generally recognized clinically until 5 to 6 weeks after the last menstrual period, but before this time β-human chorionic gonadotropin (β-hCG) assays can detect preclinical pregnancies. At least 25 percent if not 50 percent or more preimplantation embryos never implant. Of pregnancies that do implant's and are detected by β-hCG assays around the expected time of implantation (day 20 of gestation) 31 percent are lost.

Clinically recognized first-trimester fetal loss rates of 10 to 12 percent overall are well documented in both retrospective and prospective cohort studies.[4] Loss rates reflect many factors but two associations are worth emphasizing here. First, maternal age greatly increases risk, a 40-year-old woman carrying twice the risk of a 20 year-old woman. Second, prior pregnancy history is pivotal. As will be discussed below, loss rates are lowest (6 percent) among nulliparous women who have never experienced a loss[5] rising to 25 to 30 percent after three or more losses.

Fetal demise occurs before overt clinical signs are manifested. This conclusion is based on cohort studies showing that only 3 percent of viable pregnancies are lost after 8 weeks' gestation.[9] Given an accepted clinical loss rate of 10 to 12 percent, fetal viability must cease weeks before maternal symptoms appear; thus, most fetuses aborting clinically at 9 to 12 weeks must have died weeks previously. Most pregnancy losses after 8 weeks likely occur in the next 2 gestational months, as loss rates are only 1 percent in women confirmed by ultrasound to have viable pregnancies at 16 weeks. Overall, almost all losses are "missed abortions" (retained in utero for an interval prior to clinical recognition); thus, the term is archaic.

CYTOGENETIC ETIOLOGY IN CLINICALLY RECOGNIZED LOSSES

The major cause of clinically recognized pregnancy losses is chromosomal abnormalities. At least 50 percent of clinically recognized pregnancy losses result from a chromosomal abnormality.[21-23] The frequency is probably even higher.

Among third-trimester losses (stillborn infants) the frequency of chromosomal abnormalities is approximately 5 percent.[26] This frequency is less than that observed in earlier abortuses, but still higher than found among liveborns (0.6 percent).

Autosomal Trisomy

Autosomal trisomies comprise the largest (approximately 50 percent) single class of chromosomal complements in cytogenetically abnormal spontaneous abortions. Frequencies of these trisomies are listed in Table 17–1. The most common trisomy is trisomy 16. Most trisomies show a maternal age effect, but the effect is variably marked among certain chromosomes.

Various attempts have been made to correlate morphologic abnormalities with specific trisomies,[28,29] but relationships are imprecise. Trisomies incompatible with life predictably show slower growth than trisomies compatible with life (trisomies 13, 18, and 21). Potentially viable trisomies tend to show anomalies consistent with those found in full-term liveborn trisomic infants.[28,29] The malformations present have been said to be more severe than these found in induced abortuses detected after prenatal diagnosis.

Most trisomies are accounted for by maternal meiotic errors. In trisomy 13 and trisomy 21, 90 percent of these maternal cases arise at meiosis I; almost all trisomy 16 cases arise in maternal meiosis I.[30] Trisomy 18, is an exception, often arising at meiosis II.[31,32] Errors of maternal meiosis I are associated with advanced maternal age and in turn correlate with decreased to absent meiotic recombination.[31-33]

Table 17-1. CHROMOSOMAL COMPLEMENTS IN SPONTANEOUS ABORTIONS: RECOGNIZED CLINICALLY IN THE FIRST TRIMSESTER*

Complement		(%)
Normal 46,XX or 46,XY		54.1
Triploidy		7.7
69,XXX	2.7	
69,XYX	0.2	
69,XXY	4.0	
Other	0.8	
Tetraploidy		2.6
92,XXX	1.5	
92,XXYY	0.55	
Not Stated	0.55	
Monsomy X		18.6
Structural abnormalities		1.5
Sex chromosomal polysomy		0.2
47,XXX	0.55	
47,XXY	0.15	
Autosomal monosomy (G)		0.1
Autosomal trisomy for chromosomes		22.3
1	0	
2	1.11	
3	0.25	
4	0.64	
5	0.04	
6	0.14	
7	0.89	
8	0.79	
9	0.72	
10	0.36	
11	0.04	
12	0.18	
13	1.07	
14	0.82	
15	1.68	
16	7.27	
17	0.18	
18	1.15	
19	0.01	
20	0.61	
21	2.11	
22	2.26	

Table continued on following page

Table 17–1. CHROMOSOMAL COMPLEMENTS IN
SPONTANEOUS ABORTIONS: RECOGNIZED CLINICALLY
IN THE FIRST TRIMSESTER* *Continued*

Complement	(%)
Double trisomy	0.7
Mosaic trisomy	1.3
Other abnormalities or not specified	0.9
	100.0

*Pooled data from several series, as referenced elsewhere by Simpson and Bombard.[23]

Polyploidy

In polyploidy, more than two haploid chromosomal complements
exist. Triploidy (3n = 69) and tetraploidy (4n = 92) occur often
in abortuses. Triploid abortuses are usually 69,XXY or 69,XXX,
resulting from dispermy.[39,40] Pathologic findings in triploid placentas
include a disproportionately large gestational sac, cystic degeneration of placental villi, intrachorial hemorrhage, and hydropic trophoblasts (pseudomolar degeneration).[28,29] Malformations include
neural tube defects and omphaloceles, anomalies reminiscent of
those observed in triploid conceptuses progressing to term. Facial
dysmorphia and limb abnormalities have also been reported. An
association exists between triploidy and hydatidiform mole, a
"partial mole" said to exist if molar tissue and fetal parts coexist.
The more common "complete" hydatidiform mole is 46,XX, of
androgenetic origin.[40]

Tetraploidy is uncommon, rarely progressing beyond 2 to 3
weeks of embryonic life.

Monosomy X

Monosomy X is the single most common chromosomal abnormality among spontaneous abortions, accounting for 15 to 20
percent of abnormal specimens. Monosomy X embryos usually
consist of only an umbilical cord stump. Later in gestation,
anomalies characteristic of the Turner syndrome may be seen,
specifically cystic hygromas and generalized edema. Although
liveborn 45,X individuals usually lack germ cells, 45,X abortuses
show germ cells; however, these germ cells rarely develop beyond
the primordial germ cell stage.

Monosomy X usually (80 percent) occurs as a result of paternal
sex chromosome loss.[44]

Structural Chromosomal Rearrangement

Structural chromosomal rearrangement account for 1.5 percent of all abortuses (Table 17–1). Rearrangements (e.g., translocation) may either arise de novo during gametogenesis or be inherited from a parent carrying a "balanced" translocation or inversion. Phenotypic consequences depend on the specific duplicated or deficient chromosomal segments. Although not a common cause of sporadic losses, inherited translocations are an important cause of *repeated* fetal wastage.

MENDELIAN AND POLYGENIC/ MULTIFACTORIAL ETIOLOGY

The 30 to 50 percent of first-trimester abortuses that show no chromosomal abnormalities could still have undergone fetal demise as a result of other genetic etiologies. Neither mendelian nor polygenic/multifactorial disorders show chromosomal abnormalities. Many excellent anatomic studies of abortuses have demonstrated structural abnormalities, but lack of cytogenetic data on the dissected specimens makes it nearly impossible to determine the precise role of noncytogenetic mechanisms in early embryonic maldevelopment. Doubtless pivotal to early development are many mendeliam genes, mutation of which would be expected to result in embryonic death and pregnancy loss.

GENETIC COUNSELING AND RECURRENT RISKS

The obstetrician faced with a couple experiencing spontaneous abortion has several immediate obligations: (1) inform the couple concerning the frequency of fetal wastage (10 to 12 percent clinically recognized pregnancies) and its likely etiology (at least 50 percent cytogenetic), (2) provide recurrence risk rates, and (3) determine the necessity of a formal clinical evaluation.

Recurrence Risks

Loss rates are increased among women who have experienced previous losses, but not nearly to the extent once thought (Table 17–2). For decades, obstetricians fervently believed in the concept of "habitual abortion." After three losses, the risk of subsequent losses was thought to rise sharply. Such beliefs were based on theoretical calculations, and are now no longer accepted.

Table 17-2. APPROXIMATE RECURRENCE RISK
FIGURES USEFUL FOR COUNSELING WOMEN
WITH REPEATED SPONTANEOUS ABORTIONS*

	Prior Abortions	Risk (%)
Women with liveborn infants	0	5-10
	1	20-25
	2	25
	3	30
	4	30
Women without liveborn infants	3	30-40

*Recurrence risks are slightly higher for older women and for those who smoke cigarettes or drink alcohol and for those exposed to high levels of selected chemical toxins.
Based on data from Warbuton and Fraser, [49] Poland et al.,[50] and Regan[5].

One lingering consequence, however, is that these erroneous risk figures (80-70 percent) were unfortunately used as "controls" for clinical studies evaluating various treatment plans. This practice led to unwarranted acceptance of certain interventions, the most famous of which was diethylstilbestrol (DES) treatment.

Table 17-2 shows appropriate figures. Lowest risks (5 percent) are observed in nulliparous women with no prior losses.[5] Women who smoke cigarettes or drink alcohol moderately are probably at slightly higher risk.[51] Recurrence risks are higher if the abortus is cytogenetically normal than cytogenetically abnormal.[52]

Applying these risk figures, the prognosis is reasonably good even without therapy. The success rate should be 70 percent. Thus, Vlaanderen and Treffers[53] reported successful pregnancies in each of 21 women having unexplained prior repetitive losses but subjected to no intervention. Other groups reached similar conclusions, including the control (placebo) group in a recent well-publicized immunotherapy study.[54,55] To be judged efficacious, therapeutic regimens must achieve successes greater than 70 percent.

Necessity of Formal Evaluation

Every couple experiencing a fetal loss should be counseled and provided recurrence risk rates, but not every couple requires formal assessment. Infertile couples who are in their fourth decade may choose to be evaluated after only two losses. After three losses, all couples should be offered formal evaluation. Once a couple enters evaluation, they should undergo all tests standard for a given practitioner. There is no scientific rationale for performing some studies after three losses but deferring others until after four losses. Any couple having a stillborn or anomalous liveborn infant should undergo cytogenetic studies unless the stillborn was known to have a normal chromosome complement. Parental chromosomal rearrangements (i.e., translocations or inversions) should be excluded.

ETIOLOGY AND CLINICAL EVALUATION OR REPETITIVE ABORTIONS

Translocations

Structural chromosomal abnormalities are generally accepted as one explanation for repetitive abortions. The most common structural rearrangement encountered is a translocation, found in about 5 percent of couples experiencing repeated losses.[56-58] Individuals with balanced translocations are phenotypically normal, but abortuses or abnormal liveborns may show chromosomal duplications or deficiencies as a result of normal meiotic segregation. About 60 percent of the translocations detected are reciprocal (Fig. 17–1), and 40 percent are robertsonian. Females are about twice as likely as males to show a balanced translocation.[56]

The clinical significance of translocations is illustrated in Figure 4–4. If a child has Down syndrome as a result of such a translocation, the rearrangement will prove to have originated de novo in 50 to 75 percent of cases. That is, a balanced translocation will not exist in either parent. The likelihood of Down syndrome recurring in subsequent offspring is minimal. On the other hand, the risk is significant in the 25 to 50 percent of families in which individuals have Down syndrome as the result of a balanced parental translocation (e.g., parental complement 45,XX, −14, −21, + t[14q;21q]). The theoretical risk of having a child with Down syndrome is 33 percent, but empirical risks are considerably less. The likelihood is only 2 percent if the father carries the translocation and 10 percent if the mother carries the translocation.[59,60] If robertsonian (centric-fusion) translocations involve other chromosomes, empirical risks are lower. In t(13q;14q), the risk for liveborn trisomy 13 is 1 percent or less.

Reciprocal translocations do not involve centromeric fusion. Empirical data for specific translocations are usually not available, but useful generalizations can be made on the basis of pooled data derived from many different translocations. Studies of sperm chromosomes[61] theoretically might provide data specific for a given

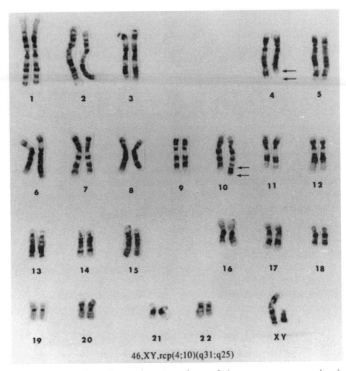

46,XY,rcp(4;10)(q31;q25)

Figure 17–1. Balanced translocation detected in a woman experiencing multiple abortions. (From Simpson JL, Tharapel AT: Principles of cytogenetics. *In* Philip E, Barnes J [eds]: Scientific Foundations of Obstetrics and Gynaecology, 4th ed. London, Heinemann Medical Books, 1991, p 27, with permission.)

translocation in a specific individual, but this is not readily available. Of interest is that sperm of fathers experiencing repeated losses show no more than the expected 10 percent of cytogenetic abnormalities.[62]

Theoretical risks for abnormal offspring (unbalanced reciprocal translocations) are far greater than empirical risks. Overall, the risk is 12 percent for offspring of either female heterozygotes or male heterozygotes.[59,60] Detecting a parental chromosomal rearrangement thus profoundly affects subsequent pregnancy management. Antenatal cytogenetic studies should be offered in subsequent pregnancies. The frequency of unbalanced fetuses is lower if parental balanced translocations are ascertained through repetitive abortions (3 percent) than through anomalous liveborns (nearly 20 percent).[59]

A few translocations preclude the possibility of normal liveborn infants, namely, translocations involving homologous chromosomes (e.g., t[13q13q] or t[21q21q]). If the father carries such a structural rearrangement, artificial insemination may be appropriate. If the mother carries the rearrangement, donor oocytes or donor embryos (assisted reproductive technologies) should be considered.

Recurrent Aneuploidy

Numerical chromosomal abnormalities (aneuploidy) may be responsible for both recurrent as well as sporadic losses. This deduction is made on the basis of observations that the complements of successive abortuses in a given family are more likely to be either recurrently normal or recurrently abnormal (Table 17–3). If the complement of the first abortus is abnormal, the likelihood is 80 percent that the complement of the second abortus also will be abnormal.[65] The recurrent abnormality usually is trisomy.

Certain couples seem predisposed toward chromosomally abnormal conceptions. Although it can be argued that corrections for maternal age render the ostensible nonrandom distribution nonsignificant, this author counsels increased risks compared with normal women of comparable age. If couples are predisposed to recurrent aneuploidy, they might logically be at increased risk not only for aneuploid abortuses but also for aneuploid liveborns. The trisomic autosome in a subsequent pregnancy might not always confer lethality, but rather might be compatible with life (e.g., trisomy 21). Indeed, the risk of liveborn trisomy 21 following an aneuploid abortus is about 1 percent.[66]

Information concerning fetal chromosomal status may be lacking for couples having repetitive abortions. Antenatal diagnosis then may or may not be appropriate. Risks for abnormal offspring are probably increased, but the risk of amniocentesis or CVS is especially troublesome to couples who have had difficulty achieving pregnancy. Finally, there is some evidence that abortion rates are *lowest* in couples with prior losses when conception occurred in midcycle.[52] Midcycle fertilization is recommended in subsequent pregnancies.

Luteal Phase Defects

Luteal phase defects (LPDs) is the term used to describe the endometrium manifesting an inadequate progesterone effect. Progesterone secreted by the corpus luteum is necessary to support the endometrium until the trophoblast produces sufficient progesterone

Table 17–3. RECURRENT ANEUPLOIDY: THE RELATIONSHIP BETWEEN KARYOTYPES OF
SUCCESSIVE ABORTUSES*

Complement of First Abortus	Complement of Second Abortus					
	Normal	Trisomy	Monosomy	Triploidy	Tetraploid	De Novo Rearrangement
Normal	142	18	5	7	3	2
Trisomy	31	30	1	4	3	1
Monosomy X	7	5	3	3	0	0
Triploidy	7	4	1	4	0	0
Tetraploidy	3	1	0	2	0	0
De novo rearrangement	1	3	0	0	0	0

*Tabulation by Warburton et al.[65]

to maintain pregnancy, an event occurring around 7 gestational (menstrual) weeks or 5 weeks after conception.

Once almost universally accepted as a common cause for fetal wastage, LPD now seems to be considered an uncommon cause. Although plausible clinically, there are no randomized studies verifying efficacy of treatment.

Diabetes Mellitus

Women whose diabetes mellitus is poorly controlled are at increased risk for fetal loss.[3] Women whose glycosylated hemoglobin level was greater than 4 SD above the mean show higher pregnancy loss rates than women with lower glycosylated hemoglobin levels. Although poorly controlled diabetes mellitus should be considered one cause for early pregnancy loss, well-controlled or subclinical diabetes is not a cause of early miscarriage.

Intrauterine Adhesions (Synechiae)

Intrauterine adhesions could interfere with implantation or early embryonic development. Adhesions may follow overzealous uterine curettage during the postpartum period, intrauterine surgery (e.g., myomectomy), or endometritis. Curettage is the usual explanation, with adhesions most likely to develop if curettage is performed 3 or 4 weeks after delivery. Individuals with uterine synechiae usually manifest hypomenorrhea or amenorrhea, but 15 to 30 percent show repeated abortions. If adhesions are detected in a woman experiencing repetitive losses, lysis under direct hyperoscopic visualization should be performed. An intrauterine device or inflated Foley catheter inserted postoperatively in the uterus may discourage reapposition of healing uterine surfaces. Estrogen administration should also be initiated.

Incomplete Müllerian Fusion

Müllerian fusion defects (Fig. 17–2) are an accepted cause of *second*-trimester losses and pregnancy complications. Low birth weight, breech presentation, and uterine bleeding are other abnormalities associated with müllerian fusion defects. A few studies claim that the worst outcomes are associated with either septate uteri[99] or T-shaped uteri,[98] but others discern few differences among various anomalies.[102]

The major problem in attributing cause and effect for second-trimester complications and uterine anomalies is that the latter are so frequent that adverse outcomes could often be coincidental.

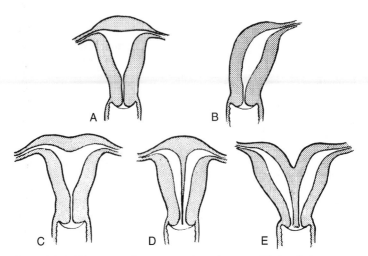

Figure 17–2. Diagrammatic representation of some müllerian fusion anomalies. *A,* Normal uterus, fallopian tubes, and cervix. *B,* Uterus unicornis (absence of one uterine horn). *C,* Uterus arcuatus (broadening and medial depression of a portion of the uterine septum). *D,* Uterus septus (persistence of a complete uterine septum). *E,* Uterus bicornis unicollis (two hemiuteri, each leading to same cervix). (From Simpson JL: Disorders of Sexual Differentiation, Etiology and Clinical Delineation. San Diego, Academic Press, 1976, with permission.)

Treatment has traditionally involved surgical correction, such as metroplasty. Women experiencing second-trimester abortions can be assumed to benefit from uterine reconstruction.

First-trimester abortions might also be caused by müllerian fusion defects, If implantation occurs on a poorly vascularized and inhospitable surface. However, reconstructive surgery is not necessarily advisable if losses are restricted to the first trimester.

Incompetent Internal Cervical Os

A functionally intact cervix and lower uterine cavity are obvious prerequisites for a successful intrauterine pregnancy. Characterized by painless dilation and effacement, cervical incompetence usually occurs during the middle second or early third trimester. This condition frequently follows traumatic events like cervical amputation, cervical lacerations, forceful cervical dilatation, or conization. A relationship to various connective tissue disorders is plausible but yet unproved. The various surgical techniques to correct cervical incompetence are discussed in Chapter 18.

Infections

Infections are accepted causes of late fetal wastage and logically could be responsible for early fetal loss as well. Microorganisms reported to be associated with spontaneous abortion include variola, vaccinia, *Salmonella typhi, Vibrio fetus,* malaria, Cytomegalovirus, *Brucella, Toxoplasma, Mycoplasma hominis, Chlamydia trachomatis,* and *Ureaplasma urealyticum.* Transplacental infection doubtless occurs with each of these microorganisms, and sporadic losses could logically be caused by any. However, verification at these logical deductions has not been forthcoming. Other studies have found no difference in outcome between women treated and not treated with antibiotics. Unanswered also is whether the infectious agents were causative in the fetal losses or merely arose secondarily after demise caused by a noninfectious etiology.

Of all organisms mentioned, *Ureaplasma* and *Chlamydia* are not only the most commonly implicated in *repetitive* abortion but also fulfill certain prerequisites necessary to assume a causal relationship. Both can exist in an asymptomatic state, and neither necessarily is so severe as to cause infertility.

Evaluation and management should consist of culturing the endometrium for *U. urealyticum* and treating culture-positive women. Alternatively, easier, tetracycline therapy can be reasoned to be so innocuous that empiric treatment with doxycycline (100 mg orally twice a day for 10 days, both husband and nonpregnant wife) could be recommended.

Antifetal Antibodies

Perturbations of the immune system can be responsible for fetal wastage. However, the nature of the immunologic process responsible for maintaining pregnancy has proved to be complex. Several different immunologic processes may play a role.

In one immunologic process, an otherwise normal mother produces antibodies against her fetus on the basis of genetic dissimilarities. Fetal loss is well documented in Rh-negative (D-negative) women having anti-D antibodies. More apropos for early pregnancy loss is the presence of anti-P antibodies. Most individuals are genotype Pp or PP, but one may be homozygous for p (pp). If a woman of genotype pp has a Pp or PP mate, resulting offspring may or must be Pp. If the mother develops anti-P antibodies, Pp fetuses will be rejected (aborted) early in gestation. Plasmapheresis and other modalities may be therapeutically efficacious.[119,120]

Hill and colleagues[121] proposed that perturbations of cytokines cause repetitive abortions in women through T-helper cell abnormalities. The rationale is based on T-helper 1 (Th1) cytokines being deleterious, but Th2 cytokines not. The former includes tumor necrosis factor (TNF), interleukin (IL) -2, and interferon (IFN)-γ; the latter includes IL-4, IL-5, IL-6, and IL-10. In women with recurrent loss, immune cell responsiveness could become activated to produce increased IFN-γ and TNF.[122]

Autoimmune Disease

An association between second-trimester pregnancy loss and certain autoimmune disease is generally accepted.[125,126] Antiphospholipid antibodies these represent a broad category that encompasses lupus anticoagulant (LAC) antibodies and anticardiolipin antibodies (aCL). Most investigators[127] agree that midtrimester fetal death is increased in women with LAC or aCL; in fact, dramatically so. Controversy centers on the role of these antibodies in first-trimester losses.

Descriptive studies initially seemed to show increased anticardiolipin antibodies in women with first-trimester pregnancy losses. However, frequencies of various antiphospholipid antibodies (LAC, aCL, aPL) soon were shown to be similar in women who experience and who do not experience first-trimester abortions.[128-131] A pitfall in assessing the role of these antibodies in first-trimester losses is the unavoidable selection bias in studying couples only after they have presented with spontaneous abortions. Perhaps antibodies arise until *after* the pregnancy loss can not be excluded in most experimental designs. To address this pitfall, Simpson et al.[132] analyzed sera prospectively obtained from women within 21 days of conception. A total of 93 women who later experienced pregnancy loss were matched 2:1 with 190 controls who subsequently had a normal liveborn offspring.[132] No association was observed between pregnancy loss and presence of either aPL or aCL.

Although neither aCL nor aPL would seem to contribute greatly, if at all, to first-trimester pregnancy loss in the general population, the issue remains open in the opinion of some. Power calculations are inadequate to exclude an effect limited to selected subsets, such as women with three or more repetitive losses.

Given the uncertainty of a relationship between first-trimester loss and aPL and aCL, treatment regimens should be offered hesitantly and only with nontoxic agents (e.g., aspirin and heparin, but not steroids). Treating aborters with intravenous immunoglobulin is not recommended.[139]

Alloimmune Disease (Shared Parental Antigens)

If fetal rejection occurs as a result of diminished fetal–maternal immunologic interaction (alloimmune factors), immunotherapy might be beneficial to stimulate beneficial blocking antibodies generated at the few loci differing from father and mother and, hence, potentially fetus. Initial studies produced impressive results,[140] but later studies were far less so. In 1994 a multicenter U.S. effort pooling results of immunotherapy by injection of paternal leukocytes into the mother reported a scant 11 percent increased pregnancy rate in the immunized group.[141] Meta-analysis by Fraser et al.[142] found the odds ratio to be only 1.3 in favor of a beneficial effect. In 1999, Ober et al.[143] reported the definitive study, a NICHD collaborative effort involving six U.S. and Canadian centers. Women with three or more spontaneous abortions of unknown cause were randomized into one arm ($n = 91$) that underwent immunization with paternal mononuclear cells; women in the other arm were given saline (controls) ($n = 92$). Pregnancy beyond 28 weeks occurred in 46 percent (31 of 68) of the immunized group versus 65 percent (41 of 63) in the nonimmunized group. These findings were the opposite of expectation if immunotherapy were salutary.

In conclusion, parental human leukocyte antigen (HLA) sharing leading to fetal rejection seems to be valid, with HLA-B the locus showing the strongest association. However, the attributable role of HLA sharing in pregnancy losses in the general population must be low, and immunotherapy is clearly not useful.

Drugs, Chemicals, and Noxious Agents

Various exogenous agents have been implicated in fetal losses. Indeed, women are exposed frequently to relatively low doses of ubiquitous agents. However, few agents can be implicated with confidence. Rarely are data adequate to determine the true role of these exogenous factors in early pregnancy losses.

Outcomes following exposures to exogenous agents are usually deduced on the basis of case-control studies. In such studies, women who aborted claimed exposure to the agent in question more often than controls. However, case-control studies suffer certain inherent biases. The primary bias is that controls have less incentive to recall antecedent events than subjects experiencing an abnormal outcome (recall bias). Employers attempt to limit exposure of women in the reproductive age group; thus, exposures to potentially dangerous chemicals are usually unwitting and, hence, poorly documented. Moreover, pregnant women usually are exposed to many agents concurrently, making it nearly impossible to attribute adverse effects to a single agent. Given these caveats, physicians should be cautious about attributing pregnancy loss to exogenous agents. On the other hand, common sense dictates that exposure to potentially noxious agents be minimized.

X-Irradiation

Irradiation and antineoplastic agents in high doses are acknowledged abortifacients. Of course, therapeutic x-rays or chemotherapeutic drugs are administered during pregnancy only to seriously ill women whose pregnancies often must be terminated for maternal indications. On the other hand, pelvic x-ray exposure of up to perhaps 10 rad places a woman at little to no increased risk. Exposure doses are usually far less (1 to 2 rad). Still, it is prudent for pregnant hospital workers to avoid handling chemotherapeutic agents and minimize potential exposures during diagnostic x-ray procedures.

Cigarette Smoking

Smoking during pregnancy is accepted as associated with spontaneous abortion, but this could be explained partly on the basis of confounding variables. Kline et al.[144] found increased abortion rates in smokers, independent of maternal age and independent of alcohol consumption. Ness et al.[145] studied the relationship between pregnancy loss and tobacco use, as assessed by urinary cotinine levels. Four hundred women with spontaneous abortions were compared with 570 who experienced ongoing pregnancies. Women with urinary cotinine had increased risk of abortion, but the odds ratio only reached 1.8 (95 percent confidence interval [CI] 1.3 to 2.6).

Caffeine

The consensus has long been that no deleterious effects of caffeine exist. Mills et al.[146] found an odds ratio for an association between caffeine (coffee and other dietary forms) to be only 1.15 (95 percent CI 0.89 to 1.49).[146] This did not exclude an effect a very high levels (>300 mg caffeine daily). Klebanoff et al.[147] showed an association between pregnancy losses and caffeine ingestion, 7 mg daily. A problem with the latter studies is difficulty in being able to separate the effects of nausea, which typically is more common in successful pregnancies. However, in general reassurance can be given concerning moderate caffeine exposure and pregnancy loss.

Alcohol

An association between alcohol consumption and fetal loss once seemed generally accepted. However, more recent studies have not reported a relationship in moderate drinkers. Halmesmärki et al.[149] found that alcohol consumption was nearly identical in women who did and did not experience an abortion; 13 percent of aborters and 11 percent of control women drank on average three to four drinks per week; other investigations have reached a similar conclusion.[145,150]

Alcohol consumption should be avoided or minimized during pregnancy for many reasons, but abstinence may only minimally if at all decrease pregnancy loss rate.

Environmental Chemicals

Limiting exposure to potential toxins in the workplace is recognized as prudent for pregnant women. The difficulty lies in defining the precise effect of lower exposures and attributing a specific risk. False alarms concerning potential toxins are frequent. Among the many chemical agents variously claimed to be associated with fetal losses, consensus seems to be evolving around a selected few.[151] These include anesthetic gases, arsenic, aniline dyes, benzene, solvents, ethylene oxide, formaldehyde, pesticides, and certain divalent cations (lead, mercury, cadmium). Workers in rubber industries, battery factories, and chemical production plants are among those at potential risk.

Trauma

Women commonly attribute pregnancy losses to trauma, such as a fall or blow to the abdomen. However, fetuses are actually well protected from external trauma by intervening maternal structures and amniotic fluid. The temptation to attribute a loss to minor traumatic events should be avoided.

Psychological Factors

That impaired psychological well-being predisposes to early fetal losses has been claimed but never firmly established.

Investigations cited as proving a benefit of psychological well-being are those of Stray-Pedersen et al.[152] Pregnant women previously having experienced repetitive abortions received increased attention but no specific medical therapy ("tender loving care"), and are proved more likely to complete their pregnancy than women not offered such close attention. A pitfall was that only women living "close" to the university were eligible to be placed in the increased-attention group. Women living farther away served as "controls"; however, these women may have differed from the experimental group in other ways as well.

Severe Maternal Illness

Many debilitating maternal diseases have been implicated in early abortion. Pathogenesis is not necessarily independent of mechanisms discussed previously, specifically endocrinologic or immunologic. Symptomatic maternal diseases established as causes of fetal wastage include Wilson disease, maternal phenylketonuria, cyanotic heart disease, hemoglobinopathies, and inflammatory bowel disease. Actually, any life-threatening disease would be expected to be associated with an increased abortion rate.

ECTOPIC PREGNANCY

In ectopic pregnancy, implantation occurs at a site other than the endometrium. Ectopic pregnancies are responsible for approximately 10 percent of all maternal mortality.[157] The prognosis for future reproduction is poor. Only one half of women having an ectopic pregnancy are eventually delivered of a liveborn infant. Most of these never become pregnant, and up to 25 percent of those who do suffer a repeat ectopic pregnancy.[158] Various factors contribute to ectopic pregnancies, the most common being infection. Unlike intrauterine spontaneous abortions, genetic factors are not paramount in the etiology of ectopic pregnancy. Ectopic embryos show chromosomal abnormalities no more often than predicted on the basis of embryonic age.[159]

Incidence

The incidence of recorded ectopic gestation is increasing. Some of this increase seems real and some spurious. A true increase can be hypothesized as a result of (1) improved treatment for pelvic inflammatory disease, a condition that in the past would have conferred sterility; (2) an increase in surgical corrections of fallopian tube occlusion; and (3) a greater number of elective sterilizations, some of which are later reversed surgically. However, there is also an artificial increase related to improved diagnostic techniques. Ectopic pregnancies that in the past would have been mislabeled as unexplained abdominal pain or bleeding are readily recognized today because pregnancy tests have become very sensitive.

Most ectopic pregnancies (96 percent) are tubal. The remainder are interstitial uterine ectopic pregnancies and, rarely, cervical, abdominal, or ovarian pregnancies.[160] Most tubal pregnancies are located in the distal (ampullary) two thirds of the tube. A few ectopic pregnancies are isthmic, located in the proximal portion of the extrauterine part of the tube.

Signs and Symptoms

Abdominal pain and irregular vaginal bleeding are the most common presenting symptoms in ectopic pregnancy.[161,162] In an older report of 328 patients presenting with ectopic pregnancy, 94 percent had pain, 89 percent had a missed menstrual period, 80 percent had vaginal bleeding, and 20 percent had hypotension.[163] An abdominal mass is palpable in only one half of patients with an ectopic pregnancy. Of course, passage of a decidual cast in association with vaginal bleeding nearly unequivocally indicates ectopic pregnancy, but this is uncommon. The Arias-Stella phenomenon is frequently found in the endometrium in association with ectopic pregnancies; however, this phenomenon is also seen in 70 to 80 percent of therapeutic and spontaneous abortions,[164] so it is not specific for ectopic gestation.

Ectopic pregnancies should be diagnosed before the onset of hypotension, bleeding, pain, and overt rupture. Patients with a history of tubal surgery, pelvic inflammatory disease, tubal disease, or previous ectopic pregnancy are at special risk for ectopic pregnancy and would benefit not only from their physicians' vigilance but also from routine hormone screening of the type discussed below. *Early* diagnosis of ectopic gestation is now quite feasible, by 6 weeks' gestation and often as early as at 4 $1/2$ gestational weeks.

Chronic ectopic pregnancy is a distinct entity. Diagnosis may be difficult because normal anatomic landmarks are distorted by the formation of adhesions resulting from chronic inflammatory processes. Chronic ectopic pregnancies present a management quandary because the significance of the associated declining β-hCG levels is difficult to determine. The dilemma is whether resolution will occur spontaneously or require surgical intervention to prevent catastrophic hemorrhage and permanent adhesion formation resulting in tubal damage.

Diagnosis

Direct vision by laparoscopy has been the diagnostic standard for ectopic pregnancy. However, if the pregnancy is early and the gestational sac small, the gestation may not be visualized. Thus, algorithms incorporating a single measurement of serum progesterone, serial measurement of the β-subunit of hCG, pelvic ultrasonography, and uterine curettage are accepted.[164] Figure 17–3 shows a useful approach.

Single Measurement of Serum Progesterone

Ectopic pregnancy can be excluded and viable intrauterine pregnancy diagnosed with at least 98 percent sensitivity if serum progesterone levels are 25 ng/ml ($\geq$79.5 nmol/L) or higher, obviating the need for further testing. Conversely, serum progesterone can identify nonviable pregnancies with 100 percent sensitivity if progesterone levels are 5 ng/ml ($\leq$15.9 nmol/L) or lower.[165–168] If a single progesterone level is 5 ng/ml or lower, diagnostic uterine evacuation

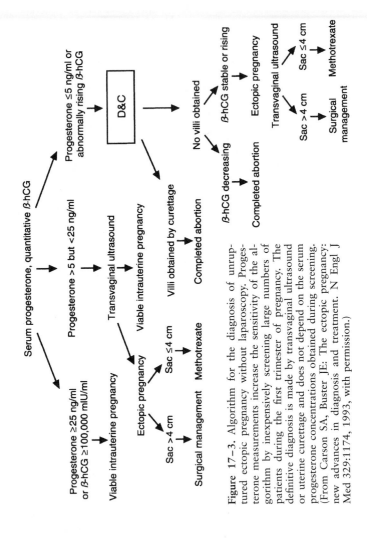

Figure 17-3. Algorithm for the diagnosis of unruptured ectopic pregnancy without laparoscopy. Progesterone measurements increase the sensitivity of the algorithm by inexpensively screening large numbers of patients during the first trimester of pregnancy. The definitive diagnosis is made by transvaginal ultrasound or uterine curettage and does not depend on the serum progesterone concentrations obtained during screening. (From Carson SA, Buster JE: The ectopic pregnancy: new advances in diagnosis and treatment. N Engl J Med 329:1174, 1993, with permission.)

can be performed even if ectopic pregnancy cannot otherwise be distinguished from a spontaneous intrauterine abortion. Progesterone values above 5 but below 25 ng/ml necessitate establishing viability by ultrasonography.

Serial Serum β-hCG Measurements

Produced by trophoblastic cells, β-hCG concentration increases 67 percent over a 2-day interval in normal pregnancies.[169] Abnormal intrauterine or ectopic pregnancies have impaired β-hCG production and, hence, a prolonged hCG doubling time. Thus, serial β-hCG measurements can be used to assess the viability of pregnancy, signal the optimal time for ultrasonography, and document the effectiveness of diagnostic curettage.

Transvaginal Ultrasound

If β-hCG is greater than 1,500 mIU/ml and the pregnancy is intrauterine, a gestational sac should be visualized by transvaginal ultrasound. By transabdominal ultrasound the gestational sac may not be identified until β-hCG reaches 6,000 mIU/ml. If β-hCG is greater than these levels but the gestational sac cannot be visualized, an ectopic location should be assumed.

Uterine Curettage

Villi float in saline, a characteristic permitting identification of tissue obtained by curettage. If no villi are recognized and a decrease in the β-hCG level of 15 percent or more 8 to 12 hours occurs after curettage, a completed abortion can be assumed to exist. If villi are not visualized and β-hCG titers plateau or rise, trophoblasts can be assumed *not* to have been removed by the uterine curettage; thus, an ectopic pregnancy can be presumed to be present.

Surgical Treatment

Salpingectomy by laparotomy has long offered almost a 100 percent cure. However, current emphasis is not just to prevent death but also to facilitate rapid recovery, preserve fertility, and reduce costs. Laparoscopic salpingostomy and partial salpingectomy are thus rapidly replacing laparotomy. Laparotomy should be performed only when a laparoscopic approach is too difficult, the surgeon is not trained in operative laparoscopy, or the patient is hemodynamically unstable.

Linear salpingostomy is the standard laparoscopic operation when an ectopic mass is unruptured yet more than 4 cm in length by ultrasound.[165,171–175] Over the bulging antimesenteric border of the implantation site, a longitudinal incision is made by electrocautery, scissors, or laser. The products of conception are removed by forceps or suction. After hemostasis is achieved, the incision is allowed to heal by secondary intention. Alternatively, sutures can be placed. Approximately 95 percent of laparoscopic salpingostomies are successful (i.e., no additional procedures are needed).[165] Of the 93 women evaluated in one study, 86 percent were later shown to have patent oviducts; 66 percent of 430 women who were followed subsequently became pregnant, with 23 percent of those pregnancies being ectopic.[176]

If segmental resection is necessary, subsequent laparotomy is then required for reanastomosis of the surgically divided oviduct. Laparoscopic salpingectomy is also desirable for patients who do not wish to become pregnant again.

Postoperative bleeding, elevated β-hCG levels indicative of persistent viable trophoblastic tissue, and other symptoms occur in up to 20 percent of cases after conservative laparoscopic surgery. Excision of the involved oviduct or medical therapy may then be necessary.

Medical Treatment

Although operative laparoscopy has substantially fewer complications than laparotomy, there remains irreducible morbidity intrinsic to surgery and anesthesia. Medical treatments can greatly reduce this morbidity. To supplant surgery, however, medical therapies must match the high success rates, low complication rates, and good reproductive potential achieved with laparoscopic operations. This appears to be true.[165,177] The agent used is the folic acid antagonist methotrexate, which inhibits synthesis of purines and pyrimidines and thus interferes with DNA synthesis and cell multiplication.

Hemodynamically stable patients with ectopic pregnancies are eligible for treatment with methotrexate if the mass is unruptured and measures 4 cm or less in diameter by ultrasound.[165] Patients with larger ectopic masses, embryonic cardiac activity, or evidence of acute intra-abdominal bleeding (acute abdomen, hypotension, or falling hematocrit) are not eligible for methotrexate therapy.[165] Outcome of treatment with systemic methotrexate.[165,178] favorably with that of laparoscopic salpingostomy; 94 percent of women successfully treated with systemic methotrexate needed no subsequent therapy. Of women tested, 81 percent had patent oviducts; 71 percent subsequently became pregnant, with 11 percent of those being ectopic.

High doses of methotrexate can cause bone marrow suppression, acute and chronic hepatotoxicity, stomatitis, pulmonary fibrosis, alopecia, and photosensitivity. Fortunately, these side effects are not only infrequent but can be mitigated against by the administration of leucovorin (citrovorum factor).

Safeguards are necessary to enhance the success and minimize the toxicity of systemic methotrexate. First, the patient should undergo a pelvic examination by only a single examiner and then infrequently. Self-control concerning this part of management should be similar to that employed with placenta previa. Second, both physician and patient must recognize that transient pain is common, usually occurring 3 to 7 days after initiation of methotrexate therapy. The pain, presumably caused by tubal abortion, normally lasts 4 to 12 hours. Perhaps the most difficult aspect of methotrexate therapy is distinguishing the transient abdominal pain associated with successful therapy from that of rupturing ectopic pregnancy. Surgical intervention becomes necessary only when pain is accompanied by orthostatic tachycardia, hypotension, or a falling hematocrit. If uncertainty exists concerning the patient's hemodynamic stability, physicians may prefer to hospitalize the patient with pain for observation. Because colicky abdominal pain is common during the first 2 or 3 days of methotrexate therapy, patients should also be warned to avoid gas-producing foods such as leeks and cabbage. Patients should also avoid exposure to the sun because of the photosensitivity methotrexate produces.

Finally, few medical advances evolve without negative consequences. As ectopic pregnancy is detected earlier and more efficiently, some pregnancies that would otherwise have been spontaneously absorbed are now treated, in retrospect, needlessly. Identifying early ectopic pregnancies that are destined for spontaneous remission would thus be useful, although efforts to do so have so far been unsuccessful. "Overtreatment" of ectopic pregnancy will thus be the inevitable corollary of early intervention.

Relative Benefits of Surgical Versus Medical Therapy

Conservative laparoscopic surgery is very efficacious, as is systemic methotrexate therapy. Systemic methotrexate therapy is less expensive than operative laparoscopy, and patients lose less time from work. On the other hand, some patients prefer surgical therapy because they wish to avoid the possible side effects of systemic chemotherapy and a more protracted counsel of treatment. However, even after laparoscopic removal of ectopic tissue, residual tissue remains to cause hemorrhage and other complications in 20 percent of cases. With either surgical or medical treatment, weekly blood tests are necessary until β-hCG becomes undetectable.

In conclusion, we recommend systemic methotrexate when laparoscopy is not required for diagnosis. Laparoscopic surgery is also preferable when the ectopic mass is larger than 4.0 cm. A laparotomy is performed only for catastrophic hemorrhage or hemodynamic instability.

RECOMMENDED EVALUATION FOR RECURRENT PREGNANCY LOSSES

1. Couples experiencing only one first-trimester abortion should receive pertinent information, but not necessarily be evaluated formally. Mention the relatively high (10 to 15 percent) pregnancy loss rate in the general population and the beneficial effects of abortion in eliminating abnormal conceptuses. Provide the relevant recurrence risks, usually 20 to 25 percent subsequent loss in the presence of a prior liveborn and somewhat higher in the absence of a prior liveborn. Risks are higher for older women. If a specific medical illness exists, treatment is obviously necessary. Intrauterine adhesions should be lysed. Otherwise, no further evaluation need be undertaken, even if uterine anomalies or leiomyomas are detected. On the other hand, occurrence of an anomalous stillborn or liveborn warrants genetic evaluation irrespective of the number of pregnancy losses.

2. Investigation may or may not be necessary after two spontaneous abortions, but after three spontaneous abortions, evaluation is usually indicated. One should then (a) obtain a detailed family history, (b) perform a complete physical examination, (c) discuss recurrence risks, and (d) order the selected tests cited below.

3. Parental chromosomal studies should be performed on all couples having repetitive losses. Antenatal chromosomal studies should be offered if a balanced chromosomal rearrangement is detected in either parent or if autosomal trisomy occurred in any previous abortus.

4. Detection of a trisomic abortus suggests the phenomenon of recurrent aneuploidy, justifying prenatal cytogenetic studies in future pregnancies. Performing prenatal cytogenetic studies solely on the basis of repeated losses is more arguable, but not unreasonable among women aged 30 to 34 years.

5. The validity of LPD as a discrete entity seems arguable.

6. Other endocrine causes for repeated fetal losses include poorly controlled diabetes mellitus (hyperglycemia) and possibly thyroid dysfunction.

7. To determine the role of infectious agents, the endometrium may be cultured for *Ureaplasma urealyticum* or a couple treated empirically with doxycycline (100 mg two times per day for 10 days) before pregnancy. Of other infections agents, only *Chlamydia trachomatis* seems plausible. Other agents are more likely to cause sporadic than repetitive losses.

8. If a müllerian fusion defect (septate or bicornuate uterus) is detected in a woman experiencing one or more second-trimester spontaneous abortions, surgical correction may be warranted. However, the same statements do not necessarily apply following *first*-trimester losses. Cervical incompetence should be managed by surgical cerclage during the next pregnancy.

9. To exclude autoimmune disease involving antiphospholipid antibodies, assessment should include aPL and aCL. Women with antibodies who experience midtrimester losses may benefit from treatment with heparin and aspirin, but the same does not necessarily hold when these antibodies are detected in asymptomatic women having first-trimester pregnancy losses. This recommendation also holds for women undergoing assisted reproductive technologies (ART). Testing for other autoantibodies (e.g., DNA) is not indicated.

10. There is some deleterious effect of HLA sharing (HLA-B), but determining parental HLA types in the absence of other immunologic testing is not recommended. Immunotherapy (by inoculation of the mother with her husband's leukocytes) has been unequivocally shown to be ineffective.

11. One should discourage exposure to cigarettes and alcohol, yet remain cautious in ascribing cause and effect in individual cases. Similar counsel should apply for exposures to other potential toxins.

Key Points

➤ Approximately 22 percent of all pregnancies detected on the basis of urinary hCG assays are lost, usually before clinical recognition.

➤ The clinical loss rate is 10 to 12 percent. Most of these pregnancies are lost before 8 weeks' gestation. Only 3 percent of pregnancies are lost after an ultrasonographically viable pregnancy at 8 to 9 weeks, and only 1 percent are lost after 16 weeks' gestation.

➤ Pregnancy losses may be recurrent. Although increasing after one loss, the recurrence risk generally reaches no more than 25 percent after three or four losses. Loss rates for 40-year-old women are approximately twice that of 20-year-old women.

Box continued on following page

Key Points *Continued*

➤ The most common causes of pregnancy losses are chromosomal abnormalities. At least 50 percent of clinically recognized pregnancy losses show a chromosomal abnormality. The types of chromosomal abnormalities differ from those found in liveborns, but autosomal trisomy still accounts for 50 percent of abnormalities. A balanced translocation is present in about 5 percent of couples having repeated spontaneous abortions.

➤ Many nongenetic causes of repetitive abortions have been proposed, but few are proved. It is reasonable to evaluate couples for these conditions, but efficacy of treatment remains uncertain and relatively few pregnancy losses are caused by these factors.

➤ Uterine anomalies are accepted causes of second-trimester pregnancies. Couples experiencing such losses may benefit from metroplasty or hysteroscopic resection of a uterine septum. Uterine anomalies are less common causes of first-trimester losses.

➤ Drugs, toxins, and physical agents are associated with spontaneous abortion, but usually not in repetitive pregnancies. Avoiding potential toxins is obviously desirable, but one should not assume that such exposures explain repetitive losses.

➤ LAC antibodies, aPL, and aCL are clearly associated with second-trimester losses, but their role in first-trimester losses is more arguable.

➤ Over recent years management of ectopic pregnancy is less commonly an acute emergency and more easily diagnosed early in gestation on the basis of maternal serum progesterone, maternal b-hCG, transvaginal ultrasound, and uterine curettage. The earlier detection of an unruptured ectopic pregnancy has greatly modified treatment. Laparotomy is now rarely necessary. Laparoscopic procedures (linear salpingostomy) are commonly used, with an increase in subsequent pregnancy rates and a decrease in repeat ectopic gestations. About one third of women with ectopic pregnancies prove eligible for medical treatment (methotrexate). Patients at high risk for ectopic pregnancy may benefit from a screening serum progesterone determination at the time of initial pregnancy test.

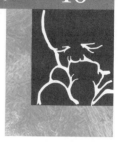

Chapter 18

Preterm Birth

JAY D. IAMS

Premature birth counts for the majority of perinatal mortality and morbidity in nonanomalous infants. In the United States, prematurity-related disorders cause more than 70 percent of fetal and neonatal deaths.[1] Long-term sequelae of prematurity disproportionately contribute to developmental delay, visual and hearing impairment, chronic lung disease, and cerebral palsy.[2]

Advances in neonatal care have led to increased survival and reduced short- and long-term morbidity for infants born before 37 weeks of pregnancy, but the rate of low-birth-weight deliveries actually increased between 1989 and 1997[3]. In 1997, 11.4 percent of births occurred before 37 weeks. An important trend is the increased number and rate of preterm births among multiple gestations. In the United States, the rate of preterm birth in 1997 was 10.0 percent for singletons, 54.9 percent for twins, and 93.6 percent for higher order multiples.[3]

Efforts to identify and treat the conditions leading to prematurity have been largely disappointing, fulfilling the prophetic words of Nicholson Eastman in 1947: "Only when the factors underlying prematurity are completely understood can any intelligent attempt at prevention be made."[6]

THE PROBLEM OF PREMATURITY

Definitions

- *Preterm or premature:* Infants born before 37 weeks' gestation (259 days from the first day of the mother's last menstrual period, or 245 days after conception).
- *Low birth weight (LBW):* Infants who weigh less than 2,500 g at birth, regardless of gestational age.
- *Very low birth weight (VLBW):* Infants who weigh less than 1,500 g at birth.
- *Extremely low birth weight (ELBW):* Infants who weigh less than 1,000 g at birth

453

Because gestational age and birth weight are directly correlated throughout most of gestation, birth weight has been used as an indirect indicator of gestational age in many studies, especially when gestational age is determined retrospectively. Interchanging the two measures may lead to erroneous interpretation of clinical and epidemiologic data because the problems of LBW infants may be the result of prematurity in some instances, of poor intrauterine growth in others, and of both in still others. Similarly, problems due to prematurity in preterm infants whose birth weight exceeds 2,500 g may go unrecognized because of their apparently "full-term" appearance.

The incidences of LBW and VLBW deliveries have changed little since 1970.[3] The LBW rate was 6.00 percent of liveborn infants in 1989, 5.93 percent in 1992, and 6.08 percent in 1997. The rate of VLBW (<1,500 g) was 1.15 percent in 1980 and increased slowly to 1.42 percent in 1997. Rates of LBW and VLBW newborns in blacks are consistently about twice as high as corresponding rates in nonblacks. Even when corrected for age and educational level, black women continue to deliver more LBW infants than do white women.

Perinatal Mortality and Morbidity

Analysis of perinatal mortality and morbidity statistics has long been confounded by the various definitions of fetal, perinatal, neonatal, and infant time periods that have been used across the United States and around the world. The definitions endorsed by the American College of Obstetricians and Gynecologists (ACOG) are used here[8] (see Chapter 7).

Significant improvements in survival rates for all preterm infants have been documented for the past 40 years, and have been especially important for infants born before 28 weeks. Data from 1982 to 1986, before the introduction of neonatal artificial surfactant, show survival rates of only 1.8 percent at 23 weeks', 9.9 percent at 24 weeks', 15.5 percent at 25 weeks', and 54.7 percent at 26 weeks' gestation.[9] After the introduction of neonatal surfactant therapy, recent data show survival to hospital discharge rates of greater than 20 percent for infants born at 23 weeks', 50 percent at 24 weeks', 60 percent at 25 weeks', and 80 percent at 26 weeks' gestation for infants born in 1993 to 1994[10] (Fig. 18–1).

The survival rates cited in these studies come from tertiary perinatal care centers, and do not necessarily reflect the experience in the general population.

Despite marked improvements in neonatal survival, the United States compares relatively unfavorably with other developed countries with respect to neonatal mortality. However, a study[21] of linked birth and perinatal death records from Norwegian and

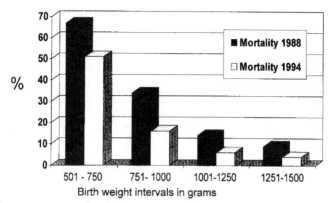

Figure 18–1. Mortality for very low birth weight infants born in 1988 and 1994 in the NICHD NICU Network. (Data from Stevenson DK, Wright LL, Lemons JA, et al: Very low birth weight outcomes of the National Institute of Child Health and Human Development Neonatal Research Network, January 1993 through December 1994. Am J Obstet Gynecol 179:1632, 1998.)

American births found that the higher rate of perinatal death in the United States is due almost entirely to a small excess of preterm births in the United States (2.9 percent) versus Norway (2.1 percent). The authors noted that a reduction in preterm delivery in the United States to the rate observed in Norway would produce the same perinatal mortality rate in both countries. They concluded that prevention of perinatal mortality in the United States depends more on prevention of prematurity, especially extreme prematurity, than of low birth weight.

Common complications in premature infants include respiratory distress syndrome (RDS); intraventricular hemorrhage (IVH); bronchopulmonary dysplasia (BPD); patent ductus arteriosus (PDA); necrotizing enterocolitis (NEC); and sepsis, apnea, and retinopathy of prematurity (ROP). Extremely preterm infants are at greatest risk.

The proportion of survivors within each birth weight group who have serious handicaps has not increased since the introduction of neonatal intensive care.

Long-term outcomes for infants with birth weights below 1,000 g have been reported as these children have reached adolescence (Fig. 18–2). A 1994 study of school-age outcomes found higher rates of cerebral palsy, severe visual impairment, and reduced head size and height for children with birth weights under 750 g when compared with children with birth weights 750 to 1,499 g and children born

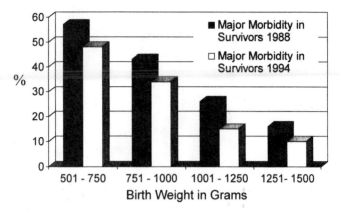

Figure 18–2. Major morbidity among survivors for very low birth weight infants born in 1988 and 1994 in the NICHD NICU Network. (Data from Stevenson DK, Wright LL, Lemons JA, et al: Very low birth weight outcomes of the National Institute of Child Health and Human Development Neonatal Research Network, January 1993 through December 1994. Am J Obstet Gynecol 179:1632, 1998.)

at term.[2] Abnormal cognitive, academic, visual motor, gross motor, and adaptive performance was also more frequent among children with birth weights below 750 g (Fig. 18–3).

The relationship between prematurity and long-term morbidity is apparently more complex than can be explained only by immature organ systems. Recent clinical and pathologic studies have linked chorioamnionitis to neonatal morbidities other than neonatal infections, especially including cerebral palsy and bronchopulmonary dysplasia.[29–39]

In addition to prolonged hospitalization at birth, many VLBW infants are rehospitalized during the first year of life.[40] Sudden infant death syndrome is also more frequent among prematurely born infants.

OVERVIEW OF THE PATHOGENESIS OF PREMATURITY

The Epidemiology of Preterm Birth

The list of maternal and fetal diagnoses antecedent to preterm deliveries is both long and diverse. Preterm labor, preterm ruptured membranes, preeclampsia, abruptio placentae, multiple gestation, placenta previa, fetal growth restriction, excessive or inadequate

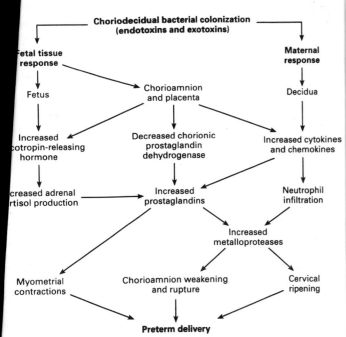

Figure 18–4. Potential pathways from choriodecidual bacterial colonization
to preterm delivery. (From Goldenberg RL, Hauth JC, Andrews WW:
Intrauterine infection and preterm delivery. N Engl J Med 342:1500, 2000,
with permission.)

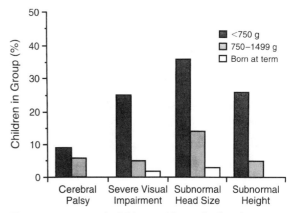

Figure 18–3. Percentage of children with cerebral palsy, severe visual impairment, subnormal head size, and subnormal height in infants born less than 750 g birth weight, 750 to 1499 g birth weight, and at term. (From Hack M, Taylor HG, Klein N, et al: School-age outcomes in children with birth weights under 750 g. N Engl J Med 331:756, 1994, with permission.)

preterm birth in both singleton[99] and multiple gestations.[100] The shorter the cervical length at 18 to 28 weeks' gestation, the greater the risk of spontaneous prematurity[99,101,102] (Fig. 18–5). This relationship has been observed throughout the entire range of cervical length, not only for cervical length below the 10th percentile (Fig. 18–6). Cervical length is strongly related to a history of spontaneous preterm birth, especially before 32 weeks' gestation.[60] Cervical length is also related to the risk of recurrent preterm birth.[61,103]

The correlation between cervical length and preterm birth risk may be explained by the physical strength or resistance of the cervix to factors such as intrauterine weight or volume, biochemical influences arising from infectious or other inflammatory stimuli,[71,105,106] or biophysical effects of uterine activity. Whatever the explanation, these investigations indicate that cervical length is a marker for cervical competence, and that cervical competence operates as a continuum. These data contradict the previous understanding of the

amniotic fluid volume, fetal anomalies amnionitis, and incompetent cervix. Maternal medical problems such as diabetes mellitus, asthma, drug abuse, and pyelonephritis may all lead to preterm delivery. Maternal characteristics associated with preterm delivery are equally numerous: maternal race (black greater than nonblack), a history of previous preterm birth, low socioeconomic status, poor nutrition, low prepregnancy weight, absent or inadequate prenatal care, age less than 18 or over 40, strenuous work, high personal stress, anemia, cigarette smoking, bacteriuria, genital colonization or infection (e.g., bacterial vaginosis, *Neisseria gonorrhoeae, Chlamydia trachomatis, Mycoplasma,* and *Ureaplasma*), cervical injury or abnormality (e.g., in utero exposure to diethylstilbestrol, a history of cervical conization, or second-trimester induced abortion), uterine anomaly or fibroids, excessive uterine contractility, and premature cervical dilation of more than 1 cm or effacement greater than 80 percent. The list of risk factors is so long that it is hard to see any common thread.

Approximately 75 percent of preterm births occur "spontaneously" after preterm labor (PTL), preterm premature rupture of membranes (preterm PROM), or related diagnoses such as amnionitis and incompetent cervix (PROM refers to rupture of membranes before the onset of labor at any gestational age, hence the apparently redundant "preterm PROM"). Complications of PTL and preterm PROM may lead to an "indication" for delivery (e.g., intrauterine infection), but these births are nevertheless termed "spontaneous" because they follow spontaneous preterm labor or preterm PROM. Risk factors for PTL and preterm PROM are similar, with a few exceptions. Women with preterm PROM are more likely to be indigent,[41] to smoke,[45] and to have experienced bleeding in the current pregnancy[46] than are women who present with preterm labor.

Indicated preterm births follow medical or obstetric disorders that place the fetus at risk (e.g., acute or chronic maternal hypertension, diabetes mellitus, placenta previa or abruption, and intrauterine growth restriction). Indicated preterm births account for 20 to 30 percent of births before 37 weeks in most series.[42,43]

Fetal stress may initiate preterm labor by uteroplacental production of corticotropin-releasing hormone (CRH), a peptide produced by the placenta, amniochorion, and decidua and known to enhance prostanoid production in these same cells.[54] These reports provide a biologically plausible mechanism by which abnormalities of the placenta and uteroplacental blood flow may lead to spontaneous preterm birth, either directly, through decidual and/or membrane injury, or indirectly by inducing fetal stress.

The Epidemiology and Pathogenesis of Spontaneous Preterm Birth

Whether preterm parturition is just normal labor that is initiated too soon, or follows a distinctly different pathway until the final stages of labor, has been the subject of great debate. Increasingly, the evidence favors the latter interpretation, with several pathologic processes capable of initiating the process.

The epidemiology of preterm birth reveals several major trends. The first is that early preterm birth (<32 weeks) and late preterm birth (>32 weeks) have a different epidemiology. Another is that some risk factors are associated with recurrent preterm birth, while others appear to be unique to the affected pregnancy.[44] Early preterm birth is more likely to recur, is more strongly associated with a short cervix and the presence of fetal fibronectin in cervicovaginal secretions, and is more often accompanied by clinical or subclinical evidence of infection and by long-term morbidity for the infant.[44] Later preterm birth is more likely to be associated with increased uterine contraction frequency and with a rise in maternal excretion of estriol (an indicator of increasing maturation of the fetal hypothalamic-pituitary-adrenal axis), and thus to mimic normal labor at term.[55]

Risk factors for nonrecurrent spontaneous preterm birth include second-trimester bleeding, abnormal amniotic fluid volume, multiple gestation, substance abuse, and trauma.

The risk of spontaneous preterm birth is increased by a history of prior preterm delivery. The recurrence risk rises as the number

of prior preterm births increases.[64] The biolog_ sistently related to recurrent spontaneous pre_ length when measured by transvaginal son_ reports suggest that cervical function is at l_ stitutional factor that influences preterm birt_ pregnancies.

The Preterm Prediction Study[44] revealed tha_ between preterm birth, black race, and bacter_ were mediated by fetal fibronectin. The relation_ birth before 32 weeks and bacterial vaginosis w_ in black women, where the population-attributabl_ 40 percent for births before 32 weeks. In contr_ women, a low body mass index (<19.8 kg/m^2) h_ association with early preterm birth.[44]

Infection and Prematurity

The association between preterm birth and infec_ reported for more than 50 years.[73,74] Numerous m_ including Ureaplasma urealyticum, Mycoplasma spec_ trachomatis, Trichomonas, Escherichia coli, group B _ and especially anaerobes such as Fusobacterium, _ anaerobic streptococci, and Mobiluncus, have been re_ the lower and upper genital tract and amniotic flui_ with preterm labor and preterm ruptured membranes.[7_

The strength of the association between both clini_ and histologic amnionitis increases as the gestational age_ decreases, especially before 30 to 32 weeks. Positive am_ cultures have been reported in 20 to 30 percent of w_ preterm labor, especially before 30 weeks' gestation and _ labor is refractory to tocolytic drugs.[75-77,83]

Infections outside the genital tract have also been _ preterm birth, most commonly urinary tract and intra-a_ infections (e.g., pyelonephritis and appendicitis). Recently, _ periodontal infections have been associated with increase_ spontaneous preterm birth.[85]

The relationship between infection and prematurity is mo_ plex than can be explained by the ascent of organisms fr_ lower to the upper genital tract during pregnancy. Recent r_ has examined the roles played by host defense, including the_ and the maternal and fetal immune response, in the occurre_ preterm birth. The pathways by which intrauterine infection_ lead to spontaneous preterm birth are indicated in Figure 18_

Cervical Length

The length of the uterine cervix as measured by transvaginal u_ sonography is inversely and continuously related to the risk

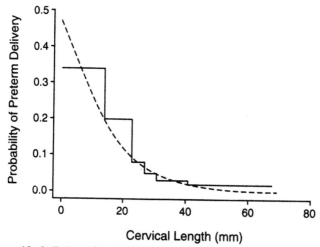

Figure 18-5. Estimated probability of spontaneous preterm delivery before 35 weeks' gestation from the logistic regression analysis *(dashed line)* and observed frequency of spontaneous preterm delivery *(solid line)* according to cervical length measured by transvaginal ultrasonography at 24 weeks. (From Iams JD, Goldenberg RL, Meis PJ, et al: The length of the cervix and the risk of spontaneous premature delivery. N Engl J Med 334:567, 1996, with permission.)

cervix as a categorical rather than a continuous variable (i.e., either competent or incompetent). If the cervix has degrees of "competence," then cervical incompetence is simply the lowermost end of a spectrum.[60] That cervical length is related to gestational age at delivery in both previous and future pregnancies indicates that cervical length is an independent risk factor for prematurity.[104]

Fibronectin

Fibronectin is an extracellular matrix protein that is best described as the "glue" that attaches the fetal membranes to the underlying uterine decidua.[107] Fibronectin is normally found in the cervicovaginal secretions before 20 to 22 weeks of pregnancy, and again at the end of normal pregnancy as labor approaches. It is not normally present in cervicovaginal secretions between 22 and 37 weeks. The presence of fibronectin in cervicovaginal secretions after 22 weeks is a marker of disruption of the decidual–chorionic interface. In the NICHD Preterm Prediction Study, multivariate analysis revealed that the strongest predictors of spontaneous preterm birth (SPTB) were cervicovaginal fibronectin,[108] transvaginal sonographic cervical

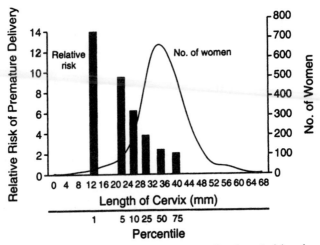

Figure 18-6. Distribution of subjects by percentile of cervical length measured by transvaginal sonography at 24 weeks *(solid line)* and relative risk of spontaneous preterm birth before 35 weeks according to percentiles of cervical length *(bars)*. Relative risk of spontaneous preterm delivery for women at the 1st, 5th, 10th, 25th, 50th, and 75th percentiles are compared with the risks among women with cervical lengths above the 75th percentile. (From Iams JD, Goldenberg RL, Meis PJ, et al: The length of the cervix and the risk of spontaneous premature delivery. N Engl J Med 334:567, 1996, with permission.)

length,[99] an obstetric history of previous preterm birth,[109] and presence of BV,[91] respectively.

The Spontaneous Preterm Birth Syndrome

When information about fibronectin, cervical length, maternal infection, and second-trimester amniotic fluid cytokines are considered together with data about intrauterine infection and neonatal morbidity, a model of early preterm birth as an indolent rather than acute process emerges.[119] Romero et al. have termed this the "preterm labor syndrome".[120] In response to a chronic intrauterine inflammatory insult (usually infectious or ischemic), and influenced by both the maternal and fetal immune response,[30] the fetal membranes and decidua produce cytokines (tumor necrosis factor-α [TNF-α], IL-1, and IL-6). This cytokine-mediated process ultimately leads to one or more of the following: (1) continued leakage of fetal fibronectin from the decidua–membrane interface, (2) elaboration of uterotonic bioactive lipids (prostaglandin E_2 [PGE$_2$], prostaglandin $F_{2\alpha}$ [PGF$_{2\alpha}$], thromboxane A_2, leukotrienes B_4 and C_4,[121] hydroperoxyeicosatetraenoic acid [5-HETE] and others) that (3) stimulate myometrial contractions and (4) initiate release of proteases that are capable of injuring the membranes and underlying decidua that (5) incites prostaglandin stimulation that results in (6) cervical ripening, dilation, and/or membrane rupture, and (7) in utero injury to the fetal brain, lung, or gut.

In this model, most women with microorganisms in the lower or upper tract or other sources of inflammation experience neither preterm birth nor neonatal morbidity. That some do while most do not may be attributed to differences in behavioral (physical or sexual activity, smoking) and/or genetic (e.g., cervical length, immune response) factors or both.

Other potential initiators of the process may include premature activation of the maternal–fetal hypothalamic- pituitary axis and/or pathologic uterine distention[122] both of which are more likely to cause later preterm births and less likely to cause major neonatal neurologic morbidity.

PREVENTION AND TREATMENT OF PRETERM BIRTH

Prevention and treatment strategies for prematurity may be described according to the public health concepts of primary, secondary, and tertiary care.[119,123] *Primary* care or prevention is the elimination or reduction of risk in an entire population. Effective primary care requires a good understanding of the pathophysiology of the disease, and public health educational efforts to modify behaviors and eliminate risk factors. For preterm birth, the target population is clear (preteens and women of childbearing age), but effective primary interventions have not been demonstrated. A primary program to reduce the incidence of prematurity might include efforts to prevent smoking and sexually transmitted diseases, to avoid unplanned pregnancies through use of birth control, to plan pregnancy to reduce stress and improve nutrition, to avoid higher order multifetal gestation, and to foster employment policies that promote the needs of pregnancy over the workplace.[124,125] *Secondary* care selects individuals with increased risk for surveillance and/or prophylactic treatment. Effective secondary care requires both accurate screening tests and effective interventions to prevent or reduce risk. Examples of secondary care for preterm birth are screening for preterm birth risk, early diagnosis and patient education programs, prophylactic medications (e.g., tocolytic drugs, progesterone supplementation, or antibiotics) and lifestyle changes such as reduced physical or sexual activity. Unfortunately, none of these has led to a decline in prematurity.[126] *Tertiary* care is treatment of an individual patient after an index illness has occurred. Tertiary care has no effect on the incidence of the disease, but rather is aimed at reducing morbidity and mortality after the diagnosis has been made. For preterm birth, tertiary care includes prompt and accurate diagnosis, referral to an appropriate care site, and specific treatment (e.g., tocolytic drugs to arrest preterm labor, antibiotics for group B β-hemolytic streptococcal sepsis prophylaxis or amnionitis, and corticosteroids to reduce neonatal mortality and morbidity).

Clinical Risk Factors for Preterm Birth

Because clinical risk factors for spontaneous preterm birth have relatively high prevalence but low sensitivity and positive predictive value, efforts to create scoring systems to identify pregnancies at risk have faltered.[133–136] Nevertheless, women with these major risk factors should be considered to be at risk of preterm birth:

1. *Prior preterm delivery.*[63,109]
2. *Multiple gestation.*
3. *Low prepregnancy weight* manifested by a body mass index below 19.8 kg/m^2.[44,136,138]
4. *Vaginal bleeding in the second or third trimester*

These historical risk factors are easily elicited, but identify less than half of women who will deliver prematurely. Just as screening for preeclampsia is part of routine prenatal care, all pregnant women should receive care and education aimed at the problem of prematurity. Other possible risk factors that have been studied as screening tests for preterm birth risk include uterine contraction frequency, digital and ultrasound examination of the cervix, vaginal microbiology, serologic markers, and the presence of fetal fibronectin in cervicovaginal secretions.

Diagnosis and Treatment of Spontaneous Preterm Birth

Clinical management of preterm labor is based on a careful assessment of the risks for mother and infant of continuing the pregnancy versus delivery.

Diagnosis of Preterm Labor

The diagnosis of preterm labor is traditionally made when persistent uterine contractions are accompanied by dilation and/or effacement of the cervix detected by digital examination.[185] Symptoms of preterm labor are nonspecific and are not necessarily those of labor at term. Women treated for preterm labor report symptoms of pelvic pressure, increased vaginal discharge, backache, and menstrual-like cramps, all of which may occur in normal pregnancy. Contractions may be painful or painless, and are distinguished from the benign contractions of normal pregnancy (called Braxton-Hicks contractions) only by their persistence. Randomized trials of drugs to arrest preterm labor have found that approximately 40 percent of subjects treated with placebo will deliver at term.[186] Conversely, other studies have found rates of preterm birth of 20 percent in women who were sent home without treatment after evaluation for possible preterm labor.[187] Difficulty in accurate diagnosis is the product of the high prevalence of the symptoms and signs of early preterm labor among normal healthy women, and the imprecision of the digital examination of the cervix. Uterine contraction frequency varies considerably in normal pregnancy according to gestational age, time of day, and maternal activity[140]. Contraction frequency alone is therefore insufficient to establish the diagnosis of preterm labor. The practice of initiating tocolytic drugs for contraction frequency without additional diagnostic criteria results in unnecessary treatment of women who do not actually have preterm labor.[189] Overdiagnosis might be acceptable if treatment were clearly effective, but that is not the case. Although digital assessment of cervical dilation of 3 cm or more is straightforward, the reproducibility of digital examination when dilation is less than 3 cm and/or effacement is less than 80 percent is low.[190] Despite their imprecision, these symptoms and subtle changes in the cervix remain the basis of the early diagnosis of preterm labor.[185]

Among symptomatic women, the best clinical predictors of preterm delivery within 24 hours to 7 days include initial cervical dilation greater than 3 cm or effacement of 80 percent or more, vaginal bleeding, and ruptured membranes.[189,191,192] Surprisingly, contraction frequency of 4 or more per hour has low positive predictive value for preterm birth within 7 to 14 days of presentation.[193,194] For this reason, symptomatic women whose cervical dilation is less than 2 cm and/or whose effacement is less than 80 percent present a diagnostic challenge. Diagnostic accuracy may be improved in these patients with transvaginal sonographic measurement of cervical length,[195–200] and/or testing for fetal fibronectin in cervicovaginal fluid.[193,194,201] Cervical sonography is useful to exclude preterm labor in some patients, and may add sensitivity to the diagnosis in others. In a review of cervical sonography as a marker for preterm birth, a sonographic cervical length of 18 mm had the optimal positive predictive value, and 30 mm the optimal negative predictive value for the diagnosis of preterm labor in symptomatic women.[200] These studies were performed with transvaginal sonography. Transabdominal sonography has poor reproducibility for cervical measurement and should not be used clinically without confirmation by a transvaginal ultrasound[159,202]. (Fig. 18–7) Cervical sonography may also be useful to evaluate patients whose contractions are accompanied by vaginal bleeding of uncertain origin (Fig. 18–8).

As the gestational sac implants and attaches to decidua in the first half of pregnancy, fibronectin is normally present in cervicovaginal fluid. The presence of fibronectin in the cervix or vagina after the 22nd week is uncommon (<5 percent of pregnancies),[108] and indicates disruption of the attachment of the membranes to the decidua. Fibronectin commonly reappears in cervicovaginal secretions as labor approaches at term. A positive fibronectin test between 22 and 37 weeks is associated with an increased risk of preterm birth, especially in symptomatic women.[193,194,203] A positive test result in a patient with persistent contractions and cervical dilation of less than 3 cm has better sensitivity (90 percent) and positive predictive value for delivery less than 7 to 14 days than standard clinical markers, but the positive predictive value is just 18 percent in accumulated series, depending on the population studied (Table 18–1)[193,194,203–206] The clinical value of the test in symptomatic women is primarily its high negative predictive value, as a test to avoid overdiagnosis and unnecessary treatment, (e.g., similar to cardiac enzymes in the evaluation of chest pain).

The suggested protocol for evaluation and treatment of women with possible preterm labor in the box incorporates fibronectin into current clinical care patterns. An evaluation of the etiology of spontaneous preterm labor is essential before treatment is initiated. Transvaginal sonography can be used as an adjunctive test in patients with persistent contractions and cervical dilation of 2 cm or less. Because of variation introduced by maternal bladder filling, transabdominal sonography is not sufficiently reproducible to be useful.[202]

To summarize, the diagnosis of preterm labor is often uncertain, and as can be seen in the next section, the treatment is not always benign. In order to increase the sensitivity of diagnosis without treating unnecessarily, it is best to be *liberal* in looking

---

Figure 18–7. *A,* Transvaginal ultrasound image of the cervix at 28 weeks in a normal pregnancy. Calipers (+) are placed at the notches marking the internal and external os where the anterior and posterior walls of the cervical canal touch. *B,* Transvaginal ultrasound image of the cervix at 28 weeks in a patient with preterm labor. The (X) calipers mark the length of the cervical canal that is used for clinical evaluation. The (+) calipers are placed at the outer edges of the cervix; this length is not useful clinically because of wide variation among patients.

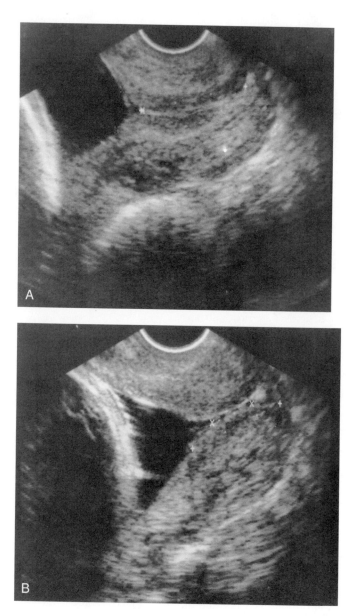

Figure 18-7. *See legend on opposite page*

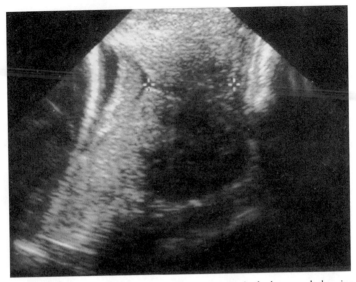

Figure 18–8. Midline sagittal image from transvaginal ultrasound showing a blood clot at the internal cervical os in a patient with contractions and vaginal bleeding.

for preterm labor, but *conservative* in diagnosis and treatment. The goal of first contact with a patient who may have preterm labor should be sensitivity, while the goal of evaluation in labor and delivery should be specificity. We recommend the following maxims:

1. Invite any patient complaining of possible symptoms of preterm labor to come in for contraction monitoring and cervical exam. Severity of symptoms bears little relation to their clinical significance.
2. Wait for cervical change of at least 1 cm in dilation, dilation of 2 cm or more, or a positive fibronectin before accepting the diagnosis of preterm labor in a patient with persistent contractions.
3. Use cervical sonography (cervix ≥30 mm) as a test to support continued observation.
4. Be wary of "incidental" diagnosis of preterm labor, especially in the afternoon and early evening. Remember the wide range of contraction frequency and the normal increase in contractions in the late afternoon and evening in normal pregnancy.

Clinical Evaluation of Patients with Possible Preterm Labor

1. Patient presents with signs/symptoms of preterm labor:
   - Persistent contractions (painful or painless)
   - Intermittent abdominal cramping, pelvic pressure, or backache
   - Increase or change in vaginal discharge
   - Vaginal spotting or bleeding
2. General physical examination:
   - Sitting pulse and blood pressure
   - Temperature
   - External fetal heart rate and contraction monitor
3. Sterile speculum examination
   - pH
   - Fern
   - Pooled fluid
   - Fibronectin swab (posterior fornix or external cervical os, avoiding areas with bleeding)
   - Cultures for *Chlamydia* (cervix), and *N. gonorrhoeae* (cervix), and group B *Streptococcus* (outer one third of vagina and perineum)
4. Transabdominal ultrasound examination:
   - Placental location
   - Amniotic fluid volume
   - Estimated fetal weight and presentation
   - Fetal well-being
5. Cervical examination (after ruptured membranes excluded):
   - Cervix ≥3 cm dilation / 80 percent effaced—Preterm labor diagnosis confirmed. Evaluate for tocolysis
   - Cervix 2 to 3 cm dilation and <80 percent effaced— Preterm labor likely but not established. Monitor contraction frequency and repeat digital examination in 30 to 60 minutes. Preterm labor diagnosis if cervical change. If not, send fibronectin or obtain transvaginal cervical ultrasound. Evaluate for tocolysis if any cervical change, cervical length <20 mm or positive fibronectin.
   - Cervix <2 cm dilation and <80 percent effaced— Preterm labor diagnosis uncertain. Monitor contraction frequency, send fibronectin and/or obtain cervical sonography, and repeat digital examination in 1 to 2 hours. Evaluate for tocolysis if there is a 1-cm change in cervical dilation, effacement >80 percent, cervical length <20 mm or positive fibronectin.

Box continued on following page

Clinical Evaluation of Patients with Possible Preterm Labor *Continued*

6. Use of Cervical Ultrasound:
   - Cervical length <20 mm and contraction criteria met = preterm labor
   - Cervical length 20 to 30 mm and contraction criteria met = probable preterm labor
   - Cervical length >30 mm = preterm labor very unlikely regardless of contraction frequency
7. Treatment of Symptomatic Fibronectin-Positive Patients:
   - Parenteral tocolysis
   - Steroids
   - Maternal transfer if appropriate
   - Group B *Streptococcus* prophylaxis
8. Care for Symptomatic Fibronectin-Negative Patients:
   - When tocolysis initiated before fibronectin returned (risk of delivery ≤7 days = 1.7 to 3.5 percent)
       Conclude course of tocolysis
       Reduce hospital stay
   - When tocolysis not initiated (risk of delivery ≤7 days = 0 to 1.8 percent)
       Observe in outpatient setting
   - Cervical sonography should be considered in these patients to assess risk of SPTD

Premature Birth and Assessment of Fetal Maturity

Amniotic fluid studies of fetal pulmonary maturity are important in two settings: (1) when dates are uncertain (e.g., fetal size larger

Table 18–1. SENSITIVITY OF TESTS TO PREDICT DELIVERY WITHIN 7 DAYS

Characteristic	Sensitivity
Fibronectin positive	90%
Cervix > 1 cm dilated	35%
Contractions > 4/hr	55%
Bleeding	40%

Combined data from Iams JD, Casal D, McGregor JA, et al: Fetal fibronectin improves the accuracy of diagnosis of preterm labor. Am J Obstet Gynecol 173:141, 1995; and Peaceman AM, Andrews WW, Thorp JM, et al: Fetal fibronectin as a predictor of preterm birth in patients with sumptoms: A multicenter trial. Am J Obstet Gynecol 177:13, 1997.

than expected for dates, suggesting a more advanced gestation or maternal glucose intolerance, or size less than expected, suggesting fetal growth restriction); and (2) when fetal jeopardy is not now present (prompt delivery would be indicated) but may occur during the remaining days or weeks of pregnancy (e.g., when membranes have ruptured, fetal heart patterns are nonreassuring, or growth restriction is suspected) (see Chapter 7). Occasionally, amniocentesis may be indicated for other studies such as fetal karyotype in patients with polyhydramnios, or culture, glucose, and Gram stain when amnionitis is suspected (see Chapter 25).

Treatment of Preterm Labor: Goals and Efficacy of Treatment

The ultimate goal for pregnancies complicated by preterm labor is delivery of an infant who suffers none of the sequelae of prematurity. Given the uncertain accuracy of the diagnosis, the treatment of women without true preterm labor in studies of tocolysis, and the relative infrequency of serious neonatal morbidity after 32 to 34 weeks, it has been difficult to demonstrate that treatment of preterm labor achieves this end point. Tocolytics do not prevent preterm birth but can delay delivery for at least 48 hours, an important interval during which effective antenatal interventions to reduce neonatal morbidity and mortality may be accomplished:

1. Antepartum transfer of the mother and fetus to the most appropriate hospital, especially when the estimated birth weight is expected to be less than 1,500 g.[214,215]
2. Antibiotic prophylaxis of neonatal group B streptococcal infection.[216]
3. Antepartum administration of corticosteroids to the mother to reduce the risk of death, respiratory distress syndrome, and intraventricular hemorrhage in the preterm neonate.[217]

A recent meta-analysis of the effect of acute treatment of preterm labor[213] evaluated the results of 16 randomized controlled trials that enrolled women with intact membranes and focused on three outcome measures: prolongation of pregnancy in days, gestational age at delivery, and birth weight. Studies of agents from each major class of tocolytic drugs (β-mimetics, calcium channel blockers, magnesium sulfate, and the nonsteroidal anti-inflammatory drugs [NSAIDs]) were combined in a meta-analysis suggesting that all four are associated with a decline in the occurrence of birth before 37 weeks.

Initial Evaluation of Preterm Labor

The initial evaluation of the patient in preterm labor is focused on the risks and benefits of continuing the pregnancy for both mother

---

Contraindications to Tocolysis

Maternal Contraindications to Tocolysis
- Significant hypertension (eclampsia, severe preeclampsia, chronic hypertension)
- Antepartum hemorrhage
- Cardiac disease
- Any medical or obstetric condition that contraindicates prolongation of pregnancy
- Hypersensitivity to a specific tocolytic agent

Fetal Contraindications to Tocolysis
- Gestational age <37 weeks
- Advanced dilation effacement
- Demise or lethal anomaly
- Chorioamnionitis
- In utero fetal compromise
    Acute: fetal distress
    Chronic: IUGR or substance abuse

---

and fetus. Common maternal contraindications to tocolysis include hypertension, bleeding, and cardiac disease (see the box "Contraindications to Tocolysis").

Potential causes of preterm labor should be sought in the initial evaluation and reassessed during the course of treatment. An underlying cause of preterm labor may be found that requires delivery (e.g., abruptio placentae or chorioamnionitis), that may affect the choice of tocolytic (e.g., a degenerating myoma often responds best to a prostaglandin synthetase inhibitor), or that requires adjunctive treatment (e.g., antibiotics for pyelonephritis or therapeutic amniocentesis for polyhydramnios).

Choosing a Tocolytic Agent

Tocolytic drugs are reasonably safe when used according to standard protocols. However, their apparent safety is due more to the youth and general good health of the patients treated than to the inherent safety of the drugs. The choice of tocolytic requires consideration of the efficacy, risks, and side effects for each individual patient.

Magnesium Sulfate

Because of its safety and familiarity, magnesium has displaced the β-mimetic drugs ritodrine and terbutaline to become the most commonly used tocolytic. The mechanism of tocolytic activity of magnesium is unclear. In vitro studies of uterine muscle strips show reduced contractility in the presence of magnesium ion. It has been suggested that magnesium acts by competition with calcium either at the motor end plate, reducing excitation, or at the cell membrane, reducing calcium influx into the cell at depolarization.

Efficacy of Magnesium Sulfate

Magnesium has become the first choice for tocolysis more because of its relative safety than for its efficacy.

Maternal Side Effects

Magnesium has a low rate of serious side effects compared with other tocolytic drugs.[224] However, flushing, nausea, vomiting, headache, generalized muscle weakness, diplopia, and shortness of breath are not rare. Major and life-threatening complications, including chest pain and pulmonary edema, also occur rarely. Side effects are significantly more common when magnesium and β-mimetics are administered simultaneously.[221] Most centers avoid combined use for this reason.

Neonatal Side Effects

Although magnesium crosses the placenta and achieves serum levels comparable to maternal levels, serious neonatal complications are uncommon. Lethargy, hypotonia, and even respiratory depression may occur. A case-control study found that maternal magnesium treatment for either preeclampsia or preterm labor was associated with lower rates of cerebral palsy (CP).[226]

Dosage of Magnesium Sulfate

Magnesium sulfate must be given parenterally to elevate serum levels above the normal range. Therapeutic dosage and serum levels have not been formally established but empirically are similar to those used for intravenous treatment of preeclampsia. A loading dose of 4 to 6 g is given over 20 to 30 minutes, followed by an infusion of 2 to 4 g/hr.[220] Serum magnesium levels alone should not serve as the end point of therapy. The drug should be titrated on the basis of clinical efficacy and toxicity.

Provided renal function is normal, the kidney rapidly excretes excess magnesium. In patients with evidence of renal impairment (e.g., oliguria or serum creatinine levels >0.9 mg/dl), magnesium therapy should be approached cautiously, and the patient should be followed with serum levels, and doses adjusted accordingly. Magnesium sulfate should not be used in patients with myasthenia gravis.

A clinical protocol for magnesium sulfate as a tocolytic is shown in the box.

Protocol for Magnesium Sulfate Tocolysis

1. Administer loading dose of 6 g magnesium sulfate in 10 to 20 percent solution over 20 to 30 minutes.
2. Maintenance dose of 2 g/hr (40 g of magnesium sulfate added to 1 L D5 0.9 normal saline or lactated Ringer's at 50 ml/hr.
3. Increase magnesium sulfate by 1 g/hr until the patient has one or less contraction per 10 minutes or a maximum dose of 4 to 5 g/hr is reached.
4. Limit intravenous fluid to 125 ml/hr. Follow fluid status closely with an indwelling urinary catheter if needed.
5. Maintain magnesium sulfate tocolysis for 12 hours after contractions have stopped or decreased to less than one per 15 minutes. Therapy may be stopped without tapering the dose.
6. Recurrent contractions require reevaluation to look for an underlying cause of the preterm labor such as amnionitis or occult abruption. Amniocentesis should be considered. The accuracy of the original diagnosis of preterm labor should be reconsidered with cervical sonography or fibronectin.
7. Patients treated with magnesium sulfate should be followed with
   a. Deep tendon reflexes and vital signs hourly.
   b. Intake and output every 2 to 4 hours.
   c. Magnesium levels if infusion exceeds 4 g/hr or if clinical concern about toxicity.

Indomethacin

Prostaglandins are mediators of the final pathways of uterine muscle contraction. Inhibition of prostaglandin synthetase by NSAIDs leads to reduced synthesis of prostaglandins. Indomethacin is the most widely used agent in this class.

Efficacy of Indomethacin

Indomethacin has been reported to delay delivery by 48 hours in over 80 percent of treated subjects.[231] The indomethacin group had significantly fewer maternal side effects when compared to ritodrine.

Maternal Side Effects of Indomethacin

The principal advantage of this agent is the relative infrequency of serious maternal side effects when the agent is used in a brief course of tocolysis. Gastrointestinal side effects such as nausea, heartburn, and vomiting are the most common, but usually mild. More serious complications include gastrointestinal bleeding, alterations in coagulation, thrombocytopenia, and asthma in aspirin-sensitive patients. Prolonged treatment can lead to renal injury, especially when other nephrotoxic drugs are employed. Hypertensive women may rarely experience acute increased blood pressure after indomethacin treatment. Drugs of this class are antipyretic agents and may obscure a clinically significant fever. Maternal contraindications to indomethacin tocolysis include renal disease including diabetic nephropathy, hepatic disease, active peptic ulcer disease, poorly controlled hypertension, asthma, and coagulation disorders.

Fetal and Neonatal Side Effects

The potential for fetal and neonatal complications of indomethacin tocolysis is worrisome. In actual practice, serious complications have been rare. Tricuspid regurgitation occurs in some fetuses, but ductal abnormalities resolve within 24 hours after the medication is discontinued. The likelihood of ductal constriction increases after 32 weeks of pregnancy.[239] Persistent ductal constriction and irreversible right heart failure have been reported after prolonged treatment.[241]

Oligohydramnios associated with indomethacin tocolysis is common, dose related, and reversible, but there is a report of neonatal renal insufficiency and death after prolonged administration.[243] Oligohydramnios is a consequence of reduced fetal urine production, due to reduction by indomethacin of the normal prostaglandin inhibition of antidiuretic hormone, and by direct effects on fetal renal blood flow.

Primary pulmonary hypertension in the neonate is a potentially fatal illness that has also been associated with prolonged (>48 hours) indomethacin therapy.[244,245] Primary neonatal pulmonary hypertension has not been reported with 24 to 48 hours of therapy, but the incidence may be as high as 5 to 10 percent with long-term therapy.[235]

Other complications, including necrotizing enterocolitis, small bowel perforation, patent ductus arteriosus, jaundice, and intraventricular hemorrhage, have been observed when indomethacin was outside of standardized protocols that did not limit the duration of treatment and/or employed the drug after 32 weeks.[246] Fetuses treated in utero with indomethacin have been followed in childhood without evidence of significant long- term effects.[247–249]

Because of the effect on fetal urine production and amniotic fluid volume, indomethacin may be an appropriate tocolytic when preterm labor is associated with polyhydramnios. Uterine activity and pain associated with degenerating uterine fibroids in pregnancy also respond well to indomethacin.

Dosage of Indomethacin

Indomethacin is well absorbed orally or per rectum. The usual dose is a 50-mg loading dose by mouth or 50 to 100 mg per rectum. Subsequently, 25 to 50 mg is administered orally every 6 hours, depending on the response. Therapy is usually limited to 2 to 4 days because of concern about side effects of oligohydramnios and neonatal pulmonary hypertension (see the box "A Protocol For Indomethacin Tocolysis").

The β-Mimetic Tocolytics

Ritodrine is the only agent approved by the FDA as a tocolytic. Terbutaline use continues despite not only the lack of FDA approval but also the specific FDA disapproval of its use as a tocolytic.[255] The concern expressed by the FDA Advisory is related specifically to subcutaneous infusion of terbutaline for prevention and treatment of preterm labor.

Efficacy of β-Mimetics

There is evidence that the β-mimetic agents are successful in prolonging pregnancy for at least 48 hours and perhaps longer. A Canadian trial of ritodrine compared with placebo reported a reduction in deliveries within 2 to 7 days of diagnosis but no significant

---

A Protocol for Indomethacin Tocolysis

1. Limit use to preterm labor before 32 weeks' gestation in subjects with normal amniotic fluid volume and normal renal function.
2. Loading dose of 50 mg rectally or orally; repeated in 1 hour if no decrease in contractions.
3. Give 25 to 50 mg every 6 hours for 48 hours.
4. Check amniotic fluid volume prior to initiation and at 48 to 72 hours. If oligohydramnios is present, the drug should be discontinued.
5. Use the drug for no longer than 48 to 72 consecutive hours. Treatment for >48 hours requires extraordinary circumstances. Ductal flow should be evaluated with Doppler echocardiography.
6. Discontinue therapy promptly if delivery seems imminent.
7. Fetal contraindications to use of indomethacin include growth restriction, renal anomalies, chorioamnionitis, oligohydramnios, ductal dependent cardiac defects, and twin–twin transfusion syndrome.

difference in births before 37 week or before 32 weeks. Any benefit of tocolysis evident in these analyses would seem to be conferred by the opportunity to administer steroids, antibiotics, and the like, and not by prolongation of pregnancy to allow further intrauterine growth and maturation of the fetus.

Pharmacology of β-Mimetics

Sympathomimetic drugs act through either α- or β-receptors. Stimulation of α-receptors leads to contraction of smooth muscles, while β-receptor stimulation carries the opposite effect, leading to smooth muscle relaxation at all sites: vascular, gastrointestinal, and uterine. The presence of β-receptors in other tissues (e.g., the heart) accounts for the side effects of β-mimetics. β- Receptors are divided into $β_1$- and $β_2$-subtypes. The $β_1$-receptors are largely responsible for the cardiac effects, while $β_2$-receptors mediate the smooth muscle relaxation as well as hepatic glycogen production and islet cell release of insulin.

Pharmacokinetics

Terbutaline has a longer half-life than ritodrine, and as a result has been associated with fewer side effects. Currently published protocols often employ subcutaneous administration, with a usual dose of 0.25 mg (250 μg) every 3 to 4 hours.[266] A single subcutaneous dose of terbutaline to arrest contractions during the initial evaluation of preterm contractions was found in one report to be an efficient method of evaluating women presenting with possible preterm labor.[262] Intravenous administration of terbutaline has been employed in some centers, beginning at 2.5 μg/min and increasing by 2.5 μg/min every 20 minutes in a manner similar to ritodrine until a maximum of 17.5 to 20 μg/min is reached.[267]

Tachyphylaxis with β-Mimetic Drugs

Tachyphylaxis or desensitization of the adrenergic receptor occurs throughout the body after prolonged exposure to β-agonists, and affects the clinical use as tocolytics. Animal studies suggest that contractions resume after only several hours of *continuous* intravenous therapy with high-dose β-mimetic therapy; the myometrium remains quiescent longer with *pulsatile* administration of lower doses of the same tocolytic agent.[268]

Side Effects and Complications of Parenteral β-Mimetic Tocolysis

Most side effects are mild and of limited duration, but serious maternal cardiopulmonary and metabolic complications have been reported, including maternal death when β-adrenergic agents were given to mothers with unrecognized or occult cardiac disease. A thorough history and review of possible cardiac symptoms before initiating treatment should be performed. Prompt attention to any patient with persistent symptoms during treatment is important to prevent complications.

Cardiopulmonary Complications

The β-mimetic drugs have the potential for serious complications, but have an acceptable margin of safety if used with care and contraindications are strictly observed. Side effects are frequent with high-dose therapy. More than 50 percent of patients develop tachycardia greater than 120 bpm.[267,271] Pulmonary edema is serious but can often be prevented.[272] Pulmonary edema in association with tocolysis was once thought to be secondary to volume overload with left heart failure. However, evaluation of cardiac function with Swan-Ganz catheters and echocardiography has failed to demonstrate left ventricular failure in all but a few cases of pulmonary edema, most of which were associated with underlying hypertension.[273] Noncardiogenic contributing causes include decreased colloid oncotic pressure and increased pulmonary vascular permeability, especially when premature labor is associated with amnionitis.[274] Most patients with pulmonary edema have received either physiologic saline solutions or lactated Ringer's solution, which further decreases colloid oncotic pressure and expands vascular volume. A patient treated with β-mimetics should be considered as having a compromised cardiovascular system and should not receive large amounts of saline or lactated Ringer's solution.

It is uncommon for pulmonary edema to develop in the first 24 hours of β-mimetic therapy. More than 90 percent of reported cases of pulmonary edema occur after 24 hours of β-mimetic therapy. Pulmonary edema has been reported without concomitant use of corticosteroids, and with tocolytics other than the β-mimetics.

Symptomatic cardiac arrhythmias and myocardial ischemia have occurred during β-agonist tocolytic therapy. Myocardial infarction with resultant maternal death has also been reported.[271] If a patient develops chest pain during tocolytic therapy, tocolysis should be discontinued and oxygen administered.

The β-mimetic agents produce a mild (5 to 10 mm Hg) fall in diastolic blood pressure, and the extensive peripheral vasodilatation makes it difficult for the patient to mount a normal response to hypovolemia. This is one of the reasons β-mimetics may be dangerous in women with antepartum hemorrhage. Another is that the important early signs of excessive blood loss (e.g., maternal and fetal tachycardia) are masked by these drugs.[271]

Metabolic Complications

β-Mimetic agents may induce transient mild hyperglycemia in non-diabetic pregnant women,[267] lead to gestational diabetes with prolonged oral use,[276,277] elevate blood glucose sufficiently to require insulin patients with diet-controlled gestational diabetes, and seriously compromise glucose control in type 1 and type 2 maternal diabetes. These drugs should in general be avoided in women with diabetes. If it is absolutely necessary to use β-mimetics, a simultaneous intravenous insulin infusion should be employed to avoid ketoacidosis. Measurement of glucose before initiating therapy and on occasion during the first 24 hours of treatment is appropriate.

Neonatal Side Effects of β-Mimetics

β-Mimetic tocolysis has been linked to an increased risk of neonatal intraventricular hemorrhage.[282] Neonatal hypoglycemia and ileus have also been reported with β-mimetics, and can be clinically significant if the maternal infusion is not discontinued more than 2 hours before delivery.[283] With all tocolytic drugs, and particularly β-mimetics and magnesium sulfate, adverse neonatal effects are greatest when the fetus is born close to a period of high-dose parenteral therapy. These drugs must be used with great caution if at all when there is advanced cervical dilatation and delivery appears inevitable.

Calcium Channel Blockers

Inhibitors of intracellular calcium entry affect the contraction of smooth muscle, and thus have potential use as tocolytics. Nifedipine and nicardipine have been studied as tocolytic agents because they selectively inhibit uterine contractions compared to others such as verapamil. Unlike other tocolytics, calcium channel blockers are rapidly absorbed after oral administration. The duration of action of a single dose can be as long as 6 hours.

Efficacy

There are no placebo-controlled trials of calcium channel blockers. When nifedipine has been compared with β-mimetics,[286-289] its efficacy has been comparable or superior, and side effects lower than with β-mimetics.

Side Effects

Maternal side effects are less common with nifedipine and nicardipine than β-mimetics. A decrease in blood pressure and rise in pulse have been noted, with occasional cases of significant hypotension.[286] Modest increases in glucose have been observed. Maternal symptoms are often related to hypotension and include headache (20 percent), flushing (8 percent), dizziness, and nausea (6 percent). Pretreatment with fluids may reduce their incidence. Reports described skeletal muscle blockade when used in conjunction with magnesium sulfate,[293,294] so this combination therapy should be avoided. Both reports describe a prompt response to cessation of magnesium and/or treatment with calcium gluconate.

Dosage

Nifedipine is usually given as a 10- to 20-mg dose every 6 to 8 hours by mouth. *Sublingual administration is not recommended* for general medical or obstetric patients because of reports of profound hypotension and myocardial ischemia.[292, 299]

Clinical Use of Tocolytic Drugs

Tocolytic therapy is employed in several clinical circumstances. In a patient who presents in active labor with advanced cervical effacement, the diagnosis is not in question, and the goal is prompt treatment to allow maternal transfer and time for corticosteroids and GBS prophylaxis. In this setting, oral nifedipine or subcutaneous terbutaline may be the best initial choice to stop contractions promptly, with either additional nifedipine or magnesium to suppress contractions for 8 to 24 hours. When the clinical presentation is more indolent, with persistent contractions and cervical effacement less than 80 percent, a slower acting agent such as magnesium is often chosen as the initial drug. Acute treatment for preterm labor is typically continued for some period of time, usually 6 to 12 hours, after contractions have stopped, or occur less than four times per hour without additional cervical change. When labor has been difficult to stop in a patient with complete cervical effacement, acute treatment is sometimes continued until a full course of steroid therapy is completed (48 hours). Evaluation of the preterm labor patient whose contractions do not respond promptly to tocolysis, especially before 30 weeks' gestation is described in the box "Management of Persistent Contractions Despite 12 to 24 Hours of Tocolysis".

Amniocentesis can be helpful in the management of some women with preterm labor. In addition to evaluation for infection, amniotic fluid studies for fetal pulmonary maturity may be helpful in the following circumstances:

1. When the gestational age is in doubt.
2. When the size of the fetus suggests poor or excessive intrauterine growth.
3. When there is any question of a chronic hostile intrauterine environment (e.g., maternal hypertension, decreased amniotic fluid volume, substance abuse).
4. When the gestational age is between 34 and 37 weeks.[307,308]

> ### Management of Persistent Contractions Despite 12 to 24 Hours of Tocolysis
>
> 1. Is the patient infected? Repeat clinical exam, white blood cell counts, and fetal assessment. Consider amniocentesis for glucose, Gram stain, and culture.
> 2. Is the fetal compromised? Review the fetal heart tracings and do a biophysical assessment.
> 3. Is there evidence of abruption? Is there a suspicion of uterine anomaly with implantation of the placenta on the septum? Repeat hemoglobin, hematocrit, and coagulation profile, and abdominal sonography for placental implantation site.
> 4. Is the diagnosis of preterm labor correct? Is the cervix changing? Perform a transvaginal cervical ultrasound to measure cervical length and look for funneling or separation of the membranes from the lower segment. Send a fibronectin swab.
> 5. If infection, fetal compromise, and abruption can be excluded, stop parenteral tocolysis for 24 hours and observe. Most patients will stop contracting spontaneously.

Continued suppression of contractions after acute tocolysis has been studied in multiple placebo-controlled trials[310-314], none of which found a significant reduction in the rate of preterm birth. None of three randomized trials of home contraction monitoring after acute treatment of preterm labor report a benefit for the monitored group.[323-325]

The duration of hospitalization for an episode of preterm labor will vary according to several factors including the dilation, effacement, and sonographic length of the cervix; ease of tocolysis; gestational age, obstetric history; distance from hospital; and the availability of home care and family support.

Adjunctive Treatment for Women with Preterm Labor

The initial goal of treatment of women with preterm labor is to delay delivery long enough to allow three adjunctive interventions that have been shown to reduce the neonatal morbidity and mortality related to prematurity:

1. Transfer of mother and fetus to a hospital equipped to care for a premature infant.[214,215]

2. Administration of glucocorticoids to decrease neonatal morbidity and mortality.[217,326]
3. Administration of antibiotic prophylaxis to prevent neonatal GBS infection.[216,327]

Maternal and Neonatal Transfer

Regionalized neonatal and maternal care has been shown to improve the rates of morbidity and mortality for LBW and especially for VLBW infants. Transfer of the mother with the fetus in utero is the preferred alternative whenever possible.

Antenatal Corticosteroids

Many studies have confirmed the benefit of maternal steroid treatment to reduce the incidence and severity of RDS and other neonatal morbidity including intraventricular hemorrhage, necrotizing enterocolitis, and patent ductus arteriosus. Most important, meta-analyses indicate that antenatal glucocorticoid treatment has led to decreased perinatal mortality, with odds ratios ranging from 0.32 to 0.9[217,329]. Antenatal steroids enhance cell differentiation and maturation rather than cell growth.

Physiologic Effects of Antenatal Corticosteroids

A 50 percent reduction in RDS occurs in steroid-treated neonates.[328] However, two principal unresolved issues about clinical use of antenatal steroids remain: (1) appropriate use of multiple courses of steroids, and (2) use in women with preterm PROM.

DOSAGE OF CORTICOSTEROIDS. Two glucocorticoid regimens have been found effective: *betamethasone,* given as a mixture of 6 mg each of betamethasone phosphate and betamethasone acetate (Celestone) 12 mg intramuscularly every 24 hours for 2 doses, and *dexamethasone* (Decadron) 6 mg, also given intramuscularly, every 12 hours for 4 doses. The oral preparation of dexamethasone should not be used.

RISKS OF ANTENATAL CORTICOSTEROID TREATMENT. In women with insulin-dependent diabetes mellitus, steroid treatment virtually always results in 48 to 96 hours of increased blood glucose that can be difficult to control with standard insulin regimens. Intravenous infusion of insulin is often necessary. In women without diabetes, impairment of maternal glucose tolerance may also occur, especially in women treated with β-mimetic drugs[280] or when traditional risk factors for gestational diabetes such as maternal age, obesity, or family history are present. Therefore, maternal glucose testing should be considered when repeated courses of glucocorticoids are administered.

Maternal treatment with betamethasone[357] but not dexamethasone[346,347] has been associated with transient reduction in fetal heart rate variability and body and breathing movements in several studies. When it occurs, typically between 48 and 72 hours after the first dose, the alteration in fetal biophysical behavior is striking. Both short- and long-term heart rate variability is reduced, and fetal body and breathing motion may be absent or significantly reduced. The effects resolve spontaneously by the 4th day.

Concern about long-term fetal effects is founded upon the observation that corticosteroids act to accelerate fetal cellular and organ maturation at the expense of cell and organ growth.[359] Data about long-term risks are mostly but not wholly reassuring, and must be viewed against the overwhelming evidence of neonatal benefit. Additional concern about repeated courses has been raised by reports in humans of reduced growth associated with multiple courses of antenatal steroids. An Australian study found that 17 percent of infants who received a single in utero course of antenatal steroids had birth weights below the 10th percentile, compared with 35 percent of infants exposed to more than three antenatal courses.[365] There was also a significant association between multiple courses and reduced head circumference in this study. It is reassuring to note that the original cohorts of infants treated in 1972 with a single course of antenatal steroids have displayed no differences when compared with gestational age-matched controls in physical or mental function.[352,366]

Clinical Use of Antenatal Corticosteroids

Both NICHD and ACOG recommend antenatal steroids for mothers expected to deliver before 32 weeks' gestation to reduce mortality and the incidence of RDS and IVH, regardless of the status of the fetal membranes. At 32 to 34 weeks, both recommend antenatal steroid treatment for mothers with intact membranes who were likely to deliver within 7 days, but noted that the benefit for infants born to women with ruptured membranes after 32 weeks is still controversial. The 1994 NICHD Consensus Panel reconvened in August 2000 and recommended that repeat dosing not be used in clinical practice pending data from ongoing research studies.

Antibiotics for Women with Preterm Labor

There are two potential uses for antibiotics in women with preterm labor. The first is prophylaxis of neonatal GBS infection, an intervention that is clearly effective (see Chapter 25). The second is antibiotic therapy aimed at prolonging gestation in women with preterm labor by targeting a broad range of microorganisms that have been implicated in the pathogenesis of spontaneous preterm birth. Administration of antibiotics to women being treated for preterm labor has been studied extensively with disappointing results.[372-377]

ABNORMAL CERVICAL COMPETENCE

See Chapter 14.

Diagnosis

A useful acronym to describe the process of effacement as seen by transvaginal sonography: TYVU. These letters form, in chronologic sequence, the sonographic appearance of the cervical canal and lower segment as it changes from the uneffaced *T* to the beginning funnel *Y*, with further shortening to *V*, and finally to a fully developed lower uterine segment, *U*. Because of the variation of the appearance of the upper funneled portion of the cervix, we have concentrated on accurate measurement of the residual lower cervical length as the most consistent measurement, both serially for each woman and for comparison with other centers.

A diagnosis of reduced cervical competence may be made prior to pregnancy or in the first trimester, if a typical history of painless dilatation and effacement of the cervix in a prior pregnancy can be documented. Women with a history of a previous second-trimester loss in which cervical sonography documented the classic picture of funneling and shortened cervical length are also candidates for prophylactic cerclage sutures. However, when the history is atypical or uncertain, it is more appropriate to follow the patient closely with frequent transvaginal ultrasound examinations beginning at 16 to 18 weeks' gestation, looking for the criteria noted above, and for funneling in response to fundal pressure.[393] Without a history of early preterm birth, the appearance of spontaneous or induced funneling after 24 weeks of pregnancy does not establish a diagnosis of cervical incompetence, nor does it require a cerclage. The obstetric history and the cervical length exclusive of any funneling are the most predictive. The appearance of a funnel with a normal residual length has little import.

PRETERM PREMATURE RUPTURE OF THE MEMBRANES

Spontaneous rupture of the fetal membranes before the onset of labor is called premature rupture of the membranes (PROM) regardless of gestational age. Preterm PROM is defined as PROM that occurs before 37 weeks' gestation.

Etiology

Clinical risk factors that have been linked to the occurrence of preterm PROM, include connective tissue disorders (e.g., Ehlers-Danlos syndrome), genital tract infection or colonization with various microorganisms,[412] coitus,[413] low socioeconomic status,[41] uterine overdistention,[414] second- and third-trimester bleeding,[46] nutritional deficiencies of copper and ascorbic acid,[409] and maternal smoking.[46,409,415] One study[416] found that a short cervical length (≤25 mm) at 24 weeks was associated with preterm PROM that occurred weeks later. This suggests that the process leading to preterm PROM is chronic rather than acute in many cases. Histologic studies of the membranes after preterm PROM often demonstrate significant bacterial contamination along the choriodecidual interface with minimal involvement of the amnion. This suggests spread of the organisms along the maternal–fetal surfaces *before* membrane rupture.[418]

Specific genital tract pathogens have also been correlated with the occurrence of PROM. The organisms include *B. fragilis* and other anaerobes, *N. gonorrhoeae, C. trachomatis, T. vaginalis,* and group B β-hemolytic streptococci.[418] Group B streptococcal colonization was not associated with PROM in the Preterm Prediction Study.[416] A consistent association has been found between bacterial vaginosis and spontaneous preterm births, including those following preterm PROM.

Diagnosis

The most common presentation is a gush of fluid from the vagina followed by persistent, uncontrolled leakage, but some patients report only intermittent leakage or perineal wetness. Any history of passing fluid through the vagina should be evaluated by a sterile speculum examination to collect fluid for confirmatory tests. Digital examination of the cervix in women with possible preterm labor or preterm PROM should be avoided until the diagnosis of ruptured membranes has been excluded. Because of the risk of introducing bacteria into the endocervix, digital examination for women with preterm PROM should not be performed until labor occurs or delivery is anticipated within 24 hours. To avoid a digital exam, a visual estimate at the time of sterile speculum examination can sometimes identify women with advanced dilation.[422] The sterile speculum examination may also reveal a collection or "pool" of fluid that can be tested for pH with nitrazine paper. Since amniotic fluid is slightly alkaline (the pH is about 7.15), vaginal secretions containing amniotic fluid will usually result in pH changes in the blue-green range, 6.5 to 7.5. Nitrazine testing is accurate in 90 to 98 percent of cases.[423] False-positive values can result from infections that raise vaginal pH (e.g., *T. vaginalis*), the presence of blood, or rarely, cervical mucus. False-negative reactions are frequent when only a scant amount of fluid is present.

When placed on a clean slide and allowed to air dry, amniotic fluid produces a microscopic crystallization in a "fern" pattern. This phenomenon is due to the interaction of amniotic fluid proteins and salts and accurately confirms PROM in 85 to 98 percent of cases. False-positive tests can result from the collection of cervical mucus, which also "ferns," but usually in a more floral pattern. The fern test is unaffected by meconium, changes in vaginal pH, and blood/amniotic fluid ratios of up to 1:5. The fern pattern in samples heavily contaminated with blood is atypical and appears more "skeletonized."[424,425]

An ultrasound evaluation for amniotic fluid volume should be performed in women with preterm PROM to determine fetal presentation, fetal weight, and gestational age. If the diagnosis of membrane rupture is equivocal, a finding of decreased or absent fluid by ultrasound supports a diagnosis of ruptured membranes. When abundant residual fluid is observed in women after a confirmed diagnosis of PROM, the possibility of polyhydramnios prior to rupture should be considered. In uncertain cases, a repeat sterile speculum examination after the patient has rested in a semiupright position for approximately 1 hour to allow the pooling of secretions in the posterior vagina may be helpful. During this time, the woman may be monitored to evaluate fetal well-being and uterine contractions. Variable decelerations suggest umbilical cord compression secondary to reduced amniotic fluid volume. When all other tests are equivocal in a patient with reduced fluid and a good history, a vaginal swab for fetal fibronectin (fibronectin is abundant in amniotic fluid) may be helpful to exclude the diagnosis. In rare instances, an amniocentesis to inject a dilute solution of indigo carmine dye to look for transcervical leakage onto a tampon can be used to make an absolute diagnosis. Methylene blue dye has been associated with hemolytic anemia and hyperbilirubinemia in the infant and should not be used.

Natural History

For women with preterm PROM between 20 and 34 weeks, the duration of pregnancy after PROM is inversely related to the gestational age at time of membrane rupture. When PROM occurs prior to 26 weeks' gestation, 30 to 40 percent of cases will gain at least 1 additional week before delivery and 20 percent will gain over 4 weeks.[426] By contrast, 70 to 80 percent of patients who experience PROM between 28 and 36 weeks' gestation deliver within the first week after PROM and more than one half of these within the first

4 days.[427] Between 32 and 34 weeks, the mean interval between rupture and delivery is 4 days.[428] At term, 80 percent enter labor within 24 hours after rupture of the membranes.

Maternal Risks

Whether a cause or result of preterm PROM, intrauterine infection is a potentially serous complication to the mother. Clinical chorioamnionitis accompanies preterm PROM in approximately 10 percent of cases. Regardless of clinical signs of infection, as many as 25 to 30 percent of women with preterm PROM will have a positive amniotic fluid culture. Most instances of amnionitis respond well to antibiotic treatment and delivery, but maternal deaths from sepsis can occur.[431] Amnionitis is more common when PROM occurs before 30–32 weeks.

Fetal and Neonatal Risks

Infection is a major potential complication for the fetus and neonate. The same organisms responsible for maternal infection can result in congenital pneumonia, sepsis, or meningitis. In published series, the range of neonatal sepsis in cases of preterm PROM with or without clinical amnionitis is 2 to 19 percent. Neonatal deaths caused by infection are reported in 1 to 7 percent of infants born to women with chorioamnionitis.

There is a higher risk of frank or occult cord prolapse, particularly if the fetus is not in a cephalic presentation. The risks of fetal distress in labor leading to cesarean delivery are significantly higher with preterm PROM than with isolated preterm labor.[432] Usually due to severe variable decelerations.

Placental abruption occurs in 4 to 6 percent of cases of preterm PROM, especially when PROM is accompanied by bleeding.[433,434] A 15 percent rate of abruption has been observed when patients with prolonged preterm PROM manifest vaginal bleeding in addition to fluid leakage.

Pulmonary hypoplasia is a particular concern when fetal membranes are ruptured prior to 26 weeks' gestation. About 25 percent of babies delivered after 26 weeks' gestation following PROM that occurred before 26 weeks' gestation were found to have pulmonary hypoplasia following birth.[426] The duration and degree of oligohydramnios are associated with the chance of pulmonary hypoplasia. The frequency of pulmonary hypoplasia is most consistently correlated with gestational age at rupture.[436,437]

Skeletal deformities may occur due to compression but usually resolve within 12 months. Twenty-Seven percent of fetuses born after prolonged PROM before 26 weeks developed skeletal deformations.[438]

Initial Evaluation and Management

After the diagnosis of preterm PROM has been confirmed, maternal and fetal indications for immediate delivery should be ruled out before considering other management options. The most dangerous fetal complications of PROM at any gestational age are prolapse of the umbilical cord, and fetal bradycardia caused by cord compression. The principal maternal indication for delivery is chorioamnionitis. If a firm diagnosis of chorioamnionitis can be made by the presence of maternal fever greater than or equal to 101 °F, uterine tenderness, and leukocytosis greater than or equal to 20,000/mm^3, delivery should be undertaken promptly regardless of the gestational age. In the absence of indications for immediate delivery, gestational age should be carefully assessed to estimate the relative risks for the fetus of delivery versus expectant management. All clinical and ultrasound dating criteria should be reviewed. Because oligohydramnios may flatten the fetal head, biparietal diameter measurements to estimate fetal weight by ultrasound may be inaccurate in women with preterm PROM.[439] Fetal tables based on head circumference, femur length, or cerebellar diameter are more reliable indicators of gestational age and fetal weight in these situations.

Before 30 to 32 weeks' gestation, the neonatal risks of prematurity will usually outweigh the in utero risks of infection and fetal compromise caused by oligohydramnios, while the reverse is usually the case after 34 to 35 weeks' gestation.[440] Consideration of individual risks forms the basis for management for women with preterm PROM and is among the most challenging tasks in obstetrics. The relative risks of prematurity, infection, and fetal well-being must be repeatedly evaluated for expectantly managed patients with preterm PROM.

Amniocentesis for Women with Preterm PROM

Assessment of amniotic fluid for infection and maturity studies should always be considered in women with preterm PROM. Expectant management requires repeated assessment of mother and fetus for evidence of maternal and fetal infection, cord prolapse, and abruption. Demonstration of either fetal pulmonary maturity or intra- amniotic bacteria may allow a decision for delivery, thus obviating the difficulties of fetal and maternal surveillance. Amniotic fluid may be obtained from either free-flowing vaginal fluid or amniocentesis for studies of fetal maturity, but amniocentesis is required to obtain fluid for culture, Gram stain, and glucose tests for infection. Placing the patient in the Trendelenburg position prior to the amniocentesis may facilitate the procedure by favoring intrauterine retention of fluid. Although the amniotic fluid pocket may be small, amniocentesis is reasonably safe when performed with ultrasound guidance.

Tests for Infection in Patients with Preterm PROM

Expectant management of preterm PROM requires initial and continued surveillance for infection. Ultimately, the end point for tests of "infection" in this clinical setting should be clinically important maternal or fetal/neonatal infection. Intermediate end points (e.g., amniotic fluid bacteria, white blood cells, glucose, and even culture), while associated with perinatal infection, do not equate uniformly with clinical infectious morbidity or mortality. The incidence of clinical amnionitis approximates 10 percent in women with preterm PROM. Of infants born to mothers with clinical amnionitis, only 1 to 15 percent will have positive cultures that confirm a diagnosis of neonatal sepsis. Finally, the rate of perinatal mortality caused by infection has ranged from 0 to 13 percent in studies of infants born after preterm PROM. The principal causes of perinatal morbidity and mortality after preterm PROM are still more often related to prematurity than to infection. Nevertheless, when it occurs, neonatal infection can be devastating. It is important to make an early diagnosis of infection because a two- to fourfold increase in perinatal mortality, intraventricular hemorrhage, and neonatal sepsis has been reported in infants born after amnionitis compared with gestational age-matched controls born to noninfected mothers.[448] Importantly, antepartum treatment of maternal amnionitis clearly decreases the incidence of neonatal sepsis.

Clinical surveillance of expectantly managed patients with preterm PROM includes frequent examinations for maternal heart rate, contractions, uterine tenderness, fever greater than or equal to 38 °C, and biophysical profile or nonstress testing, looking for variable decelerations, tachycardia, and absent fetal movement. An extensive review of laboratory tests to detect intrauterine infection concluded that none was wholly satisfactory.[452] White blood cell counts are customary in patients with preterm PROM, but are not always predictive of the presence or absence of chorioamnionitis. An elevated maternal leukocyte count has a reported sensitivity of 23 to 80 percent, a specificity of 60 to 95 percent, a positive predictive value of 50 to 75 percent, and a negative predictive value of 40 to 90 percent to predict clinical or histologic amnionitis.[453]

Amniotic fluid obtained by amniocentesis can be used to detect amnionitis, based on demonstration of bacteria on a Gram stain of unspun fluid, amniotic fluid glucose levels, or the presence of IL-6 (see Chapter 25). Approximately 10^5 organisms/ml are needed before a Gram stain will be positive. Thus, not all culture-positive fluids have positive Gram stains, though virtually all positive Gram stains result from culture-positive fluids. The Gram stain for bacteria has reported sensitivity ranging from 36 to 80 percent, and a specificity of 80 to 97 percent to predict a subsequent positive culture. Amniotic fluid culture has a reported sensitivity of 65 to 85 percent and a specificity of 85 percent to predict clinical chorioamnionitis. The presence of white blood cells in amniotic fluid has not proven helpful in predicting infection, but a low amniotic fluid glucose (≤ 16 to 20 mg/dl) has been found to correlate well with a positive fluid culture, with sensitivity and specificity of approximately 80 to 90 percent. The amniotic fluid glucose is simple, rapid, and available around the clock.

Management Strategies

When a thorough assessment reveals no evidence of fetal distress or infection, and fetal pulmonary maturity cannot be confirmed, three management options remain. The first is conservative or expectant management, in which the patient is hospitalized for intensive surveillance for signs of fetal compromise or infection, at which time labor is allowed or induced if necessary. This approach is associated with a low rate of cesarean delivery, but relies upon methods of fetal assessment that must be performed at least daily and, as noted, are not always accurate. An alternate choice is immediate delivery for pregnancies beyond a certain gestational age (e.g., ≥ 32 weeks) or estimated fetal weight (e.g., $\geq 1,500$ to 1,800 g). This strategy avoids the need for ongoing surveillance for fetal well-being and infection, but commits to delivery some women who might have continued the pregnancy long enough to allow additional fetal development and reduced neonatal morbidity. This strategy has a high rate of cesarean delivery for failed induction. The third strategy is an attempt to delay delivery in order to influence the relative risks of prematurity and infection. For example, antibiotics have been found to reduce morbidity and prolong pregnancy[458] and corticosteroids are effective for reducing fetal morbidity, (especially intraventricular hemorrhage) and mortality, when given to women with PROM before 32 weeks. Any of the three strategies may be an appropriate choice, depending on the gestational age and individual assessments of the risk of infection and prematurity.

Corticosteroids and Antibiotics

Antenatal corticosteroids appear to reduce the risk of intraventricular hemorrhage for infants born before 32 weeks, regardless of the status of the membranes before delivery. Because grades III and IV intraventricular hemorrhages are rare after 32 weeks, the decision to use steroids after 32 weeks depends on analyses of the effect of steroids on morbidity other than IVH. As noted above, randomized trials of the effect of corticosteroids on RDS in the presence of PROM have revealed conflicting results. The 1994 NICHD Consensus Conference encouraged more study of steroids for reduction of RDS in preterm PROM after 32 weeks.[370] The ACOG also advocates caution in using steroids for preterm PROM after 32 weeks.[326] At our center, we currently administer a single course of antenatal steroids to expectantly managed patients with preterm PROM up to 34 weeks.

Because the risk of perinatal group B streptococcal infection is associated with both premature birth and duration of membrane rupture before delivery, women with preterm PROM prior to 37 weeks should be treated presumptively with an appropriate antibiotic. The importance of maternal antibiotics for group B streptococcal prophylaxis in preterm PROM has been well established and is endorsed by both the ACOG[327] and by the American Academy of Pediatrics.[461]

Antibiotic prophylaxis has also been studied as a method of prolonging the interval from rupture to delivery in an effort to reduce perinatal morbidity and mortality due to infection and prematurity. A multicenter trial enrolled 614 women with preterm PROM between 24 and 32 weeks in a study that compared combined neonatal morbidity and mortality in subjects randomly assigned to receive treatment with either antibiotics or placebo within 72 hours of amniorrhexis[458]. The antibiotic group received 48 hours of intravenous ampicillin and erythromycin, followed by oral amoxicillin and erythromycin for 5 days or until delivery. Erythromycin was combined with ampicillin to treat *Mycoplasma* and *Ureaplasma urealyticum*. None of the subjects in this trial received antenatal corticosteroids. Women in both groups who were colonized with group B streptococcus were treated with open-label ampicillin or erythromycin in addition to their assigned study regimen; these 118 subjects were analyzed separately. The primary outcome was composite mortality and morbidity including sepsis within 72 hours of birth, RDS, grade III to IV intraventricular hemorrhage, and stage 2 to 3 necrotizing enterocolitis. The mortality rate was 5 percent in both groups, but the antibiotic group had significantly less morbidity. Latency was also prolonged in the antibiotic group. Infants born to women who were treated for positive group B streptococcus cultures did as well as the antibiotic study group. As might be expected in a study that enrolled a largely indigent population, chorioamnionitis was relatively common in both groups.

The combined use of antibiotics and corticosteroids appears to confer greater benefit than either treatment alone for women with preterm PROM.

In summary, prophylactic antibiotics should be given to all women with preterm PROM to reduce the risk of neonatal group B streptococcal infection. Significant reductions in composite neonatal morbidity can also be achieved with broad-spectrum antibiotic treatment, especially in populations with a high prevalence of chorioamnionitis. Furthermore, combined treatment with corticosteroids benefits infants born after preterm PROM before 32 weeks of pregnancy.

Use of Tocolytics

There is currently little evidence to support routine use of tocolytic agents in women with preterm PROM. Prospective randomized trials of prophylactic tocolysis revealed no consistent benefit to adjunctive tocolytics for these patients.[465,466] However, the studies cited above that suggest benefit for adjunctive antibiotics and steroids have raised anew the question of short-term tocolysis in order to allow a course of steroids and antibiotics.

Preterm PROM in Special Circumstances

Preterm PROM before 26 weeks of pregnancy has diverse etiologies that may alter management. For instance, PROM may occur following amniocentesis. If the amniocentesis was performed for genetic studies or evaluation of Rhesus disease, a good outcome should be expected. A brief course of bed rest and expectant management until the leakage stops and does not resume is usually all that is required. However, infection and/or delivery are likely if the amniocentesis was performed to evaluate a patient with advanced cervical dilation or preterm labor. When preterm PROM occurs in a woman who has experienced persistent second-trimester bleeding, especially when accompanied as well by a history of prerupture oligohydramnios and/or an elevated maternal serum α-fetoprotein, the prognosis for a surviving infant is poor. These patients often have had abnormal placental implantation noted on ultrasound evaluation. Management of these patients should include a thorough history and placental evaluation, to detect placental trauma or loss of a blighted twin, and an attempt to obtain both placental and fetal samples for karyotype. Other possible diagnoses for second-trimester losses (e.g., fetal anomaly or aneuploidy, uterine anomalies, DES, incompetent cervix, and maternal trauma), both exogenous and self induced, should all be considered.

When preterm PROM occurs before 26 weeks, risks for both mother and fetus are higher than for PROM later in pregnancy and decisions are more difficult. Because neonatal outcome for infants born before 24 to 25 weeks is poor, immediate delivery is not an easy choice. On the other hand, expectant management carries concern about maternal risks and an uncertain outcome for the fetus. Maternal risk is the first concern. A review[467] of 898 women with early preterm PROM reported in 11 observational studies found that only six women (0.7 percent) developed sepsis; however, there was a single maternal death. Other maternal risks of expectant management include the consequences of activity restriction: muscle wasting, bone demineralization, venous thromboembolism, and its prophylaxis (e.g., heparin-induced thrombocytopenia). In the collected series cited above, 15 percent of infants were stillborn, 39 percent died before 28 days of life, and 46 percent (417 of 914) survived the neonatal period. Among 195 infants who were followed for 3 to 36 months, 119 (61 percent) had normal neurologic examinations.[467]

CONDUCT OF LABOR AND DELIVERY FOR THE PRETERM INFANT

Estimation of Gestational Age-Specific Neonatal Mortality and Morbidity

Infants born after 26 weeks experience intact survival rates in excess of 60 percent, but concerns about both the likelihood and quality of survival are important in the conduct of labor before 26 weeks. As neonatal and perinatal care has improved, the lower limit of "viability" has been a progressively earlier gestational age. Regionalized perinatal care, broader use of antenatal corticosteroids, and advances in neonatal care (e.g., surfactant treatment) have led to steady improvements in perinatal, neonatal, and infant morbidity and mortality. As many as 15 percent of infants born at 23 weeks, 56 percent at 24 weeks, and 80 percent at 25 weeks may now survive to hospital discharge in the postsurfactant era.[470] Several studies have reported that the expectation by the medical team of survival for the ELBW infant actually influences the likelihood of survival. Health care providers should encourage parental and family participation in the decisions surrounding the birth of an extremely preterm infant.[474]

These observations underscore the importance of accurate information about neonatal outcome during labor management before 26 weeks of pregnancy. The "best obstetric estimate of gestational age," combining menstrual history and laboratory confirmation of pregnancy with earliest ultrasound biometry, is a more reliable antenatal predictor of neonatal survival than either estimated fetal weight or biparietal diameter (BPD).[475,476] One study identified ultrasound biometric thresholds (femur length <40 mm, BPD <54 mm, estimated weight <382 g, or estimated gestational age <22 weeks) below which there were no survivors, regardless of gestational age.[476] Unfortunately, infants who survived to 120 days with markers of serious long-term morbidity could not be distinguished before delivery from those who survived without morbidity markers by any antenatal information. Each patient's situation is unique. Kilpatrick and Piecuch developed a useful algorithm based on both literature and experience to begin discussions of intrapartum care and neonatal resuscitation, as shown in Table 18–2.[12,13] Information available after delivery (e.g., actual birth weight) more accurately predicts outcome than information before

Table 18-2 INTRAPARTUM CARE AND NEONATAL RESUSCITATION AT 23 TO 25 WEEKS

Gestational Age	Cesarean for Distress?	Pediatrics at Delivery?
≤23 w, 6 d	No	No
24 to 24 w + 6 d	Advise against, but OK if family insists	Yes
≥25 w, 0 d	Yes	Weigh in delivery room

Data from Kilpatrick SJ, Schleuter MA, Piecuch R, et al: Outcome of infants born at 24–26 weeks' gestation: I. Survival and cost. Obstet Gynecol 90:803, 1997.

birth, so it is always important to remind parents that a neonatal reassessment of the very preterm infant's prognosis is appropriate.

Intrapartum Fetal Assessment

Fetal monitoring is especially important when the fetus is premature. The preterm fetus may tolerate labor poorly, and the cause of the preterm birth may create additional intrapartum risk. Careful fetal surveillance has been associated with significantly improved outcome. Ominous heart rate tracings have the same associations with fetal acidosis as they do later in gestation. Prompt intervention can minimize their effect on perinatal morbidity and mortality.[479,480]

Anesthesia and Analgesia

There is no one method of anesthesia or analgesia in labor with a preterm fetus that is superior for all conditions. The goal of intrapartum care is to provide the neonatologist with the least traumatized, least depressed, and least acidotic fetus consistent with maternal health. Epidural anesthesia offers the advantage of pelvic floor and outlet muscle relaxation, minimizing an important source of resistance to the soft premature fetal head.

Anesthesia for cesarean delivery creates special concerns for each potential method when the fetus is preterm. The epidural technique requires a deeper, more intense block, involving more spinal segments than vaginal delivery. This may increase the chance of hypotension. General anesthesia is quicker to administer in an emergency situation and usually involves fewer changes in uteroplacental perfusion. However, it does entail greater risks to the mother, can lead to fetal depression if the surgery is difficult, and deprives the mother of perhaps her only chance to see and bond with a sick premature infant during its first hours of life.

Labor

The course of labor in a preterm gestation is often significantly shorter than that of term pregnancy. Of particular importance are the rapidity of the active phase and the short second stage of labor. Care should be taken to ensure that the fetus does not have a precipitous delivery without control of the fetal head.

Delivery

The principal goals of intrapartum management of the preterm infant are avoidance of perinatal acidosis and birth trauma. Although a generous episiotomy has been recommended to minimize the effect of perineal resistance on the small soft fetal head, data that demonstrate improved outcome associated with the use of episiotomy are difficult to find.[482] When delivering a VLBW infant, an early episiotomy is appropriate if there is perineal resistance. Few multiparous women will be in this group. Forceps may be employed for premature infants for the customary indications, but should not be used prophylactically.

Cesarean Delivery

Routine cesarean delivery of all preterm or VLBW infants is not justified by current literature.[483,484,485] Several large studies have failed to note improvement in perinatal morbidity or mortality with cesarean birth for indications other than classic obstetric ones.[483,485]

For infants in breech presentation, there are intuitive reasons for cesarean birth, particularly to avoid trapping of the aftercoming head and other manipulations that could lead to trauma or hypoxia. Older retrospective studies that suggested a benefit for cesarean delivery led to the current custom of cesarean delivery for preterm breech fetuses, but support for this practice remains weak.

When cesarean delivery for the preterm breech is chosen, it is illogical to avoid a traumatic vaginal delivery only to encounter a difficult cesarean birth because of an undeveloped lower uterine segment or an inadequate incision. Clearly, the operation must be carried out in a way that will fulfill its purpose: atraumatic delivery through a generous incision. While some have recommended routine use of a low vertical or classic incision, the exact uterine incision can depend on the fetal position and on the anatomy of the individual patient. If the lower uterine segment is well developed and the fetus is in the lower one third of the uterus, a transverse incision is reasonable.

Key Points

➤ Preterm birth is the single greatest cause of perinatal morbidity and mortality in nonanomlaous infants, responsible for 70 percent of fetal, neonatal, and infant deaths.

➤ The outcome for premature and low-birth-weight infants is better than most medical professionals believe it to be.

➤ Spontaneous preterm birth is a syndrome in which multiple risk factors operate collaboratively via injury to the maternal–fetal interface to produce several related clinical disorders.

➤ Preterm labor may be initiated by infection, ischemia/hemorrhage, uterine distention, or endocrine factors.

➤ Major risk factors for preterm birth are a prior history of preterm delivery, multifetal gestation, bleeding after the first trimester of pregnancy, and a low maternal body mass index (BMI), but these factors precede no more than 50 percent of preterm births. Every pregnancy is potentially at risk.

➤ Cervical "competence" is not an absolute or categorical property of the cervix, but rather is a continuum. The risk of spontaneous preterm birth increases as the length of the cervix decreases.

➤ Accurate early diagnosis of preterm labor is a major problem. Up to 50 percent of patients diagnosed with preterm labor do not actually have preterm labor, yet as many as 20 percent of symptomatic patients diagnosed as not being in labor will deliver prematurely.

➤ Effective therapies that can reduce perinatal morbidity and mortality are (1) transfer of the mother and fetus to an appropriate hospital, (2) administration of antibiotics to prevent neonatal group B streptococcus infection, (3) administration of corticosteroids to reduce neonatal respiratory distress syndrome and intraventricular hemorrhage, a treatment that has been underutilized in the past, and (4) administration of labor-arresting (tocolytic) medications to allow the above to occur.

➤ There is no truly reliable test for fetal well-being or infection in women with preterm PROM.

➤ Prevention of preterm birth will require prevention of risk in the population.

Chapter 19

Multiple Gestations

USHA CHITKARA AND
RICHARD L. BERKOWITZ

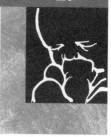

Pregnancies complicated by twinning are by their very nature at higher risk than those of most singletons. Twins are either monozygotic (MZ) or dizygotic (DZ). In the former case, a single fertilized ovum splits into two distinct individuals after a variable number of divisions. Such twins are almost always genetically identical and therefore of the same sex. When two separate ova are fertilized, DZ twins result. These individuals are as genetically distinct as any other children born to the same couple. DZ half-siblings have been reported in which two ova were fertilized by different fathers. In most cases, DZ twins are genetically dissimilar true siblings, while MZ twins are genetically identical.

The frequency of MZ twins is fairly constant throughout the world at a rate of approximately 4 per 1,000 births. This rate does not seem to vary with maternal characteristics such as age or parity. DZ twinning, however, is associated with multiple ovulation, and its frequency varies between races. In general, the frequency of DZ twins is low in Asians, intermediate in whites, and high in blacks.

The frequency of DZ births is affected by maternal age, increasing from a rate of 3 in 1,000 in women under age 20, to 14 in 1,000 at ages 35 to 40. Between 1980 to 1987, the greatest increase in U.S. birth rates of triplets and higher order multiple pregnancies occurred in women aged 30 to 39—an almost sevenfold increase in that time period.[3] Above age 40, the rate declines.

Infertility patients treated with menopausal urinary gonadotropins (Pergonal) or clomiphene citrate are well known to have a dose-dependent increase in multiple births. The use of in vitro fertilization (IVF) and embryo transfer has further increased the incidence of multiple pregnancies, and reports suggest that the incidence of multiple gestations in IVF patients may be as high as 22 percent.[4,5]

PLACENTATION

Twin placentas are described in terms of their membranes (Fig. 19–1). The sac of a singleton pregnancy consists of an outer chorion and an inner amnion. Each DZ twin develops within a similar sac because both blastocysts generate their own placentas. If implantation of these blastocysts is not proximal to each other, two separate placentas will result, each of which will have a chorion and an amnion. Should they implant side by side, intimate fusion of the placental disks will occur, but these placentas are always diamniotic and dichorionic, and vascular anastomoses rarely occur. While MZ twins may also have placentas with two amnions and two chorions, this generally is not the case. Monochorionic placentas have a single chorion that usually surrounds two amnions, but occasionally there is only a single amnion. Triplets and quadruplets have also been delivered with monochorial placentas and shown to be MZ. Almost all monochorial placentas have blood vessel communications between the fetal circulations.

The type of placenta that develops in an MZ pregnancy is determined by the timing of cleavage of the fertilized ovum. If twinning is accomplished during the first 2 to 3 days, it precedes the setting aside of cells that eventually become the chorion. In that case, two chorions and two amnions will be formed. After approximately 3 days, however, twinning cannot split the chorionic cavity, and from that time on a monochorial placenta must result. If the split occurs between the third and eighth days, a diamniotic monochorial placenta will develop. Between the 8th and 13th days, the amnion has already formed, and the placenta will therefore be monoamniotic and monochorionic. Embryonic cleavage between the 13th and 15th days will result in conjoined twins within a single amnion and chorion; beyond that point, the process of twinning cannot occur.

Because monochorial placentas can only occur in MZ pregnancies, study of the membranes will establish zygosity in 20 percent of cases in the United States. In approximately 35 percent of cases the twins will be of opposite sex and therefore necessarily DZ. This leaves only 45 percent of cases (twins of like sex having dichorionic placentas) in which further studies are necessary in order to determine zygosity. This 45 percent breaks down into 8 percent MZ and 37 percent DZ. The more genotypic markers that are studied, the greater the likelihood of demonstrating dizygosity. The most accurate method for determination of twin zygosity is by analysis of DNA polymorphism.[10,11]

PERINATAL MORBIDITY AND MORTALITY

Perinatal morbidity and mortality are greater in twins than in singletons, approximately three times greater than that of comparable singletons at the same institutions. Both preterm delivery and intrauterine growth restriction (IUGR) contribute to this problem. Twins also have an increased frequency of congenital anomalies, placenta previa, abruptio placentae, preeclampsia, cord accidents, and malpresentations.

A decline in perinatal mortality has been reported over the past two decades. Most of the improved neonatal outcome is due to increased survival rates in neonates weighing 1,000 to 1,500 g at birth.

In one series, more than 70 percent of the deaths occurred before 30 weeks' gestation, either in utero or during the neonatal period. If obstetricians are to have a major impact on the perinatal survival of twins, they must concentrate on the period between 25 and 30 weeks' gestation.

Although perinatal mortality rates have decreased, the risk of prematurity in multifetal gestations has not changed significantly over the past 20 to 30 years. The average gestational age at delivery for triplets consistently seems to be 33 weeks. Approximately 75 percent of these patients deliver prior to 37 weeks, and at least 20 percent deliver prior to 32 weeks.

Among survivors, the incidence of severe handicap is significantly higher among multiple births, 1.7-fold and 2.9-fold higher rate among twins and triplets compared with singletons.

DIAGNOSIS

Before common use of ultrasound, 50 percent of twins remained undiagnosed until the time of delivery.[30] Multiple gestations should be suspected whenever the uterus seems to be larger than dates, hydramnios or unexplained maternal anemia develops, or the pregnancy has occurred following ovulation induction.

Separate gestational sacs can be identified ultrasonically as early as 6 weeks from the first day of the last menstrual period. With transabdominal scanning, an embryo within each sac should be visible by 7 weeks, and beating fetal hearts should be seen by 7.5 to 8 weeks.[35] With good equipment, the fetal cranial pole is also identifiable during this period, but the intracranial landmarks used for accurate biparietal diameter measurements are usually not seen

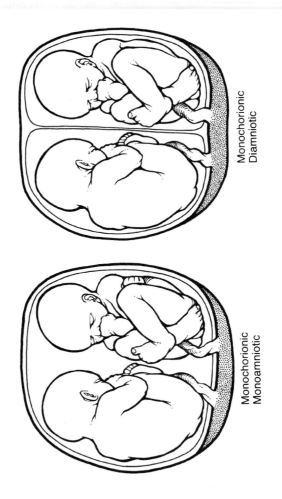

Monochorionic
Diamniotic

Monochorionic
Monoamniotic

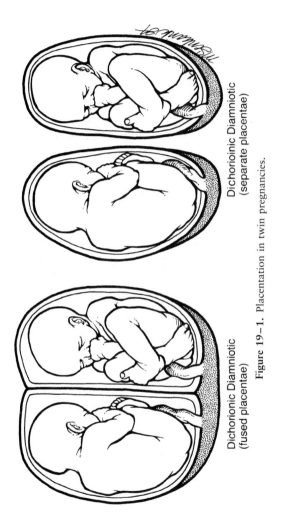

Dichorionic Diamniotic
(fused placentae)

Dichorioinic Diamniotic
(separate placentae)

Figure 19–1. Placentation in twin pregnancies.

until 14 to 16 weeks. Increasing sophistication in the development and use of endovaginal scanning has made it possible to visualize these developmental landmarks 1 to 2 weeks earlier than with abdominal scanning techniques so that the embryonic pole and fetal heart can be seen by 6 weeks and the intracranial landmarks are visible by 10 to 12 weeks' gestation.[36]

It is mandatory to visualize separate fetuses. Retromembranous collections of blood or fluid or a prominent fetal yolk sac should not be confused with a twin gestation. Demonstration of the viability of each fetus at the time of the examination requires visualization of independent cardiac activity. The ultrasonologist must be compulsive in examining the entire uterine cavity. A scan should not be completed until the orientation of all the visualized fetal parts is understood.[37]

EARLY WASTAGE IN MULTIPLE GESTATIONS

The incidence of multiple gestations in humans is higher than is usually appreciated and a significant amount of early wastage occurs. This has led to the concept of the "vanishing twin".

One explanation for the disappearance of a gestational sac is resorption, which has been ultra-sonically described in human multiple gestations between 7 and 12 weeks. Another explanation is the presence of a blighted ovum or anembryonic pregnancy, a gestational sac having a volume of 2.5 ml or more in which no fetus can be identified on ultrasound examination. The only complication of regression of a blighted ovum is slight vaginal bleeding. A coexisting normal pregnancy has a good prognosis for carrying to term.

GROWTH AND DEVELOPMENT

Normal individual twins grow at the same rate as singletons up to 32 weeks' gestation. After that time, they do not gain weight as rapidly as singletons of the same gestational age.[47] Twins' birth weights drop below the mean for singletons by 32 weeks, but remain within the low normal range until the 36th week, after which time they fall progressively below the tenth percentile. Twin birth lengths and head circumferences remain within the low normal range for singletons throughout the entire pregnancy. Alterations in twin growth occur primarily in the third trimester, worsen as gestational age progresses, and are usually asymmetric in nature. Discrepancies in birth weight could be due, in part, to constitutional factors especially in DZ twins. There are also several pathologic situations in which twins may be born with substantial weight differences. These include the twin-to-twin transfusion syndrome, the combination of an anomalous fetus with a normal co-twin, and growth restriction affecting only one twin because of local placental factors.[37] IUGR, on the other hand, can affect both twins relatively equally, in which case they would both be small, but not discordant in size. Charts derived from singleton pregnancies may be reliably used to estimate gestational age of twins. As the difference between twin BPDs increases, the likelihood that the smaller fetus will be growth restricted increases.

Crane et al.[58] defined discordance in utero as an intrapair difference in BPD of 5 mm or more and a fall in BPD below 2 SD for gestational age on their normal twin curve. They suggested that head circumference (HC) be measured if BPD intrapair differences exceed 5 mm. Since HC is less likely to be affected by molding in utero, an intrapair HC difference of less than 5 percent suggests that true discrepancy does not exist.

A survey of multiple parameters on serial ultrasound examinations provides the most accurate assessment of the size of each individual fetus in twin gestations. The highest accuracy for predicting either appropriate or restricted growth is obtained by estimating the fetal weight. Among individual parameters, abdominal circumference is the single most sensitive measurement in predicting both IUGR and growth discordance.[65,66,69,70] An intrapair difference in abdominal circumference measurement of 2 cm or more can be effectively used as a screening test for discordant fetal growth and IUGR in the smaller twin.[66,69,70] However, individual measurements of BPD, HC, or femur length are relatively poor predictors for either IUGR or growth discordance.[65,69,70] We recommend that women with twins be scanned every 3 to 4 weeks after the 26th week.

Ultrasonographic Prediction of Amnionicity and Chorionicity

The incidences of IUGR and fetal death are higher in monochorionic than dichorionic twins, and the twin-to-twin transfusion syndrome (TTS) occurs only in monochorionic twins.

The sonographic prediction of chorionicity and amnionicity should be systematically approached by determining the number of placentas visualized and the sex of each fetus and then by assessing the membranes that divide the sacs. The pregnancy is clearly dichorionic if two separate placental disks are seen or if the twins are of different sex. When a single placenta is present and the twins are of the same sex, careful sonographic examination of the dividing membrane will usually result in a correct diagnosis. Evaluation should be done of three features in the intertwin membrane: (1) thickness of the intertwin membrane, (2) the number of layers visualized in the membrane, and (3) assessment of the junction of the membrane with the placental site the "twin peak" sign.[71] In dichorionic diamniotic pregnancies, the dividing membrane appears "thick"[72–74] and has a measured diameter of greater than or equal to 2 mm,[75] and either three or four layers can often be identified (Fig. 19–2).[76,77] With a monochorionic diamniotic pregnancy, only two layers of membranes will be identified, and the

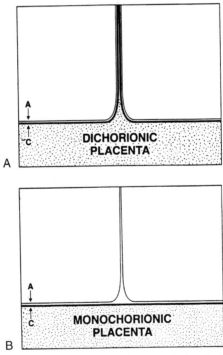

Figure 19–2. In a dichorionic pregnancy with fused placentas, both the amnions (A) and the chorions (C) reflect away from the placental surface at the point of origin of the septum. This creates a potential space in direct continuity with the chorionic villi and into which they can extend. *B,* In a monochorionic twin pregnancy, the septum is formed by reflection of the two amnions away from the placenta. There is a continuous single chorion, which provides an intact barrier, preventing extension of placental villi into the potential interamniotic space.

membrane appears to be "thin and hairlike"[76] A floating monochorionic diamniotic membrane may fold back upon itself and give a false impression of having four layers. Inspection of the membranes near their placental insertion will reduce this artifact. Significant magnification of the image is helpful in counting the number of layers. Determination of membrane thickness allows correct identification of di- or monochorionic gestation in 80 to 90 percent of cases,[71-73] and counting the number of layers can increase the predictive accuracy to almost 100 percent.[76,77]

The twin peak sign which identifies dichorionic pregnancies is a triangular projection of tissue with the same echogenicity as the placenta extending beyond the chorionic surface of the placenta. This tissue is insinuated between the layers of the intertwin membrane, wider at the chorionic surface and tapering to a point at some distance inward from that surface (Fig. 19-2). This space exists only in a dichorionic pregnancy and is produced by reflection of each chorion away from its placenta at the place where it encounters the chorion and placenta of the co-twin. The twin peak sign cannot occur in monochorionic placentation because the single continuous chorion does not extend into the potential interamniotic space of the monochorionic diamniotic twin membrane. The absence of the twin peak sign alone does not guarantee that the pregnancy is monochorionic.

In some pregnancies with monochorionic diamniotic placentation, the dividing membranes may not be sonographically visualized because they are very thin. In other cases they may not be seen because severe oligohydramnios causes them to be closely apposed to the fetus in that sac. This results in a "stuck twin" appearance, where the trapped fetus remains firmly held against the uterine wall despite changes in maternal position.[71] Diagnosis of this condition confirms the presence of a diamniotic gestation. In monoamniotic twins, free movement of both twins and occasionally entanglement of their umbilical cords can be demonstrated.[84]

Doppler Studies in Multiple Gestation

Several studies in singleton pregnancies have demonstrated that abnormal Doppler velocimetry in the umbilical artery (UA) and other fetal vessels is often associated with fetal IUGR, pregnancy complications, and adverse perinatal outcome.[85-88] Although some investigators favor continuous wave systems, we think that Doppler studies in multiple gestations are best performed using a pulsed Doppler duplex system to be certain that the vessel being studied belongs to a targeted fetus.

Umbilical artery S/D ratios in normal twins decrease with advancing gestation the same as in singletons. Umbilical artery S/D ratios in fetuses of a twin gestation can be evaluated as if two singleton fetuses were being assessed.

Abnormal Doppler studies may precede documentation of the IUGR by sonographic biometry or abnormalities in other tests of fetal well-being.[88] Abnormal umbilical artery wave-forms may reflect vascular lesions in the placenta, which can increase resistance to blood flow through the umbilical arteries.[91] An S/D ratio difference of 0.4 or more is a better predictor than ultrasound for birth weight discordancy in the SGA/AGA twin pairs, but is poor in predicting discordant weight in the SGA/SGA, AGA/AGA, or AGA/LGA twin pairs.

While the overall sensitivity of Doppler alone for predicting an SGA fetus is only 58 percent, abnormal Doppler findings precede sonographic diagnosis of SGA by about 3.7 weeks. A combination of sonographic and Doppler parameters improves the sensitivity to 84 percent, suggesting that Doppler velocimetry complements real-time ultrasonography in the early detection of abnormal growth in twin pregnancies.

Our routine for the surveillance of patients with multiple gestations is as follows:

1. Ideally, an initial ultrasound is performed at 10 to 14 weeks' gestation to determine the number of fetuses and the amnionicity/chorionicity.
2. The second ultrasound evaluation is scheduled at 18 to 20 weeks' gestation. This includes standard biometry to confirm gestational age, assessment of amniotic fluid volume in each sac, and an anatomic survey of each fetus to rule out morphologic anomalies. If the patient did not have a first-trimester ultrasound, an attempt is made to determine chorionicity by examining fetal gender, the number of placentas, the thickness as well as number of layers in the membrane separating the sacs, and the presence or absence of the lambda or twin peak sign.
3. If the first two scans are normal and suggestive of a DC/DA twinning, subsequent scans for fetal growth are performed at 24 to 26 weeks and every 3 to 4 weeks thereafter as long as fetal growth and amniotic fluid volume in each sac remains normal.
4. If the initial ultrasound is suggestive of a MC/DA placentation, and therefore a potential risk for developing TTS, subsequent scans are repeated at a minimum of 2-week intervals.
5. If there is evidence of IUGR, discordant fetal growth, or discordant fluid volumes, fetal surveillance is intensified and includes frequent nonstress testing along with biophysical profile and Doppler velocimetry studies.

ABNORMALITIES ASSOCIATED WITH MULTIPLE GESTATION

Twin-to-Twin Transfusion Syndrome

TTS in humans has only been reported in association with mono-chorionic placentas. The potential for the transfusion syndrome occurs when the arterial circulation of one twin is in communication with the venous circulation of the other through arteriovenous shunts. In this situation, one fetus becomes a donor that transfuses its co-twin. The donor becomes anemic and growth restricted. Although occasionally it may become hydropic as a result of high-output failure, more frequently this twin is significantly smaller than the other. The recipient twin, on the other hand, becomes polycythemic and can suffer from congestive heart failure as a result of circulatory overload. The perinatal mortality associated with TTS is as high as 70 percent. Antenatal factors that predict a poor outcome in these pregnancies include (1) an early gestational age at diagnosis with delivery before 28 weeks, (2) severe polyhydramnios requiring multiple therapeutic amniocenteses, (3) fetal hydrops, and (4) absent or reversed diastolic flow on umbilical artery Doppler studies.

When severe, the syndrome usually manifests itself clinically as a result of polyhydramnios that is almost always found to exist in the sac of the larger twin. Sonographic criteria that provide an antenatal diagnosis of TTS include (1) the presence of same-sex twins with a single placenta; (2) thin (two-layer) separating membrane between the sacs; (3) significant discordance in fetal growth; (4) discordant amniotic fluid volume with polyhydramnios in the sac of the larger recipient twin and often a "stuck twin" appearance as a result of oligohydramnios in the sac of the donor twin; and (5) signs of hydrops or cardiac failure in either fetus, more frequently in the larger twin.

When twins of unequal size are discovered on ultrasound examination, it is important to distinguish TTS from a pregnancy in which one fetus is growth restricted but the other is developing normally. In the latter situation the normal twin is usually surrounded by an appropriate quantity of amniotic fluid, and oligohydramnios may or may not be present in the other sac. In TTS, however, the donor is smaller than it should be and not simply smaller than its larger sibling. This latter point may be useful in ruling out a third uncommon situation, namely, that of a normal fetus and a larger hydropic co-twin that is anomalous or erythroblastotic.

Various therapeutic maneuvers have been attempted in an effort to improve pregnancy outcome in severe cases of TTS. These approaches include therapeutic amniocenteses,[102,119-122] laser ablation of vascular anastomoses,[123-125] selective feticide,[126,127] puncture of the intertwin membrane, and maternal treatment with digoxin or indomethacin.[128-130]

Iatrogenic or spontaneous disruption of the intertwin membrane can result in subsequent cord entanglement and fetal death.[134-136] Isolated maternal treatment with either digoxin or indomethacin for TTS has not proven beneficial in improving fetal outcome.[128-130] Selective feticide of one twin in the presence of the placental vascular communications expected in TTS can have devastating consequences, including death of the co-twin or survival with permanent damage.[137] Fetoscopically directed Yttrium-aluminum-garnet (YAG) laser occlusion of placental vascular communications has been reported by a few centers[124,125,132].

Repeated therapeutic amniocenteses provide the best option for treatment until delivery is possible.[119-121] The total number and frequency of amniocenteses must be individualized, since some patients show improvement following one or two procedures, whereas others may require that it be performed far more frequently. The volume of fluid aspirated at any one time should again be individualized, with an aim to removing as much fluid as possible from the polyhydramniotic sac and attaining a relatively "normal" fluid volume.

CONGENITAL ANOMALIES IN MULTIPLE GESTATIONS

Anomalies occur more frequently in twins than in singletons. One series reported a rate of anomalies of 1.4 percent for singletons, 2.7 percent for twins, and 6.1 percent for triplets. Among cases of twins in which anomalies were detected, both twins were affected in 14.8 percent.

Anomalies Related to Twinning

Acardia and conjoined twins are directly related to the twinning process. *Acardia* is a malformation that occurs in one fetus of MZ pregnancies with a frequency of approximately 1 per 30,000 deliveries.[6] These pregnancies always have monochorial placentas and vascular anastomoses that sustain the life of the acardiac twin.

There is also a high incidence of chromosomal abnormalities in these pregnancies. By ultrasound the anomalous twin may appear to be an amorphous mass or may show a wide range of abnormalities. The pump twin, although structurally normal, is at increased risk for in utero cardiac failure, and mortality rates of 50 percent or higher have been reported.[145]

Conjoined twins occur with a frequency of about 1 per 50,000 deliveries and in approximately 1 per 600 twin births.[155–157] Dystocia, may be a frequent and serious complication if vaginal delivery is attempted at term. It is therefore recommended that conjoined twins except craniopagus twins be delivered by cesarean section.[156] If they are considered to have a poor chance of surviving and are small enough to pass through the birth canal without damaging the mother, vaginal delivery might be on option.

DEATH OF ONE TWIN IN UTERO

The death of one twin in utero occurs in 2.2 to 6.8 percent of twins. When only one twin dies in utero, it may become a fetus papyraceous. In that condition, the fluid is resorbed from the dead twin's body, and it is compressed into the adjacent membranes by the growth of the living fetus.

When a dead twin remains undelivered, a legitimate medical concern is the potential for disseminated intravascular coagulation (DIC) in the mother, but this is rare in twins. In selected situations it may be possible to treat the chronic maternal coagulopathy associated with a retained dead twin in order to allow a premature living co-twin to continue to develop in utero. When death in utero of one twin is detected before 34 weeks, conservative management is the wisest course. This should include weekly maternal clotting profiles and serial assessments of fetal growth and well-being. No coagulation disorders have been observed after spontaneous or induced first-trimester death of one or more fetuses in a multiple gestation.

Successful reversal of a consumption coagulopathy within the maternal circulation does not ensure that the surviving fetus will be unaffected by the process. If vascular anastomoses exist within a monochorial placenta, the shared circulation may permit volume and blood pressure changes in the other twin. Cortical necrosis,[186] multicystic encephalomalacia,[187] and other structural abnormalities[188,190] have been reported in liveborn MZ twins with stillborn macerated co-twins. Damage to the survivor occurs far less frequently in the case of DZ twins or MZ twins with dichorionic placentas. There is a 17 percent chance that the surviving twin in a monochorionic gestation will either die or suffer major morbidity.

SELECTIVE TERMINATION OF AN ANOMALOUS FETUS

Intracardiac injection of potassium chloride[199] is the procedure of choice because of its safety and is currently preferred both for selective termination procedures in the second trimester and for elective reduction of fetal numbers in the first trimester.[40-42,139,185,198] Before initiating the procedure, it is critical that the abnormal fetus be correctly identified.

The overall results are excellent, with delivery of a viable infant or infants in over 90 percent of cases. There were no cases of DIC or serious maternal complications.

In considering selective termination of an abnormal twin, particular caution must be exercised to exclude the possibility of a monochorionic gestation. Vascular connections between fetal circulations occur in approximately 70 percent of MZ twins. In this situation, a lethal agent injected into the anomalous twin could enter the circulation of its normal sibling and result in death or permanent damage.[137] This has led perinatologists to attempt to occlude completely the circulation of the anomalous monochorionic twin at the time of the procedure by performing cord ligation with surgical removal of the fetus by hysterotomy[137,202,203] or cord ligation by fetoscopy,[140] use of a helical metal coil,[151] or surgical silk suture soaked in 96 percent ethanol[204] to induce thrombosis.

FIRST-TRIMESTER MULTIFETAL PREGNANCY REDUCTION

The increasingly successful use of ovulatory drugs, in vitro fertilization, and related therapies has resulted in a growing incidence of multifetal pregnancies with three or more fetuses. Because of a high risk of perinatal morbidity and mortality from premature delivery in these pregnancies, first-trimester reduction[36-38] of the number of fetuses has been advocated as a method to improve outcome. The overall loss rate is 9.6 percent, with early premature deliveries (25-28 weeks) occurring in 3.7 percent. The miscarriage and severe preterm delivery rates were related to both the starting and finishing numbers of fetuses. The rates of prematurity, however, correlated directly with the finishing number.

Perinatal morbidity and mortality are likely to improve when pregnancies with four or more fetuses are reduced to smaller numbers. The advantages of reducing triplets to twins remains far more controversial. A first-trimester reduction from three to two fetuses cannot be justified on the basis of improving perinatal mortality. However, a reduction in the morbidity associated with severe prematurity may result from reducing triplets to twins.

PROBLEMS RELATED TO PLACENTATION

Prolapse of the cord and rupture of a vasa previa with fetal exsanguination are more common in twins than in singletons. A velamentous cord insertion occurs in 7 percent of twin placentas as opposed to 1 percent in singletons.

Monoamniotic twins are rare and have a high risk of fetal mortality, with double survival rates of 40 percent.[215] The high fetal mortality associated with a single amniotic sac is due to prematurity, vascular anastomoses in the placenta and, most commonly, entanglement of the umbilical cords which occurs in as many as 70 percent of monoamniotic twins. Inability to visualize a membrane separating two sacs in a twin gestation is suggestive of a monoamniotic pregnancy but is not diagnostic because occasionally the membrane can remain undetected even though it is present. The observation of entangled umbilical cords in the absence of a membrane separating twin fetuses provides a reliable sign for the sonographic diagnosis of monoamniotic twin gestation. It is essential to trace both cords into the entangled mass before making this diagnosis. Another uncommon mishap that can result from this type of placentation is inadvertant clamping of the undelivered twin's cord after delivery of the first twin, such as when a tight cord around the neck of twin A was clamped and divided and then found to belong to twin B. Division of a cord around the first twin's neck should be avoided.

The optimal management of monoamniotic twin pregnancies with respect to timing and route of delivery remains controversial. Because of an impression of increasing morbidity and mortality rates in monoamniotic twins with advancing gestations, prophylactic preterm delivery by 32 to 34 weeks has been advocated to prevent cord-related deaths late in pregnancy.[219] Cesarean delivery is recommended in all viable monoamniotic twin pregnancies.

AMNIOCENTESIS IN MULTIPLE GESTATIONS

When Should Both Sacs Be Tapped?

In some situations, it is obviously necessary to perform amniocentesis on each twin sac. Two series have found a close correlation between lecithin/sphingomyelin (L/S) ratios in amniotic fluid samples from twin sets.

However, the firstborn of triplets and quadruplets have higher pharyngeal L/S ratios and less severe respiratory distress than those of their siblings delivered subsequently.

In patients not in labor at the time of delivery, no significant intrapair differences in L/S ratio are found. In labor, however, there may be a significant increase in the L/S ratio of the presenting twin when compared with its sibling.

In most cases of nonlaboring patients with twins, an L/S ratio from one sac will accurately reflect the status of both fetuses. If one twin appears to be abnormal for any reason, however, or if the patient is in premature labor, both sacs should be tapped to assess pulmonary maturity. Should the operator elect to tap only one sac in these situations, it should be that of the twin who appears to be normal in the former case and that of the second twin in the latter. The stressed twin, or the presenting twin in these two instances, can be assumed to have an L/S ratio at least as mature as that of its sibling.

The Technique of Tapping Multiple Sacs

An amniocentesis needle is introduced into one sac. After some fluid is aspirated, indigo carmine or Evan's blue is injected to serve as a marker, and then the needle is removed. A different needle is then inserted and the aspiration of untinged fluid indicates that the second sac has been successfully entered.

Several points should be stressed:

1. A thorough ultrasound examination should precede the amniocentesis, at which time the viability of all fetuses should be verified and their gestational ages and relative sizes assessed. It is particularly important to note the position of one fetus relative to the other(s) and to label the aspirated fluids appropriately, as well as placing a drawing in the patient's chart so that at a later date it is possible to correlate a particular fetus with its fluid specimen. This becomes critically important in the case of genetic studies if at a later date selective termination of one fetus is to be considered.
2. Direct ultrasonic visualization of the needle tip during its insertion allows for much greater precision in guiding the needle to an optimal sampling site.

Second-trimester amniocentesis in twin pregnancies is not associated with excess pregnancy loss.

The Antepartum Period

No benefit of bed rest in the hospital for a patient carrying twins has been confirmed, and in one study preterm delivery was more common among the hospitalized group.

Bed rest in the hospital is expensive and disrupts normal family life. Since there is no evidence to suggest that elective hospitalization is beneficial for patients with twins, we feel that these women should only be hospitalized for the same indications that would be used to admit women with singletons. Prophylactic administration of tocolytic agents to women with twins has not prevented preterm birth.

Results of studies using prophylactic cervical cerclage in women with multiple gestations have been disappointing.[2] Since this surgical procedure may be associated with adverse sequelae for both the mother and her fetuses, it is recommended that cerclage placement be limited to women with either a strong suggestive history or with objectively documented cervical incompetence.

Ultrasonographic assessment of cervical length, and fetal fibronectin (FFN)—are useful adjuvant tests in the prediction of preterm labor in multiple gestations.[252-255]

Premature cervical shortening on ultrasound has good predictive ability for preterm labor and delivery in patients with multiple gestations. A cervical length measurement of greater than or equal to 35 mm by transvaginal ultrasound at 24 to 26 weeks in twin gestation will identify patients who are at low risk for delivery prior to 34 weeks' gestation. On the other hand, a cervical length of 25 mm or less at 24 to 26 weeks' gestation predicts a high risk for preterm labor and delivery.[253-255] A positive FFN test at 28 weeks is a significant predictor of spontaneous preterm labor prior to 32 weeks' gestation. It would be reasonable to incorporate these two tests (i.e., FFN test and vaginal ultrasound for cervical length at 24 to 28 gestational weeks), as a screening test for all multiple gestations in order to identify those at high risk for preterm delivery before 34 weeks' gestation (see Chapter 18).

Ambulatory home monitoring of uterine contractions with a mobile tocodynamometer has not proven to be of benefit. Nonstress tests in twins, whether reactive or nonreactive, appear to be prognostically comparable to those previously reported in singleton third-trimester pregnancies.

Gonen et al.[22] reported the outcome and follow-up data of 30 multiple gestations (24 triplets, 5 quadruplets, and 1 quintuplet) managed over a 10-year period from 1978 to 1988. In their study, the early neonatal mortality rate was 31.6 per 1,000, late neonatal mortality was 21 per 1,000, and the perinatal mortality was 51.5 per 1,000 live births. The incidence of respiratory distress syndrome was 43 percent, bronchopulmonary dysplasia 6 percent, retinopathy of prematurity 3 percent, intraventricular hemorrhage 4 percent, and cerebral palsy 2 percent. Follow-up of 84 infants for a period of 1 to 10 years showed 75 percent of them to be free from any neurologic or developmental handicap, 22 percent had mild functional delay, one infant was mildly handicapped, and one was moderately handicapped.

Management of multifetal gestations with three or more fetuses can be achieved on an outpatient basis in most cases, but must include intensified surveillance of the mother and fetuses. Our protocol includes (1) modified bed rest at home initiated at 16 weeks' gestation; (2) frequent prenatal visits with cervical assessment for evidence of effacement or dilatation and measurement of cervical length by ultrasound (routine cerclage is not recommended, but is offered to patients with clinical documentation or historical evidence of cervical incompetence); (3) serial ultrasound studies for evaluation of fetal growth; (4) early initiation of weekly nonstress tests at 26 to 28 weeks' gestation; (5) hospitalization for any evidence of preterm labor or other obstetric/medical complications; (6) tocolytic agents and betamethasome restricted to patients with documented preterm labor; and (7) elective cesarean delivery recommended in all cases either at onset of labor near term or at 36 completed weeks' gestation following documentation of lung maturity.

The Intrapartum Period

Intrapartum twin presentations can be classified into three groups: twin A vertex, twin B vertex; (43 percent) twin A vertex, twin B nonvertex; (38 percent) and twin A nonvertex, twin B either vertex or nonvertex (19 percent). When both twins are in vertex presentation, a cesarean delivery should only be performed for the same indications applied to singletons. Currently, cesarean delivery is the method of choice when the presenting twin is in a nonvertex position. If the second twin is in a vertex presentation and faces its sibling, the potential for locking exists. The frequency of locking is approximately 1 per 1,000 twin deliveries, with an associated fetal mortality of 31 percent. This condition occurs most commonly in breech-vertex presentations when the fetal chins overlie each other. It is usually not recognized until the body of the presenting twin is out of the vagina and the aftercoming head cannot be delivered. Eventually it becomes clear that entry of the first twin's head into the pelvis is being obstructed by that of the second twin.

In external cephalic versions performed on transverse and breech malpositioned second twins,[269] version to vertex presentation is successful in 46 to 73 percent of cases. External version is associated with a higher failure rate than breech extraction, and also a higher rate of fetal distress, cord prolapse, and compound presentation.

We currently feel that elective cesarean delivery is the safest mode for triplets or higher order multiple pregrancies.

TIME INTERVAL BETWEEN DELIVERIES

Another variable important in the outcome of twin pregnancies is the time interval between their deliveries. After delivery of the first twin, uterine inertia may develop, the second twin's cord can prolapse, and partial separation of its placenta may render the second twin hypoxic. In addition, the cervix can clamp down, making rapid delivery of the second twin extremely difficult if fetal distress develops. The interval between deliveries should ideally be within 15 minutes and certainly not more than 30 minutes,[6,13,30,285,286] although these data were obtained before the advent of intrapartum fetal monitoring. While some second twins may require rapid delivery, others can be safely followed with fetal heart rate surveillance beyond 30 minutes and remain undelivered for substantial periods of time. This less hurried approach when twin B is not in distress may reduce the incidence of both maternal and fetal trauma associated with difficult deliveries performed to meet arbitrary deadlines.

There are obviously situations in which expeditious delivery of the second twin is desirable shortly after the birth of the first, but this is not always the case. The total number of reported cases in which delayed delivery of the retained twin, triplets, or quadruplets has been attempted are limited. The goal was to delay delivery of very premature infants to allow more maturation. A management protocol for these patients includes high ligation of the umbilical cord of the delivered twin with an absorbable suture, prophylactic use of tocolytics, bed rest, ongoing monitoring of the patient for evidence of infection and/or coagulation disorders, and serial monitoring for growth and well-being of the viable fetus(es). Three areas that still remain controversial are the routine use of cervical cerclage, prophylactic antibiotics, and corticosteriods for enhancement of fetal lung maturity of the viable fetus(es). This type of management, however, should not be considered "standard of care."

ULTRASOUND AND THE INTRAPARTUM MANAGEMENT OF MULTIPLE GESTATIONS

Ultrasound can also be useful during labor and delivery. On admission to the delivery floor, the position and sizes of each twin can be quickly and accurately assessed. It is also possible to rule out extension of the head when a fetus is in breech presentation. There is an incidence of more than 70 percent for spinal cord transection when breeches with extended heads are delivered vaginally compared with no cord injuries when infants with extended heads are delivered by cesarean section.

When a patient with twins or triplets is taken to the delivery room, the real-time scanner should accompany her. After delivery of the first infant, real-time examination immediately and precisely establishes the position of the second fetus. Visualization of the fetal heart allows the second fetus to be monitored for evidence of bradycardia until one fetal pole settles into the pelvis, membranes are ruptured, and a scalp electrode is applied.

In addition to monitoring heart rate, visualization of the second twin permits both external and internal manipulations to be performed in a more controlled fashion. Externally, it is often possible to guide the vertex over the inlet by directing pressure from the ultrasound transducer over the fetal head while pushing the buttocks toward the fundus with the other hand.[294] If this is unsuccessful, an internal version can be made less difficult by visualizing the operator's hand within the uterus and directing it toward the fetal feet.

Key Points

- ➤ Perinatal/neonatal morbidity and mortality are significantly higher in multiple gestations than singleton pregnancies.

- ➤ Any patient with a multiple gestation should be clinically managed as a high-risk pregnancy.

- ➤ The incidence of congenital structural malformations is two to three times higher in fetuses of multiple gestations when compared with those of singleton gestations.

- ➤ Ultrasound evaluation is the single most important diagnostic test in multiple gestations.

- ➤ All patients with multiple gestations should have a thorough first- and second-trimester ultrasound examination to assess for chorionicity, amnionicity, individual fetal growth, and congenital malformations.

- ➤ Twin-to-twin transfusion syndrome is a serious potential complication in monozygotic twins, with a high fetal mortality rate.

Box continued on following page

Key Points *Continued*

➤ Prophylactic cerclage, tocolytics, or hospitalization for bed rest do not have any proven advantage in the management of multiple gestations.

➤ In twin pregnancies with discordant growth, fetal lung maturity studies obtained from amniotic fluid of the larger twin will usually also represent similar or greater lung maturity of the smaller twin.

➤ The presentation of each fetus must be sonographically verified as soon as a patient with twin pregnancy presents in labor.

➤ As a general rule, mode of delivery should be vaginal when both twins are vertex, individualized for vertex-nonvertex twins, and cesarean section when the first twin is nonvertex. For triplets or more, the safest mode of delivery is by cesarean section.

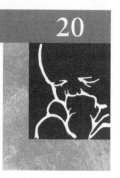

20

Intrauterine Growth Restriction

IRA BERNSTEIN, STEVEN G. GABBE,
AND KATHRYN L. REED

Intrauterine growth restriction (IUGR) is the second leading contributor to the perinatal mortality rate.[1] The perinatal mortality rate for these infants is 6 to 10 times greater than that for a normally grown population, 120 per 1,000 for all cases of growth restriction and 60 to 80 per 1,000 if anomalous infants are excluded. As many as 40 percent of all stillborns are growth restricted.[63] This includes 53 percent of preterm stillbirths and 26 percent of term stillbirths. The incidence of intrapartum asphyxia in cases complicated by IUGR has been reported to be 50 percent.[2] A portion of these perinatal complications are preventable. If the growth-restricted fetus is appropriately identified and managed, the perinatal mortality can be lowered.

DEFINITION

A commonly used classification has developed that reserves the obstetric label of IUGR for the fetus who suffers morbidity and/or mortality associated with the failure to reach growth potential (Fig. 20–1) and the pediatric term "small for gestational age" as the more general term for the small fetus for whom no pathology is identified. For the purposes of this chapter, we have chosen the terms "fetal" or "intrauterine growth restriction" and apply the label in the prenatal period based on estimates of fetal size alone. We believe that this term appropriately characterizes the syndrome and eliminates the negative cognitive associations of the term "retardation."

Ultrasound criteria have emerged as the diagnostic standard used in the identification of fetal growth restriction. Two patterns of altered head growth were originally described. In "late flattening," which represents approximately two thirds of all cases of IUGR, the biparietal diameter (BPD) increases normally until late pregnancy and then lags behind. In the "low-profile" or symmetric type,

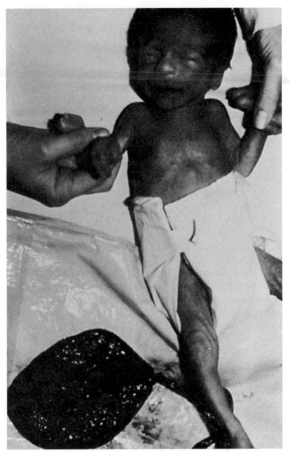

Figure 20–1. A growth-restricted infant exhibiting subcutaneous wasting.

impaired head growth occurs much earlier in gestation. These abnormal growth patterns were later labeled types 1 (late flattening) and 2 (low profile), and these concepts would become generalized to describe asymmetric and symmetric growth deficiencies, respectively.

As an individual parameter, abdominal circumference (AC) has demonstrated the greatest sensitivity in the identification of the small child. The use of AC, a directly measurable fetal parameter, in combination with head circumference has been widely adopted. The most common assessment of fetal size in the United States is the estimation of fetal weight. Investigators have identified distinct fetal parameters identifiable by ultrasound that are useful in the estimation of fetal size.[13-15] All of the techniques incorporate an index of abdominal size as a variable contributing to the estimation of fetal weight. These techniques generally have 95 percent confidence limits that deviate approximately 15 percent around the actual value.

An absolute threshold used for the definition of growth restriction can be applied to any of the parameters evaluated (BPD, AC, or estimated fetal weight [EFW]). Birth weight below the population 10th percentile, corrected for gestational age, has been the most widely used criterion for defining growth restriction at birth, and this has been generalized to imply a sonographically estimated fetal weight below the 10th percentile for appropriate population-based cross-sectional growth charts.

Using the birth weight 10th percentile cutoff, approximately 70 percent of the infants thus identified as growth restricted are normally or constitutionally small, so-called light for gestational age or small for gestational age (SGA).[17] These neonates are *not* at increased risk for poor outcome, but represent one end of the spectrum of normal neonatal size. The remaining 30 percent of this group, does include infants who are truly growth restricted and who are at risk for increased perinatal morbidity and mortality.

ETIOLOGY

Etiologies for fetal growth restriction can be crudely separated into fetoplacental and maternal in origin (see the boxes "Fetoplacental Etiologies of Fetal Growth Retardation" and "Risk Factors for Fetal Growth Restriction"). The fetoplacental origins of growth restriction include those etiologies that have been traditionally ascribed to the fetus, including the chromosomal abnormalities, the genetic syndromes, and the infectious etiologies, as well as those secondary to placental abnormalities.

Fetoplacental Origins

Intrauterine infection, though long recognized as a cause of growth restriction, accounts for less than 10 percent of all cases. Herpes, cytomegalovirus, rubella, and toxoplasmosis are well documented, and other intrauterine infections are strongly suspected (see Chapter 25). The infectious process produces early disruption of fetal growth during the stage of cell hyperplasia and is, therefore, associated with a poor prognosis for normal development. For the agents associated with IUGR, prevention of the infection is the most important therapy.

Ectoplacental Etiologies of Fetal Growth Retardation

Chromosomal abnormalities
    Trisomies (13, 18, 21)
    Trisomy 9 mosaicism
    Trisomy 4p
    4p-, 5p-, 11p-, 13q- syndromes
    Partial trisomy 10q

Genetic syndromes
    Cretinism (hypothyroidism)
    Russell-Silver
    Bloom's
    Lowe's
    De Lange's
    Progeria
    Leprechaunism

Congenital malformations
Infectious diseases
    Cytomegalovirus
    Toxoplasmosis
    Rubella

Placental pathology
    Previa
    Abruption
    Circumvallate
    Mosaicism
    Infarctions
    Twins

Chromosomal abnormalities, congenital malformations, and genetic syndromes have been associated with less than 10 percent of cases of IUGR. Abnormalities in cell replication and reduced cell number produce a pattern of impaired growth that is early in onset and symmetric. Neonatal prognosis in these cases is determined by the specific abnormality identified.

An absolute or relative decrease in placental mass affects the quantity of substrate the fetus receives and has been recognized ultrasonographically to antedate fetal growth restriction. Thus, a circumvallate placenta, partial placental abruption, placenta accreta, placental infarction, or hemangioma may result in growth restriction. An elevated maternal serum α-fetoprotein (MSAFP) or human chorionic gonadotropin (hCG) level in the second trimester has been associated with an increased risk for IUGR and may result from abnormal placentation.[21-24] Intrinsic placental pathology has

Risk Factors for Fetal Growth Restriction: Indications for Ultrasound

History of fetal growth restriction
Hypertension
Diabetes mellitus
Elevated MSAFP/hCG
Antiphospholipid syndrome
Chronic medical illnesses
Low maternal prepregnancy weight (<90% IBW)
Poor maternal weight gain
Twin gestation
Substance abuse (tobacco, alcohol, drugs)
Preterm labor
Abnormalities of placentation
Vaginal bleeding
Maternal anemia (Hgb < 10)
Maternal hypoxia (cyanotic cardiac or pulmonary disease, altitude)
Maternal hemoglobinopathies
Drug ingestion (hydantoin, coumarin)

been identified in some cases of growth restriction, including the presence of a single umbilical artery or the presence of placental mosaicism, either of which may act to impair normal fetoplacental exchange mechanisms.[26] Placental location has also been linked to growth restriction. Placenta previa without bleeding has been suggested as a risk factor, because the low implantation site may not be optimal for nutrient transfer.[27]

Twin gestation is often associated with IUGR as confirmed by an incidence of 17.5 percent in one study (see Chapter 19).[29] This finding implies relative placental insufficiency as opposed to intrinsic fetal compromise and suggests that the longer the twin pregnancy continues, the greater the delay in intrauterine growth, with "catch-up" growth.

Maternal Origins

Decreased uteroplacental blood flow with its associated reduction in transfer of nutrients to the fetus is responsible for the majority of clinically recognized cases of IUGR. Maternal vascular disease, whether chronic hypertension, preeclampsia, or diabetes with vasculopathy, has been associated with impaired fetal growth. Preeclampsia is generally marked by asymmetric IUGR with maintenance of normal fetal head growth and reduction in the size of the fetal liver, heart, thymus, spleen, pancreas, and adrenal glands.

Poor maternal weight gain has long been recognized as a risk factor for growth restriction. Maternal prepregnancy weight and weight gain in pregnancy are two of the most important variables contributing to birth weight.

Maternal drug ingestion may result in IUGR by a direct effect on fetal growth as well as through inadequate dietary intake. Smoking produces a symmetrically smaller fetus through reduced uterine blood flow and impaired fetal oxygenation and is a major cause of growth restriction in developed countries. The consumption of alcohol and the use of coumarin or hydantoin derivatives are now well known to produce particular dysmorphic features in association with impaired fetal growth. Maternal use of cocaine has been associated with not only IUGR but also reduced head circumference growth.[46]

A history of poor pregnancy outcome is clearly correlated with the subsequent delivery of a growth-restricted infant. Prior birth of an IUGR infant is the obstetric factor most often associated with the subsequent birth of a growth-restricted infant. Women whose first pregnancy results in a growth-restricted infant have a one in four risk of delivering a second infant below the 10th percentile. After two pregnancies complicated by IUGR, there is a fourfold increase in the risk of a subsequent growth-restricted infant.[52] When all indices of risk have been applied, the one third of the population considered at highest risk accounts for two thirds of the infants identified as growth restricted. Two thirds of pregnancies, although not judged to be "at risk" for IUGR, yield one third of neonates below the 10th percentile.[49] Most of these babies are constitutionally small.

In summary, á framework does exist for considering the causes of growth restriction. Is the fetus abnormal? Is the delivery system disrupted? Is the maternal supply line compromised? These questions categorize the source of the problem without explaining the mechanism by which the growth process is disturbed.

DIAGNOSIS

In the past, clinical parameters such as maternal weight gain and measurement of fundal height were used to reflect fetal growth. Curvilinear fundal height measurements in centimeters from the symphysis pubis can be correlated with gestational age: a lag of 4 cm or more suggests growth restriction. However, studies have confirmed the lack of sensitivity of fundal height measurements for detecting fetal growth restriction. The presence of risk factors should therefore prompt ultrasound estimation of fetal size independent of maternal weight gain or fundal height growth.

Fetal Measurements

The use of fetal weight has been the most common method for characterizing fetal size and thereby growth abnormalities. An accurate sonographic estimate of fetal weight is essential in detecting and follow patients suspected of having a growth-restricted infant.[55]

Fetal growth as opposed to fetal size is a dynamic process and requires more than a single evaluation for its estimation. The absence of fetal growth over a sustained period is a concern. The routine clinical evaluation of fetal growth is based on fundal height enlargement during the course of pregnancy. In pregnancies at risk or in those in whom fetal size is already estimated to be below the 10th percentile, serial ultrasound estimations of fetal size are performed. The recommended interval between evaluations is 3 weeks, as shorter intervals increase the likelihood of a false-positive diagnosis.[65,66]

In an attempt to increase detection of the fetus with asymmetric growth restriction, head circumference (HC)/AC ratios can be assessed (Figs. 20–2 and 20–3).[69,70] In the normally growing fetus, the HC/AC ratio exceeds 1.0 before 32 weeks' gestation, is approximately 1.0 at 32 to 34 weeks' gestation, and falls below 1.0 after 34 weeks' gestation. In fetuses affected by asymmetric growth restriction, the HC remains larger than that of the body (Fig. 20–2). The HC/AC ratio is then elevated. In symmetric IUGR, both the HC and the AC are reduced, and the HC/AC ratio remains normal (Fig. 20–3). Using the HC/AC ratio, 85 percent of growth-restricted fetuses are detected, with a reduction in false-negative diagnoses.

In some cases, measurement of the HC may be difficult as a result of fetal position. One can then compare the FL, which is relatively spared in asymmetric IUGR, to the AC.[71] The FL/AC is 22 at all gestational ages from 21 weeks to term and so can be applied without knowledge of the number of weeks gestation. An FL/AC ratio greater than 23.5 suggests IUGR.

In summary, the ability to determine appropriate fetal growth using fundal height measurements in a normal population is limited. Fundal height measurements lack both sensitivity and specificity in the identification of the small fetus. It is therefore reasonable to use ultrasound whenever clinical circumstances point to an increased risk for a growth-restricted fetus. A number of clinical conditions that increase the risk for a small child were listed earlier. In the absence of routine clinical indications,

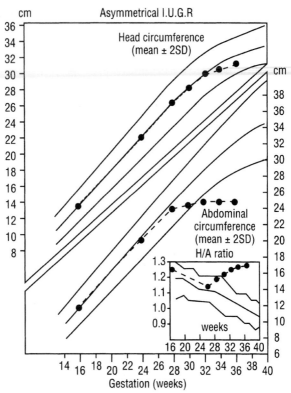

Figure 20–2. Growth chart in a case of asymmetric IUGR. Although head circumference is preserved, AC growth falls off early in the third trimester. For this reason, the H/A ratio shown in the lower right corner of the graph becomes elevated. IUGR, intrauterine growth restriction. (From Chudleigh P, Pearce JM: Obstetric Ultrasound. Edinburgh, Churchill Livingstone, 1986, with permission.)

ultrasound screening of these high-risk pregnancies should be performed at 16 to 18 weeks for dating (if not otherwise established) and again at 32 to 34 weeks.

Oligohydramnios

Decreased amniotic fluid volume has been associated clinically with IUGR and may be the earliest sign detected on ultrasonography,

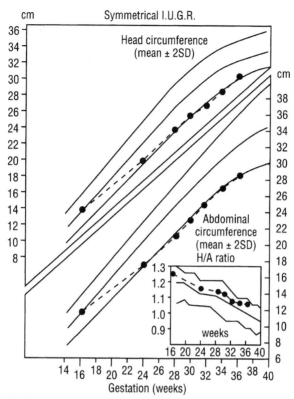

Figure 20–3. Growth chart in a case of symmetric IUGR. Note the early onset of both HC and AC growth restriction. For this reason, the H/A ratio shown in the lower right corner remains normal. IUGR, intrauterine growth restriction. (From Chudleigh P, Pearce JM: Obstetric Ultrasound. Edinburgh, Churchill Livingstone, 1986, with permission.)

preceding an elevation in HC/AC ratio and lagging fetal growth. Decreased perfusion of the fetal kidneys and reduced urine production explain this observation.[72]

The patient with an uncertain gestational age who presents late in pregnancy poses a difficult diagnostic dilemma because interpretation of BPD and HC/AC ratios must be related to accurate gestational age. Under these conditions, measuring an amniotic fluid pocket, or an FL/AC ratio, may be helpful, as these do not rely on knowledge of the gestational age. A 2-cm vertical pocket is considered normal, 1 to 2 cm marginal, and less than 1 cm decreased.

One may also use the amniotic fluid index to quantitate amniotic fluid volume (see Chapter 5), although this technique requires a knowledge of gestational age.

MANAGEMENT

In developing a plan for the management of suspected growth restriction, it is important to remember the major etiologic groups. Most infants thought to be growth restricted are constitutionally small and require no intervention. Approximately 15 percent exhibit symmetric growth restriction attributable to an early fetal insult for which there is no effective therapy. Here, an accurate diagnosis is essential. Finally, approximately 15 percent have growth restriction or extrinsic growth failure because of placental disease or reduced uteroplacental blood flow. In such cases, antepartum fetal monitoring and carefully timed delivery may be critical.

Once growth restriction is suspected, a well-organized approach to management should be undertaken. The clinician should evaluate and treat problems that may be contributing to growth restriction. Therapy of growth restriction is often nonspecific but should be directed at the underlying cause of poor fetal growth if one can be determined. When a maternal medical problem such as inflammatory bowel disease is contributing to poor growth, specific therapy should be instituted. Alleviation of hypoxia, therapy of high blood pressure and anemia, and hyperalimentation are three examples. Certainly, mothers should be counseled to stop smoking and ingesting alcohol. Nonspecific therapies include bed rest in the left lateral decubitus position to increase placental blood flow. Although an inadequate diet has not been clearly established as a cause of growth restriction in this country, dietary supplementation may be helpful in those with poor weight gain or low prepregnancy weight.

Antepartum Evaluation

Fetal Growth

Serial evaluations of fetal growth should be instituted as soon as the diagnosis of growth restriction is confirmed or for patients in whom the suspicion for growth restriction is high. Ultrasound examinations should be scheduled every 3 to 4 weeks and should include determinations of the BPD, HC/AC, fetal weight, and amniotic fluid volume. Arrested head growth is of great concern, especially in light of the most recent data available on ultimate developmental potential for the growth-restricted infant. Clear documentation of arrested head growth over a 4-week period is alarming, and the feasibility and safety of delivery should be reviewed.[110]

Ultrasound should be used not only to document abnormal growth but also to detect lethal congenital malformations such as renal agenesis. In cases of severe symmetric growth restriction, amniocentesis, placental biopsy, or cordocentesis should be considered to rule out a chromosomal abnormality such as trisomy 13, 18, or 21.[19]

Fetal Well-Being

Fetal well-being should also be assessed regularly once the diagnosis of growth restriction is entertained. These infants have an increased incidence of intrauterine demise, presumably from cord compression as well as placental insufficiency. Monitoring these infants decreases the stillbirth rate by detecting the compromised fetus and allowing timely intervention.

Experience with the nonstress test (NST) in cases of growth restriction has confirmed that a reactive NST correlates highly with a fetus that is not in immediate danger of intrauterine demise. Twice-weekly nonstress testing is an appropriate interval.[111] The appearance of spontaneous decelerations during the NST may reflect oligohydramnios and cord compression and has been associated with a high perinatal mortality rate.[113] The addition of a measure of amniotic fluid volume to the NST has been called a "modified biophysical profile." When compared with a weekly contraction stress test, the twice-weekly modified biophysical profile results in similar perinatal outcome.[114] An assessment of amniotic fluid volume at least weekly is advised in cases of suspected IUGR.

Nonreactive NST results are often falsely positive and should be further evaluated before any management decision is made. Contraction stress testing (CST) is one option for additional testing. A negative CST result, even when the CST is performed early in the third trimester, is an indication of adequate placental respiratory reserve.[115] Conversely, positive CST results occur in 30 percent of the pregnancies complicated by proven growth restriction. Information from antepartum fetal heart rate testing must always be reviewed in concert with the gestational age of the fetus, as well as other indices of fetal well-being and fetal growth.

The fetal biophysical profile score can provide appropriate follow-up to nonreassuring fetal heart rate testing or can be used as an alternative method for primary antenatal surveillance. Several studies have demonstrated good correlation between these test results and the level of fetal acidemia as determined by percutaneous umbilical blood sampling in the growth-restricted fetus without anomalies.[118,119] As a backup test for nonreassuring fetal heart rate testing the biophysical profile leads to lower rates of intervention when compared with the CST, with no impact on perinatal outcome.[121]

Maternal monitoring of fetal activity has been used extensively for the assessment of pregnancies complicated by IUGR. In a study of 50 cases. The techniques available for monitoring fetal movement are reviewed in Chapter 7.

Doppler flow studies of the fetal circulation have been used to identify and manage the fetus with suspected growth restriction. Doppler studies of fetal internal carotid and intracerebral arterial blood flow have shown a decrease in pulsatility index in these vessels in fetuses with IUGR.[123,124] The mechanism would be consistent with an increase in blood flow that results from vasodilation in response to hypoxia. Renal and aortic blood flow velocity waveforms show evidence of increased pulsatility indices, consistent with increases in resistance.[125,126] These findings have confirmed some of the basic fetal responses to growth restriction, including the preservation of brain growth and oligohydramnios observed in asymmetric IUGR.

The major focus of Doppler studies for the assessment of fetal health has been the umbilical circulation. The association between an increase in Doppler blood flow indices in the umbilical artery and increased resistance in the placental circulation has been demonstrated by many investigators. The small arterial vessel count in the tertiary stem villi of the placenta is significantly lower in patients with high umbilical artery S/D ratios than in those with normal S/D ratios. Therefore, the increased resistance to flow indicated by a high S/D ratio appears to be associated with a failure to develop, or an obliteration, of the small muscular arteries in the tertiary stem villi.

Absent or reversed end-diastolic velocity in the umbilical artery has repeatedly been associated with poor perinatal outcome (see Chapter 7). In 904 fetuses with absent or reversed end-diastolic flow velocities in the umbilical artery,[136] eighty percent were growth-restricted, and the perinatal mortality was 36 percent. The time between the discovery of the absence of end-diastolic blood flow in the umbilical artery and an indication for delivery, such as abnormal fetal heart rate testing, averaged 6 to 8 days and ranged from 0 to 49 days.

Fetuses with absent end-diastolic umbilical flow velocity should undergo intensive antenatal surveillance at a level greater than that usually provided for the small fetus. Reversed end-diastolic flow in the umbilical artery reflects severe fetal compromise and is an ominous finding. Fetuses with this finding should be monitored immediately, and delivery should be considered.

In summary, Doppler velocimetry of fetal vessels has improved our understanding of the pathophysiology of fetal growth restriction.

Weekly evaluation of umbilical artery Doppler velocimetry has been used in combination with the modified biophysical profile in fetuses exhibiting poor growth. A small fetus with normal umbilical artery Doppler studies is probably constitutionally small and is at low risk for morbidity. However, a small fetus with abnormal umbilical artery waveforms is at greater risk for neonatal morbidity and mortality.[66,140] In controlled trials, the use of fetal Doppler waveform analysis has been associated with improved perinatal outcome.

Timing of Delivery

Proper timing of delivery is often the critical management issue when dealing with the growth-restricted fetus. The crux of management is to balance the hazards of prematurity with the threat of intrauterine demise. Careful consideration should be given to the reliability of the information on which the gestational age of the fetus has been established, the fetal growth curve, and the results of antepartum fetal monitoring.

Amniocentesis may be an important adjunct to this decision-making process. The lecithin/sphingomyelin (L/S) ratio may also provide information that allows more accurate dating of the pregnancy. A surprisingly low L/S ratio would suggest an earlier gestational age rather than fetal growth restriction. In cases of symmetric growth restriction, a late amniocentesis may also be used to obtain amniotic fluid for a fetal karyotype.

To review, if growth restriction is suspected or anticipated, appropriate fetal testing and daily maternal assessment of fetal activity should be instituted. Ultrasound examinations to assess fetal growth should be scheduled every 3 weeks. As long as studies show continued fetal head growth and test results remain reassuring, no intervention is required. If the patient fails a primary surveillance tool such as the NST or fetal Doppler surveillance, follow-up evaluation may be appropriate. If the CST result is positive, or the fetal biophysical profile score is either 6 with oligohydramnios or 4 or less or reversed end-diastolic flow is observed, delivery should be considered. An assessment of fetal lung maturity should be made if possible. In the face of a mature L/S ratio and ominous antepartum test results, delivery should be effected. If the patient has an immature L/S ratio and abnormal test findings, then consideration can be given to corticosteroid administration with continuous heart rate monitoring and oxygen supplementation until delivery or until antepartum test results improve. If amniotic fluid cannot be obtained for an L/S ratio as a result of oligohydramnios and the clinical picture supports the diagnosis of severe IUGR, early delivery should be considered. In these difficult cases, the pediatricians who will care for the baby should be included in the decision making process.

Because a large proportion of growth-restricted infants suffer intrapartum asphyxia, intrapartum management demands continuous fetal heart rate monitoring. During labor, a tracing without late decelerations is predictive of a good outcome in cases complicated by IUGR. However, with late decelerations, the incidence of asphyxia in growth-restricted infants is far greater than in normally grown infants. Therefore, earlier intervention may be indicated.[150] As many growth-restricted fetuses require preterm delivery, an unfavorable cervix is not uncommon. The presence of IUGR has been considered a relative contraindication to the use of prostaglandin for cervical preparation by some authors.[151] An unfavorable cervix may also preclude internal fetal heart rate monitoring. In the face of an inadequate external tracing, cesarean delivery may be necessary.

NEONATAL OUTCOME

Immediate Morbidity

Neonatal morbidity must be anticipated when the growth-restricted fetus is delivered. These infants suffer more frequently from meconium aspiration than do appropriately grown infants. At delivery, careful suctioning of the nasopharynx and oropharynx with the DeLee catheter decreases the incidence of this complication.[159] Further clearing of the airway can be accomplished at delivery by direct laryngoscopy and aspiration by an experienced pediatrician. Because immediate attention to the many neonatal problems experienced by these infants is essential, appropriate pediatric support should be present in the delivery room when an infant suspected of being growth restricted is to be delivered.

Hypoglycemia is a frequent problem in growth-restricted infants, a result of both inadequate glycogen reserves secondary to intrauterine malnutrition and a gluconeogenic pathway that is less responsive to hypoglycemia than that of the normally grown infant.[160] Hypoglycemia should be anticipated in all growth-restricted infants and frequent blood glucose monitoring instituted. Hypocalcemia, another well-recognized problem in growth-restricted babies, may be caused by relative hypoparathyroidism, a result of acidosis associated with intrauterine asphyxia.[161] Frequent calcium monitoring is essential, as symptoms are nonspecific and similar to those associated with hypoglycemia.

Polycythemia is observed three to four times more frequently in the growth-restricted infant than in weight-matched controls. Polycythemia results from hypoxia, which leads to increased production of red blood cells, and from transfer of blood volume from the placental circulation to the fetal circulation in the face of intrauterine asphyxia.[160] Polycythemia leads to increased red blood cell breakdown, accounting in part for the high incidence of hyperbilirubinemia in these infants. Polycythemia is a criterion for, but does not necessarily lead to, hyperviscosity, which can result in capillary bed sludging and thrombosis. Multiple organ systems can be affected, leading to pulmonary hypertension, cerebral infarction, and necrotizing enterocolitis.

Hypothermia, another common problem for the growth-restricted infant, results from decreased body fat stores secondary to intrauterine malnourishment.[160] If unrecognized and untreated, hypothermia can contribute to the metabolic deterioration of an already unstable growth-restricted infant.

Long-Term Morbidity

Have improvements in obstetric and pediatric care favorably affected the outcome of the growth-restricted infant? The perinatal mortality rate for those infants who receive optimal intrapartum and neonatal management is decreased when compared with that for age-matched controls who did not have intensive care.[162] The ultimate growth potential for growth-restricted infants appears to be good. The degree of catch-up growth observed in several longitudinal studies suggests that these infants can be expected to have normal growth curves and normal albeit slightly reduced size as adults. In general, those infants suffering growth restriction near the time of delivery do tend to catch up. However, those neonates with earlier onset and more longstanding growth restriction in utero continue to lag behind.

Neurologic outcome depends on the degree of growth restriction, especially the impact on head growth, its time of onset, the gestational age of the infant at birth, and the postnatal environment. An early intrauterine insult, between 10 and 17 weeks' gestation, could limit neuronal cellular multiplication and would obviously have a profound effect on neurologic function.[172] In the third trimester, brain development is characterized by glial multiplication, dendritic arborization, establishment of synaptic connections, and myelinization, all of which continue during the first 2 years of life. Recovery after a period of impaired growth in the third trimester is, therefore, more likely to occur. Thus, the preterm appropriately grown infant has more normal neurologic development and fewer severe neurologic deficits than its preterm growth-restricted counterpart. Developmental milestones and neurologic development of mature infants with IUGR and mature infants of normal birth weight are similar. Presumably, this also reflects heightened physician awareness of the growth-restricted infant that allows detection, appropriate antepartum management, intrapartum therapy, and early pediatric intervention. The premature growth-restricted infant suffers from increased susceptibility to intrauterine asphyxia and all of the neonatal complications of the premature, as well as those of the infant with IUGR. If growth restriction is associated with lagging head growth before 26 weeks, even mature infants have significant developmental delay at 4 years of age.[173]

There has been significant interest in the hypothesis that diseases commonly associated with adulthood may have their origins during fetal life, the "Barker Hypothesis." Dr. David Barker, an epidemiologist from Southampton, England, first proposed that intrauterine conditions could program the development of the cardiovascular system later in life.[174] Examining birth records that included not only the infant's birth weight but its birth length, abdominal and head circumference measurements, and placental weight, he and his colleagues found that infants with a birth weight of less than 5.5 lb had a threefold increase in death attributable to coronary artery disease later in life.[175] The risks for stroke and hypertension were also greater. The infants at greatest risk were those who not only were low birth weight but had a smaller head circumference, were shorter, and had an increased placenta/birth weight ratio.

Epidemiologic data support a link between IUGR, low birth weight and an increased risk of developing cardiovascular disease, abdominal obesity, type 2 diabetes mellitus, and hyperlipidemia.[176–179] Proposed mechanisms for this association include congenital pancreatic deficiency, which manifests in later life as insulin resistance,[180,181] as well as alterations in sympathetic nervous activity[182] or adrenocortical function.[183–185]

Key Points

➤ Fetal growth restriction is a major cause of perinatal morbidity and mortality. Intrauterine growth restriction is currently defined by fetal size alone.

➤ Characterization of fetal size should be performed using growth curves that are population specific and appropriate.

➤ The definition of fetal growth restriction has not been based on correlations with short- and long-term morbidity.

➤ Preterm delivery is associated with an increased incidence of fetal growth restriction.

➤ Fundal height measurements have low sensitivity in the identification of fetal growth restriction.

Box continued on opposite page

Key Points *Continued*

➤ Mortality resulting from fetal growth restriction can be reduced with appropriate antenatal surveillance strategies, which may include early delivery.

➤ Low-dose aspirin therapy can prevent recurrent IUGR.

➤ The use of fetal umbilical Doppler flow studies in the management of the growth-restricted fetus reduces perinatal morbidity and mortality.

➤ Fetal growth restriction is associated with high rates of intrapartum asphyxia.

➤ Intrauterine growth restriction can result in both short-term and lifelong morbidities.

Prolonged Pregnancy

MICHAEL Y. DIVON

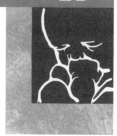

In 1902, Ballantyne questioned the ability of the placenta to support the fetus that "has stayed too long in intrauterine surroundings."[1] In 1954, Clifford recognized that prolonged pregnancy could result in fetal growth restriction when he described the "postmaturity with placental dysfunction syndrome."[2] Clifford suggested that these neonates appeared malnourished due to recent weight loss with loose, peeling skin and meconium staining. Birth asphyxia, meconium aspiration, and perinatal death were reported in severe cases.

In the 1970s that it became apparent that perinatal mortality was significantly increased in prolonged pregnancies, and that fetal surveillance combined with selective use of induction of labor might result in improved perinatal outcome.

DEFINITION

The standard definition of a prolonged pregnancy is 42 completed weeks of gestation (i.e., 294 days after the first day of the last menstrual period [LMP] or more). This definition is endorsed by the American College of Obstetricians and Gynecologists (ACOG), The World Health Organization (WHO), and the International Federation of Gynecology and Obstetrics (FIGO).[3–5] It is based on data derived prior to the widespread use of fetal surveillance modalities and the use of ultrasound for pregnancy dating. In view of more recent perinatal mortality data that were derived from accurately dated pregnancies, it would be reasonable to conclude that prolonged pregnancy should be defined as a gestational age at birth of greater than or equal to 41 weeks of gestation (see section Perinatal Morbidity and Mortality, below).

The incidence of prolonged pregnancy varies depending on the criteria used to define gestational age at birth. It is estimated that 4 to 19 percent of pregnancies reach or exceed 42 weeks' gestation and 2 to 7 percent complete 43 weeks of gestation.

ETIOLOGY

It is clear that the most common cause of prolonged gestation is an error in determining the patient's due date. Using the LMP for the determination of gestational age is fraught with inaccuracy. When prolongation of pregnancy is adequately documented, its cause is often undetermined and the most likely etiology is biologic variability of the duration of pregnancy.

Various fetal and placental abnormalities may predispose to prolongation of pregnancy. The increase in the incidence of fetal anomalies among women who deliver beyond their due date is generally explained by abnormalities of the fetal hypothalamic-pituitary-adrenal axis.[8] Indeed, major central nervous system (CNS) abnormalities (such as anencephaly) have long been associated with loss of the normal mechanisms that initiate labor at term.

Additional evidence regarding the complexity of the mechanisms involved with initiation of labor is provided by the X-linked recessive deficiency of placental sulfatase, which leads to abnormally low estrogen production in affected male fetuses with a subsequent prolongation of pregnancy and difficulties in both cervical ripening and labor induction.[11]

Primiparity has been identified as the only maternal variable, which has a small but significant association with prolonged pregnancies of greater than or equal to 294 days. Women who have previously delivered beyond term have a 50 percent chance of experiencing a subsequent prolonged pregnancy.[13] Thus, history of a previous delivery beyond term is a strong predictor of a subsequent late delivery.

DIAGNOSIS

The term "prolonged pregnancy" represents a diagnosis that is based on the best available estimation of the duration of gestation at the time of delivery. Optimal diagnosis of gestational age at the time of delivery is hindered by inaccuracy in pregnancy dating. Recently, it has become apparent that clinical methods for estimation of gestational age are inferior to sonographic measurements obtained early in pregnancy.[14] Several studies have demonstrated that the use of more accurate estimates of gestational age based on early ultrasound or known conception dates results in a significantly lower frequency of prolonged pregnancies.

PERINATAL MORTALITY AND MORBIDITY

Recent studies using very large computerized databases of well-dated pregnancies provide new insights into the true incidence and nature of adverse perinatal outcome in prolonged pregnancy. Divon et al. evaluated fetal and neonatal mortality rates in 181,524 accurately dated term and prolonged pregnancies.[21] A significant increase in fetal mortality was detected from 41 weeks' gestation onward. Fetal growth restriction (i.e., birthweight of <2 SD below the mean for gestational age) was associated with significantly higher odds ratios for both fetal and neonatal mortality rates at every gestational age examined with odds ratios ranging from 7.1 to 10.0 for fetal death and from 3.4 to 9.4 for neonatal death. Thus, this study documented a small but significant increase in fetal mortality in accurately dated pregnancies that extend beyond 41 weeks' gestation and demonstrated that fetal growth restriction is independently associated with a large increase in perinatal mortality in these pregnancies.

Recent studies have evaluated the association of perinatal morbidity with prolonged pregnancy. Fetal compromise was more common in the SGA fetuses, whereas shoulder dystocia, labor dysfunction, obstetric trauma, and maternal hemorrhage were more common in the LGA fetus. A large Swedish database of term and postterm (defined as ≥294 days) singleton, normally formed neonates showed that prolonged pregnancies were associated with an increased frequency of neonatal convulsions, meconium aspiration syndrome, and Apgar scores of less than 4 at 5 minutes. Again, morbidity in postterm SGA infants was higher than in postterm AGA infants.

It is reasonable to conclude that in the absence of perinatal asphyxia, growth restriction, or meconium aspiration, prolonged pregnancy is associated with normal, long-term neonatal developmental outcome.

ABERRANT FETAL GROWTH

The incidence of fetal macrosomia increases with advancing gestational age. A 23 percent incidence of infants whose birthweight was greater than 4,000 g and a 4 percent incidence of birthweights greater than 4,500 g have been documented at greater than or equal to 41 weeks' gestation.[31] Prolonged pregnancy is not only associated with an increased incidence of macrosomia, but a doubling of the cesarean delivery rate for protraction or descent disorders as well.[32]

Despite many years of research and debate, the management of suspected fetal macrosomia is still controversial. A reasonable policy for management of macrosomia would entail a conservative approach awaiting the onset of spontaneous labor in the absence of a favorable uterine cervix, adequate intrapartum management such as assessment of the adequacy of the maternal pelvis, assessment of the progress of labor and careful use of oxytocin, avoidance of vaginal operative deliveries, and avoidance of excessive traction on the impacted shoulder in favor of the maneuvers described for the management of shoulder dystocia (see Chapter 11).

FETAL SURVEILLANCE

Fetal surveillance may be used in an attempt to observe the prolonged pregnancy safely while awaiting the onset of labor or spontaneous ripening of the cervix prior to elective induction. The optimal gestational age for the initiation of fetal testing has not been established. Data presented earlier in this chapter indicate that perinatal mortality is significantly increased as early as 41 weeks' gestation. Thus, it would seem prudent to initiate fetal testing at 41 weeks of gestation.

Extensive experience with biophysical profile testing in high-risk populations indicates a perinatal mortality rate of 0.73 per 1,000 tested pregnancies within 1 week of a normal test, provided that the amniotic fluid volume is normal.[42] Twice-weekly testing with the biophysical profile in a series of 293 patients followed beyond 42 weeks of gestation has been reported. No stillbirths were observed in this small series.[43]

The primary disadvantages of biophysical profile scoring are the time required to perform the test and the need for an experienced sonographer. Recently, investigators have examined the efficacy of using the nonstress test as a primary testing modality with the addition of a sonographic assessment of amniotic fluid volume. Vibroacoustic stimulation may be used to shorten the duration of the nonstress test.[45] Amniotic fluid volume assessment was performed by measurement of the AFI, with induction of labor reserved for an AFI of 5 cm or less. Twice-weekly testing was performed in a subset of 279 prolonged pregnancies. No stillbirths were recorded.

More recently, Miller et al. reported the use of a similar protocol in 15,482 high-risk pregnancies for which 54,617 tests were performed.[47] The false-negative rate of this test was 0.8 per 1,000 women tested—a rate that favorably compares with those reported for the contraction stress test or the complete biophysical profile.[42,48] Of note, 6,390 patients were assessed in this study for prolonged pregnancy. These patients were first evaluated in the 41st week of gestation and twice-weekly testing was initiated after 42 weeks of gestation. Five stillbirths were reported in this subpopulation. An analysis of all false-positive tests showed that the routine use of nonstress testing combined with the AFI resulted in a 60 percent false-positive rate in the prediction of intrapartum fetal compromise compared with a 40 percent false-positive rate using the complete biophysical profile. This increase in false-positive tests was felt to be partly a result of poor specificity of the AFI in predicting fetal compromise.

Oligohydramnios

The majority of pregnancies at greater than or equal to 41 weeks' gestation have a normal volume of amniotic fluid, as measured with ultrasound.

The presence of sonographically diagnosed oligohydramnios is often used as an indication for delivery of pregnancies that reach term gestation or extend beyond term. One should realize, however, that up to 50 percent of patients who are diagnosed as having oligohydramnios by ultrasound will have a normal volume of amniotic fluid upon artificial rupture of the membranes.[68] In addition, there are no large-scale, prospective, randomized studies documenting the benefits of delivery once oligohydramnios has been detected. In the absence of such studies, it would seem prudent to deliver patients at or beyond 41 weeks' gestation who demonstrate oligohydramnios primarily because of the large body of data that documents an association between diminished amniotic fluid volume and adverse perinatal outcome, due, in part, to umbilical cord compression.

MANAGEMENT

Antenatal testing may be used in an attempt to observe the prolonged pregnancy safely while awaiting the spontaneous onset of labor or for ripening of the cervix prior to labor induction. Other opinions argue in favor of induction of labor regardless of the cervical status.

Sweeping the Membranes

Membrane sweeping or stripping is an age-old method of inducing labor that is still in common use. This intervention results in a local increase in prostaglandin production and is believed to hasten the onset of labor. A meta-analysis of the use of sweeping of the membranes to induce labor or to prevent prolonged pregnancy showed that sweeping of the membranes in term pregnancies shortens the duration of pregnancy by a mean of 4 days. Consequently, it decreases the frequency of patients reaching 41 or 42 weeks' gestation. Thus intervention had no significant impact on mode of delivery or the incidence of maternal or neonatal infections. Vaginal bleeding, painful uterine contractions not leading to delivery, and discomfort during vaginal examination are significantly more common in women allocated to sweeping of the membranes.

Induction of Labor

A major concern in the management of the prolonged pregnancy is the balance between the likelihood of a successful induction of labor and the risks of expectant management. The October 1997 ACOG Practice Patterns states that there is insufficient information to determine whether either labor induction or expectant management result in the best outcome in women with a prolonged pregnancy and a favorable cervix.[3] This publication does state that "according to current obstetric practice, labor is induced in most of these women." Accordingly, most practitioners feel that if the likelihood of a successful vaginal delivery is sufficiently high, there is no reason to expose the patient to the added risks associated with prolongation of pregnancy. Thus, in the absence of randomized controlled trials, induction of labor in women with prolonged pregnancy and a favorable cervix is a reasonable approach.

The management of the patient who presents with an unfavorable cervix is much more controversial. It consists of either expectant management (i.e., antenatal surveillance until there are signs of fetal jeopardy, or until the patient presents in either spontaneous labor or with a favorable cervix) or induction of labor any time after 41 weeks' gestation.

Oxytocin in combination with amniotomy remains the method of choice for inducing labor in women with a favorable cervix. The use of cervical ripening agents such as prostaglandins in patients with an unfavorable cervix certainly results in a significant increase in cervical dilation and effacement. However, the use of these agents is still associated with a high cesarean delivery rate subsequent to a failed induction of labor. Relative to women who present in spontaneous labor, the cesarean delivery rate is approximately doubled when induction of labor is attempted in nulliparous women at term.[85]

Induction of Labor versus Expectant Management

Although most authors agree that induction of labor is indicated in women with an "inducible" uterine cervix, there is lack of agreement as to the management of the patient whose cervix is deemed "unfavorable." Induction of labor in all women at 42 weeks' gestation is one option. Another option is serial fetal surveillance to assess well-being in women with an unfavorable cervix. These surveillance programs have focused on the detection of fetal hypoxia associated with uteroplacental insufficiency. To this end, fetal heart rate monitoring, biophysical profile, and ultra-sonographic assessment of amniotic fluid volume have been utilized. Delivery is undertaken when signs of fetal or maternal compromise are detected. In a recent study, Hanna et al. random-ized 3,407 women with uncomplicated pregnancies of 41 or more weeks' gestation to two management protocols: induction of labor or serial fetal monitoring.[86] They concluded that the rates of peri-natal morbidity and mortality were the same with the two approaches; however, the cesarean section rate was lower in the induction group. In contrast, Almstrom et al., who also random-ized patients into active and conservative management protocols, concluded that serial fetal monitoring resulted in a lower cesarean section rate.[87] A recent meta-analysis of 11 prospective studies demonstrated that induction of labor resulted in a slightly lower cesarean section rate compared with expectant management.[88] The randomized controlled trial ($n = 440$) conducted by the National Institute of Child Health and Human Development Network of Maternal-Fetal Medicine Units reported no fetal or maternal advantages to elective induction of labor at 41 weeks of gestation relative to serial fetal monitoring and indicated that either man-agement approach was acceptable.[83]

SUMMARY AND RECOMMENDATION

Management of the prolonged pregnancy is primarily determined by the interplay of three factors: certainty of gestational dating, the risks associated with expectant management, and the likeli-hood of spontaneous vaginal delivery following an induction of labor.

Key Points

➤ Whenever possible, gestational age should be established by a first- or an early second-trimester ultrasound examination.

➤ Sweeping of the membranes at term decreases slightly the number of pregnancies reaching either 41 or 42 weeks' gestation.

➤ Consider induction of labor at or beyond 41 weeks' gestation in patients with a favorable cervix.

➤ Initiate semiweekly fetal testing (nonstress test and AFI) at 41 weeks' gestation.

➤ Conservative management (i.e., semiweekly fetal testing) or active management (i.e., induction of labor) are equally reasonable options for patients with an unfavorable cervix.

➤ Perinatal morbidity and mortality are significantly increased when gestational age at birth is 41 weeks or more.

Alloimmunization in Pregnancy

MARC JACKSON AND
D. WARE BRANCH

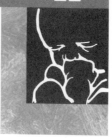

This chapter reviews the causes and management of alloimmunization in pregnancy. Topics included are Rh alloimmunization, sensitization caused by other erythrocyte antigens, and platelet alloimmunization. Rh alloimmunization is emphasized because it remains a leading cause of perinatal death from hemolytic disease. Also, to a great degree, the principles of pathophysiology and management discussed under Rh alloimmunization apply to the other causes of alloimmunization. With regard to Rh alloimmunization, the following are discussed: the genetics and biochemistry of the Rh antigen, the causes of Rh alloimmunization, the use of Rh immune globulin, and the assessment and management of the Rh-alloimmunized pregnancy. Throughout this chapter, the traditional term *sensitization* is used interchangeably with *alloimmunization*.

GENETICS AND BIOCHEMISTRY OF THE Rh ANTIGEN

The Rh gene complex involves several closely linked genes. Eight gene complexes exist (listed in decreasing order of frequency in the white population): CDe, cde, cDE, cDe, Cde, cdE, CDE, and CdE. Genotypes are indicated as pairs of gene complexes, such as CDe/cde. Certain genotypes, and thus certain phenotypes, are more prevalent than others. The genotypes CDe/cde and CDe/CDe are the most common, with approximately 55 percent of all whites having the CcDe or CDe phenotype (Table 22–1).[8] The genotype CdE has never been demonstrated.[7] Although the alleles are always written in the order C(c), D, E(e), the actual order for the genes on chromosome 1 coding for the antigens is D, C(c), E(e).

Table 22–1. FREQUENCY OF RH PHENOTYPES AND GENOTYPES AMONG WHITES*

Phenotype (genes expressed)	Population Frequency (%)	Frequency Within Genotype	(%)
CcDe	35	CDe/cde (R^1/r)	94
		CDe/cDe (R^1/R^0)	6
		cDe/Cde (R^0/r')	<1
CDe	20	CDe/CDe (R^1/R^1)	95
		CDe/Cde (R^1/r')	5
cde	16	cde/cde (r/r)	100
CcDEe	13	CDe/cDE (R^1/R^2)	189
		CDe/cdE (R^1/r″)	7
		cDE/Cde (R^2/r')	2
		CDE/cde (R^z/r)	1
		CDE/cDe (R^z/R^0)	<1
cDEe	10	cDE/cde (R^2/r)	93
		cDE/cDe (R^2/R^0)	6
		cDe/cdE (R^0/r″)	1
cDE	3	cDE/cDE (R^2/R^2)	86
		cDE/cdE (R^2/r″)	14
cDe	2	cDe/cde (R^0/r)	97
		cDe/cDe (R^0/R^0)	3
Cde	1	Cde/cde (r'/r)	100

*Genotyped results from deletion of D and thus is not an expressed gene product.

Genetic Expression

The genetic locus for the Rh antigen complex is on the short arm of chromosome 1.[11,12] Within the Rh locus are two distinct structural genes adjacent to one another, RhCcEe and RhD. These two genes likely share a single genetic ancestor, as they are identical in more than 95 percent of their coding sequences.[13] The first gene codes for the C/c and E/e antigens, and the second gene codes for the D antigen.

Expression of the D antigen occurs if one (heterozygous) or both (homozygous) chromosome 1 contains a normal RhD gene sequence. Patients who are D-negative (dd) lack the normal RhD gene sequence on both their chromosomes. Therefore, they cannot transcribe this region, which is responsible for producing the D antigen. The d phenotype occurs when there is deletion of the D allele; no sequence codes for d per se.

There is a relatively constant number of Rh antigen sites available on the erythrocyte surface, totaling about 100,000 sites per cell; these sites appear to be approximately evenly divided between C(c), D, and E(e) antigens.[14,15]

Allelic interaction on Rh antigen sites has been described: erythrocytes of genotype CDe/cde express less D antigen than do the erythrocytes of genotype cDE/cde.[18] Thus, the presence of the C antigen seems to affect the expression of the D antigen. Similarly, individuals of genotype CDe/cDE express less C antigen than individuals of genotype CDe/cde.[8] In addition, genes other than those coding for the Rh antigen may affect the final antigenic expression; two independently segregating regulator genes have been described.[10]

The precise function of the Rh antigens is unknown, although they probably have a role in maintaining red cell membrane integrity. Rh_{null} erythrocytes, which lack all of the Rh antigens, manifest several membrane defects. The Rh antigens may interact with a membrane adenosine triphosphatase,[23] possibly functioning as part of a proton or cation pump that controls volume or electrolyte flux across the erythrocyte membrane. Supporting this hypothesis, Rh_{null} erythrocytes have increased osmotic fragility and abnormal shapes.[31] It has also been proposed that Rh antigens regulate the asymmetric distribution of different phospholipids through the red cell membrane as a component of the enzyme phosphatidyl flippase.[32,33]

CAUSES OF Rh ALLOIMMUNIZATION

For Rh alloimmunization to occur in a pregnancy, at least three circumstances must exist:

1. The fetus must have Rh-positive erythrocytes, and the mother must have Rh-negative erythrocytes.
2. A sufficient number of fetal erythrocytes must gain access to the maternal circulation.
3. The mother must have the immunogenic capacity to produce antibody directed against the D antigen.

Incidence of Rh-Incompatible Pregnancy

About 15 percent of whites of European extraction are Rh-negative; only 5 to 8 percent of American blacks and 1 to 2 percent of Asians and Native Americans are Rh-negative. In the white population, an Rh-negative woman has about an 85 percent chance of mating with an Rh-positive man. About 60 percent of Rh-positive men are heterozygous and 40 percent are homozygous at the D locus. Given that one half of conceptions due to heterozygous men will be Rh-positive, the overall chance of an Rh-positive man producing an Rh-positive fetus is about 70 percent. Thus, without knowing the father's blood type, an Rh-negative woman has about a 60 percent chance of bearing an Rh-positive fetus (0.85 × 0.70). Among whites, the net result is that about 10 percent of pregnancies are Rh incompatible (0.15 × 0.60). However, because sufficient feto-maternal hemorrhage and a subsequent maternal antibody response do not occur in every case, less than 20 percent of incompatible pregnancies eventuate in maternal sensitization. Thus, in the era before Rh-immune globulin prophylaxis, about 1 percent of pregnant women had anti-D antibody.

Fetomaternal Hemorrhage

Fetal red cells gain access to the maternal circulation during pregnancy and the immediate postpartum period. Fetomaternal hemorrhage in a volume sufficient to cause alloimmunization is most common at delivery, occurring in about 15 to 50 percent of births.[34-37] In more than half of these intrapartum fetomaternal bleeds, the amount of fetal blood entering the maternal circulation is 0.1 ml or less.[37,38] However, in 0.2 to 1 percent of cases, the estimated volume of fetomaternal hemorrhage is 30 ml or more.[35, 39, 40] Clinical factors such as cesarean delivery, multiple gestation, bleeding placenta previa or abruption, manual removal of the placenta, and intrauterine manipulation may increase the chance of substantial hemorrhage. However, the majority of excessive fetomaternal hemorrhages occur in patients without risk factors who have an uncomplicated vaginal delivery.[40,41]

The amount of fetomaternal hemorrhage necessary to cause alloimmunization varies from patient to patient, probably due to the immunogenic capacity of the Rh-positive erythrocytes and the immune responsiveness of the mother. As little as 0.1 ml of Rh-positive red blood cells has been shown to sensitize some Rh-negative volunteers, and about 3 percent of women found to have 0.1 ml of fetal erythrocytes in their circulation after an Rh-incompatible delivery develop anti-D antibodies within 6 to 12 months.[37]

Overall, about 16 percent of Rh-negative women will become alloimmunized by their first Rh-incompatible (ABO-compatible) pregnancy if not treated with Rh-immune globulin.[38] Half of these women respond with the production of sufficient anti-D antibody to be detectable within the first 6 months after delivery; in the remainder, anti-D is not detected until early in the next incompatible pregnancy. In this latter group, sensitization likely occurred during the first pregnancy, but the primary immune response was too slight for detectable antibody levels to develop. Though not all Rh-negative women bearing Rh-positive infants will become sensitized, the risk of sensitization approaches 50 percent after several incompatible pregnancies.

Even without labor or obvious disruption of the choriodecidual junction, antepartum fetomaternal hemorrhage occurs in sufficient volume to result in alloimmunization in a small percentage of cases. In one large series, fetomaternal hemorrhage was detected in the first trimester in 7 percent of patients, in 16 percent of patients during the second trimester, and in 29 percent of the third-trimester determinations.[34] The result of this antepartum fetomaternal hemorrhage is an overall rate of Rh sensitization of about 1 to 2 percent before delivery.[42] However, antepartum sensitization rarely occurs before the third trimester.

Fetomaternal hemorrhage leading to alloimmunization has also been described with abortion and tubal pregnancy.[43-46] Fetal Rh antigens are present at least by the 38th day after conception and, assuming that as little as 0.1 ml of fetal blood can cause alloimmunization, a fetomaternal hemorrhage leading to sensitization could occur by the seventh week after the last menses.[47]

Between 5 and 25 percent of spontaneous abortions result in detectable fetomaternal hemorrhage.[36] For the unsensitized Rh-negative woman, a spontaneous first-trimester abortion carries a 3 to 4 percent risk of alloimmunization.[49] Induced abortions are also likely to produce detectable fetomaternal hemorrhage (in 7 to 27 percent of cases); the overall risk of sensitization is about 5 percent.[46] In the second trimester, pregnancy termination by either saline injection or hysterotomy is associated with significant fetomaternal hemorrhage.[45,46]

Threatened abortion in the first trimester may also increase the risk of sensitization. Fetomaternal hemorrhage can be demonstrated in 11 to 45 percent of such patients,[50,51] and a case of apparent sensitization following threatened first-trimester miscarriage has been reported.[52]

All Rh-negative unsensitized women should receive 50 μg of Rh-immune globulin within 72 hours of induced or spontaneous first-trimester abortion. Patients in the second trimester, 13 weeks or more, are routinely given a full dose, 300 μg.

Ectopic pregnancy can result in alloimmunization in a susceptible woman.[43] The risk of significant fetomaternal hemorrhage may be greater in cases of ruptured tubal pregnancy, presumably because of the absorption of fetal erythrocytes into the maternal circulation across the peritoneum.[53]

Amniocentesis in the second and third trimesters is associated with fetomaternal hemorrhage in 15 to 25 percent of cases, even when ultrasound is used to identify placental location.[54,55] Alloimmunization occurring after amniocentesis has been reported.[56]

Maternal Immunologic Response

Two characteristics affect whether alloimmunization will occur in a susceptible Rh-negative woman. First, as many as 30 percent of Rh-negative individuals appear to be immunologic "nonresponders" who will not become sensitized, even when challenged with large volumes of Rh-positive blood.[57,58] Second, ABO incompatibility exerts a protective effect against the development of Rh sensitization.[59]

ABO incompatibility diminishes the risk of alloimmunization to about 1.5 to 2 percent after the delivery of an Rh-positive fetus.[61] This effect is most pronounced in matings in which the mother is type O and the father is type A, type B, or type AB.[62]

THE USE OF Rh-IMMUNE GLOBULIN

The principle that a passively administered antibody will prevent active immunization by its specific antigen is termed *antibody-mediated immune suppression* (AMIS) and was well known to immunologists for decades before being applied to the prevention of Rh disease. During the early 1960s, Freda et al.[63] in the United States and Clarke et al.[64] in Great Britain simultaneously undertook to evaluate AMIS in humans. Both groups achieved a high degree of protection from alloimmunization by administering anti-D immune globulin (Rh-immune globulin) to Rh-negative male volunteers who had been infused with Rh-positive red cells.[63,64] In 1963, Pollack et al.[65] established that 300 μg of Rh-immune globulin would reliably prevent alloimmunization in male volunteers who had received 10 ml of Rh-positive cells. By extrapolation Pollack et al. showed that 20 μg of Rh-immune globulin per milliliter of fetal erythrocytes or 10 μg/ml of whole fetal blood was required to prevent alloimmunization. Thus, 10 μg Rh-immune globulin was recommended for every 1 ml of fetal blood in the maternal circulation.

Although 300 μg or more of Rh-immune globulin was used initially, it has subsequently been shown that a dose of 100 to 150 μg is probably adequate for routine use.[68,69] Nonetheless, the standard approved dose for Rh prophylaxis in the United States remains 300 μg.

The 72-hour time limit set for the postpartum administration of Rh-immune globulin is an artifact of the design of the early male prisoner volunteer studies. Prison officials would only allow the investigators to visit the volunteers at 3-day intervals[70]; thus, the use of Rh-immune globulin at intervals of more than 3 days after a challenge with Rh-positive cells was never extensively evaluated. However, to be effective, Rh-immune globulin must be given before the primary immune response is established. The time required to mount a primary immune response doubtlessly varies from case to case, and it is prudent to administer Rh-immune globulin to appropriate mothers as soon as possible after delivery. If for some reason the neonatal Rh status is unknown by the third day after delivery, it is preferable to administer Rh-immune globulin to an Rh-negative mother rather than to continue to await the neonatal results. Finally, if an Rh-negative mother who is a candidate for Rh-immune prophylaxis is mistakenly not treated within the recommended 72 hours following delivery, she may be given Rh-immune globulin up to 14 to 28 days after delivery in an effort to avoid sensitization.[71]

Antepartum Prophylaxis

Early trials showed that 1 to 2 percent of susceptible women became sensitized in spite of postpartum Rh-immune prophylaxis. The majority of these "prophylaxis failures" resulted from antepartum fetomaternal hemorrhage. In an effort to address this problem, Bowman and colleagues[72] in Canada conducted an antepartum Rh prophylaxis trial in which 300 μg of Rh-immune globulin was given at 28 and 34 weeks' gestation. Antenatal sensitization was reduced from 1.8 to 0.1 percent. Subsequently, it was shown that 300 μg of Rh-immune globulin given only at 28 weeks' gestation is nearly as effective.[73]

MANAGEMENT OF THE UNSENSITIZED Rh-NEGATIVE PREGNANT WOMAN

At the first prenatal visit of each pregnancy, every patient should have her ABO blood group, Rh type, and antibody screen checked (Fig. 22–1). It is essential that these determinations are made in each subsequent pregnancy, as previous maternal antibody screening is not an adequate assessment.

If the patient is Rh-negative, weak D-negative, and has no demonstrable antibody, she is a candidate for 300 μg Rh-immune globulin as prophylaxis at 28 weeks' gestation and again immediately after birth. It is the recommendation of the American Association of Blood Banks that a second antibody screen be obtained before administration of Rh-immune globulin at the beginning of the third trimester,[84] to ensure that the patient is not already sensitized and producing anti-D, but this second screen is probably clinically unnecessary.[85] Similarly, a repeat antepartum antibody screen at 35 to 36 weeks' gestation is unnecessary. Routine screening of Rh-positive patients for irregular antibodies at the beginning of the third trimester is not warranted.[86]

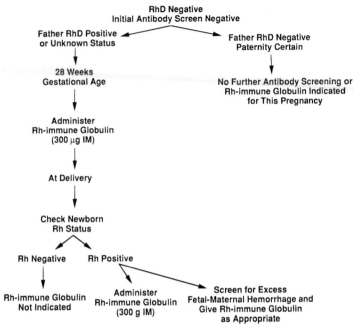

Figure 22–1. Flow diagram outlining the management of Rh-negative, non-immunized pregnancies.

When the Rh-negative, unsensitized patient is admitted for delivery, an antibody screen is routinely done. If the antibody screen is negative and the newborn is Rh-positive or weak D-positive, the patient should again be given Rh-immune globulin.

Because up to 1 percent of deliveries result in a fetomaternal hemorrhage of greater than 30 ml (the largest volume of fetal blood adequately covered by a standard 300 μg dose of Rh-immune globulin), Rh-negative patients with an Rh-positive or weak D–positive newborn should be screened for "excessive" fetomaternal hemorrhage immediately postpartum.[84] For patients with a positive screen, Kleihauer-Betke testing can be used to quantitate the volume of fetal red cells in the maternal circulation. In this way, the appropriate dose of Rh-immune globulin can be calculated. If the volume of hemorrhage is estimated to be greater than 30 ml whole blood, a dose of Rh-immune globulin calculated at 10 μg/ml of whole fetal blood should be administered.

Management of the weak D–positive patient is sometimes confusing. A weak D–positive mother who delivers an Rh-positive infant is not at significant risk of Rh sensitization, probably because the weak D antigen is actually an incompletely expressed

D antigen. Thus, weak D–positive mothers are clinically treated as if they were Rh-positive, and they do not require Rh-immune globulin. However, occasionally a woman previously typed as Rh-negative is unexpectedly found to be weak D–positive during pregnancy or after delivery. In this situation, the clinician should be suspicious that the patient's "new" weak D–positive status is actually due to a large number of Rh-positive fetal cells in the maternal circulation. Appropriate diagnostic studies should be performed, and if fetomaternal hemorrhage is found, the mother should be treated with Rh-immune globulin.

Because of the risk of significant fetomaternal hemorrhage with abortion or ectopic pregnancy, Rh-immune globulin prophylaxis is indicated if the patient is Rh-negative and unsensitized. If the pregnancy loss occurs at 12 weeks' gestation or less, a 50-μg dose of Rh-immune globulin is adequate to cover the entire fetal blood volume[87] (Table 22–2). If the gestational age is unknown or beyond 12 weeks, a full 300 μg dose of Rh-immune globulin is indicated.

Management of the Rh-negative patient with threatened miscarriage in the first trimester is controversial, and there is no clear consensus or evidence-based recommendation on use of Rh-immune

Table 22–2. RECOMMENDED DOSES OF RH-IMMUNE GLOBULIN

Indication	Dose (μg) of Rh-Immune Globulin
First-trimester spontaneous or induced abortion	50
First-trimester chorionic villus sampling	50
Ectopic pregnancy	
Prior to 12 weeks' gestation	50
After 12 weeks' gestation	300
Amniocentesis, second-trimester chorionic villus sampling, or other intrauterine procedures	300
Abdominal trauma or fetal death in the second or third trimester	300
Fetomaternal hemorrhage	10 per estimated ml of whole fetal blood

From American College of Obstetricians and Gynecologists: Prevention of RhD alloimmunization. ACOG Practice Bulletin 4. Washington, DC, American College of Obstetricians and Gynecologists, 1999.

globulin.[85] Even though fetal–maternal hemorrhage can occur with threatened abortion before 12 weeks,[51] documented sensitization is extremely uncommon. In the United Kingdom, current recommendations are that Rh-immune globulin is unnecessary with threatened miscarriage before 12 weeks, although anti-D can be considered for patients with heavy or repeated bleeding late in the first trimester.[88]

An Rh-negative, unsensitized patient who has antepartum bleeding or suffers an unexplained second- or third-trimester fetal death should receive 300 µg Rh-immune globulin and be evaluated for the possibility of massive fetomaternal hemorrhage. If fetal cells are found in the maternal circulation, Rh-immune globulin is indicated at a dose of 10 µg per estimated milliliter of whole fetal blood (Table 22–2).

Antenatal Rh-immune globulin is indicated at the time of chorionic villus sampling or amniocentesis in an Rh-negative, unsensitized patient. For first-trimester procedures, 50 µg of Rh-immune globulin is protective. For second- or third-trimester procedures, a full 300-µg dose is indicated even if the procedure is not associated with detectable hemorrhage (Table 22–2). When amniocentesis is performed within 72 hours of delivery, such as for the determination of fetal pulmonary maturity, Rh-immune globulin may be withheld and administered immediately postpartum if the infant is found to be Rh-positive or D^u positive; if delivery is to be delayed for more than 72 hours, Rh-immune globulin should be given.

Since Rh-immune globulin became available in the United States in the late 1960s, the incidence of Rh alloimmunization has been drastically reduced. Antepartum sensitizations have markedly declined with the now widespread practice of antepartum prophylaxis; however, postpartum prophylaxis failures still represent a significant problem.[89] The routine use of postpartum screening programs to detect "excessive" fetomaternal hemorrhage will likely avoid the majority of these postpartum sensitizations.

Failure to administer Rh-immune globulin when it is indicated also remains a problem.[89] In one study, nearly one fourth of the cases of new sensitization were due to this inexcusable oversight.[90]

THE Rh-ALLOIMMUNIZED PREGNANCY: ASSESSMENT OF THE FETUS

Any patient with an anti-D antibody titer of greater than 1:4 should be considered Rh sensitized and her pregnancies managed accordingly. The eventual goal of management is to minimize fetal and neonatal morbidity and mortality. Patients (fetuses) can be roughly categorized as (1) those who are unlikely to require intrauterine intervention and who can be delivered when they achieve pulmonary maturity and (2) those who, will likely have moderate to severe hemolytic disease and require intrauterine transfusion and early delivery. An accurate assignment of gestational age using menstrual dates and early ultrasound is crucial in management of the Rh-alloimmunized pregnancy, as the timing of amniocentesis, umbilical cord blood sampling, in utero treatment, and delivery will depend on it.

Determination of the Fetal Antigen Status

When first confronted with an Rh-immunized pregnancy, the possibility that the fetus might be Rh-negative and therefore not need expensive and potentially hazardous procedures should be considered. If the woman might have become sensitized during a pregnancy fathered by another partner or by a mismatched blood transfusion, determining the paternal Rh antigen status is especially reasonable, since the father of the current pregnancy might be Rh-negative. If he is Rh-negative (and it is certain that he is the father of the fetus), further assessment and intervention are unnecessary. If the father is Rh-positive, the blood bank laboratory can reliably estimate the probability that he is heterozygous for the D antigen by using Rh antisera to determine his most likely genotype (Table 22–1). Alternatively, DNA analysis can be used to determine his status with a high degree of certainty.[91] Of course, if the man has fathered Rh-negative children, he is a known heterozygote.

If the father is homozygous for the D antigen, all his children will be Rh-positive; if he is heterozygous, there is a 50 percent likelihood that each pregnancy will have an Rh-negative fetus who is at no risk of anemia and does not require further assessment or treatment.

In the past, cordocentesis with analysis of fetal red blood cells was required to determine fetal antigen status. Some authors advocated routine umbilical cord blood sampling for fetal Rh antigen status at 18 to 20 weeks' gestation in all Rh-immunized pregnancies with a heterozygous father.[92] However, this approach never gained widespread acceptance, at least in part because of the increased risks of fetal loss and fetomaternal hemorrhage associated with cordocentesis.[93]

Recently, advances in molecular genetics have made it possible to determine fetal Rh status without direct analysis of fetal red blood cells. The Rh locus on chromosome 1p34-p36 has been cloned,[94] and polymerase chain reaction (PCR) now allows determination of fetal Rh status from the uncultured amniocytes in 2 ml of amniotic fluid or as little as 5 mg of chorionic villi.[95,96]

Because of the possibility of severe fetal anemia and death, it is most important that an Rh-positive fetus not be misidentified as Rh-negative. Van den Veyver et al.[103] pointed out that such a misdiagnosis can occur when an Rh-positive father carries a gene rearrangement near the RhD locus which would prevent binding of the primer and yield a negative result with PCR. They recommended that paternal blood be analyzed simultaneously with amniotic fluid, using the same primers and PCR technique.

At most centers in the United States, DNA analysis of fetal cells is routinely included in the Rh assessment protocol. If an Rh-sensitized patient (with a partner who is heterozygous or whose status is unknown) is having a chorionic villus sampling or second-trimester amniocentesis for another, unrelated indication, fetal RhD typing is performed at that time. In other cases, fetal Rh typing is performed at the time of the first amniocentesis for amniotic fluid bilirubin analysis. When PCR results indicate an Rh-negative fetus, patients are offered surveillance with fetal kick counts and serial ultrasounds, after a full discussion and explanation of the small likelihood of a misdiagnosis.

In the future, it seems likely that fetal Rh status may be routinely available from analysis of maternal blood. Favorable early experience with prenatal diagnosis of fetal antigen status has been reported using maternal blood,[104] fetal DNA extracted from maternal plasma,[105] and fetal mRNA in maternal blood.[106] Preimplantation genetic diagnosis of RhD type on single blastomeres has also been described.[99]

Antibody Titer

In the first sensitized pregnancy, the level of the anti-D antibody titer determines the need for amniocentesis. A number of authors have noted that severe erythroblastosis or perinatal death does not occur when the antibody levels remain below a certain "critical titer."[60,107,108] This titer varies between laboratories but is usually 1:16 or 1:32.

An anti-D titer of 1:8 or greater is considered at many centers to be an indication for amniocentesis to manage the sensitized pregnancy (Fig. 22–2). If the initial anti-D titer is less than 1:8, and if the patient does not have a history of a previously affected infant, the pregnancy may be followed with anti-D titers every 2 to 4 weeks and serial ultrasound assessment of the fetus.

Except for using the "critical titer" to establish the need for amniocentesis in the first sensitized pregnancy. Indeed, titers may remain stable throughout gestation in as many as 80 percent of severely affected pregnancies.[104] Variability between maternal antibody levels and severity of fetal disease is explained by the fact that antibody concentration is only one factor influencing the degree of anemia.

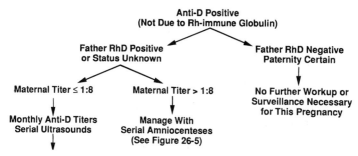

Figure 22–2. Flow diagram outlining the management of a first Rh-sensitized pregnancy.

Obstetric History

A well-documented obstetric history can be an important management guide for the Rh-alloimmunized patient. Fetal hemolytic disease tends to be either as severe, or more severe, in subsequent pregnancies. A history of previous intrauterine or neonatal death from hemolytic disease carries a particularly grave prognosis.[107,115] As a general rule of thumb, if a mother has had a hydropic fetus, the chance that the next Rh-incompatible fetus will become hydropic (if left untreated) is more than 80 percent. Only occasionally will an Rh-incompatible fetus be less severely affected than its previous sibling.

In general, hemolysis and hydrops develop at about the same time or somewhat earlier in subsequent pregnancies; this can be used as a rough guide for timing initial fetal studies and transfusions. However, the history is not particularly helpful if the previous pregnancy was the first sensitized pregnancy, since relatively few fetuses develop hydrops in a first sensitized pregnancy.

Amniotic Fluid Analysis

Assessment of amniotic fluid in Rh immunization is based on the original observations of Bevis[116] that spectrophotometric determinations of amniotic fluid bilirubin correlated with the severity of fetal hemolysis. The bilirubin in amniotic fluid is a by-product of fetal hemolysis that reaches the amniotic fluid primarily by excretion into fetal pulmonary and tracheal secretions and diffusion across the fetal membranes and the umbilical cord. Using a semilogarithmic plot, the curve of optical density of normal amniotic fluid is approximately linear between wavelengths of 525 and 375 nm. Bilirubin causes a shift in the spectrophotometric density with a peak at a wavelength of 450 nm. The amount of shift in optical density from linearity at 450 nm (the ΔOD_{450}) is used to estimate the degree of fetal red cell hemolysis (Fig. 22–3).

Liley[117] correlated amniotic fluid ΔOD_{450} values with newborn outcome by dividing a semilogarithmic graph of gestational age versus ΔOD_{450} into three zones. Unaffected fetuses and those with mild anemia had ΔOD_{450} values in zone I (the lowest zone), whereas severely affected fetuses had ΔOD_{450} values in zone III (the highest zone). Fetuses with zone II values (the middle zone) had disease ranging from mild to severe, indicated primarily by the trend of the amniotic fluid bilirubin determinations. There is a normal tendency for amniotic fluid bilirubin to decrease as pregnancy advances; thus, the boundaries of the zones slope downward as gestational age increases (Fig. 22–4).

A single measurement of ΔOD_{450} was poorly predictive of fetal condition unless it is very high or very low.[11] Queenan[119] subsequently analyzed serial amniotic fluid ΔOD_{450} values in patients delivering unaffected (Rh-negative), mildly affected (cord hemoglobin >14 g/dl), severely affected (cord blood hemoglobin <10 g/dl), and stillborn infants. There was a clear downward trend in the ΔOD_{450} values in unaffected and mildly affected infants, and values from the severely affected fetuses showed a mixed pattern of higher values. The amniotic fluid ΔOD_{450} values from infants who died in utero from erythroblastosis showed upward trends except in a single case that was complicated by polyhydramnios. Thus, a horizontal or rising trend is ominous and indicates the need for intervention either by intrauterine transfusion or delivery. Clinical management now includes serial amniocenteses to determine the trend of ΔOD_{450} values over time.[119,120]

The usefulness of the late second- and early third-trimester amniotic fluid ΔOD_{450} determinations for the management of Rh-immunized pregnancies has been confirmed by decades of experience in many centers. However, several practical caveats deserve emphasis. First, a single ΔOD_{450} value is often insufficient for management purposes; the ΔOD_{450} trend, as established by serial amniocenteses, provides more reliable information about the fetal status. Second, amniotic fluid bilirubin levels are an indirect measure of fetal anemia, and relying solely on the ΔOD_{450} values occasionally leads to the false impression that a mildly or moderately involved fetus is severely anemic or vice versa. Finally, the fairly common practice of extrapolating Liley's original graph for use prior to 27 weeks' gestation is controversial.

In analysis of amniotic fluid bilirubin levels obtained between 14 and 40 weeks' gestation, Queenan et al.[126] plotted 520 ΔOD_{450} values from unaffected fetuses and 163 ΔOD_{450} values from Rh-immunized pregnancies, using a nonlogarithmic graph. In unaffected pregnancies, normal amniotic fluid ΔOD_{450} values trended upward between 14 and 22 weeks, leveled off until 26 weeks, then

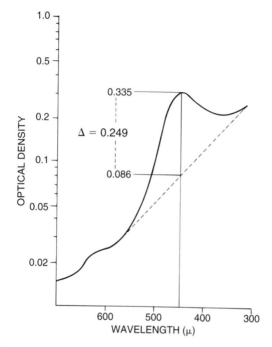

Figure 22–3. Graph of spectrophotometric analysis of amniotic fluid taken from an Rh-sensitized pregnancy with fetal hydrops. The *solid line* is the plot of the optical density of the bilirubin-containing fluid across the wavelengths on the x-axis. The interrupted line represents the curve expected from amniotic fluid without increased bilirubin. The difference between the optical density of the *solid line* and the *interrupted line* at 450 nm is the ΔOD_{450} value.

declined steadily until term. Using the mean and standard deviation of values across the gestational age range, these authors proposed a new graphic framework for assessment of ΔOD_{450} values in Rh-sensitized pregnancies, with four zones instead of Liley's three.

Recognizing that this issue is not completely settled, we currently use a standard semilogarithmic Liley curve for amniotic fluid assessment, extrapolated linearly back to 24 weeks' gestational age (Fig. 22–4). We emphasize trends rather than single ΔOD_{450} values, especially before the third trimester, taking history and gestational age into consideration in clinical management.

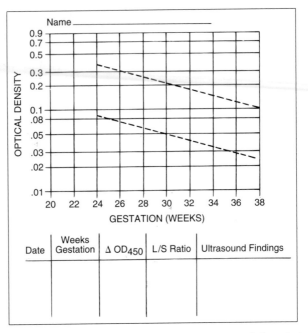

Figure 22–4. Liley graph with linear extrapolation of boundaries to 24 weeks' gestation.

Fetal Blood Analysis

Fetal blood sampling was the first method to determine reliably fetal antigen status when the zygosity of the father was unknown or uncertain. As a result, fetal blood sampling was considered by many to be the first step in the assessment of the fetus at risk for severe hemolytic disease.

The fetal hematocrit and the amniotic fluid ΔOD_{450} values are in agreement in 80 percent of cases. However, the amniotic fluid ΔOD_{450} value underestimates the degree of fetal anemia in 10 percent of comparisons and overestimates the degree of fetal anemia in 10 percent.

Adoption of routine umbilical cord blood sampling has also not been universal because of concern for potential fetal and maternal morbidity. The procedure is successful in greater than 95 percent of cases, but attributable fetal loss rates between 0.5 and 2 percent per procedure have been reported by experienced investigators.[133–135] In 5 percent of patients, other morbidity occurs; complications such as acute refractory fetal distress, umbilical cord hematoma, amnionitis with maternal adult respiratory distress syndrome, and placental abruption have been described.[136-138]

Additionally, there appears to be a significant risk (25–50%) of fetomaternal bleeding with umbilical cord blood sampling, with the potential for worsened maternal sensitization and fetal involvement.[139-141]

The need for cordocentesis to determine fetal antigen status has been obviated by the availability of DNA analysis of amniotic fluid. Thus, the role of umbilical cord blood sampling in the management of alloimmunization is limited to assessment of those fetuses already known to be antigen-positive and who are suspected of having moderate to severe anemia.

Ultrasound and Doppler Studies

Ultrasonographic examination of the fetus has become an extremely important adjunct in the management of the Rh-sensitized pregnancy, primarily as a guide to amniocentesis, fetal blood sampling, and intrauterine transfusion. Ultrasound has also been studied in an effort to identify sonographic findings that might predict the severity of erythroblastosis fetalis and reduce the need for invasive assessments. Polyhydramnios, placental thickness greater than 4 cm, pericardial effusion, dilation of the cardiac chambers, chronic enlargement of the spleen and liver, visualization of both sides of the fetal bowel wall, and dilation of the umbilical vein have all been proposed as indicators of significant prehydropic fetal anemia.[142-151]

Sonographic findings other than hydrops are not sufficiently reliable in distinguishing mild from severe hemolytic disease, even in experienced hands, and the role of ultrasound in the monitoring of fetuses with severe Rh immunization is still limited to the establishment of gestational age; monitoring for hydropic changes; and guidance for amniocentesis, umbilical cord blood sampling, and transfusion.

Doppler flow velocity waveforms have also been extensively investigated as noninvasive predictors of fetal anemia[152-161] and acidosis.[162,163] However, because of the large overlap in values between anemic and nonanemic fetuses, Doppler measurements cannot accurately predict the degree of fetal anemia.

Fetal blood flow velocity waveforms have also not been predictive of acid–base status in Rh-alloimmunized pregnancies. Again the wide range and overlap of values in both groups of patients have limited the clinical utility of Doppler technology.

However, ultrasound and Doppler ultrasound technology continue to advance rapidly, and it seems likely that these noninvasive tools may one day be used to reliably determine the degree of fetal anemia and, hence, to direct fetal management. However, at present, neither ultrasound nor Doppler blood flow analysis can be recommended in

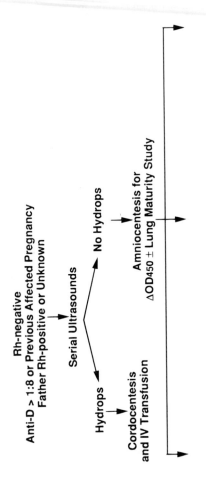

Rh-negative
Anti-D > 1:8 or Previous Affected Pregnancy
Father Rh-positive or Unknown

Serial Ultrasounds

No Hydrops

Hydrops

Cordocentesis
and IV Transfusion

Amniocentesis for
$\Delta OD450 \pm$ Lung Maturity Study

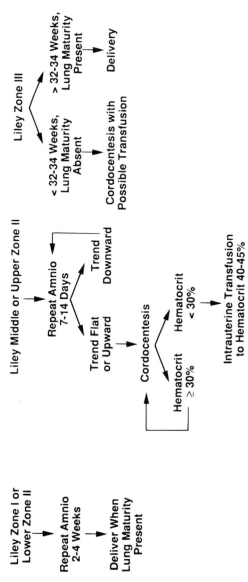

Figure 22–5. Flow diagram outlining the management of an Rh-sensitized pregnancy. The timing of the first amniocentesis is based on the history, maternal titer, and gestational age. At the first amniocentesis, fluid should be sent for determination of fetal antigen status, and if negative, a noninvasive surveillance protocol is continued. In incompatible pregnancies, all patients monitor fetal movements on a daily basis after 26 to 28 weeks and have nonstress tests one to two times weekly and ultrasound exams every 1 to 2 weeks, in addition to assessment of amniotic fluid bilirubin or umbilical cord hematocrit.

lieu of amniotic fluid ΔOD_{450} determinations or fetal blood sampling for intrauterine transfusion or delivery in Rh-immunized pregnancies.

Determining the Need for Intrauterine Transfusion

About one half of susceptible infants of Rh-immunized pregnancies never require intrauterine transfusion or extensive extrauterine therapy. Such fetuses are considered to have mild to moderate hemolytic disease. In general, mild to moderate fetal hemolysis is expected when (1) the involved pregnancy is the first sensitized pregnancy or (2) previously delivered Rh-positive infants have been mildly to moderately affected (mild to moderate anemia without hydrops). In such cases, ultrasound examinations is performed on the fetus every 2 to 4 weeks from 20 weeks' gestation until delivery. If the fetus shows no signs of hydrops, amniotic fluid ΔOD_{450} determinations are used for the initial management, performing the first amniocentesis at 24 to 28 weeks' gestation. Timing of repeat amniocenteses and determination of the need for intrauterine transfusion or delivery are based on the ΔOD_{450} values and trend (Fig. 22–5). If the values fall within the low zone or the lower half of the middle zone on the Liley graph, amniocentesis is repeated every 2 to 4 weeks, depending on the ΔOD_{450} trend. Severe anemia requiring intrauterine transfusion is suspected when the ΔOD_{450} values rise into the upper quarter of the middle zone or into zone III, especially before 30 weeks' gestation. Depending on the clinical situation, a single ΔOD_{450} value in zone III also may be taken as an indication of severe anemia. If at any time the fetus has evidence of hydrops by ultrasound, one can assume a fetal hematocrit less than about 15 percent,[146,147] and fetal blood sampling and transfusion should be arranged immediately.

There is no proven advantage to cordocentesis and intravascular transfusion in nonhydropic fetuses, and experienced practitioners have described excellent perinatal outcomes using amniotic fluid ΔOD_{450} values with intraperitoneal transfusions.[164–166] However, because of the morbidity associated with fetal transfusion regardless of route, it seems appropriate to obtain umbilical cord blood when practical to confirm anemia prior to transfusion. The optimum management in any individual case will be determined by the clinical presentation and the experience and expertise of the physicians involved.

When the obstetric history suggests that the fetus is at risk for moderate to severe hemolysis and hydrops, we are more likely to begin the search for fetal anemia earlier in the pregnancy. In this situation, we usually follow the trend of ΔOD_{450} values, using an extrapolation of the Liley curve, with the understanding that interpretation of ΔOD_{450} values before 24 weeks is difficult. Between 18 and 24 weeks, we stress ΔOD_{450} trends over single values and typically use Queenan's horizontal zones,[125] with ΔOD_{450} values below 0.09 suggesting an unaffected or mildly affected infant and ΔOD_{450} values above 0.15 suggesting fetal anemia. In some cases, especially those with a history of severe second-trimester disease or previous severe disease with misleading ΔOD_{450} values, cordocentesis to determine the fetal hematocrit is a reasonable first step. Again, the optimum management in an individual case will be determined by history, clinical findings, and the experience and expertise of the management team.

At any gestational age, the presence of fetal hydrops should be taken as evidence of severe fetal anemia, and cordocentesis with immediate intravascular transfusion is indicated.

Timing of Delivery

If the history and antenatal studies indicate only mild fetal hemolysis, we undertake delivery by induction of labor at 37 to 38 weeks' gestation, unless fetal pulmonary maturity is documented earlier by amniocentesis. In these cases, fetal pulmonary maturation does not seem to be either delayed or accelerated by disease, and amniotic fluid studies accurately reflect fetal maturity.[215,216] If the cervix is not ripe, we typically use intracervical prostaglandin gel prior to oxytocin induction.

With severely sensitized pregnancies, the risks of continued cord blood sampling and transfusions must be weighed against the expected neonatal morbidity and mortality associated with early delivery. Because the overall neonatal survival rate in most neonatal intensive care nurseries is greater than 95 percent after 32 weeks, procedures have generally been timed so that the last transfusion is performed at around 30 to 32 weeks' gestation, with patients then delivered at 32 to 34 weeks after maternal steroid administration to enhance fetal pulmonary maturity.

If delivery can be carried out at about 34 to 36 weeks, overall neonatal survival approaches 100 percent at this gestational age and long-term morbidity from prematurity is exceedingly low. Re-gardless of the usual institutional practices, individual case circumstances need to be carefully weighed when making the decision as to when the fetus should be delivered.

SENSITIZATION CAUSED BY MINOR ANTIGENS

In addition to the D antigen, hundreds of other distinct antigens exist on the red blood cell surface. Known as "minor," "atypical," or "irregular" antigens, they have different frequencies in different ethnic populations. For instance, about 30 percent of blacks are positive for the Duffy antigen, whereas less than 5 percent of whites are Duffy positive.

In the past, minor antigens were a relatively infrequent cause of maternal sensitization and fetal or neonatal hemolytic disease. Because of the reduction in Rh disease brought about by Rh-immune globulin prophylaxis, minor antigen sensitization has become relatively more frequent in pregnancy. In fact, antibodies to minor antigens are much more common in the general population than antibodies to the D antigen.[90]

The large majority of cases of minor antigen sensitization are caused by incompatible blood transfusion. Overall, antibodies to minor antigens occur in about 1.5 to 2.5 percent of obstetric patients.[219,220] Fortunately, some of the most common atypical antibodies, such as anti-Le^a, anti-Le^b, and anti-I, do not cause fetal or neonatal hemolysis. Le^a and Le^b, the Lewis antigens are not true erythrocyte antigens, but are secreted by other tissues and then adsorbed onto the red cell surface.[221] Fetal erythrocytes acquire very little antigen in utero and thus react only weakly to anti-Lewis.

However, antibodies to a number of the minor antigens can result in fetal anemia and hydrops. Of the potentially serious antibodies, anti-E, anti-Kell, anti-c, anti-c + E, and anti-Fy^a (Duffy) are the most common.[90]

In general, management of the pregnant patient with antibody to one of the significant minor antigens is much the same as for RhD immunization. Pregnancies are followed using previous history as a guide, paternal antigen and zygosity testing to determine risk, frequent measurement of maternal antibody levels until a critical titer is reached, then serial amniocenteses with assessment of fetal antigen status and amniotic fluid bilirubin levels, and transfusion or delivery based on the ΔOD_{450} values and trends.[120,222] However, few centers have experience with a large number of pregnancies affected by minor antigen sensitization; thus, establishment of a critical maternal titer is difficult, and it is uncertain whether amniotic fluid bilirubin studies are as reliable as with RhD alloimmunization.

MNSs

Of the minor antigens, special mention is given to MNS. The M antigen is part of the MNSs blood group system and is one of the commonly encountered minor antigens, since approximately 20 to 25 percent of the population is M negative. Improvements in antibody screening techniques have improved the sensitivity of detection of anti-M, and the frequency of identification of maternal anti-M is apparently increasing. In general there is limited benefit to following serial anti-M titers, and if there is no previous history of an affected fetus and the initial titer is 1:4 or less, no further assessment of anti-M titers is necessary.

There are case reports of severe fetal and neonatal hemolytic disease due to M sensitization.[230,231] It has been suggested that although most anti-M is an IgM antibody with no implications for the fetus, some sensitized women produce a potent anti-M IgG which can cross the placenta and result in fetal anemia and hydrops.

We assess paternal M antigen status and perform serial anti-M titers in sensitized pregnancies without a history of an affected fetus. If the titer rises unexpectedly, amniocentesis is performed for amniotic fluid bilirubin studies and determination of fetal M status. Because anti-M does not seem to be as aggressive or as serious as most of the other antigens, our threshold for amniocentesis is generally higher than for the other serious antigens, although we consider each case on an individual basis.

Kell

The Kell antigen also requires additional discussion. Pregnancy with Kell sensitization can result in severe fetal anemia, hydrops, and fetal death. In common usage, "Kell" refers to the K or K1 antigen of the Kell blood group system. Only about 9 percent of whites are positive for the Kell antigen; the population frequency of kk (Kell negative) is 91.1 percent, Kk (heterozygous positive) 8.7 percent, and KK (homozygous positive) 0.2 percent.[7] About 0.2 percent of pregnant women are positive for anti-Kell. As mentioned above, most cases of immunization are the result of Kell-incompatible transfusion.

A number of investigators have suggested that the fetal anemia associated with Kell sensitization is qualitatively different from that of Rh disease and requires a different management protocol.[232,238] Maternal titers and amniotic fluid ΔOD_{450} values may not be as predictive of the degree of fetal anemia as with RhD sensitization.

Recognizing that amniotic fluid bilirubin studies may be misleading in some pregnancies and that more liberal use of umbilical cord blood sampling is appropriate, we still use serial ΔOD_{450} measurements. When the father is known to be Kell negative, the fetus will also be Kell negative, and no surveillance or testing is necessary. When the father is Kell positive or of uncertain status and there is no history of severe fetal involvement, we follow maternal anti-Kell titers, track fetal movements, and perform serial ultrasounds as long as the maternal titer remains below 1:8. For patients whose titers rise above 1:8 or who have a history of fetal involvement, we perform serial amniocenteses every 1 to 4 weeks unless the fetus is known to be Kell negative, beginning at 20 to 28 weeks depending on history, maternal titer, and previous ΔOD_{450} value. At the first amniocentesis, we determine fetal Kell antigen status by DNA testing. As with RhD disease, we use a modified Liley curve extrapolated back to 24 weeks (Fig. 22–4); before 24 weeks' gestation, we typically use Queenan's boundaries[125] with an emphasis on ΔOD_{450} trends. If ΔOD_{450} levels rise into or above the middle of zone II, we recommend umbilical cord blood sampling for hematocrit, with blood ready for transfusion if necessary. Between amniocenteses and/or fetal blood samplings, we perform nonstress tests and frequent ultrasounds, watching for any signs of developing hydrops.

Key Points

➤ To reduce the incidence of Rh sensitization, Rh-immune globulin should be given to Rh-negative unsensitized women at 28 weeks' gestational age and again after delivery if the newborn is Rh-positive. Rh-immune globulin is also indicated for these patients in cases of miscarriage; ectopic pregnancy; chorionic villus sampling, amniocentesis, or other intrauterine procedures; abdominal trauma or fetal death in the second or third trimester; or fetomaternal hemorrhage.

➤ The gene coding for the D antigen has been identified, and prenatal determination of fetal Rh status is routinely available from uncultured amniocytes obtained at amniocentesis.

➤ Measurement of amniotic fluid bilirubin remains the standard for assessment of pregnancies at risk for significant fetal anemia. Neither ultrasound alone nor Doppler studies are adequately sensitive to identify anemic fetuses.

➤ The timing of the first amniocentesis is based on history, maternal anti-D titers, gestational age, and ultrasound findings. The timing of subsequent amniocenteses is based on the ΔOD_{450} values and trends.

➤ Analysis of amniotic fluid bilirubin before 26 weeks is controversial. Although most data suggest that ΔOD_{450} values and trends are accurate before the third trimester, more liberal use of cordocentesis may be appropriate.

➤ With the reduction in Rh disease brought about by widespread use of Rh-immune globulin prophylaxis, sensitization to the minor or atypical antigens has become relatively more common. A number of these minor antigens can cause several fetal anemia.

➤ Management of pregnancies complicated by sensitization to one of the serious minor antigens (such as Kell) is based on analogy to Rh disease; determination of fetal antigen status from uncultured amniocytes is available for the most common antigens. However, amniotic fluid bilirubin analysis may not be as accurate an indicator of fetal anemia with Kell sensitization as with Rh disease, and a more frequent use of cordocentesis is probably appropriate.

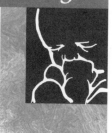

Pregnancy and Coexisting Disease

Chapter 23

Hypertension in Pregnancy

BAHA M. SIBAI

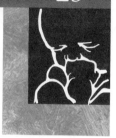

Hypertensive disorders are the most common medical complications of pregnancy, with a reported incidence between 5 and 10 percent.[1] The term *hypertension in pregnancy* is usually used to describe a wide spectrum of patients who may have only mild elevations in blood pressure or severe hypertension with various organ dysfunctions.

DEFINITIONS

Women with hypertension may be classified into one of three categories: gestational hypertension, preeclampsia/eclampsia, or chronic hypertension.

Gestational Hypertension

Gestational hypertension is the development of an elevated blood pressure ≥140/90 mm Hg, on at least two occasions 4 hours apart, during pregnancy or in the first 24 hours postpartum without other signs or symptoms of preeclampsia or preexisting hypertension. The blood pressure must return to normal within 6 weeks after delivery.

Preeclampsia and Eclampsia

The so-called classic triad of preeclampsia includes hypertension, proteinuria, and edema. However, there is now universal agreement that edema should not be considered as part of the diagnosis of preeclampsia.[5-7] Indeed, edema is neither sufficient nor necessary to confirm the diagnosis of preeclampsia, since edema is a common finding in normal pregnancy and approximately one third of

> ### Criteria for Severe Preeclampsia
>
> 1. Blood pressure of ≥160 mm Hg systolic or ≥110 mm Hg diastolic, recorded on at least two occasions at least 6 hours apart with patient at bed rest
> 2. Proteinuria of ≥5 g in 24 hours
> 3. Oliguria (≤400 ml in 24 hours)
> 4. Cerebral visual disturbances
> 5. Epigastric pain, nausea, and vomiting
> 6. Pulmonary edema
> 7. Impaired liver function of unclear etiology
> 8. Thrombocytopenia
> 9. IUGR or oligohydramaios

eclamptic women never demonstrate the presence of edema.[8] At present, preeclampsia is primarily defined as gestational hypertension plus proteinuria. Proteinuria is defined as a concentration of 0.1 g/L or more in at least two random urine specimens collected 4 hours or more apart or 0.3 g in a 24-hour period. In the absence of proteinuria, the syndrome of preeclampsia should be considered when gestational hypertension is present in association with persistent cerebral symptoms, epigastric or right upper quadrant pain plus nausea or vomiting, fetal growth restriction, or with abnormal laboratory tests such as thrombocytopenia and abnormal liver enzymes.[3,9] In mild preeclampsia, the diastolic blood pressure remains below 110 mm Hg and the systolic blood pressure remains below 160 mm Hg (see the box "Criteria for Severe Preeclampsia"). Eclampsia is the occurrence of seizures not attributable to other causes.

Chronic Hypertension

Chronic hypertension is defined as hypertension present before the pregnancy or that diagnosed before the 20th week of gestation. Hypertension that persists for more than 42 days postpartum is also classified as chronic hypertension.

Chronic Hypertension with Superimposed Preeclampsia

Women with chronic hypertension may develop superimposed preeclampsia. The diagnosis of superimposed preeclampsia is based on one or more of the following findings: in women with hypertension and no proteinuria prior to 20 weeks' gestation, development of new-onset proteinuria is defined as the urinary excretion of 0.5 g protein or greater in a 24-hour specimen; in women with hypertension and proteinuria before 20 weeks, the diagnosis requires severe exacerbation in hypertension plus development of symptoms and/or thrombocytopenia and abnormal liver enzymes.[10]

PREECLAMPSIA

The incidence of preeclampsia ranges between 3 and 7 percent in nulliparas[3,11-13] and between 0.8 and 5.0 percent in multiparas.[12,20] The incidence is significantly increased in patients with twin pregnancies, a family history, preeclampsia in a previous pregnancy, preexisting hypertension, renal disease, or diabetes mellitus.

The etiology of preeclampsia is unknown. Many theories have been suggested, but most of them have not withstood the test of time.

Laboratory Abnormalities in Preeclampsia

Women with preeclampsia may exhibit a symptom complex ranging from minimal blood pressure elevation to derangements of multiple organ systems. The renal, hematologic, and hepatic systems are most likely to be involved.

Renal Function

In preeclampsia, vasospasm and glomerular capillary endothelial swelling (glomerular endotheliosis) lead to an average reduction in GFR of 25 percent below the rate for normal pregnancy.[129] Serum creatinine is rarely elevated in preeclampsia, but uric acid is commonly increased.[130]

Hepatic Function

Hepatic involvement is observed in only 10 percent of women with severe preeclampsia.[134] When liver dysfunction occurs in preeclampsia, mild elevation of serum transaminase is most common,[136] and bilirubin is rarely increased. Elevated liver enzymes are part of the syndrome of hemolysis, elevated liver enzymes, and low platelets (HELLP), a variant of severe preeclampsia.

Hematologic Changes

Thrombocytopenia is the most common hematologic abnormality in women with preeclampsia.

Leduc and associates[140] studied the coagulation profile (platelet count, fibrinogen, prothrombin time, and partial thromboplastin time) in 100 consecutive women with severe preeclampsia.

A platelet count less than $150,000/mm^3$ is found in 50 percent and a count of less than $100,000/mm^3$ in 36 percent of women with severe preeclampsia. The admission platelet count is an excellent predictor of subsequent coagulation studies, and fibrinogen levels, prothrombin time, and partial thromboplastin time should be obtained only in women with a platelet count of less than $100,000/mm^3$.

The HELLP Syndrome

The syndrome of hemolysis, elevated liver enzymes and low platelets (HELLP) is a variant of severe preeclampsia. Thrombocytopenia, a platelet count less than $100,000/mm^3$, has been the most consistent finding. There is a strong association between the presence of HELLP syndrome and eclampsia, with HELLP syndrome present in 30 percent of patients.

Hemolysis, defined as the presence of microangiopathic hemolytic anemia, is the hallmark of the HELLP syndrome. The HELLP syndrome is not a variant of DIC, since coagulation parameters such as prothrombin time, partial thromboplastin time, and serum fibrinogen are normal.[143] DIC is defined as the presence of thrombocytopenia, low fibrinogen levels (plasma fibrinogen <300 mg/dl), and fibrin split products above 40 mg/ml. DIC is seen in 20 percent of patients with HELLP syndrome. The majority of cases occur in women who have antecedent abruptio placentae, peripartum hemorrhage, or subcapsular liver hematomas. In the absence of these complications, the frequency of DIC is only 5 percent.[153]

Laboratory criteria to establish the diagnosis are presented in the box "Criteria to Establish the Diagnosis of HELLP Syndrome."

The patient is usually seen remote from term complaining of epigastric or right upper quadrant pain (65 percent), nausea or vomiting (50 percent), or nonspecific viral syndrome-like symptoms. The majority of patients will give a history of malaise for the past few days

---

Criteria to Establish the Diagnosis of HELLP Syndrome

Hemolysis
  Abnormal peripheral blood smear
  Increased bilirubin >1.2 mg/dl
  Increased lactic dehydrogenase >600 IU/L

Elevated liver enzymes
  Increased SGOT ≥72 IU/L
  Increased lactic dehydrogenase >600 IU/L

Thrombocytopenia
  Platelet count <$100,000/mm^3$

before presentation; some may present with hematuria or gastrointestinal bleeding. Hypertension and proteinuria may be absent or slightly abnormal.[153-155] Physical examination will demonstrate right upper quadrant tenderness and significant weight gain with edema.

Severe hypertension is not a constant or even a frequent finding in HELLP syndrome. Patients are often misdiagnosed as having various medical and surgical disorders (see the box "Medical and Surgical Disorders Confused with the HELLP Syndrome"). A rare but interesting complication of HELLP syndrome is transient nephrogenic diabetes insipidus. It is postulated that elevated circulating vasopressinase may result from impaired hepatic metabolism of the enzyme.

Pregnant women with probable preeclampsia presenting with atypical symptoms should have a complete blood count, a platelet count, and liver enzyme determinations irrespective of maternal blood pressure.[146]

Management of preeclamptic patients presenting with the HELLP syndrome is similar to that used in the management of severe preeclampsia remote from term. The majority of these patients will experience deterioration in either maternal or fetal condition within 1 to 10 days after conservative management. It is doubtful that such limited pregnancy prolongation will result in improved perinatal outcome, and maternal and fetal risks are substantial.

The reported perinatal mortality has ranged from 7.7 to 60 percent and maternal mortality from 0 to 24 percent. Maternal

Medical and Surgical Disorders Confused with the HELLP Syndrome

Acute fatty liver of pregnancy
Appendicitis
Diabetes mellitus
Gallbladder disease
Gastroenteritis
Glomerulonephritis
Hemolytic uremic syndrome
Hepatic encephalopathy
Hyperemesis gravidarum
Idiopathic thrombocytopenia
Kidney stones
Peptic ulcer
Pyelonephritis
Systemic lupus erythematosus
Thrombotic thrombocytopenic purpura
Viral hepatitis

morbidity is common. Most of these patients have required transfusions of blood and blood products and are at increased risk for the development of acute renal failure, pulmonary edema, ascites, pleural effusions, and hepatic rupture,[151,153,164,167–170] and abruptio placentae with DIC.

Seventy percent of patients have the syndrome antepartum, and 30 percent postpartum, with the majority developing it within 48 hours postpartum. Eighty percent of the postpartum patients have preeclampsia prior to delivery, whereas 20 percent have no evidence of preeclampsia before delivery. The differential diagnosis should include exacerbation of systemic lupus erythematosus, thrombotic thrombocytopenic purpura, and hemolytic uremic syndrome.

Patients with the HELLP syndrome who are remote from term should be referred to a tertiary care center, and their initial management should be the same as that for any patient with severe preeclampsia. The first priority is to assess and stabilize maternal condition, particularly coagulation abnormalities. The next step is to evaluate fetal well-being using the nonstress test and biophysical profile. Then, a decision must be made as to whether delivery is indicated. The patient may be given steroids to accelerate fetal lung maturity and then delivered 24 hours later. During this time, both maternal and fetal conditions should be monitored closely. This syndrome is not an indication for immediate cesarean delivery. Patients presenting with well-established labor should be allowed to deliver vaginally as indicated. In addition, labor may be induced as indicated.

The majority of these patients will have spontaneous resolution of their disease. Some have recommended that a trial of plasma exchange with fresh frozen plasma be considered in HELLP syndrome that persists past 72 hours postpartum and in which there is evidence of a life-threatening microangiopathy, but plasmapheresis is not usually needed in the management of such patients.[153,170]

Subcapsular Hematoma of the Liver in HELLP Syndrome

Because it occurs so rarely, the diagnosis of a subcapsular hematoma of the liver in pregnancy is often overlooked. The differential diagnosis should include acute cholecystitis with sepsis, acute fatty liver of pregnancy, ruptured uterus, placental abruption with DIC, and thrombotic thrombocytopenia purpura (TTP). In addition to the signs and symptoms of preeclampsia, physical findings consistent with peritoneal irritation, epigastric pain and hepatomegaly may be present. Profound hypovolemic shock with hypotension in a previously hypertensive patient is a hallmark of rupture of the hematoma. Laboratory evaluation is often consistent with DIC.

Rupture of a subcapsular hematoma of the liver is a life-threatening complication of HELLP syndrome. An ultrasound or computed axial tomographic (CAT) scan of the liver should be performed to rule out subcapsular hematoma and detect the presence of intraperitoneal bleeding.[172] Paracentesis can confirm intraperitoneal hemorrhage suspected by radiographic imaging.

Surgical repair has been recommended for hepatic hemorrhage without liver rupture. More recent experience suggests, however, that this complication can be managed conservatively in patients who remain hemodynamically stable.[172-174] Serial assessment of the subcapsular hematoma with ultrasound or computed tomographic (CT) scan is necessary with immediate intervention for rupture or worsening maternal status. It is important with conservative management to avoid exogenous sources of trauma to the liver such as abdominal palpation, convulsions, or emesis and to use care in transportation of the patient.

There is an 82 percent overall survival for the patients managed by packing and drainage, whereas only 25 percent of gravidas undergoing hepatic lobectomy survived.

The Management of Preeclampsia

Definitive therapy in the form of delivery is the only cure for preeclampsia. The decision between immediate delivery and expectant management will depend on the severity of the disease process, maternal and fetal status at the time of initial evaluation, and fetal gestational age.

Mild Preeclampsia

Patients with diagnosed preeclampsia should ideally be hospitalized at the time of diagnosis for evaluation of maternal and fetal conditions. These pregnancies may be associated with reduced uteroplacental blood flow jeopardizing the fetus. The mother is at a increased risk for the development of abruptio placentae or convulsions, particularly in cases remote from term. Thus, women with mild disease who have a favorable cervix at or near term should undergo induction of labor. The pregnancy should not continue past 40 weeks' gestation, even if conditions for induction of labor are unfavorable.

The optimal management of mild preeclampsia less than 37 weeks' gestation is hospitalization for the duration of pregnancy, because this approach enhances fetal survival and diminishes the frequency of progression to severe disease.[199,200] Patients who have only mild gestational hypertension without proteinuria can be safely managed on an ambulatory basis.

At our institution, women with mild preeclampsia are hospitalized at the time of their diagnosis. During hospitalization, patients receive a regular diet with no salt restriction and no activity limits. Diuretics and antihypertensive drugs are not prescribed, and sedatives are not used. Patients initially undergo evaluation of maternal and fetal well-being. The frequency of subsequent testing usually depends on the gestational age and maternal response following hospitalization. Subsequent fetal evaluation includes serial ultrasonography for fetal growth every 3 weeks, daily fetal movement count, nonstress testing every week, and a biophysical profile if needed. Maternal evaluation includes blood pressure monitoring (every 4 hours during the day) and daily assessment of maternal weight to detect excessive weight gain. In addition, women are questioned regarding symptoms of impending eclampsia (persistent headache, visual disturbances, or epigastric pain). Laboratory evaluation includes measurements of 24 hour urine protein, hematocrit, platelet count, and liver function tests once or twice weekly, as patients may develop thrombocytopenia and elevated liver enzymes with minimal blood pressure elevation.[155]

Severe Preeclampsia

The clinical course of severe preeclampsia may be characterized by progressive deterioration in both maternal and fetal conditions. All such patients should be delivered if the disease develops after 34 weeks' gestation or prior to that time if there is evidence of maternal or fetal distress.[209] There is also agreement on delivery of such patients prior to 35 weeks' gestation in the presence of any of the following: premature rupture of membranes, labor, or severe fetal growth restriction.

There is considerable disagreement about management of patients with severe disease prior to 34 weeks' gestation. Some authors consider delivery as the definitive therapy for all cases, regardless of gestational age, whereas others recommend prolonging pregnancy in all severe preeclamptic gestations remote from term until development of fetal lung maturity, fetal or maternal distress, or a gestational age of 34 weeks is achieved.[169,170,209-213]

Severe Preeclampsia at 28 to 32 Weeks' Gestation

Studies describing expectant management of women with severe preeclampsia at 28 to 32 weeks' gestation[209] suggest that expectant management can improve outcome in selected patients.[209] Patients managed expectantly with intensive monitoring and nifedipine had a safer perinatal outcome than those delivered within 72 hours.

Mid-Trimester Severe Preeclampsia

Aggressive management with immediate delivery will result in high neonatal mortality. However, attempts to prolong pregnancy may result in fetal demise or asphyxial damage in utero and severe maternal morbidity and even mortality. All patients are first admitted to labor and delivery and are evaluated carefully for the presence of either maternal or fetal compromise. Pregnancy termination is recommended for patients with gestational ages of 24 weeks or less whereas expectant management is recommended for patients with gestational age over 24 weeks. The latter patients are managed with bed rest, magnesium sulfate, antihypertensive drugs, and frequent evaluation of maternal and fetal well-being. Expectant management for women with severe preeclampsia should be selective and done only in a tertiary care center with adequate intensive care facilities.[218] Neonatal survival is 65 percent in expectantly managed patients compared with 24 percent who are given steroids and delivered 48 hours later.

Patients with resistant severe hypertension or other signs of maternal or fetal deterioration are delivered within 24 hours, irrespective of gestational age or fetal lung maturity.[209] In addition, patients in labor, or those with fetuses with a gestational age greater than 34 weeks, and those with evidence of fetal lung maturity by amniocentesis are also are delivered within 24 hours.[209] Patients at 32 to 34 weeks gestation with immature fluid receive steroids to accelerate fetal lung maturity and are delivered 24 hours after the last dose of steroids in the absence of any change in maternal or fetal condition.

Corticosteroids are safe and effective drugs for preventing respiratory distress syndrome, treating thrombocytopenia, and improving perinatal outcome in severe preeclampsia. We administer betamethasone 12 mg as soon as possible and the dose is repeated 24 hours later.

Patients at 28 to 32 weeks' gestation receive individualized management based on their clinical response during the observation period. All of these patients receive steroids to accelerate fetal lung maturity, as there is still benefit even if the delivery occurs in less than 24 hours or more than 1 week later. If the blood pressure remains below 100 mm Hg diastolic without antihypertensive therapy after the observation period, magnesium sulfate is discontinued, and the patients are followed closely on the antepartum high-risk ward until fetal maturity is achieved. During hospitalization, they receive antihypertensive drugs, usually oral nifedipine 40 to 120 mg/day, to keep their diastolic blood pressure between 90 and 100 mm Hg, with daily evaluation of maternal and fetal well-being.

All women with severe preeclampsia should receive magnesium sulfate to prevent eclampsia. Magnesium sulfate is administered by a controlled continuous intravenous infusion with a loading dose of 6 g in 100 ml over 15 to 20 minutes. The intravenous route for magnesium therapy permits more precise control of the patient's blood level and avoids the pain of intramuscular injections. Maintenance therapy is given at a rate of 2 g in 100 ml of fluid per hour. Treatment is continued for 12 to 24 hours after delivery.

Magnesium is excreted in the urine, so, an accurate record of maternal urine output must be maintained. In patients with normal renal function, the half-life for magnesium excretion is about 4 hours. In the therapeutic range (4.8 to 9.6 mg/dl), magnesium sulfate slows neuromuscular conduction and depresses central nervous system irritability. For this reason, maternal respiratory rate, deep tendon reflexes, and state of consciousness must be frequently monitored to detect magnesium toxicity. An ampule of calcium gluconate, 1 g (10 ml of 10 percent solution) should be drawn up in a syringe, clearly labeled, and kept at the bedside in case of magnesium toxicity. If respiratory depression occurs, the magnesium sulphate should be stopped and the calcium gluconate should be given intravenously over 3 minutes. (see the box "Magnesium Toxicity").

We carefully monitor the volume of intravenous fluids used in women with preeclampsia or eclampsia. Intake and output should be assessed hourly. Our goal is to maintain the urine output at 30 ml/h. If urine output drops below 100 ml in 4 hours, the dose of magnesium sulfate and intravenous fluids should be reduced accordingly. Another cause of decreased urine output is a drop in maternal blood pressure due to repeated injections of hydralazine. Hydralazine has a relatively long duration of action and, when multiple bolus injections of hydralazine are used to control blood pressure, the diastolic blood pressure may be reduced more than intended, which will reduce urine output for 2 to 3 hours. One of the potential problems when attempting to limit intravenous fluids to 125 ml/h is that high concentrations of drugs must be used if the woman is receiving intravenous magnesium sulfate, oxytocin, and hydralazine.

To control severe maternal hypertension intrapartum, we use bolus injections of hydralazine 5 to 10 mg every 20 to 30 minutes to lower the diastolic blood pressure to the 90 to 100 mm Hg

Magnesium Toxicity	
Loss of patellar reflex	8–12 mg/dl
Feelings of warmth, flushing	9–12 mg/dl
Somnolence	10–12 mg/dl
Slurred speech	10–12 mg/dl
Muscular paralysis	15–17 mg/dl
Respiratory difficulty	15–17 mg/dl
Cardiac arrest	30–35 mg/dl

range. This requires monitoring of blood pressure every 5 minutes for at least 30 minutes after the drug is given. An alternative regimen is to use bolus injections of labetalol hydrochloride, 20 to 80 mg. Unlike hydralazine, labetalol does not cause maternal tachycardia, flushing, or headaches. Oral nifedipine in doses of 10 to 20 mg every 4 to 6 hours may also be used.

Counseling Women Who Have Had Preeclampsia in Prior Pregnancies

There is a strong familial predisposition for preeclampsia. In 273 primigravidas whose sisters did not have preeclampsia, the incidence of severe preeclampsia was 4.5 percent. The incidence of severe preeclampsia was 13.8 percent for women whose sisters had severe preeclampsia during their first pregnancies. The incidence of severe preeclampsia was 15.9 percent in the 126 mothers of primigravidas who had severe preeclampsia compared with 4.4 percent in the 136 mothers-in-law.

We have examined the pregnancy outcomes and incidences of preeclampsia in subsequent pregnancies, as well as the frequency of chronic hypertension and diabetes mellitus in women who had severe preeclampsia or eclampsia in their first pregnancies compared with 409 women who remained normotensive during their first pregnancies. The incidence of chronic hypertension was significantly higher in the preeclampsia patients (14.8 vs. 5.6 percent; $p < 0.001$). This difference became even greater for those women followed for more than 10 years (51 vs. 14 percent; $p < 0.001$). The incidence of severe preeclampsia was also significantly higher in the second pregnancies (26 to 5 percent) as well as in the subsequent pregnancies (12 to 5 percent) of women with preeclampsia.[239]

In women who had severe preeclampsia in the second trimester,[240] 65 percent of subsequent pregnancies were complicated by preeclampsia. Overall, 21 percent of all subsequent pregnancies were complicated by severe preeclampsia in the second trimester. In addition, these women have a high rate of chronic hypertension on follow-up, with the highest incidence being in those who had recurrent severe preeclampsia in the second trimester (55 percent).

The risk of abruptio placentae increases significantly in those with severe preeclampsia before 34 weeks' gestation and particularly in those who have severe preeclampsia in the second trimester.[241] The risk of subsequent abruptio ranges from 5 to 20 percent.

Women with severe preeclampsia remote from term may have underlying renal disease for which they should be evaluated after delivery.

ECLAMPSIA

Eclampsia is the occurrence of convulsions or coma unrelated to other cerebral conditions with signs and symptoms of preeclampsia. Magnesium sulfate is the drug of choice for eclampsia. Women in whom eclampsia develops exhibit a wide spectrum of signs and symptoms, ranging from extremely high blood pressure, 4+ proteinuria, generalized edema, and 4+ patellar reflexes to minimal blood pressure elevation, no proteinuria or edema, and normal reflexes.

Eclampsia usually begins with rapid weight gain and ends with the onset of generalized convulsions or coma. Hypertension is the hallmark of eclampsia and excess weight gain or edema are not necessary for the diagnosis.[8] Eclampsia is usually associated with significant proteinuria. In eclamptic women, headache, visual disturbances, and right upper quadrant/epigastric pain are the most common premonitory symptoms before convulsions. Of interest was the absence of edema (26 percent) and proteinuria (14 percent) in 399 eclamptic women.

Convulsions may occur antepartum, intrapartum, or postpartum. Half of all cases of eclampsia usually occur before the onset of labor, with the other 50 percent equally divided between the intrapartum and postpartum periods. Maternal death occurs in approximately 1/250 eclamptic women, either from magnesium toxicity or cardiorespiratory arrest after multpile seizures. The main risks to the fetus are abruptio placentae, prematurity, IUGR, and sequalae of hypoxia during the convulsions. CAT scans and other imaging studies have not proven helpful in patient care.

Management of Labor and Delivery in Eclampsia

The woman with eclampsia should undergo continuous intensive monitoring. The guard rails should be up on the bed and a padded tongue blade kept at the bedside. A large-bore peripheral intravenous line should be in place. No other anticonvulsants should be left at the bedside except for a syringe containing 2 to 4 g magnesium sulfate. No more than 8 g magnesium sulfate should be given over a short period of time to control convulsions.

We previously recommended only a complete blood count including blood smear and platelet count, clot observation, and serum creatinine in women with eclampsia.[275] Liver function tests were obtained only in women with upper abdominal pain. However, because of an increase in the number of women with HELLP syndrome and eclampsia as well as those with serious medical problems, we have expanded the laboratory tests ordered in eclamptic women to include fibrinogen, electrolytes, and arterial blood gases.

Once convulsions have been controlled and the woman has regained consciousness, her general medical condition is assessed. When she is stable, induction of labor with oxytocin is initiated. Delivery is the treatment for eclampsia. Fetal heart rate and intensity of uterine contractions should be closely monitored. There is a high intrapartum complication rate in eclampsia that develops before 30 weeks' gestation,[276] including fetal growth restriction (30 percent), abruption (23 percent), and fetal distress during labor (65 percent), so elective cesarean section may be appropriate in this group.

Fetal bradycardia can occur during an eclamptic seizure, with fetal tachycardia occurring frequently after the prolonged bradycardia. Loss of beat-to-beat variability with transitory late decelerations occur during the recovery phase. Uterine hyperactivity demonstrated by both increased uterine tone and increased frequency of uterine contractions occurs during an eclamptic seizure. The duration of the increased uterine activity varies from 2 to 14 minutes.

Fetal outcome is generally good after an eclamptic convulsion. The mechanism for the transitory fetal bradycardia may be a decrease in uterine blood flow caused by intense vasospasm and uterine hyperactivity, or the absence of maternal respiration during the convulsion. Since the fetal heart rate pattern usually returns to normal after a convulsion, other conditions should be considered if an abnormal pattern persists, such as IUGR or placental abruption.

Treatment of Eclamptic Convulsions

Eclamptic convulsions are a life-threatening emergency and are tonic-clonic in type. The woman usually bites her tongue unless it is protected. Respirations are absent throughout the seizure. Coma follows the convulsion, and the woman usually remembers nothing of the recent events. If she has repeated convulsions, some degree of consciousness returns after each convulsion. She may enter a combative state and be agitated and difficult to control. Rapid and deep respirations usually begin as soon as the convulsions end. Maintenance of oxygenation is usually not a problem after a single convulsion; the risk of aspiration is low in the well-managed patient.

Several steps should be taken in managing an eclamptic convulsion:

1. *Do not attempt to shorten or abolish the initial convulsion:* Drugs such as diazepam should not be given in an attempt to stop or shorten the convulsion, especially if the patient does not have an intravenous line in place and someone skilled in intubation is not immediately available. Rapid administration of diazepam may lead to apnea or cardiac arrest, or both.[278]
2. *Prevent maternal injury during the convulsion:* A padded tongue blade should be inserted between the patient's teeth to prevent

biting of the tongue. Place the woman on her left side and then suction the foam and secretions from her mouth.

3. *Maintain adequate oxygenation:* After the convulsion has ceased, the patient begins to breathe again and oxygenation is rarely a problem. Difficulty with oxygenation may occur in women who have had repetitive convulsions or who have received drugs in an attempt to abolish the convulsions.

4. *Minimize the risk of aspiration:* Aspiration should be a rare occurrence with eclamptic convulsions. It may be caused by forcing the padded tongue blade to the back of the throat, stimulating the gag reflex with resultant vomiting and aspiration. The use of sedative drugs increases the risks of aspiration and so they should be avoided.

5. *Give adequate magnesium sulfate to control the convulsions:* As soon as the convulsion has ended, a large secure intravenous (IV) line should be inserted and a loading dose of magnesium sulfate given intravenously. In our institution, we use a 6-g intravenous loading dose given over *15 to 20 minutes.* If the patient has a convulsion after the loading dose, another bolus of 2 g magnesium sulfate can be given intravenously over 3 to 5 minutes. Approximately 10 to 15 percent of women will have a second convulsion after receiving the intravenous loading dose of magnesium sulfate.

We use serum magnesium levels in the clinical management of the eclamptic woman. If the initial level, obtained 4 hours after the loading dose, is high, over 10 mg/dl, we reduce the 2-g/hr maintenance dose of magnesium sulfate. This will occasionally occur in women with renal compromise. Similarly, in the rare patient with a brisk urine output, we give a maintenance dose of 3 g/hr to keep levels in the therapeutic range.

Fourteen percent of patients will have recurrent convulsions while receiving therapeutic doses of magnesium sulfate. In these cases, a short-acting barbiturate such as sodium amobarbital can be given in a dose of up to 250 mg IV over 3 to 5 minutes or an intravenous sodium pentothal drip can be used.

Magnesium toxicity should be considered in those women who do not regain consciousness as accidental overdoses have been reproted.

6. *Maternal acidemia should be corrected:* Blood oxygenation and pH should be in the normal range. Patients who have had repeated convulsions may be acidotic and a low PO_2 may indicate aspiration pneumonitis. Sodium bicarbonate is not given unless the pH is below 7.10. Abnormal blood gases may be the result of respiratory depression.

7. *Avoid polypharmacy:* Polypharmacy is extremely hazardous in the woman with eclampsia, as addition of diazepam or phenytoin may lead to respiratory depression or respiratory arrest.

No alternate drug has been proven to be as effective as magnesium sulfate in treating eclamptic convulsions.[18]

Atypical Eclampsia

Eclampsia occurring before the 20th week of gestation or more than 48 hours postpartum has been called *atypical eclampsia.* Eclampsia occurring before the 20th week of gestation has usually been reported with molar or hydropic degeneration of the placenta.

These women may be misdiagnosed as having hypertensive encephalopathy or a seizure disorder. Women in whom convulsions develop in association with hypertension and proteinuria during the first half of pregnancy should be considered to have eclampsia. They should be treated with parenteral magnesium sulfate to control convulsions, with termination of pregnancy as the definitive therapy.

Late postpartum eclampsia accounts for 16 percent of eclampsia cases. Because of the unusual time of occurrence of eclampsia in these women, neurologic consultations are recommended to rule out abnormalities.[251]

Can Eclampsia Be Prevented?

Eclampsia is generally considered a preventable complication of pregnancy. Severe forms of preeclampsia should be preventable by appropriate prenatal care. About 30 to 42 percent of cases of eclampsia are not preventable.

Counseling Women with Eclampsia and Their Relatives

Long-term follow-up of women who had eclampsia found no increase in hypertension in these patients above that expected in the general female population. Preeclampsia/eclampsia does not cause hypertension. Women who had eclampsia as multiparas died at a rate which was significantly higher than the expected mortality rate. Eighty-two percent of the remote deaths were due to cardiovascular/renal disease.

The prognosis for future pregnancies after eclampsia is good. Preeclampsia/eclampsia recurred in 34.5 percent of the women and in 20.6 percent of their subsequent pregnancies. When hypertension occurred in a future pregnancy, it was usually mild. Eclampsia developed in 1 percent in pregnancies beyond 20 weeks' gestation.

The sisters and daughters of eclamptic women are at increased risk for the development of preeclampsia and eclampsia.[301] Preeclampsia occurred in 25 percent, and eclampsia in 3 percent of the daughters. Preeclampsia was observed in 37 percent of first pregnancies, and eclampsia developed in 4 percent of the sisters.

The incidence of preeclampsia is much higher in future pregnancies in women who have had eclampsia remote from term.

CHRONIC HYPERTENSION

Diagnosis of Chronic Hypertension

The diagnosis of chronic hypertension in pregnancy is usually made on the basis of either of the following:

1. Documented history of high blood pressure antedating pregnancy
2. Persistent elevation of blood pressure (at least 140/90 mm Hg) on two occasions more than 24 hours apart before the 20th week of gestation

Other findings might be suggestive of the presence of chronic hypertension:

Retinal changes on funduscopic examination
Cardiac enlargement on chest radiograph and ECG
Compromised renal function
Presence of medical disorders known to lead to hypertension
Multiparity with previous history of hypertensive pregnancies
Evidence of persistent hypertension beyond the 42nd day postpartum

Sometimes the diagnosis is difficult to make because of the marked and variable changes seen with blood pressure during midpregnancy. During midpregnancy the blood pressure can be in the normal range in women who were severely hypertensive prior to pregnancy.

Etiology and Classification of Chronic Hypertension

Essential hypertension is by far the most common cause of chronic hypertension during pregnancy. Chronic hypertension in pregnancy is classified as mild or severe depending on the systolic or diastolic blood pressure reading. Hypertension is severe if either systolic pressure is more than 160 mm Hg or diastolic pressure is above 110 mm Hg.

Superimposed preeclampsia is defined as exacerbation of hypertension of at least 30 mm Hg in systolic or at least 15 mm Hg in diastolic blood pressure, together with the development of protein-uria during the course of the pregnancy (at least 500 mg/24 h), or exacerbation of preexisting proteinuria (at least 5 g/24 h), and ele-vation of serum liver enzymes, uric acid, low platelets, or develop-ment of symptoms.[10]

Maternal and Fetal Risks of Chronic Hypertension

Pregnancies complicated by chronic hypertension are at increased risk for the development of superimposed preeclampsia, abruptio placentae, IUGR and poor perinatal outcome. In women on antihy-pertensive medications where exacerbation of blood pressure is less common, the diagnosis should be based on the development of sub-stantial proteinuria and abnormal laboratory tests or symptoms.[10]

Most of the poor perinatal outcomes are associated with protein-uria. Because superimposed preeclampsia is often an indication for delivery, it is important to use strict criteria to avoid unnecessary preterm delivery.

Pregnancy Outcome in Relation to Treatment of Chronic Hypertension

There is general agreement that chronic antihypertensive therapy will decrease the incidence of cardiovascular complications and cerebrovascular accidents in patients with diastolic blood pressures exceeding 105 mm Hg. However, it is not clear if antihypertensives are equally beneficial in pregnancies with mild uncomplicated hypertension, which is seen in about 95 percent of all pregnant women with chronic hypertension. In addition, no studies have shown any reduction in the incidence of superimposed preeclampsia or abruptio placentae when antihypertensives were used.[2,310]

Superimposed preeclampsia and abruptio placentae are respon-sible for most of the poor perinatal outcome in women with mild chronic hypertension. Antihypertensive drugs do not reduce the frequency of either of these complications. Most patients with mild chronic hypertension will have a good outcome with proper obstet-ric follow-up without the use of antihypertensive agents.[2]

Antihypertensive Drugs in Pregnancy

Methyldopa

Methyldopa is the only antihypertensive drug whose long-term safety for the mother and the fetus has been adequately assessed. It is the drug most commonly used to treat hypertension during pregnancy and is the standard against which other agents are compared. No adverse fetal effects have been noted. It reduces systemic vascular resistance without causing physiologically significant changes in heart rate or cardiac output, while renal blood flow is maintained. If used in mild hypertension the usual dose is 250 mg three times daily and 1 to 4 grams per day can be used for severe hypertension. The fall in blood pressure is maximal about 4 hours after an oral dose. It is considered a weak antihypertensive best suited for cases with mild hypertension, and if adequate blood pressure control is not achieved with the maximum dosage, additional antihypertensive agents may be added.

Clonidine

Clonidine is used primarily for treatment of mild to moderate hypertension. The usual oral dose in pregnancy is 0.1 to 0.3 mg/day given in two divided doses, which can be increased up to 1.2 mg/day as needed. A randomized study in 100 pregnant hypertensive women comparing clonidine to methyldopa found no significant difference in blood pressure control or maternal and fetal outcome.

Prazosin

Prazosin reduces both systolic and diastolic blood pressures, while producing significantly less tachycardia and sodium retention than methyldopa. It causes vasodilation of both the resistance and capacitance vessels, thereby reducing cardiac preload and afterload without reducing renal blood flow or glomerular filtration rate. In addition, it produces a decrease in plasma renin activity and is probably the drug of choice for treatment of hypertension characterized by high plasma renin levels. The usual dose of prazosin is 1 mg twice daily; however, the drug has been used in doses as high as 20 mg/day. The first dose in some individuals can produce syncope due to exaggerated hypotension, which can be avoided by decreasing the first dose. In 80 women with chronic hypertension who were treated with either prazosin ($n = 40$) or methyldopa ($n = 40$), both drugs were effective in controlling hypertension, and the incidence of superimposed preeclampsia was similar. There were no differences in perinatal outcome between the two groups.

Calcium Channel Blockers

Calcium channel blockers cause vasodilation and reduction in the peripheral resistance. They have rapid onset of action following oral administration. Nifedipine has potent vasodilating properties without reduction in cardiac output.[2,130,131,213,226,227,332,333] The drug is effective in controlling maternal blood pressure, and no adverse fetal or neonatal effects have been noted. However, there is limited experience with nifedipine treatment of chronic hypertension. Care should be exercised when using nifedipine with magnesium sulfate, which is a calcium channel blocker itself, since the use of both agents together could potentiate the antihypertensive action.

Angiotensin-Converting Enzyme Inhibitors

Angiotensin-converting enzyme (ACE) inhibitors (captopril, enalapril, lisinopril) induce vasodilation without reflex increase in the cardiac output. Because of their efficacy and low side effects, these agents are becoming widely used as first-line therapy for chronic hypertension in the nonpregnant state. In human pregnancy, the chronic use of ACE inhibitors has been associated with renal tubular dysplasia in utero, renal failure, oligohydramnios, fetal growth restriction, neonatal hypotension, anuria, renal failure and death.[336-339] Thus, it is recommended that the use of these agents in pregnancy be avoided.[337] Similar recommendations apply to the use of angiotensin receptor blockers.

Hydralazine

Hydralazine is a potent vasodilator that acts directly on the vascular smooth muscle. It is the agent most commonly used to control severe hypertension in preeclampsia, when it is given intravenously in bolus injections. After its intravenous use, the hypotensive effect of this drug develops gradually over 15 to 30 minutes, peaking at 20 minutes. The usual bolus dose is 5 to 10 mg to be repeated every 20 to 30 minutes as needed. Because oral hydralazine when used as a monotherapy is a weak antihypertensive, it is usually combined with diuretics, methyldopa, or β-blockers. The usual oral dose is 10 mg given four times daily, but this can be increased up to 300 mg/day.

β-Blockers

β-blockers have been used extensively and are felt to be safe in pregnancy. Their use in pregnancy has been reportedly associated with neonatal bradycardia and hypoglycemia when given to the mother within 2 hours of delivery.

The chronic use of atenolol during pregnancy has been consistently associated with reduced fetal weights and an increased risk of growth restriction.

Thiazide Diuretics

In the first 3 to 5 days of treatment, these drugs result in a reduction of both plasma and extracellular fluid volumes with a concomitant decrease in the cardiac output and lowering of the blood pressure. However, these changes tend to return to pretreatment levels within 4 to 6 weeks. These effects are followed by a long-term reduction in peripheral resistance. A single 25-mg dose is usually given in the morning. Neonatal adverse effects are electrolyte imbalance and thrombocytopenia.

Sibai et al.[351] noted that pregnant patients with chronic hypertension treated with diuretics have a marked reduction in plasma volume. However, plasma volume expansion is normal after the discontinuation of diuretics. Prophylactic thiazide therapy does not reduce the incidence of preeclampsia.

Because the initiation of diuretic therapy causes a decrease in blood volume and cardiac output, adding a diuretic late in pregnancy is contraindicated unless it is needed for the treatment of pulmonary edema. Since plasma volume depletion is associated with poor perinatal outcome, we have cautioned against the use of diuretics in pregnancies complicated by chronic hypertension. Furthermore, when diuretics are discontinued, few patients require additional medications during the remainder of the pregnancy.[351]

Preconceptional Evaluation of Chronic Hypertension

Management of patients with chronic hypertension should ideally begin before pregnancy, when evaluation is undertaken to assess the etiology and the severity of the hypertension, the presence of other medical illnesses, and to rule out the presence of target organ damage. Diuretics, ACE inhibitors, and β blockers should be changed to others with well-documented safety.

Pregnancies in women with chronic hypertension and renal insufficiency are associated with increased perinatal loss and a higher incidence of superimposed preeclampsia, preterm delivery, and fetal growth restriction.[354-357] These risks rise in proportion to the severity of the renal insufficiency. Thus, women with renal disease desiring pregnancy should be counseled to conceive before renal insufficiency becomes severe. For women with hypertension and severe renal insufficiency in the first trimester, the decision to continue pregnancy should not be made without extensive counseling regarding the potential maternal and fetal risks.

Initial and Subsequent Prenatal Visits for Patients with Chronic Hypertension

Early prenatal care will ensure accurate determination of gestational age as well as an assessment of the severity of hypertension in the first trimester. Initial counselting should include:

1. Instruction by a nutritionist regarding nutritional requirements, weight gain, and sodium intake
2. Instruction regarding the negative impact of maternal smoking, caffeine, and drugs on maternal blood pressure and perinatal outcome

3. Counsel regarding the possible adverse effects and complications of hypertension during pregnancy
4. Counsel regarding the importance of frequent prenatal visits and their impact on preventing or minimizing the above adverse effects

If the patient is well motivated, she can be instructed in self-determination of blood pressure, which avoids the phenomenon of "white coat hypertension." It is recommended that patient-recorded measurements of blood pressure be used to supplement those recorded in the doctor's office.

Maternal evaluation should include serial measurements of hematocrit, serum creatinine, and 24-hour urinary excretion of protein once every trimester. The occurrence of one or more of the following may be an indication for hospitalization:

1. Pyelonephritis
2. Significant elevations in blood pressure with levels in the range of severe hypertension
3. Severe fetal growth restriction

Managing Low-Risk Chronic Hypertension

Most patients with uncomplicated mild chronic hypertension will have a good perinatal outcome irrespective of the use of antihypertensive drugs. Only 13 percent of patients will require antihypertensive medications for exacerbation of hypertension during the third trimester. Most poor outcomes were related to the development of superimposed preeclampsia. It is our policy to discontinue all antihypertensive medications in such patients at the time of first prenatal visit. Antihypertensive therapy is subsequently started only if the blood pressure exceeds 160 mm Hg systolic or 110 mm Hg diastolic. These patients are usually treated with methyldopa (750 mg to 4 g/day) given as needed to keep diastolic blood pressure consistently at or below 105 mm Hg. The development of exacerbated hypertension alone is not an indication for delivery. Pregnancy in these patients may be continued until term or the onset of superimposed preeclampsia. Superimposed preeclampsia or suspected fetal growth restriction is an indication for close evaluation of maternal and fetal well-being. Mild superimposed preeclampsia is an indication for delivery if the gestational age is at least 37 weeks.

There are short-term maternal benefits from treating women with mild hypertension and target organ damage such as diabetes mellitus, renal disease, and cardiac dysfunction. As a result, we recommend treating mild chronic hypertension in pregnant women with these complications, keeping diastolic blood pressure below 90 mm Hg.

Managing High-Risk Chronic Hypertension

Pregnancies in women at high risk are associated with increased maternal and perinatal complications and should be managed in consultation with a maternal–fetal medicine specialist. Patients with chronic renal disease—serum creatinine >2.5 mg/dl)—should be managed in consultation with a nephrologist as well. Antihypertensive agents should be used to keep systolic blood pressure between 140 and 160 mm Hg and diastolic blood pressure between 90 and 105 mm Hg. Maternal blood pressure can be controlled with methyldopa (1 to 4 g/day), labetalol (600 mg to 2.4 g/day), or nifedipine (40 to 120 mg/day). These women need close monitoring throughout pregnancy and may require multiple hospital admissions for control of blood pressure or associated medical complications. Fetal evaluation should be started as early as 26 weeks and repeated as needed. Superimposed preeclampsia is an indication for immediate hospitalization. Severe superimposed preeclampsia is an indication for delivery in all patients with a gestational age beyond 34 weeks. If preeclampsia develops before this time, the pregnancy may be followed conservatively with daily evaluation of maternal and fetal well-being.

Hypertensive Emergencies in Chronic Hypertension

Life-threatening clinical conditions require immediate control of blood pressure, e.g., hypertensive encephalopathy, acute left ventricular failure, acute aortic dissection, or increased circulating catecholamines (pheochromocytoma, clonidine withdrawal, cocaine ingestion). Although a diastolic blood pressure of 115 mm Hg or greater is usually considered a hypertensive emergency, this level is actually arbitrary, and the rate of change of blood pressure may be more important than the absolute level.[359]

Hypertensive encephalopathy is usually seen in patients with systolic blood pressure above 250 mm Hg or diastolic blood pressure above 150 mm Hg.[360] Patients with acute onset of hypertension may develop encephalopathy at pressure levels that are generally tolerated by those with chronic hypertension. Severe hypertension may result in abruptio placentae with resultant DIC.

Lowering Blood Pressure

There are risks associated with too rapid or excessive reduction of elevated blood pressure. The aim of therapy is to lower mean blood pressure by no more than 15 to 25 percent. Small reductions in blood pressure in the first 60 minutes, working toward a diastolic level of 100 to 110 mm Hg, have been recommended.[359,360]

Hypertension that proves increasingly difficult to control is an indication to end the pregnancy.

The drug of choice in hypertensive crisis is sodium nitroprusside. Other drugs such as nitroglycerin, nifedipine, trimetaphan, labetalol, and hydralazine can also be used.

Sodium nitroprusside causes arterial and venous relaxation and is given as an intravenous infusion of 0.25 to 8.0 µg/kg/min. The onset of action is immediate, and its effect may last 3 to 5 minutes after discontinuing the infusion. Hypotension caused by nitroprusside should resolve within a few minutes of stopping the infusion, because the drug's half-life is so short.

Nitroglycerin is an arterial but mostly venous dilator. It is given as an intravenous infusion of 5 µg/min that is gradually increased every 3 to 5 minutes to titrate blood pressure up to a maximum dose of 100 µg/min. It is the drug of choice in preeclampsia associated with pulmonary edema and for control of hypertension associated with tracheal manipulation. It is contraindicated in hypertensive encephalopathy because it increases cerebral blood flow and intracranial pressure.[360]

Key Points

➤ Hypertension is the most common medical complication during pregnancy.

➤ Preeclampsia is a leading cause of maternal mortality and morbidity worldwide.

➤ The pathophysiologic abnormalities of preeclampsia are numerous, but the etiology is unknown.

➤ At present, there is no proven method to prevent preeclampsia.

➤ The HELLP syndrome may develop in the absence of maternal hypertension.

➤ Expectant management improves perinatal outcome in a select group of women with severe preeclampsia before 32 weeks' gestation.

➤ Magnesium sulfate is the ideal agent to prevent or treat eclamptic convulsions.

➤ Rare cases of eclampsia can develop before 20 weeks' gestation and beyond 48 hours postpartum.

Box continued on following page

Key Points *Continued*

➤ Antihypertensive agents do not improve pregnancy outcome in women with mild uncomplicated chronic hypertension.

➤ Methyldopa is the drug of choice for the treatment of chronic hypertension; ACE inhibitors should be avoided due to renal dysplasia and oligohydramnios.

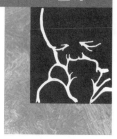

Chapter 24

Medical
Complications

The management of medical complications in pregnancy represents one of the most demanding and rewarding areas of obstetrics. The clinician must first be familiar with the normal physiologic changes brought about by pregnancy. This information must then be integrated with the pathophysiology of the disease itself. In short, one must ask how pregnancy affects this medical disorder and how this medical disorder affects pregnancy. In addition, the obstetrician must be aware of the consequences of the medical complication for both the mother and her fetus. These considerations encompass not only the consequences of the disease itself, but the risks associated with the treatment of the disorder as well.

Cardiac Disease and Critical Care

THOMAS R. EASTERLING AND
CATHERINE OTTO

Cardiovascular adaptations to pregnancy are well tolerated by healthy young women. However, these adaptations are of such magnitude that they can significantly compromise women with abnormal or damaged hearts. The best care for women with heart disease is usually achieved from a thorough understanding of maternal cardiovascular physiology, knowledge of existing literature, and extensive clinical experience brought by the clinical management team.

MATERNAL HEMODYNAMICS

Three key features of the maternal hemodynamic changes in pregnancy are particularly relevant to the management of women with cardiac disease: (1) increased cardiac output, (2) increased heart rate, and (3) reduced vascular resistance. In conditions such as mitral stenosis where cardiac output is relatively fixed, the drive to achieve an elevated cardiac output may result in pulmonary congestion. If a patient has an atrial septal defect, the incremental increase in systemic flow associated with pregnancy will be magnified in the pulmonary circulation to the extent that pulmonary flow exceeds systemic flow.

Many cardiac conditions are heart rate dependent. Flow across a stenotic mitral valve is dependent on time in diastole. Tachycardia reduces left ventricular filling and cardiac output. Coronary blood flow is also dependent on the length of diastole. Patients with aortic stenosis will have increased wall tension and therefore increased myocarial oxygen requirements. Tachycardia reduces coronary perfusion time in diastole while simultaneously further increasing myocardial oxygen requirements. The resulting imbalance between oxygen demand and supply may precipitate myocardial ischemia. Patients with complex congenital heart disease experience significant tachyarrhythmias. The increasing heart rate in pregnancy may be associated with a worsening of tachyarrhythmias.

Reduction in vascular resistance may be beneficial to some patients; afterload reduction reduces cardiac work. Cardiomyopathy, aortic regurgitation, and mitral regurgitation benefit from reduced afterload. Alternatively, patients with intracardiac shunts, where right and left ventricular pressures are nearly equal when not pregnant, may reverse their shunt during pregnancy and desaturate.

DIAGNOSIS AND EVALUATION OF HEART DISEASE

Many women with heart disease have been diagnosed and treated prior to pregnancy. For example, in women with prior surgery for congenital heart disease, detailed historical information may be available. Others only know that they have a murmur or a "hole in my heart." Alternatively, heart disease may first be diagnosed during pregnancy due to symptoms precipitated by increased cardiac demands.

The classic symptoms of cardiac disease are palpitations, shortness of breath with exertion, and chest pain. Since these symptoms also may accompany normal pregnancy, a careful history is needed to determine if the symptoms are out of proportion to the stage of pregnancy. Symptoms are of particular concern in a patient with other reasons to suspect underlying cardiac disease, such as a woman who has grown up in an area where rheumatic heart disease is prevalent.

Any diastolic murmur and any systolic murmur that is loud ($\geq$ grade 3/6) or radiates to the carotids should be considered pathologic. Careful evaluation for elevation of the jugular venous pulse, for peripheral cyanosis or clubbing, and for pulmonary crackles is needed in women with suspected cardiac disease.

Indications for further cardiac diagnostic testing in pregnant women include a history of known cardiac disease, symptoms in excess of those expected in a normal pregnancy, a pathologic murmur, evidence of heart failure on physical examination, or arterial oxygen desaturation in the absence of known pulmonary disease. The most appropriate next step in evaluation of pregnant women with suspected heart disease is transthoracic echocardiography. A chest radiograph is only helpful if congestive heart failure is suspected. An electrocardiogram (ECG) is likely to be nonspecific. If symptoms are consistent with a cardiac arrhythmia, an event monitor or 24-hour ECG monitor may be indicated.

Echocardiography provides detailed information on cardiac anatomy and physiology that allows optimal management of women with heart disease. Basic data obtained on echocardiography include left ventricular ejection fraction, pulmonary artery systolic pressure, qualitative evaluation of right ventricular systolic function, and evaluation of valve anatomy and function. When valvular stenosis is present, the pressure gradient (ΔP) across the valve is calculated from the Doppler-derived velocity (v) of flow across the valve: $\Delta P = 4v^2$.

GENERAL CARE

Deterioration in cardiac status during pregnancy is frequently insidious. Continuity of care with a single provider facilitates early intervention prior to overt decompensation. Regular visits should include particular attention to heart rate, weight gain, and oxygen saturation. An unexpected increase in weight may indicate the need for more aggressive outpatient therapy. A fall in oxygen saturation will often precede a clearly abnormal chest exam or radiograph. Regular use of a structured history of symptoms (see the box "Structured Review of Cardiac Symptoms") will alert the physician to a change in condition. Regular review educates the patient and reinforces their role as "partners in care."

The physiologic changes of pregnancy are usually continuous and therefore offer adequate time for maternal compensation despite cardiac disease. Intercurrent events superimposed on pregnancy in the context of maternal heart disease are usually responsible for acute decompensation. Antepartum, the most common significant "intercurrent events" are febrile episodes. Screening for bacteriuria and vaccination against influenza and pneumococcus are appropriate. Patients should be instructed to report symptoms of upper respiratory infection, particularly fever. Many patients with heart disease (adolescents, recent immigrants, and those living in poverty), will also be at risk for iron deficiency. Prophylaxis against anemia with iron and folate supplementation may decrease cardiac work.

Structured Review of Cardiac Symptoms

"How many flights of stairs can you walk up with ease?" —
"Two? One? None?"
"Can you walk a level block?"
"Can you sleep flat in bed?" "How many pillows?"
"Does your heart race?"
"Do you have chest pain?"
   "with exercise?"
   "when your heart races?"

Standard Cardiac Care for Labor and Delivery

1. Accurate diagnosis
2. Mode of delivery based on obstetric indications
3. Medical management initiated early in labor
   - Prolonged labor avoided.
   - Induction with a *favorable* cervix
4. Maintenance of hemodynamic stability
   - Invasive hemodynamic monitoring when required
   - Initial, compensated hemodynamic reference point
   - Specific emphasis based on particular cardiac condition
5. Avoidance of pain and hemodynamic responses
   - Epidural analgesia with narcotic/low-dose local technique
6. Prophylactic antibiotics when at risk for endocarditis
7. Avoidance of maternal pushing
   - Caudal for dense perineal anesthesia
   - Low forceps or vacuum delivery
8. Avoidance of maternal blood loss
   - Proactive management of the third stage
   - Early but appropriate fluid replacement
9. Early volume management postpartum
   - Often careful but aggressive diuresis

A strategy of "standard cardiac care" for labor and delivery is described in the box. The general principles for care are similar for most cardiac diagnoses. Physiologically, the ideal labor for a woman with heart disease is short and pain free. While induction of labor facilitates organization of care and early pain control, shortening the duration of pregnancy by 1 or 2 weeks at the cost of a 2 or 3 day induction of labor is not worthwhile. Induction of labor with a favorable cervix is therefore ideal. Some patients with severe cardiac disease will benefit from invasive hemodynamic monitoring with an arterial catheter and a pulmonary artery catheter. Cesarean section is usually reserved for obstetric indications. The American Heart Association does not recommend routine antibiotic prophylaxis for the prevention of endocarditis, although it is optional in high-risk patients having a vaginal delivery (Table 24–1). Because bacteremia is common at the time of vaginal delivery and cesarean section,[10,11] many practitioners will provide antibiotic prophylaxis in all patients at risk.

Women with significant heart disease should be counseled prior to pregnancy regarding the risk of pregnancy, interventions that may be required, and potential risks to the fetus. However, women with significant uncorrected disease may present with an ongoing pregnancy. In this situation, the risks and benefits of termination of pregnancy

Table 24–1. PROPHYLACTIC REGIMENS FOR LABOR AND DELIVERY

Patients	Regimens
High-risk patients Prosthetic valves—both biopros-thetic and homografts Complex cyanotic congenital heart disease (CHD) Surgically constructed systemic pulmonic shunts or conduits Previous bacterial endocarditis	Ampicillin + gentamicin Ampicillin 2.0 g IM or IV Gentamicin 1.5 mg/kg (not to exceed 120 mg) in active labor; 6 h later, ampicillin 1 g IM/IV or amoxicillin 1 g PO
High-risk patients allergic to ampicillin/amoxicillin	Vancomycin + gentamicin Vancomycin 1.0 g IV over 1–2 h + gentamicin as above in active labor
Moderate-risk patients Most other CHD Acquired valvular dysfunction (e.g., rheumatic heart disease) Hypertrophic cardiac myopathy Mitral valve prolapse with regurgitation	Amoxicillin or ampicillin Amoxicillin 2.0 g orally or ampicillin 2.0 g IM/IV in active labor
Moderate-risk patients allergic to ampicillin/amoxicillin	Vancomycin Vancomycin 1.0 g IV over 1–2 h in active labor

Adapted from Dajani AS, Taubert KA, Wilson W, et al: Prevention of bacterial endocarditis: recommendations by the American Heart Association. JAMA 277:1794, 1997.

versus those of continuing a pregnancy should be addressed. The decision to become pregnant or carry a pregnancy in the context of maternal disease is a balance of two forces: (1) the objective medical risk including the uncertainty of that estimate, and (2) the value of the birth of a child to an individual woman and her partner. The first goal of counseling is to educate the patient. Only a few cardiac diseases represent an overwhelming risk of maternal mortality: Eisenmenger's syndrome, pulmonary hypertension with right ventricular dysfunction, and Marfan syndrome with significant aortic dilation. Most other conditions require aggressive management and significant disruption in lifestyle. Intercurrent events such as antepartum pneumonia or obstetric hemorrhage pose the greatest risk of initiating life-threatening events. Fastidious care can reduce but not eliminate the risk of these events. Maternal congenital heart disease increases the risk of congenital heart disease in the fetus from 1 percent to approximately 4 to 6 percent.[12,13] Marfan syndrome and some forms of hypertrophic cardiomyopathy are inherited as autosomal dominant conditions; the children of these women will carry a 50 percent chance of inheriting the disease. The second goal of counseling is to help the woman integrate the medical information into her individual value system and her individual desire to be a mother. Many women with significant but manageable heart disease will choose to carry a pregnancy. The basis for their decisions must be individualized.

MITRAL STENOSIS

Mitral stenosis is nearly always due to rheumatic heart disease. Valvular dysfunction progresses continuously throughout life. Deterioration may be accelerated by recurrent episodes of rheumatic fever. Rheumatic fever itself is an immunologic response to group A β-hemolytic streptococcus infections.

Patients with asymptomatic mitral stenosis have a 10-year survival of greater than 80 percent. Once significantly symptomatic, 10-year survival without treatment is less than 15 percent. In the presence of pulmonary hypertension, mean survival is less than 3 years. Death is due to progressive pulmonary edema, right heart failure, systemic embolization, or pulmonary embolism.[14]

Stenosis of the mitral valve impedes the flow of blood from the left atrium to the left ventricle during diastole. The normal mitral valve area is 4.0 to 5.0 cm^2. Symptoms with exercise can be expected with valve areas less than or equal to 2.5 cm^2. Symptoms at rest are expected at less than or equal to 1.5 cm^2. The left ventricle responds with Starling mechanisms to increased venous return with increased performance, elevating cardiac output in response to demand. The left atrium is limited in its capacity to respond. Cardiac output is therefore limited by the relatively passive flow of blood through the valve during diastole; increased venous return results in pulmonary congestion rather than increased cardiac output. Thus, the drive for increased cardiac output in pregnancy cannot be achieved, resulting in increased pulmonary congestion. The relative tachycardia experienced in pregnancy shortens diastole, decreases left ventricular filling, and therefore further compromises cardiac output and increases pulmonary congestion. Pregnancy itself does not negatively affect the natural history of mitral stenosis.

The diagnosis of mitral stenosis in pregnancy prior to maternal decompensation is uncommon. Tiredness and dyspnea on exertion are characteristic symptoms of mitral stenosis but are also ubiquitous among pregnant women. While the presence of a diastolic rumble or jugular venous distention may suggest mitral stenosis, these findings are subtle and may be overlooked or not appreciated. Not uncommonly, an intercurrent event such as a febrile episode will result in exaggerated symptoms and the diagnosis of pulmonary edema or oxygen desaturation. Under these circumstances, particularly in the context of a patient from an at-risk group, an echocardiogram should be performed to rule out mitral stenosis.

The goal of antepartum care in the context of mitral stenosis is to achieve a balance between the drive to increase cardiac output and the limitations of flow across the stenotic valve. Most women with significant disease will require diuresis with a drug such as furosemide. In addition, β-blockade reduces heart rate, improves diastolic flow across the valve, and relieves pulmonary congestion.

Women with a history of rheumatic valvular disease who are at risk for contact with populations with a high prevalence of streptococcal infection should receive prophylaxis with daily oral penicillin G or monthly benzathine penicillin.[14] Most pregnant women will live in close contact with groups of children and will usually be considered at risk. Atrial fibrillation is a complication associated with mitral stenosis due to left atrial enlargement. Rapid ventricular response to atrial fibrillation may result in sudden decompensation. Digoxin, β-blockers, or calcium channel blockers can be used to control ventricular response. In the context of hemodynamic decompensation, electrical cardioversion may be necessary. Anticoagulation with heparin should be used before and after cardioversion to prevent systemic embolization. Patients with chronic atrial fibrillation and a history of an embolic event should also be anticoagulated.[14]

Labor and delivery can frequently precipitate decompensation in patients with critical mitral stenosis. Pain induces tachycardia. Uterine contractions increase venous return and therefore pulmonary congestion. Women frequently cannot tolerate the work of pushing in the second stage. Aggressive, anticipatory diuresis will reduce pulmonary congestion and the potential for oxygen desaturation.

The hemodynamics of women with symptomatic stenosis or a valve area of 1cm² or less should be managed with the aid of a pulmonary artery catheter. Ideally, hemodynamic parameters are assessed when the patient is well compensated, early in labor. These findings serve as a reference point to guide subsequent therapy. Pain control is achieved with an epidural. Heart rate control is maintained through pain control and β-blockade. To avoid pushing, the second stage is shortened with low forceps or vacuum delivery. Aggressive diuresis is initiated immediately postpartum. Cesarean section is reserved for obstetric indications.

Aggressive medical management including hospital bed rest will be sufficient to manage most women with mitral stenosis. The woman with uncommonly severe disease may require surgical intervention. While successful valve replacement and open commissurotomy have been reported in pregnancy,[17,18] they are now rarely needed.

MITRAL REGURGITATION

Mitral regurgitation may be due to a chronic progressive process such as rheumatic valve disease or mitral valve prolapse. As regurgitation increases over time, forward flow is maintained at the expense of left ventricular dilation with eventual impaired contractility. Left atrial enlargement may be associated with atrial fibrillation and should be managed with ventricular rate control and anticoagulation. The patient with chronic mitral regurgitation may remain asymptomatic even with exercise. Preconceptional counseling should include consideration of valve replacement in consultation with a cardiologist. In general, valve replacement is recommended for: (1) symptomatic patients, (2) atrial fibrillation, (3) ejection fraction less than 50 to 60 percent, (4) left ventricular end-diastolic dimension greater than 45 to 50 mm, or (5) pulmonary systolic pressure greater than 50 to 60 mm Hg.[14]

The hemodynamic changes associated with pregnancy can be expected to have mixed effects. A reduction in systemic vascular resistance will tend to promote forward flow. The drive to increase cardiac output will exacerbate left ventricular volume overload. Increased atrial dilation may initiate atrial fibrillation. Pulmonary congestion can be managed by careful diuresis with the knowledge that adequate forward flow is usually dependent on a high preload to achieve adequate left ventricular filling. Atrial fibrillation should be managed consistent with care outside pregnancy. An increase in systemic vascular resistance due to progressive hypertension secondary to preeclampsia may significantly impair forward flow and should be treated. Labor and delivery should be managed with "standard cardiac care." Catecholamine release due to pain or stress will impair forward low. Particular attention should be paid to left ventricular filling. Excessive preload will result in pulmonary congestion. Insufficient preload will not fill the enlarged left ventricle and will result in insufficient forward flow. A pulmonary artery catheter can be used to determine appropriate filling pressure in early labor or prior to induction. While a large v-wave may complicate the interpretation of pulmonary artery wedge pressure, the pulmonary artery diastolic pressure can be used as a reference point. Diuresis in the early postpartum period may be required.

Mitral valve prolapse is a common condition, affecting as many as 12 percent of young women.[21] In the absence of conditions of abnormal connective tissue such as Marfan and Ehler-Danlos syndromes and clinically significant mitral regurgitation, women with mitral prolapse can be expected to have uncomplicated pregnancies. They may experience an increase in tachyarrhythmias that can be treated with β-blockers. Prophylactic antibiotics are usually used at the time of delivery.

PROSTHETIC VALVES

Definitive therapy for significant valvular disease requires surgical repair, or more commonly replacement. Mechanical valves are durable but require anticoagulation. Porcine tissue valves, when used in a young woman, will usually require replacement in her lifetime. Reports of pregnancies associated with prosthetic valves suggest significant variability in outcomes. Table 24–2 summarizes a review of 151 pregnancies complicated by a prosthetic valve.[27] Mechanical valves and anticoagulation were associated with a moderate increase in miscarriage and thromboembolic events.

Decisions surrounding the timing and choice of valve replacement for a woman of reproductive age are complex. Managing a pregnancy with moderate valve disease may be less complicated than managing a pregnancy with a prosthetic valve. The durability of a mechanical valve has considerable advantages for a young person, but it is associ-

Table 24–2. PREGNANCY OUTCOMES WITH PROSTHETIC VALVES

	Mechanical	Porcine
Women	31	57
Pregnancies	56	95
Fetal loss	27.7%	12.3%
Premature birth	5.9%	7.7%
Valve deterioration	5.3%	7.0%
Thromboembolic event	5.3%	—

ated with more adverse outcomes in pregnancy. Delay in valve replacement until child bearing is completed is appropriate when the severity of heart disease is felt to be manageable in pregnancy.

Anticoagulation is required with a mechanical valve. Oral anticoagulation in the first trimester is associated with congenital anomalies; potentially serious fetal bleeding may be encountered in the second and third trimesters. The American College of Cardiology/ American Heart Association guidelines recommend consideration of subcutaneous heparin in the first trimester to avoid warfarin embryopathy, and the use of warfarin until 36 weeks, when subcutaneous heparin is substituted until after delivery.[14] These recommendations remain controversial in that they may underestimate the risk of fetal intracerebral bleeding in the absence of labor.[29] The fetus exposed to coumadin in the second and third trimesters is at risk for developmental toxicity. Individual patients should be counseled regarding the risks of either strategy and participate actively in a final choice of therapy. If heparinization is chosen, the activated partial thromboplastin time (aPTT) should be increased to two to three times control at middosing interval. Intravenous heparin can be administered on an ambulatory basis and should be considered for mitral valves, which are more likely to clot, and for patients who may be noncompliant with subcutaneous administration. Women treated for prolonged periods with heparin should be counseled regarding the risk of osteoporosis.

CONGENITAL HEART DISEASE

Congenital heart disease is present in 0.7 to 1 percent of live births, accounting for as many as 30 percent of infants with birth anomalies. Currently, congenital disease is estimated to exceed rheumatic disease by 1:4. While many will enter pregnancy with known heart disease, some women will have their disease first recognized due to the hemodynamic demands of pregnancy.

Table 24–3 summarizes the distribution of congenital heart disease in childhood and in pregnancy.[26,33] Major risks in pregnancy include (1) cyanosis, (2) left (or systemic) ventricular dysfunction, and (3) pulmonary hypertension, particularly with right ventricular dysfunction. Pregnancy outcome worsens considerably in the presence of maternal cyanosis.

Men and women with congenital heart disease are at increased risk for having children with congenital heart disease. In a prospective study with aggressive pediatric evaluation, the incidence was estimated to be as high as 14.2 percent.[13] Specific parental defects are not generally associated with the same defect in the child. The risk for cardiac maldevelopment is inherited rather than the risk for a specific defect.

Table 24–3. INCIDENCE OF CONGENITAL HEART DEFECTS IN CHILDHOOD AND IN PREGNANCY

	Childhood	Pregnancy
Ventricular septal defect	35%	13%
Atrial septal defect	9%	9%
Patent ductus arteriosis	8%	2.7%
Pulmonary stenosis	8%	8%
Aortic stenosis	6%	20%
Coarctation of the aorta	6%	8%
Tetralogy of Fallot	5%	12%
Transposition of the great vessels	4%	5.4%

Contraceptive counseling should be offered to all women with congenital heart disease. Cyanosis, pulmonary hypertension, low cardiac output, dilated cardiac chambers, sluggish venous conduits (e.g., Fontan), and atrial fibrillation place patients at risk for thrombosis. This small group of women should probably avoid combined estrogen/progestin oral contraceptives. Progestin-only pills are not associated with risk for thrombosis but require regular dosing to achieve optimal efficacy. Parenteral progestins are safe for women with cardiac disease and are extremely effective. They do cause irregular bleeding, which may be significant if the patient is anticoagulated. The intrauterine device carries a risk for pelvic inflammatory disease and therefore a theoretical risk of bacteremia and endocarditis. However, the actual risk has been estimated to be 1 per 1 million patient-years.[36]

ISOLATED SEPTAL DEFECTS

Ventricular and atrial septal defects represent greater than 40 percent of congenital heart disease identified in childhood. Many defects identified in children will close with advancing age. In adulthood, 50 percent of large ventricular septal defects (>1.5) lead to the development of Eisenmenger's syndrome. Ten percent of uncorrected atrial septal defects will also develop pulmonary hypertension.

The patient with a significant pulmonary/systemic shunt ratio can be expected to normally expand her cardiac output during pregnancy. However, the price of a normal systemic cardiac output is a high pulmonary flow. In the absence of associated anomalies, arrhythmias, and pulmonary hypertension, the presence of an atrial septal defect does not usually complicate pregnancy.

EISENMENGER'S SYNDROME

Eisenmenger's syndrome is characterized by pulmonary-to-systemic shunting associated with cyanosis and increased pulmonary pressures secondary to pulmonary vascular disease. Eisenmenger's syndrome may develop from any intracardiac shunt resulting in blood from the high-pressure systemic circulation being directed into the pulmonary circulation. The fall in systemic vascular resistance associated with pregnancy may initiate shunt reversal in a patient not previously cyanotic.

Patients with Eisenmenger's syndrome are at risk for congestive heart failure, hemoptysis due to pulmonary hemorrhage, sudden death due to arrhythmia, cerebrovascular accident, and hyperviscosity syndrome. The diagnosis should be considered in any cyanotic patient and is confirmed by echocardiography with the demonstration of increased pulmonary pressure and an intracardiac shunt. Treatment is nonspecific, and includes supportive care and avoidance of destabilizing events such as surgery and unnecessary medications.

A recent review of cases in the United Kingdom between 1991 and 1995 confirms the poor prognosis for pregnant women with Eisenmenger's syndrome despite considerable advancement in the management of cardiac disease in pregnancy.[54] Mortality remains extremely high; forty percent of the women died. In addition, 85 percent of the births were preterm.

While the risks associated with Eisenmenger's syndrome in pregnancy are clear, appropriate management is not. Decreased activity, hospital observation, and oxygen supplementation are usually employed. Reduction of pulmonary pressures and improved systemic oxygen saturation after oxygen supplementation indicates that pulmonary vascular resistance is not fixed and suggests a better prognosis. Intercurrent antepartum events such as pneumonia or urinary tract infection will be poorly tolerated. Preventing microcytosis with iron supplementation may decrease the risk of microvascular sludging.

Cesarean section is reserved for obstetric indications and is avoided whenever possible. A pulmonary artery catheter and a peripheral arterial catheter are usually used to guide hemodynamic management.

CARDIOMYOPATHY

Dilated cardiomyopathy is characterized by the development of pulmonary edema in the context of left ventricular dysfunction and dilation. Peripartum cardiomyopathy is a rare syndrome of heart failure presenting in late pregnancy or postpartum. The diagnosis is made after excluding other causes of pulmonary edema and heart failure. The cause of peripartum cardiomyopathy is unknown.

The mortality rate for peripartum cardiomyopathy is reported to be 25 to 50 percent. Death is usually due to progressive congestive heart failure, arrhythmia, or thromboembolism.[59] Within 6 months, half of patients will demonstrate resolution of left ventricular dilation. Their prognosis is very good. Of those who do not, 85 percent will die within the next 4 to 5 years.[60] The magnitude of risk for subsequent pregnancies after peripartum cardiomyopathy is unclear. A recent survey of suggests a mortality rate of 8 percent when left ventricular dysfunction has not resolved, and 2 percent in patients with normal function.[61]

CRITICAL CARE—HEMODYNAMIC MONITORING AND MANAGEMENT

Acute indications for invasive hemodynamic monitoring can be broadly categorized based on questions of physiology (see the box "Indications for Hemodynamic Monitoring"). Severe preeclampsia, sepsis, adult respiratory distress syndrome (ARDS), pneumonia, previously undiagnosed heart disease, and fluid management after resuscitation from obstetric hemorrhage are the most common conditions that will require hemodynamic monitoring.

Hemodynamic Monitoring

The objective of hemodynamic monitoring is to provide continuous assessment of systemic and intracardiac pressures and to provide the means to determine cardiac output and, therefore, to calculate systemic and pulmonary resistances. An arterial catheter is usually placed in the radial artery to measure systemic pressure. The diastolic pressure obtained will usually correlate well with noninvasive measurements. Systolic pressure may be significantly higher than noninvasive measurements due to a very brief peak in pressure in early systole. (The spike in pressure contributes little to mean arterial pressure.) The noninvasive measurement is usually more clinically relevant to the patient's condition. The arterial catheter permits easy access to arterial blood sampling and relieves the patient from the discomfort of frequent blood draws.

Measurement of intracardiac pressures and cardiac output are obtained through the insertion of a catheter into the central venous circulation and advancement into and through the right heart. Venous access is most commonly obtained through the right internal jugular vein; a subclavian approach may also be used.

Indications for Hemodynamic Monitoring

1. Why is the patient hypoxic?
   - Are pulmonary capillary pressures high due to relative volume overload? (e.g., mitral stenosis postpartum)
   - Are pulmonary capillary pressures high due to depressed cardiac function? (e.g., cardiomyopathy)
   - Is capillary membrane integrity intact? (e.g., ARDS, pneumonia)
2. Why is the patient persistently hypertensive?
   - Is vascular resistance elevated?
   - Is cardiac output elevated?
3. Why is the patient hypotensive?
   - Is left ventricular filling pressure low? (e.g., after hemorrhage)
   - Is vascular resistance low? (e.g., septic shock)
4. Why is the patient's urine output low?
   - Is left ventricular filling pressure low resulting in low cardiac output?
5. Is the patient expected to be unstable in labor?
   - Is the window of left ventricular filling narrow? (e.g., aortic stenosis)
   - Will normal physiologic changes associated with delivery be tolerated poorly? (e.g., volume loading postpartum—mitral stenosis, pulmonary hypertension)

Traditionally, insertion is guided by using the sternocleidomastoid muscle and the clavicle as landmarks. The higher frequency ultrasound transducer found on a vaginal probe can also be used to facilitate insertion under direct visualization. Once central venous access has been obtained and confirmed, a pulmonary artery catheter can be "floated" into the right heart and pulmonary artery. Success in "floating" the catheter is initially confirmed by observation of characteristic waveforms in the right ventricle, pulmonary artery, and wedged position, and subsequently with a radiograph. In experienced hands, complications from pulmonary artery catheterization are uncommon: pneumothorax (<0.1 percent), pulmonary infarction (0 to 1.3 percent), pulmonary artery rupture (<0.1 percent), and septicemia (0.5 to 2.0 percent).[105] Arrhythmias are usually transient and associated with passage of the catheter through the right ventricle. If the patient has significant pulmonary hypertension, difficulty may be encountered maintaining placement in the pulmonary artery.

Once the catheter has been successfully placed, continuous readings of central venous pressure and pulmonary artery pressures can

Table 24–4. CALCULATED HEMODYNAMIC VARIABLES

		Calculation	Units
Mean arterial pressure	MAP	$\dfrac{sBP + 2\,dBP}{3}$	mm Hg
Stroke volume	SV	$\dfrac{CO \cdot 1000}{HR}$	ml
Systemic vascular resistance	SVR	$\dfrac{(MAP - CVP) \cdot 80}{CO}$	$dyne \cdot sec \cdot cm^{-5}$
Total peripheral resistance	TPR	$\dfrac{MAP \cdot 80}{CO}$	$dyne \cdot sec \cdot cm^{-5}$
Pulmonary vascular resistance	PVR	$\dfrac{mPAP - PAWP}{CO}$	$dyne \cdot sec \cdot cm^{-5}$

sBP, systolic blood pressure; dBP, diastolic blood pressure; CO, cardiac output; CVP, central venous pressure; mPAP, mean pulmonary artery pressure; PAWP, pulmonary artery wedge pressure.

be obtained. By inflating the balloon at the catheter tip, the catheter can be wedged in the pulmonary artery to obtain a PAWP. PAWP reflects the filling pressure, preload, in the left ventricle. CVP measured in the right atrium is a measure of right ventricular filling pressure. In pregnant women, CVP cannot be assumed to accurately reflect left ventricular filling. Right atrial pressures and systolic pulmonary pressures can be measured noninvasively by echocardiography.

Table 24–4 summarizes formulas used to calculate hemodynamic parameters not directly measured.

Hemodynamic Management

Table 24–5 summarizes the most common clinical goals of therapy. To achieve each goal, a number of physiologic interventions are possible. Each of these interventions will precipitate a secondary or compensatory response. The secondary response, if excessive, may adversely affect the patient. The choice of intervention from available options will often be determined by the potential for and magnitude of adverse effect. Hemodynamic monitoring permits the physician to choose an intervention and subsequently assess the positive and negative impact.

Table 24–5. HEMODYNAMIC INTERVENTIONS

Clinical Goal	Physiological Interventions	Agents	Compensatory Response
↑ Oxygenation	↑ FIO_2 ↓ capillary pressure ↑ airway pressure ↓ resistance	O_2 Diuretic PEEP Vasodilator	 ↓ BP, ↓ CO ↓ CO ↑ CO
↓ Blood pressure	↓ cardiac output ↓ HR ↓ SV ↑ resistance	 β-Blocker Diuretic α-Agonist	 ↓ CO ↓ CO ↓ CO
↑ Blood pressure	↑ cardiac output	Ionotropic Volume	↑ CO ↑ CO_2 ↓ O_2 saturation
↑ Perfusion	↑ cardiac output ↑ contractility ↑ preload ↓ resistance	 Ionotropic Volume Vasodilator	 ↑ HR ↓ O_2 saturation ↓ BP

Key Points

➤ Hemodynamic changes in pregnancy may adversely affect maternal cardiac performance.

➤ Intercurrent events during pregnancy are usually the cause of decompensation.

➤ Women with heart disease in pregnancy frequently have unique psychosocial needs.

➤ Labor, delivery, and postpartum are times of hemodynamic instability.

➤ Invasive hemodynamic monitoring should be used to address specific clinical questions.

➤ Many maternal heart conditions can be medically managed during pregnancy. A few are associated with a very high risk of maternal mortality.

➤ Many patients with congenital heart disease can successfully complete a pregnancy.

Pulmonary Disease

JANICE E. WHITTY AND
MITCHELL P. DOMBROWSKI

PNEUMONIA IN PREGNANCY

Pneumonia is a rare complication of pregnancy, complicating pregnancy in 1 per 118 deliveries to 1 per 2,288 deliveries.[1,2] However, pneumonia contributes to considerable maternal mortality and is reportedly the most common nonobstetric infection to cause maternal mortality in the peripartum period.[3]

HIV infection is associated with an increased risk of invasive pneumococcal disease and legionnaires' disease. HIV infection further predisposes the pregnant woman to the infectious complications of the acquired immunodeficiency syndrome (AIDS).[7,8] Women with medical conditions that increase the risk of pulmonary infection, such as cystic fibrosis, are living to childbearing age more frequently than in the past. This disorder also contributes to the increased incidence of pneumonia in pregnancy.

Pneumonia can complicate pregnancy at any time during gestation and may be associated with preterm birth, poor fetal growth, and perinatal loss.

BACTERIAL PNEUMONIA

Streptococcus pneumoniae (pneumococcus) is the most common bacterial pathogen causing pneumonia in pregnancy, with *H. influenzae* being the next most common. These pneumonias typically present as an acute illness accompanied by fever, chills, purulent productive cough, and a lobar pattern on the chest radiograph. Streptococcal pneumonia produces a "rusty" sputum, with gram-positive diplococci on Gram stain and asymmetric consolidation with air bronchograms on chest radiograph.[13] *H. influenzae* is a gram-negative coccobacillus that produces consolidation with air bronchograms, often in the upper lobes.[13] Less frequent bacterial pathogens include *Klebsiella pneumoniae* which is a gram-negative rod that causes extensive tissue destruction, with air bronchograms, pleural effusion, and cavitation noted on chest radiograph.

Atypical pneumonia pathogens, such as *Mycoplasma pneumoniae, Legionella pneumophila,* and *Chlamydia pneumoniae* present with gradual onset, a lower fever, a mucoid sputum, and a patchy or interstitial infiltrate on chest radiograph. The severity of the findings on chest radiograph are usually out of proportion to the mild clinical symptoms. *Mycoplasma pneumoniae* is the most common organism responsible for atypical pneumonia and is best detected by the presence of cold agglutinins, seen in 70 percent of cases.

Any gravida suspected of having pneumonia should be managed aggressively. She should be admitted to the hospital and an investigation undertaken to determine the pathologic etiology. Work-up should include physical examination, arterial blood gases, chest radiograph, sputum Gram stain and culture, as well as blood cultures. Empiric antibiotic coverage should be started, usually with a third-generation cephalosporin such as ceftriaxone or cefotaxime. *Legionella* pneumonia has a high mortality and sometimes presents with consolidation, mimicking pneumococcal pneumonia. Therefore, it is recommended that a macrolide, such as azithromycin, be added to the empiric therapy. Once the results of the sputum culture, blood cultures, Gram stain, and serum studies are obtained and a pathogen has been identified, antibiotic therapy can be directed towards the identifiable pathogen. The third-generation cephalosporins are effective agents for the majority of pathogens causing a community-acquired pneumonia. They are also effective against penicillin-resistant *Streptococcus pneumoniae*. In addition to antibiotic therapy, oxygen supplementation should be given. Frequent arterial blood gas measurements should be obtained to maintain the PO_2 at 70 mm Hg, a level necessary to ensure adequate fetal oxygenation. Arterial saturation can be monitored with pulse oximetry as well. When the gravida is afebrile for 48 hours and has signs of clinical improvement, an oral cephalosporin can be started and intravenous therapy discontinued. A total of 10 to 14 days of treatment should be completed.

VIRAL PNEUMONIAS

Influenza Virus

In the epidemic of 1957, autopsies demonstrated that pregnant women died from fulminant viral pneumonia most commonly, while nonpregnant patients died most often from secondary bacterial infection.[16] Primary influenza pneumonia is characterized by rapid progression from a unilateral infiltrate to diffuse bilateral disease. The gravida may develop fulminant respiratory failure requiring mechanical ventilation and positive end-expiratory pressure (PEEP). When pneumonia complicates influenza in pregnancy, antibiotics should be started, directed at the likely pathogens that can cause secondary infection, including *Staphylococcus aureus,* pneumococcus, *H. influenza,* and certain enteric gram-negative bacteria. Antiviral agents, such as amantadine and ribavirin, can be considered.[17] It has been recommended that the influenza vaccine be given routinely to gravidas in the second and third trimesters of pregnancy in order to prevent the occurrence of influenza and the development of pneumonia secondary to that infection.

Varicella

Varicella pneumonia occurs most often in the third trimester, and the infection is likely to be severe.[11,19,20] The maternal mortality from varicella pneumonia may be as high as 35 to 40 percent as compared to 11 to 17 percent in nonpregnant individuals.[11,20]

Varicella pneumonia usually presents 2 to 5 days after the onset of fever, rash, and malaise and is heralded by the onset of pulmonary symptoms including cough, dyspnea, pruritic chest pain, and hemoptysis.[11] The severity of the illness may vary from asymptomatic radiographic abnormalities to fulminant pneumonitis and respiratory failure[11,21] All gravidas with varicella pneumonia should be aggressively treated with antiviral therapy and admitted to the intensive care unit for close observation or intubation if indicated. Acyclovir, a DNA polymerase inhibitor, should be started. Treatment with acyclovir is safe in pregnancy. A dose of 7.5 mg/kg intravenously every 8 hours has been recommended.[23]

TUBERCULOSIS IN PREGNANCY

From 1985 through 1991, reported cases of tuberculosis increased by 18 percent, representing approximately 39,000 more cases than expected had the previous downward trend continued. This increase is due to many factors, including the HIV epidemic, the deterioration in the health care infrastructure, and more cases among immigrants.[24] The emergence of drug-resistant tuberculosis has also become a serious concern. In New York City, in 1991, 33 percent of tuberculosis cases were resistant to at least one drug, and 19 percent were resistant to both isoniazid (INH) and rifampin (RIF).[25] Between 1985 and 1992, the number of tuberculosis cases in women of childbearing age increased by 40 percent.[26] One report noted tuberculosis-complicated pregnancies in 94.8 cases per 100,000 deliveries between 1991 and 1992.[27]

Diagnosis

The majority of gravidas diagnosed with tuberculosis in pregnancy will be asymptomatic. All gravidas at high risk for tuberculosis (see the box "High-Risk Factors for Tuberculosis") should be screened with subcutaneous administration of intermediate-strength purified protein derivative (PPD). If anergy is suspected, control antigens such as candida, mumps, or tetanus toxoids should also be placed.[28] The sensitivity of the PPD is 90 to 99 percent for exposure to tuberculosis. The tine test should not be used for screening because of its low sensitivity.

The onset of the recent tuberculosis epidemic stimulated the need for rapid diagnostic tests using molecular biology methods to detect *M. tuberculosis* in clinical specimens. Two direct amplification tests (DATs) have been approved by the Food and Drug Administration (FDA). When testing acid-fast stain smear-positive respiratory specimens, each test has a sensitivity of greater than 95 percent and a specificity of essentially 100 percent for detecting the *M. tuberculosis* complex.[30,31] When testing acid-fast stain smear-negative respiratory specimens, the specificity remains greater than 95 percent, but the sensitivity ranges from 40 to 77 percent.[30,31] To date, these tests are FDA-approved only for testing acid-fast stain smear-positive respiratory specimens obtained from untreated patients or those who have received no more than 7 days of antituberculosis therapy. The PPD remains the most commonly used screening test for tuberculosis.

Immigrants from areas where tuberculosis is endemic may have received the bacille Calmette-Guéerin (BCG) vaccine. Such individuals will likely have a positive response to the PPD. However, this

---

High-Risk Factors for Tuberculosis

HIV infection

Close contact with persons known or suspected to have tuberculosis

Medical risk factors known to increase risk of disease if infected

Birth in a country with high tuberculosis prevalence

Medically underserved status

Low income

Alcohol addiction

Intravenous drug use

Residency in a long-term care facility (e.g., correctional institutions, mental institutions, nursing homes and facilities)

Health professionals working in high-risk health care facilities

reactivity should wane over time. Therefore, the PPD should be utilized to screen these patients for tuberculosis unless their skin tests are known to be positive.[32] If the BCG vaccine was given 10 years earlier and the PPD is positive with a skin test reaction of 10 mm or more, that individual should be considered infected with tuberculosis and managed accordingly.[32]

Women with a positive PPD skin test must be evaluated for active tuberculosis with a thorough physical examination for extrapulmonary disease and a chest radiograph once they are beyond the first trimester.[13] Symptoms of active tuberculosis include cough (74 percent), weight loss (41 percent), fever (30 percent), malaise and fatigue (30 percent), and hemoptysis (19 percent).[33] Individuals with active pulmonary tuberculosis may have radiographic findings including adenopathy, multinodular infiltrates, cavitation, loss of volume in the upper lobes, and upper medial retraction of hilar markings. The finding of acid-fast bacilli in early morning sputum specimens confirms the diagnosis of pulmonary tuberculosis. At least three first-morning sputum samples should be examined for the presence of acid-fast bacilli. If sputum cannot be produced, sputum-induction, gastric washings, or diagnostic bronchoscopy may be indicated.

Prevention

The majority of gravidas with a positive PPD in pregnancy will be asymptomatic with no evidence of active disease and therefore classified as infected without active disease. The risk of progression to active disease is highest in the first 2 years of conversion. It is important to prevent the onset of active disease while minimizing maternal and fetal risk. An algorithm for management of the positive PPD is presented in Figure 24–1.[38] In women with a known recent conversion (2 years) to a positive PPD and no evidence of active disease, the recommended prophylaxis is isoniazid, 300 mg/day, starting after the first trimester and continuing for 6 to 9 months.[13] Isoniazid should be accompanied by pyridoxine (vitamin B_6) supplementation, 50 mg/day, in order to prevent the peripheral neuropathy that is associated with isoniazid treatment. Women with an unknown or prolonged duration of PPD positivity (>2 years) should receive isoniazid, 300 mg/day for 6 to 9 months after delivery. Isoniazid prophylaxis is not recommended for women older than 35 years of age who have an unknown or prolonged PPD positivity in the absence of active disease. The use of isoniazid is discouraged in this group because of an increased risk of hepatotoxicity. Isoniazid is associated with hepatitis in both pregnant and nonpregnant adults. However, monthly monitoring of liver function tests may prevent this adverse outcome. Among individuals receiving isoniazid, 10 to 20 percent will develop mildly elevated liver function tests. These changes resolve once the drug is discontinued.[39]

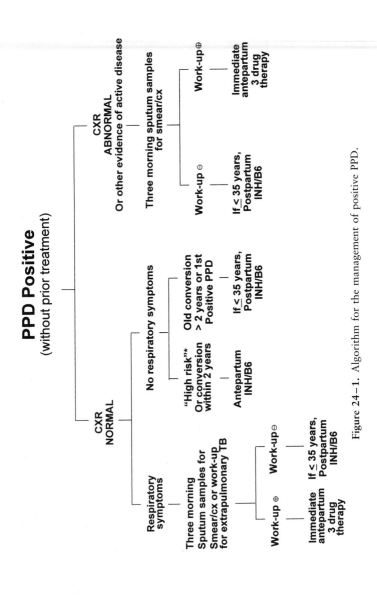

Figure 24–1. Algorithm for the management of positive PPD.

Treatment

The gravida with active tuberculosis should be treated initially with isoniazid, 300 mg/day, combined with rifampin, 600 mg/day (Table 24–6).[40] Resistant disease results from initial infection with resistant strains (33 percent) or can develop during therapy.[41] If resistance to isoniazid is identified or anticipated, ethambutol 2.5 g/day should be added and the treatment period should be extended to 18 months.[40] Ethambutol is teratogenic in animals; however, this has not been noted in humans. The most common side effect of ethambutol therapy is optic neuritis. Streptomycin should be avoided during pregnancy because it is associated with eighth nerve damage in neonates.[42] Antituberculous agents not recommended for use in pregnancy include ethionamide, streptomycin, capreomycin, kanamycin, cycloserine, and pyrazinamide.[13] Women who are being treated with antituberculous drugs may breast-feed.

In summary, high-risk gravidas should be screened for tuberculosis and treated appropriately with INH prophylaxis for infection without overt disease and with dual antituberculous therapy for active disease. In addition, the newborn should be screened for evidence of tuberculosis as well.

ASTHMA IN PREGNANCY

Asthma, which may be the most common potentially serious respiratory complication of pregnancy, is characterized by chronic airway inflammation with increased airway responsiveness to a variety of stimuli, and airway obstruction that is partially or completely reversible.[44] Approximately 4 percent of women of child-bearing age have a history of asthma, but up to 10 percent of the population appears to have nonspecific airway hyperresponsiveness.[45] In general, the prevalence, morbidity, and mortality from asthma are increasing. The effects of pregnancy on asthma are controversial.

Studies have shown that patients with more severe asthma may have the greatest risk for complications during pregnancy.[47,52] In 1993, the National Asthma Education Program (NAEP) working group defined mild, moderate, and severe asthma according to symptomatic exacerbations (wheezing, cough, and/or dyspnea) and objective tests of pulmonary function. The most commonly used parameters are the peak expiratory flow rate (PEFR) and the forced expiratory volume in 1 second (FEV_1). The NAEP guidelines did not consider the need for regular medication to be a factor for classifying asthma severity during pregnancy. In a recent prospective observational study of 1,800 pregnant women with asthma and 900 control subjects, patients with mild asthma but who required

Table 24-6. ANTITUBERCULOSIS DRUGS

Drug	Dosage Forms	Daily Dose	Weekly Dose	Major Adverse Reactions
First-line drugs (for initial treatment):				
Isoniazid	PO, IM	10 mg/kg up to 300 mg	15 mg/kg up to 900 mg	Hepatic enzyme elevation, peripheral neuropathy hepatitis, hypersensitivity
Rifampin	PO	10 mg/kg up to 600 mg	10 mg/kg up to 600 mg	Orange discoloration of secretions and urine, nausea, vomiting, hepatitis, febrile reaction, purpura (rare)
Pyrazinamide	PO	15–30 mg/kg up to 2 g	50–70 mg/kg	Hepatotoxicity, hyperuricemia, arthralgias, skin rash, gastrointestinal upset
Ethambutol	PO	15 mg/kg up to 2.5 g	50 mg/kg	Optic neuritis (decreased red-green color discrimination, decreased visual acuity), skin rash
Streptomycin	IM	15 mg/kg up to 1 g	25–30 mg/kg up to 1 g	Ototoxicity, nephrotoxicity

Second-line drugs (daily therapy):			
Capreomycin	IM	15–30 mg/kg up to 1 g	Auditory, vestibular, and renal toxicity
Kanamycin	IM	15–30 mg/kg up to 1 g	Auditory and renal toxicity, rare vestibular toxicity
Ethionamide	PO	15–20 mg/kg up to 1 g	Gastrointestinal disturbance, hepatotoxicity, hypersensitivity
Para-aminosalycylic acid	PO	150 mg/kg up to 1 g	Gastrointestinal disturbance, acidhypersensitivity, hepatotoxicity, sodium load
Cycloserine	PO	15–20 mg/kg up to 1 g	Psychosis, convulsions, rash

623

regular medications (β-agonist, theophylline, or inhaled corticosteroids) were similar to subjects with moderate asthma in respect to asthma exacerbations.[53] It seems prudent to consider pregnant patients requiring regular systemic corticosteroids to control asthma symptoms to have severe asthma (see the box "Modified NAEP Asthma Severity Classification").

Asthma Management

The ultimate goal of asthma therapy is maintaining adequate oxygenation of the fetus by preventing hypoxic episodes in the mother. The effective management of asthma during pregnancy relies on four integral components outlined below.

Objective Measures for Assessment and Monitoring

The FEV_1 following a maximal inspiration is the single best measure of pulmonary function. However, measurement of FEV_1 requires a spirometer. The PEFR correlates well with the FEV_1, and has the advantages that it can be measured reliably with inexpensive, disposable, portable peak flowmeters. Patient self-monitoring of PEFR provides valuable insight to the course of asthma throughout the day, assesses circadian variation in pulmonary function, and helps detect early signs of deterioration so that timely therapy can be instituted.

Modified NAEP Asthma Severity Classification

Mild asthma
   Brief (<1 hour) symptomatic exacerbations less than twice a week
   PEFR $\geq 80\%$ of personal best
   FEV_1 $\geq 80\%$ of predicted when asymptomatic
Moderate asthma
   Symptomatic exacerbations more than twice a week
   Exacerbations affect activity levels
   Exacerbations may last for days
   PEFR, FEV_1 range from 60 to 80% of predicted
   Regular medications necessary to control symptoms
Severe asthma
   Continuous symptoms/frequent exacerbations limit activity levels
   PEFR, FEV_1 <60% of expected, and are highly variable
   Regular oral corticosteroids necessary to control symptoms

Avoid or Control Asthma Triggers

Limiting adverse environmental exposures during pregnancy is important for controlling asthma. Irritants and allergens that provoke acute symptoms also increase airway inflammation and hyperresponsiveness.

Patient Education

Patients should be made aware that controlling asthma during pregnancy is especially important for the well-being of the fetus. The patient should have a basic understanding of strategies to reduce asthma triggers and medical management during pregnancy, including self-monitoring of PEFRs and the correct use of inhalers.

Pharmacologic Therapy

The goal of asthma therapy is multiphasic: (1) relieve bronchospasm, (2) protect the airways from irritant stimuli, (3) prevent the pulmonary and inflammatory response to an allergen exposure, and (4) resolve the inflammatory process in the airways leading to improved pulmonary function with reduced airway hyperresponsiveness. The therapeutic approach includes increasing the number and frequency of medications with increasing asthma severity.

Asthma Pharmacotherapy

Current medical treatment for asthma emphasizes reduction of airway inflammation to decrease airway hyperresponsiveness and prevent asthma symptoms. Although it is assumed that asthma medications are as effective in pregnant as in nonpregnant patients, differences in maternal physiology and pharmacokinetics may affect the absorption, distribution, metabolism and clearance of medications during pregnancy.

Three classes of inhaled anti-inflammatory asthma medications are available at the present time: inhaled corticosteroids, nedocromil sodium, and cromolyn sodium. In separate controlled studies of nongravid subjects, use of inhaled corticosteroids or cromolyn sodium led to improvement in (1) asthma symptoms,[59-61] (2) pulmonary function,[59] (3) nonspecific bronchial hyperactivity,[62] (4) emergency room relapses,[61] and (5) hospitalizations[59] (see the box "Typical Dosages of Common Asthma Medications").

Inhaled Corticosteroids

Airway inflammation is present in nearly all cases; therefore, inhaled corticosteroids have even been advocated as first-line therapy for patients with mild asthma.[63] The use of inhaled corticosteroids among nonpregnant asthmatics has been associated with a marked reduction in fatal and near-fatal asthma.[64] In addition to their anti-inflammatory effect, corticosteroids increase the effectiveness of β-adrenergic drugs by inducing formation of new β_2-receptors. Beclomethasone is the preferred agent, but other inhaled steroids may be continued in a well-controlled patient. The inhaled steroids are currently labeled FDA pregnancy class C.

Cromolyn Sodium and Nedocromil Sodium

Given the potential for systemic effects of inhaled corticosteroids, even at low doses, it is important to identify nonsteroidal anti-inflammatory medications. At the present time, cromolyn sodium and nedocromil sodium are the only approved medications that fit into this category.

Theophylline

Theophylline has anti-inflammatory actions[92] that may be mediated by the inhibition of leukotriene production and its capacity to stimulate prostaglandin E (PGE$_2$) production.[93] The NAEP Working Group on Asthma and Pregnancy recommended that theophylline be considered a second-line drug to be used to supplement inhaled corticosteroids when control is not achieved.

Inhaled β-Agonists

β-Agonists are currently recommended for use with all degrees of asthma during pregnancy.[48,51] This group of medications has evolved from those that are relatively short acting (epinephrine, iso-

Typical Dosages of Common Asthma Medications	
Cromolyn sodium	2 inhalations qid
Beclomethasone	2–5 inhalations bid–qid
Triamcinolone	2 inhalations tid–qid or 4 inhalations bid
Budesonide	2–4 inhalations bid
Fluticasone	88–220 μg bid
Flunisolide	2–4 inhalations bid
Theophylline	Maintain serum levels of 8–12 μg/ml; decrease dosage by thalf if reated with erythromycin or cimetidine
Prednisone	1 week 40 mg/day burst for active symptoms followed by 1 week taper
Albuterol	2 inhalations q 3–4 hours

proterenol) to those with a longer duration of action (albuterol, terbutaline, pirbuterol), of 4 to 6 hours.[97] Their greatest advantage is a rapid onset of effect in the relief of acute bronchospasm via smooth muscle relaxation.

While β_2-agonists are associated with tremor, tachycardia, and palpitations, recent studies have found more serious complications including an association with an increased risk of death with chronic use.[99,100]

Leukotriene Pathway Moderators

Leukotrienes are arachidonic acid metabolites that have been implicated in transducing bronchospasm, mucus secretion, and increased vascular permeability.[101] Treatment with the leukotriene receptor antagonist montelukast has been shown to significantly improve pulmonary function as measured by FEV_1.[102] The leukotriene receptor antagonists zafirlukast (Accolate), and montelukast (Singulair) are both rated FDA pregnancy category B.

Step Therapy

The step-care therapeutic approach increases the number and frequency of medications with increasing asthma severity (see the box "Step Therapy Medical Management of Asthma"). A burst of oral corticosteroids is indicated for exacerbations not responding to initial β-agonist therapy regardless of asthma severity. Additionally, patients who require increasing inhaled β_2-agonist therapy (more

---

Step Therapy Medical Management of Asthma

Mild
  Inhaled β_2-agonist as needed*

Moderate
  Inhaled β_2-agonist as needed*
  Inhaled corticosteroids (or cromolyn)
  Theophylline for nocturnal asthma or increased symptoms

Severe
  Inhaled β_2-agonist as needed*
  Inhaled corticosteroids (or cromolyn)
  Theophylline for nocturnal asthma or increased symptoms

Oral systemic corticosteroids

---

*PEFR or FEV_1 <80 percent, asthma exacerbations, or exposure to exercise or allergens (oral corticosteroid burst if inadequate response to β_2-agonist regardless of asthma severity).

than 12 puffs per day) to control their symptoms may benefit from oral corticosteroids. In such cases, a short course of oral prednisone, 40 to 60 mg/day for 1 week followed by 7 to 14 days of tapering may be effective.

Antenatal Management

Patients with moderate and severe asthma should be considered to have high-risk pregnancies. Adverse outcomes can be increased by underestimation of asthma severity and under treatment of asthma exacerbations. The first prenatal visit should include a detailed medical history with attention to medical conditions that could complicate the management of asthma, including diabetes mellitus, hypertension, cardiac disease, adrenal disorders, hyperthyroidism, HIV, hemoglobinopathies, hepatic disease, and active pulmonary problems. The patient should be questioned about the presence and severity of symptoms, episodes of nocturnal asthma, the number of days of work missed due to asthma exacerbations, history of acute asthma emergency care visits, and smoking history. The type and amount of asthma medications including the number of puffs of β_2-agonists used each day should be recorded. Asthma severity should be determined.

Gravidas with mild, well-controlled asthma may receive routine prenatal care. Moderate and severe asthmatic women should have scheduling of prenatal visits based on clinical judgment; most will need prenatal visits at least every 2 weeks, then weekly at 36 weeks' gestation. In addition to routine care, each antenatal visit should include an evaluation of (1) asthma severity and symptom frequency, nocturnal asthma; (2) FEV_1 or PEFR; (3) medications (assessing compliance and dosage); and (4) emergency visits and hospital admissions for asthma exacerbations. Patients should be instructed on proper dosing and administration of their asthma medications. The step-care therapeutic approach includes increasing the number and frequency of medications with increasing asthma severity. The lowest number of medications needed to control asthma symptoms should be used. Avoidance and control of asthma triggers are particularly important in pregnancy, since pharmacologic control of asthma potentially has adverse fetal effects.

Moderate and severe asthmatics require additional fetal surveillance in the form of ultrasound examinations and antenatal fetal testing. Because asthma has been associated with intrauterine growth restriction and preterm birth, it is critical to accurately establish pregnancy dating. Ultrasound examinations also are needed to evaluate fetal viability, anatomy, amniotic fluid volume, placental location, and interval fetal growth. Repeat ultrasound examinations are recommended for patients with suboptimally controlled asthma, and following asthma exacerbations to evaluate fetal activity, growth, and amniotic fluid volume. The intensity of antenatal fetal surveillance should be based on the severity of the asthma. All patients should be instructed to be attentive to fetal activity and keep a record of fetal kick counts. In most cases, patients with moderate and severe asthma should have fetal testing starting by 32 weeks' gestation.

Home Management of Asthma Exacerbations

An asthma exacerbation that causes minimal problems for the mother may have severe sequelae for the fetus. Indeed, an abnormal fetal heart rate tracing may be the initial manifestation of an asthmatic exacerbation. A maternal PO_2 below 60 mm Hg or hemoglobin saturation less than 90 percent may be associated with profound fetal hypoxia. Therefore, asthma exacerbations in pregnancy must be aggressively managed. Patients should be given an individualized guide for decision making and rescue management.

Patients should be educated to recognize signs and symptoms of early asthma exacerbations such as coughing, chest tightness, dyspnea, or wheezing, or by a 20 percent decrease in their PEFR. This is important so that prompt home rescue treatment may be instituted in order to avoid maternal and fetal hypoxia. In general, patients should use inhaled albuterol 2 to 4 puffs every 20 minutes up to 1 hour. A good response is considered if symptoms are resolved or become subjectively mild, normal activities can be resumed, and the PEFR is greater than 70 percent of personal best. The patient should seek further medical attention if the response is incomplete, or if fetal activity is decreased.

Hospital and Clinic Management

The principal goal should be the prevention of hypoxia. Continuous electronic fetal monitoring should be initiated if gestation has advanced to the point of potential fetal viability. Albuterol should be delivered by nebulizer (2.5 mg = 0.5 ml albuterol in 2.5 ml normal saline) driven with oxygen; treatments are given every 20 minutes.[103-105] Occasionally, nebulized treatment is not effective because the patient is moving air poorly. In such cases, terbutaline 0.25 mg can be administered subcutaneously every 15 minutes for three doses. The patient should be assessed for general level of activity, color, pulse rate, use of accessory muscles, and airflow obstruction determined by auscultation and FEV_1 and/or PEFR before and after each bronchodilator treatment. Measurement of oxygenation via pulse oximeter or arterial blood gases is essential. Arterial blood gases should be obtained if oxygen saturation remains below 95 percent. Chest x-rays are not commonly needed. Guidelines for the management of asthma exacerbations are presented in the box "Emergency Assessment and Management of Asthma Exacerbations."

Labor and Delivery Management

Asthma medications should not be discontinued during labor and delivery. Although asthma is usually quiescent during labor, consideration should be given to assessing PEFRs on admission and at 12-hour intervals. The patient should be kept hydrated and should receive adequate analgesia in order to decrease the risk of bronchospasm. If systemic corticosteroids have been used in the previous 4 weeks, then hydrocortisone (100 mg every 8 hours intravenously) should be administered during labor and for the 24-hour period following delivery to prevent adrenal crisis (NAEP).

It is rarely necessary to deliver a fetus via cesarean section for an acute asthma exacerbation. Usually, maternal and fetal compromise can be managed by aggressive medical management. Occasionally, delivery may improve the respiratory status of a patient with unstable asthma who has a mature fetus. PGE_2 or PGE_1 can be used for cervical ripening, the management of spontaneous or induced abor-

---

Emergency Assessment and Management of Asthma Exacerbations

1. **Initial evaluation:**
   History, examination, PEFR, oximetry
   Fetal monitoring if potentially viable

2. **Initial treatment**
   Inhaled α_2-agonist ×3 doses over 60–90 minutes
   O_2 to maintain saturation >95 percent
   If no wheezing and PEFR or FEV_1 >70 percent baseline, discharge with follow-up

3. **If oximetry <90 percent, FEV_1 <1.0 L, or PEFR <100 L/min on presentation:**
   Continue nebulized albuterol
   Start intravenous corticosteroids
   Consider intravenous aminophylline
   Obtain arterial blood gases
   Admit to intensive care unit
   Possible intubation

4. **If PEFR or FEV_1 >40 percent but <70 percent baseline after β_2-agonist:**
   Obtain arterial blood gases
   Continue inhaled β_2-agonist every 1–4 hours
   Start intravenous corticosteroids in most cases
   Consider intravenous aminophylline
   Hospital admission in most cases

tions, or postpartum hemorrhage; however, 15-methyl $PGF_2\alpha$ and methylergonovine can cause bronchospasm. Magnesium sulfate, which is a bronchodilator, is a safe choice for treating preterm labor. Indomethacin can induce bronchospasm in the aspirin-sensitive patient. Lumbar anesthesia has the benefit of reducing oxygen consumption and minute ventilation during labor.[106] Communication between the obstetric, anesthetic, and pediatric care givers is important for optimal care.

VENOUS THROMBOSIS AND PULMONARY EMBOLISM

Venous thromboembolic diseases, which include superficial and deep thrombophlebitis, pulmonary embolus, septic pelvic thrombophlebitis, and thrombosis account for almost one half of all obstetric morbidity.[110] The leading cause of pregnancy-related mortality in the United States, pulmonary embolism is responsible for 17 percent of maternal deaths.[111] Thromboembolic disease occurs more frequently during gestation, and the likelihood of venous thromboembolism in normal pregnancy and the puerperium is increased by a factor of 5 when compared with nonpregnant women of similar age.[112] An untreated deep vein thrombosis (DVT) is associated with a 15 to 25 percent incidence of pulmonary embolus, with a 12 to 15 percent mortality rate.[113]

Diagnosis of Deep Vein Thrombosis

The diagnosis of a DVT during pregnancy can be challenging. Clinical suspicions are aroused by signs and symptoms including pain, tenderness to palpation, and edema. Edema of the lower extremities occurs frequently in normal pregnancy, particularly in the third trimester. However, should edema be asymmetric, that is, more than 2 cm difference in circumference between the affected and normal leg, or if there is a positive Homans' sign or Lowenberg test, an investigation to rule out a DVT should be undertaken.

Venography

Ascending contrast venography is the reference standard for the diagnosis of a DVT.[148] The technique involves injection of a radiographic contrast dye into a distal, dorsal foot vein while the patient is relaxed, non–weight bearing, and in 40 percent of reversed Trendelenburg position. The diagnosis of DVT requires visualization in at least two different views of a well-defined intraluminal filling defect.

If indicated during pregnancy, a limited venogram can be performed using pelvic and abdominal shielding with lead aprons. This can protect the fetus from potential hazards of radiation exposure. Visualization of the iliac veins may be compromised, and isolated iliac vein thrombosis cannot be diagnosed.[148] If complete visualization of the entire deep venous system is indicated, a complete venogram can be done. The estimated amount of radiation absorbed by the fetus with an unshielded unilateral venogram was 0.314 rad in one study.[149] This compared with less than 0.050 rad with a limited venogram. [125]I fibrinogen scanning is not recommended for diagnosis of deep vein thrombosis in pregnancy.

Impedance Plethysmography

Impedance plethysmography (IPG) is a safe, inexpensive, and relatively sensitive and specific test for the detection of a proximal DVT. However, it is not sensitive for detecting proximal nonobstructive thrombi or calf DVT.[150] A positive IPG after 20 weeks of gestation requires confirmation by venography before initiating anticoagulant therapy.[113]

Venous Duplex Doppler Ultrasound

Venous duplex Doppler ultrasound is a safe, simple, and inexpensive method to indirectly assess the competency of the deep venous system in the lower extremities. However, this technique is subjective and requires considerable expertise.[148] Venous Doppler assessment has a sensitivity of 76 to 94 percent and a specificity of 90 to 95 percent for a proximal DVT, but has a low sensitivity for a calf DVT.[148,153]

When there is clinical suspicion of DVT, the diagnostic approach should be such that disease can be diagnosed while minimizing potentially harmful fetal irradiation. One approach is to use Doppler ultrasound as the initial diagnostic test. If the test is positive, anticoagulant therapy should be given. If the ultrasound is normal, the patient's symptoms may be due to a calf DVT, which may be undetected by ultrasound. Serial ultrasound testing may then be done to assess for progression of a calf DVT into the proximal veins.[148] If repeat ultrasound identifies a newly formed proximal DVT, anticoagulation therapy should be initiated.

If isolated iliac vein thrombosis is suspected, Doppler ultrasound or IPG can be used for diagnosis. IPG can be used as the initial test. If IPG is positive during the first or second trimester of pregnancy, then a DVT can be diagnosed and anticoagulation started.[148] A positive test in the third trimester may be falsely positive because of outflow obstruction caused by the gravid uterus. In this circumstance, further investigation with a limited venogram should be considered and, if a DVT is seen, treatment can be started. If a limited venogram does not demonstrate a thrombus, a complete venogram should be considered, given the possibility of proximal femoral vein thrombosis or isolated iliac DVT. If the initial IPG is negative and the pretest clinical likelihood of DVT is low or moderate, then serial IPG testing should be done over a 7- to 14-day period.[148] If the repeat IPG becomes positive, then this can provide sufficient basis for diagnosing a DVT. If the initial IPG is negative and the pretest clinical likelihood for a DVT is high, a limited venogram or Doppler ultrasound should be performed.[148] If either of these examinations is positive, therapy should be started.

Pulmonary Embolism

Pulmonary embolus (PE) contributes to significant maternal morbidity and mortality and, therefore, clinical suspicion should be high. Signs and symptoms may include dyspnea, tachypnea, cough, pleuritic chest pain, tachycardia, pleural friction rub, diaphoresis, cyanosis, hemoptysis, or a new murmur. Of these, the most common sign is tachypnea.[155] Any gravida presenting with signs and symptoms consistent with a pulmonary embolus requires further evaluation. An initial evaluation should include auscultation, pulse oximetry, and an arterial blood gas. Additional tests should include a chest radiograph and electrocardiogram. A PO_2 greater than 85 mm Hg on room air is reassuring; however, it does not rule out the possibility of a PE. As many as 14 percent of patients with a pulmonary embolus have a PO_2 greater than 85 mm Hg.[155] Any patient with an oxygen saturation less than 95 percent on room air without obvious clinical conditions associated with hypoxia, such as atelectasis, pneumonia, or asthma, deserves an investigation. A chest radiograph is useful to rule out pneumonia and atelectasis; however, even the presence of an infiltrate does not rule out the possibility of PE and, again, investigation should be continued if clinical suspicion is high. The most frequent electrocardiographic finding is tachycardia; however, findings consistent with acute cor pulmonale (right axis shift and nonspecific T-wave inversions) may be seen after massive pulmonary embolism. If clinical suspicion for PE is moderate to high, the gravida should be anticoagulated while the diagnosis is pursued.

When pulmonary embolus is suspected, Doppler ultrasound or IPG may be performed to identify a DVT. If these tests are diagnostic for DVT, one can assume the patient does indeed have a pulmonary embolus and anticoagulation therapy should be instituted. If the diagnosis of DVT has not been established, ventilation-perfusion (V/Q) lung scanning should be performed. The perfusion scan is performed by injecting ^{99m}Tc-labeled albumin. These particles are aggregated within the pulmonary precapillary arteriolar bed. A ventilation scan using ^{133}Xe isotope is done after the perfusion scan to document ventilatory defects. The V/Q scans are then examined for matching defects. These scans are interpreted as normal, indeterminate, or revealing low, moderate, or high suspicion of pulmonary embolus. If there are abnormalities on the chest radiograph that coincide with areas of perfusion defect, the scan is considered indeterminate. When there is V/Q mismatching or multiple defects, the probability of pulmonary embolism is considered high.

When the Doppler examination is negative, the V/Q scan is low probability, and the clinical suspicion of PE is low as well, the test can be considered negative, and therapy need not be initiated. If the V/Q scan is indeterminate, low or moderately suspicious for PE, and clinical suspicion is high, a pulmonary arteriogram should be performed. If a pulmonary arteriogram is diagnostic of PE, therapy should be instituted with heparin. If the V/Q scan is consistent with high probability, the patient can be considered as having a positive test for PE, and therapy should be instituted.

When pulmonary embolus is diagnosed, therapy should be initiated immediately. Heparin is the anticoagulant of choice during pregnancy. Because of its large molecular weight, it does not cross the placenta and is not excreted in breast milk. Heparin must be given parenterally, and intravenous therapy achieves therapeutic levels most quickly. The initial loading dose should be 70 units/kg, administered intravenously, followed by a continuous infusion of 1,000 units/h. The dose of heparin should be adjusted to keep the activated partial thromboplastin time (aPTT) approximately twice normal or the heparin level at 0.2 to 0.4 units/ml. This therapy should be continued for approximately 10 days. The patient can then be switched to subcutaneous heparin at a dose sufficient to keep the aPTT about 1 1/2 times normal and the heparin titer 0.1 to 0.2 units/ml. In general, a dose of 7,500 to 10,000 units of heparin administered every 8 to 12 hours will achieve therapeutic levels.[157] This therapy should be continued throughout gestation because the risk of a recurrent thrombus remains high. Therefore, a DVT and/or PE should be treated with full anticoagulation for at least 3 to 6 months. Subsequently, both therapeutic and prophylactic regimens of heparin have been advocated until 6 to 12 weeks postpartum.[158]

Hemorrhage is the major risk of heparin therapy. This occurs in approximately 4 percent of properly monitored nonsurgical patients receiving intravenous heparin.[159] Osteoporosis and compression fractures can occur when heparin has been administered in doses greater than 15,000 units/day for more than 6 months.[160] This side effect can be diminished by administration of adequate amounts of calcium and vitamin D and may be reversible following cessation of therapy.[158] Thrombocytopenia can also complicate heparin therapy but occurs in only 3 percent of patients treated with porcine heparin.[161] A platelet count should be obtained periodically during the first 3 weeks of therapy. Low-molecular-weight heparin has been used during gestation. Patients treated with low-molecular-weight heparin may be less likely to develop heparin-induced thrombocytopenia. Low-molecular-weight heparin has the advantage of only single daily dosing, but is 10 times more expensive than heparin therapy.[162]

In the postpartum period, treatment can be switched to warfarin (Coumadin). Coumadin does not enter breast milk in significant amounts. A starting dose of 5 mg/day for the first 2 days is followed by daily dosing adjusted to the international normalized ratio (INR) of 2.0 to 3.0. An overlap of 3 to 5 days with a therapeutic INR and aPTT is recommended. Warfarin is continued for approximately 3 months or indefinitely if risk factors are still present or if thromboembolism is recurrent.[163]

Prophylaxis

Women with a previous venous thromboembolism have a 7 to 30 percent risk of recurrence during a subsequent pregnancy.[164,165] Therefore, heparin prophylaxis is administered during pregnancy at 7,500 units every 12 hours, from 13 weeks of gestation, and 10,000 units every 12 hours from 30 weeks of gestation.[167]

Key Points

> ➤ Pneumonia is the most common nonobstetric infection to cause maternal mortality. Preterm delivery complicates pneumonia in up to 43 percent of cases. *Streptococcus pneumoniae* is the most common bacterial pathogen to cause pneumonia. Empiric antibiotic coverage should be started, including a third-generation cephalosporin and a macrolide, such as azithromycin, to cover atypical pathogens.

> ➤ High-risk gravidas should be screened for tuberculosis and treated appropriately with INH prophylaxis for infection without overt disease and with dual antituberculosis therapy for active disease. If resistant tuberculosis is identified, ethambutol 2.5 g/day should be added to therapy and the treatment period should be extended to 18 months.

> ➤ Asthma is characterized by chronic airway inflammation with increased airway responsiveness to a variety of stimuli and airway obstruction that is partially or completely reversible. Patients with severe asthma have the greatest risk for complications during pregnancy. Complications

Box continued on following page

Key Points *Continued*

include preeclampsia, asthma exacerbation, preterm rupture of the membranes, increased perinatal mortality, prematurity, and low birth weight. Therapy should include education, bronchodilators, and the addition of inhaled steroids.

➤ Asthma medications should be continued during labor and delivery. PEFR should be measured on admission and at 12-hour intervals. If systemic corticosteroids have been used in the previous 4 weeks, hydrocortisone (100 mg every 8 hours) should be administered during labor and for the 24-hour period following delivery to prevent adrenal crisis.

➤ Thromboembolic disease is the leading cause of pregnancy-related mortality in the United States. An untreated deep vein thrombosis (DVT) is associated with a 15 to 25 percent incidence of pulmonary embolus with a 12 to 15 percent mortality rate. Pregnancy is accompanied by a hypercoagulable state. Hypercoaguable conditions, such as AT-III deficiency, prothrombin 20210A allele, protein C deficiency, protein S deficiency, factor V Leiden, dysfibrinogenemia, hyperhomosystenemia, and the antiphospholipid syndrome may increase the risk of deep vein thrombosis and pulmonary embolus.

➤ Investigation for deep vein thrombosis in pregnancy should include impedance plethysmography, venous Doppler ultrasound, real-time ultrasound, and venography. ^{125}I fibrinogen scanning should be avoided during pregnancy because of high levels of fetal radiation exposure and concentration of the radiolabeled iodine in the fetal thyroid.

➤ A high index of suspicion for pulmonary embolus is necessary. Diagnosis should be undertaken with venous Doppler ultrasound of the extremities to identify a DVT and V/Q scanning and pulmonary arteriography if indicated.

➤ Therapy for thrombosis and pulmonary embolus in pregnancy should be accomplished with heparin. Coumadin may be used in the postpartum period. The aPTT and/or INR should be monitored closely.

Key Points *Continued*

➤ The interstitial lung diseases include idiopathic pulmonary fibrosis, sarcoidosis, hypersensity pneumonitis, pneumonosis, drug-induced lung disease, and connective tissue disease. Restrictive lung disease is generally well tolerated in pregnancy; however, exercise intolerance and need for oxygen supplementation may develop. Gravidas with pulmonary hypertension complicating restrictive lung disease may suffer a high mortality.

➤ An increasing number of women with cystic fibrosis are surviving to the reproductive years and usually maintain their fertility with meticulous management of pulmonary function, including pulmonary toilet and aggressive surveillance for signs of pulmonary infection and treatment of antibiotics in adequate doses. Close attention to nutrition is required secondary to maldigestion, malabsorption, and malnutrition, which can complicate cystic fibrosis. Gravidas with good clinical studies, good nutritional status, nearly normal chest radiographs, and only mild obstructive lung disease will tolerate pregnancy well. Fetal growth should be monitored closely.

Renal Disease

PHILIP SAMUELS AND DAVID F. COLOMBO

EVALUATION OF RENAL STATUS

The most frequently utilized method to evaluate the urine is the spot *urinalysis*. With the exception of the glucose, the study can be utilized as it would in the nonpregnant patient. It is, however, only a screening tool. If there is a concern that a patient has a change in her renal status or the possibility of bacteriuria, further testing is needed.

One of the best methods to evaluate kidney function is collection of a *24-hour urine sample* for total protein analysis. The nonpregnant patient will usually spill less than 150 mg/day of protein. Most investigators consider up to 260 mg/day of total urinary protein and 29 mg/day of albumin normal in the gravid patient.[10] It should be noted that when one is using serial 24-hour urine samples to evaluate a change in renal status, it is crucial that the collection is standardized. The amount a creatinine cleared in a day should remain constant during the course of a pregnancy for a given patient.

Urinalysis has been used to screen for bacteriuria. However, it is recommended that a urine culture be used as the primary method of screening all pregnant patients.

INFECTIONS OF THE URINARY TRACT

See Chapter 25.

Urolithiasis

The prevalence of urolithiasis during pregnancy is 0.03 percent, with an incidence no higher than that of the general population.[31] Colicky abdominal pain, recurrent UTI, and hematuria suggest urolithiasis. If the diagnosis is suspected, intravenous pyelography should be undertaken, limiting this study to the minimum number of exposures necessary to make the diagnosis. Ultrasound can often be used to establish the diagnosis without radiation exposure. For any patient suspected or proved to have renal stones, serum calcium and phosphorous levels should be measured to rule out hyperparathyroidism. Serum urate should also be determined.

Because of the physiologic hydroureter characteristic of pregnancy, most patients with symptomatic urolithiasis will spontaneously pass their stones. Treatment should be conservative, consisting of hydration and narcotic analgesia for pain relief.[32]

Acute Renal Failure in Pregnancy

Acute renal failure (ARF) is defined as a urine output of less than 400 ml in 24 hours. To make the diagnosis, ureteral and urethral obstruction must be excluded. The incidence of ARF during pregnancy is approximately 1 per 10,000. It is seen most frequently in septic first-trimester abortions and in cases of sudden severe volume depletion resulting from hemorrhage caused by placenta previa, placental abruption, or postpartum uterine atony.[41] It is also observed in the marked volume contraction associated with severe preeclampsia[42] and with acute fatty liver of pregnancy.[42,43] The incidence of ARF in pregnancy has decreased over the years.

Renal ischemia is the common denominator in all cases of ARF. With mild ischemia, quickly reversible prerenal failure results. With more prolonged ischemia, acute tubular necrosis occurs. This process is also reversible, as glomeruli are not affected. Severe ischemia, however, may produce acute cortical necrosis. This pathology is irreversible, although on occasion a small amount of renal function is preserved.[45]

Clinically, patients with reversible ARF first experience a period of oliguria of variable duration. Polyuria then occurs. It is important to recognize that BUN and serum creatinine levels continue to rise early in the polyuric phase. During the recovery phase, urine output approaches normal. In these patients, it is important to monitor electrolytes frequently and to treat any imbalance carefully. The urine/plasma osmolality ratio should be determined early in the course of the disease. If the ratio is 1.5 or greater, prerenal pathology is likely, and the disorder tends to be of shorter duration and less severity. A ratio near 1.0 suggests acute tubular necrosis.

The main goal of treatment is elimination of the underlying cause. Volume and electrolyte balance must receive constant scrutiny. To assess volume requirements, invasive hemodynamic monitoring is useful and lessens the need for clinical guesswork.

This is especially true during the polyuric phase. Central hyperalimentation may also be required if renal failure is prolonged.

Acidosis frequently occurs in cases of ARF. Arterial blood gases therefore should be followed regularly. Acidosis must be treated promptly to prevent hyperkalemia, which may develop rapidly and can be fatal. Absolute restriction of potassium intake should be instituted immediately. Sodium bicarbonate, used to treat acidosis, may overload the patient with sodium and water. In this case, peritoneal or hemodialysis may be instituted. The main indications for dialysis in ARF of pregnancy are hypernatremia, hyperkalemia, severe acidosis, volume overload, and worsening uremia.

Nephrotic Syndrome

The nephrotic syndrome was initially described as a 24-hour urine protein excretion of 3.5 g or more, reduced serum albumin, edema, and hyperlipidemia.[61] Currently, the syndrome is defined by massive proteinuria alone, which is often the result of damage to the glomeruli.[61] The most common etiology of nephrotic syndrome in pregnancy (especially the third trimester) is preeclampsia. Other etiologies include proliferative glomerulonephritis, minimal change disease, lupus nephropathy, hereditary nephritis, diabetic nephropathy, renal vein thrombosis, and amyloidosis.[62]

Patients with newly diagnosed or persistent nephrotic syndrome must be followed closely in pregnancy. Whenever possible, the etiology of the proteinuria should be determined. In many cases, steroid therapy may be employed; however, its use can in some cases aggravate the underlying disease process.[62] One common complication of nephrotic syndrome in pregnancy is profound edema secondary to massive protein excretion in addition to the normal decline in serum albumin associated with pregnancy.[62] A second area of concern is a possible hypercoagulable state precipitated by urinary losses of antithrombin III, reduced levels of protein C and S, hyperfibrinogenemia, and enhanced platelet aggregation.[63]

CHRONIC RENAL DISEASE IN PREGNANCY

Chronic renal disease can be silent until its advanced stages. Because obstetricians routinely examine the patient's urine for the presence of protein, glucose, and ketones, they may be the first to detect chronic renal disease.

Any gravida with more than trace proteinuria should collect a 24-hour urine specimen for creatinine clearance and total protein excretion. Creatinine clearance is elevated in pregnancy and, during the first trimester, may exceed 140 ml/min. Before pregnancy, 24-hour urinary protein excretion should not exceed 0.2 g. During gestation, quantities up to 0.3 g/day may be normal. Moderate proteinuria (<2 g/day) is seen in glomerular disease, most commonly lipoid nephrosis, systemic lupus erythematosus, and glomerulonephritis.

Microscopic examination of the urine can reveal much about the patient's renal status. If renal disease is suspected, a catheterized specimen should be obtained. More RBCs than one to two per high-power field or RBC casts are indicative of renal disease. RBCs usually indicate glomerular disease or collagen vascular disease. Less frequently, they suggest trauma or malignant hypertension. Increased numbers of white blood cells (WBCs), more than one to two per high-power field, or the appearance of WBC casts is usually indicative of acute or chronic infection. Cellular casts are found in the presence of renal tubular dysfunction, and hyaline casts suggest significant proteinuria. A single bacterium seen in an unspun catheterized urine specimen is suggestive of significant bacteriuria, and a follow-up culture should be performed.

The obstetrician can easily be misled when relying solely on the BUN and serum creatinine to assess renal function. A 70 percent decline in creatinine clearance, an indirect measure of GFR, can be seen before a significant rise in the BUN or serum creatinine occurs. In fact, little change in the serum creatinine or the BUN is seen until the creatinine clearance falls to 50 ml/min. Below that level, small decrements in creatinine clearance can lead to large increases in the BUN and creatinine. A single creatinine clearance value less than 100 ml/min is not diagnostic of renal diseases. An incomplete 24-hour urine collection is the most frequent cause of this finding. An abnormal clearance rate should therefore be restudied.

Effect of Pregnancy on Renal Function

Although baseline creatinine clearance is decreased in patients with chronic renal insufficiency, it should still rise during gestation.

The long-term effect of pregnancy on renal disease remains controversial. If the patient's serum creatinine is less than 1.5 mg/dl, pregnancy should have little effect on the long-term prognosis of the patient's kidney disease. Ideally, patients with chronic renal disease should be thoroughly counseled about the possible consequences of pregnancy before conception.

Severe hypertension is the greatest threat to the pregnant patient with chronic renal disease. Approximately 50 percent of these patients will have worsening hypertension as pregnancy progresses, and diastolic blood pressures of 110 mm Hg or greater will develop in about 20 percent of cases.[67] Blood pressure control is the cornerstone of successful treatment of chronic renal disease in pregnancy.

Worsening proteinuria is common during pregnancy complicated by chronic renal disease and often reaches the nephrotic range.[67] In general, massive proteinuria does not indicate an increased risk for mother or fetus.[68] Low serum albumin, however, has been correlated with low birth weight.[69] In late pregnancy it is often difficult to differentiate impending preeclampsia from worsening chronic renal disease.

Effect of Chronic Renal Disease on Pregnancy

More than 85 percent of women with chronic renal disease will have a surviving infant if renal function is well preserved. Antepartum fetal surveillance and advances in neonatal care have made great strides in improving perinatal outcome in these patients. Preterm births and IUGR remain important problems in these pregnancies are frequently observed in patients whose baseline creatinine level exceeds 1.5 mg/dl.

MANAGEMENT OF CHRONIC RENAL DISEASE IN PREGNANCY

A 24-hour urine collection for creatinine clearance and total protein excretion should be obtained as soon as the pregnancy is confirmed. These parameters should be monitored monthly. The patient should be seen once every 2 weeks until 32 weeks' gestation and weekly thereafter. These are general guidelines, and more frequent visits may be necessary in individual cases.

Control of hypertension is critical in managing patients with chronic renal disease. β-Blockers, calcium channel blockers, and hydralazine can be used to treat blood pressure effectively as long as the dosages are monitored carefully. Clonidine is occasionally useful in refractory patients. Doxazosin and prazosin may be used if necessary. Angiotensin-converting enzyme (ACE) inhibitors should be avoided during pregnancy. These drugs have been associated with fetal and neonatal oliguria/anuria.[85,86]

The use of diuretics in pregnancy is controversial.[87,88] For massive debilitating edema, a short course of diuretics can be helpful. Electrolytes must be monitored carefully. Salt restriction does not appear to be beneficial once edema has developed. Salt restriction, however, should be instituted without hesitation in pregnant women with true renal insufficiency.

Fetal growth should be assessed with serial ultrasonography, because growth restriction is common in women with chronic renal disease. Antepartum fetal heart rate testing should be started at 28 weeks' gestation.[89]

Obstetricians should have a low threshold for hospitalizing patients with chronic renal disease. Increasing hypertension and decreasing renal function warrant immediate hospitalization. A sudden deterioration of renal function may be due to infection, dehydration, electrolyte imbalance, or obstruction.

The timing of delivery must be individualized. Maternal indications for delivery include uncontrollable hypertension, the development of superimposed preeclampsia, and decreasing renal function after fetal viability has been reached. Fetal indications are dictated by the assessment of fetal growth and fetal well-being.

Renal biopsy is rarely indicated during pregnancy.

RENAL TRANSPLANTATION

Pregnancy following renal transplantation has become increasingly common. Many previously anovulatory patients begin ovulating postoperatively and regain fertility as renal function normalizes.[94] Many transplant recipients have failed to realize they are pregnant until well into the second trimester.

Upon learning they are pregnant, many women stop taking all medications. The importance of continuing immunosuppressive therapy cannot be emphasized strongly enough to renal allograft recipients. Glucocorticoids, especially prednisone, are metabolized in the placenta by 11 β-ol-dehydrogenase, with only limited amounts reaching the fetus.

Azathioprine cannot be activated in the fetus because of its lack of inosinate pyrophosphorylase.[96] These risks are outweighed, however, by the disastrous consequences of allograft rejection that may occur if the patient stops her medication.

Cyclosporin A appears to be relatively safe for use during gestation, but does hold some risks. Patients may develop arterial hypertension secondary to its interference with the normal hemodynamic adaptation to pregnancy.[100] Cyclosporin A crosses the placenta, but there is no evidence of teratogenesis.[101,102] The medication should be continued throughout gestation.

During pregnancy, renal allograft recipients must be carefully watched for signs of rejection. Significant episodes of rejection may occur in as many as 9 percent of transplant recipients during gestation, a figure no greater than that expected in the nonpregnant population. Unfortunately, the clinical hallmarks of rejection—fever, oliguria, tenderness, and decreasing renal function—are not always exhibited by the pregnant patient. Occasionally, rejection may mimic pyelonephritis or preeclampsia, which occurs in approximately one third of renal transplant patients. In these cases, renal biopsy is indicated to distinguish rejection from preeclampsia. Rejection has been known to occur during the puerperium, when maternal immune competence returns to its prepregnancy level.[105] Therefore, it may be advisable to increase the dose of immunosuppressive medications in the immediate postpartum period.

Infection can be disastrous for the renal allograft. Therefore, urine cultures should be obtained at least monthly during pregnancy, and any bacteriuria should be aggressively treated. Renal function, as determined by 24-hour creatinine clearance and protein excretion, should be assessed monthly. Approximately 15 percent of transplant recipients will exhibit a significant decrease in renal function in late pregnancy.[106]

As is recommended for patients with chronic renal disease, serial ultrasonography should be used to assess fetal growth, and antepartum fetal heart rate testing should be started at 28 weeks' gestation. Approximately 50 percent of renal allograft recipients will deliver preterm. Preterm labor, preterm rupture of membranes, and IUGR are common. Vaginal delivery should be accomplished when possible, with cesarean delivery reserved for obstetric indications. Allograft recipients may have an increased frequency of cephalopelvic disproportion from pelvic osteodystrophy,[107] resulting from prolonged renal disease with hypercalcemia or extended steroid use. The transplanted kidney, however, rarely obstructs vaginal delivery despite its pelvic location.

Suggested guidelines are summarized in the box "Guidelines for Renal Allograft Recipients Who Wish to Conceive."

Guidelines for Renal Allograft Recipients Who Wish to Conceive

Absolute Criteria
- Wait 2 years after cadaver transplant or 1 year after graft from living donor
- Immunosuppression should be at maintenance levels

Relative Criteria
- Plasma creatinine <1.5 mg/dl
- Absent or easily controlled hypertension
- No or minimal proteinuria
- No evidence of active graft rejection
- No pelvicalyceal distention on a recent ultrasound or intravenous pyelogram
- Prednisone dose 15 mg/day
- Azathioprine dose 2 mg/kg/day
- Cyclosporin A dose 2–4 mg/kg (available data on the use of this drug in pregnancy includes <150 patients)

Adapted from Lindheimer M, Katz A: Pregnancy in the renal transplant patient. Am J Kidney Dis 19:173, 2000.

Key Points

➤ Asymptomatic bacteriuria complicates 10 percent of pregnancies, and if left untreated will result in symptomatic urinary tract infections in 40 percent of patients.

➤ Pyelonephritis complicates 1 to 2 percent of pregnancies, making it the most frequent nonobstetric cause of hospitalization during pregnancy.

➤ Patients with glomerulonephritis can have successful pregnancies, but pregnancy loss rates increase greatly if the patient has preexisting hypertension.

➤ Creatinine clearance can decline 70 percent before significant increases are seen in the BUN or serum creatinine level. Therefore, a 24-hour urine specimen for creatinine clearance should be collected in any patient when renal disease is suspected.

➤ The chance of successful pregnancy is reduced if the creatinine clearance is less than 50 ml/min or if the serum creatinine level is more than 1.5 mg/dl.

➤ Severe hypertension is the greatest threat to the pregnant woman with chronic renal disease.

➤ Growth restriction and preeclampsia are common in women with chronic renal disease. These patients should have frequent sonograms and should start antepartum fetal surveillance at 28 weeks' gestation.

➤ Patients with chronic renal disease are often anovulatory. After transplantation, as renal function returns, they ovulate and may become pregnant unexpectedly.

➤ Patients should wait 2 years after receiving a cadaver renal allograft and 1 year after receiving a living allograft before contemplating pregnancy. Furthermore, there should be no signs of allograft rejection.

➤ Renal transplant patients should remain on their immunosuppressive medications throughout gestation.

Diabetes Mellitus

MARK B. LANDON, PATRICK M. CATALANO,
AND STEVEN G. GABBE

Management techniques have been developed over the past 30 years to prevent complications based on an understanding of the pathophysiology of the diabetic pregnancy. These advances have resulted in perinatal mortality rates in optimally managed cases that approach that of the normal population. Excluding major congenital malformations, which continue to plague pregnancies in the insulin-dependent woman, perinatal loss for the diabetic woman has fortunately become an uncommon event.

Glucose Metabolism

Normal pregnancy has been characterized as a "diabetogenic state" because of the progressive increase in postprandial glucose levels and insulin response in late gestation. These changes result from increasing levels of human placental lactogen, cortisol, progesterone, and prolactin. Early gestation can be viewed as an anabolic condition with an increase in maternal fat stores and a decrease in free fatty acid concentrations. Significant decreases in maternal insulin requirements are observed early in gestation in insulin-dependent women with optimal glucose control prior to conception. There are progressive increases in insulin secretion in response to an intravenous glucose challenge with advancing gestation. Although there is a progressive decrease in fasting glucose with advancing gestation, the decrease is most probably a result of the increase in plasma volume in early gestation and increase in fetoplacental glucose utilization in late gestation.

Placental glucose transport is a non–energy-requiring process and takes place through facilitated diffusion. Glucose transport is dependent on a family of glucose transporters referred to as the GLUT glucose transporter family. The principal glucose transporter in the placenta is GLUT 1, which is found in the syncytiotrophoblast.[23]

DIABETES MELLITUS

Diabetes mellitus is a chronic metabolic disorder characterized by either absolute or relative insulin deficiency, resulting in increased glucose concentrations. Although glucose intolerance is the common outcome of diabetes mellitus, the pathophysiology remains heterogeneous. The two major classifications of diabetes mellitus are type 1, formerly referred to as insulin-dependent diabetes or juvenile onset diabetes, and type 2, formerly referred to as non–insulin-dependent or adult-onset diabetes. During pregnancy, classification of women with diabetes has often relied on the White classification,[27] first proposed in the 1940s. This classification is based on factors such as the age of onset of diabetes and duration as well as end-organ involvement, primarily retinal and renal (see Table 24–7).

Type 2 Diabetes/Gestational Diabetes

The pathophysiology of type 2 diabetes involves abnormalities of both insulin-sensitive tissues (i.e., a decrease in skeletal muscle and hepatic sensitivity to insulin) and β-cell response as manifested by an inadequate insulin response for a given degree of glycemia. Initially in the course of development of type 2 diabetes, the insulin response to a glucose challenge may be increased relative to that of individuals with normal glucose tolerance but is inadequate to maintain normoglycemia. In women with gestational diabetes, the hormonal events of pregnancy may represent an unmasking of a genetic susceptibility to type 2 diabetes.

Type 1 Diabetes

Type 1 diabetes is usually characterized by an abrupt onset at a young age and absolute insulinopenia with lifelong requirements for insulin replacement. In some populations, the onset of type 1 diabetes may occur in individuals in the third or fourth decades of life. Patients with diabetes mellitus may have a genetic predisposition for antibodies directed against their pancreatic islet cells. Because of the complete dependence on exogenous insulin, pregnant women with type 1 diabetes are at increased risk for the development of diabetic ketoacidosis. Additionally, because intensive insulin therapy is used in women with type 1 to decrease the risk for spontaneous abortion and congenital anomalies in early gestation, these women are at greater risk of hypoglycemic reactions. Women with type 1 diabetes are at increased risk for hypoglycemic reactions during pregnancy because of diminished counterregulatory epinephrine and glucagon response to hypoglycemia. The deficiency in counterregulatory response may be in part due to an independent effect of pregnancy.

Because of maternal insulinopenia, insulin response during gestation can only be estimated relative to pregravid requirements. Insulin requirements in women with type 1 diabetes and strict glucose control either prior to conception or before 10 weeks' gestation fall 12 percent from 10 to 17 weeks' gestation and increase 50 percent from 17 weeks' until delivery as compared with pregravid requirements. After 36 weeks' gestation there is a small decrease in insulin requirements.

PERINATAL MORBIDITY AND MORTALITY

Fetal Death

In the past, sudden and unexplained stillbirth occurred in 10 to 30 percent of pregnancies complicated by type 1 (insulin-dependant) diabetes mellitus.[77,78] Although relatively uncommon today, such losses still plague the pregnancies of patients who do not receive optimal care. Stillbirths have been observed most often after the 36th week of pregnancy in patients with vascular disease, poor glycemic control, hydramnios, fetal macrosomia, or preeclampsia. Women with vascular complications may develop fetal growth restriction and intrauterine demise as early as the second trimester. In the past, prevention of intrauterine death led to a strategy of scheduled preterm deliveries for type 1 diabetic women. This empiric approach reduced the number of stillbirths, but errors in estimation of fetal size and gestational age as well as the functional immaturity characteristic of the infant of the diabetic mother (IDM) contributed to many neonatal deaths from hyaline membrane disease (HMD).

Congenital Malformations

With the reduction in intrauterine deaths and a marked decrease in neonatal mortality related to HMD and traumatic delivery, congenital malformations have emerged as the most important cause of perinatal loss in pregnancies complicated by type 1 and type 2 diabetes mellitus. In the past, these anomalies were responsible for approximately 10 percent of all perinatal deaths. At present, however, malformations account for 30 to 50 percent of perinatal mortality.[78] Neonatal deaths now exceed stillbirths in pregnancies complicated by pregestational diabetes mellitus, and fatal congenital malformations account for this changing pattern.

Most studies have documented a two- to sixfold increase in major malformations in infants of type 1 and type 2 diabetic mothers. In general, the incidence of major malformations in worldwide studies of offspring of diabetic mothers has ranged from 5 to 10 percent.

The insult that causes malformations in IDM impacts on most organ systems and must act before the seventh week of gestation.[82] Central nervous system malformations, particularly anencephaly, open spina bifida and, possibly, holoprosencephaly, are increased 10-fold.[90] Cardiac anomalies, especially ventricular septal defects and complex lesions such as transposition of the great vessels, are increased fivefold. The congenital defect thought to be most characteristic of diabetic embryopathy is sacral agenesis or caudal dysplasia, an anomaly found 200 to 400 times more often in offspring of diabetic women (Fig. 24–2).

Impaired glycemic control and associated derangements in maternal metabolism appear to contribute to abnormal embryogenesis. The profile of a woman most likely to produce an anomalous infant would include a patient with poor periconceptional control, long-standing diabetes, and vascular disease.[90]

Fetal Macrosomia

Macrosomia has been variously defined as birth weight greater than 4,000 to 4,500 g as well as large for gestational age where birth weight is above the 90th percentile for population and sex-specific growth curves. Fetal macrosomia complicates as many as 50 percent of pregnancies in women with gestational diabetes and 40 percent of pregnancies complicated by type 1 diabetes, including some women treated with intensive glycemic control (Fig. 24–3). Delivery of an infant weighing greater than 4,500 g occurs 10 times more often in women with diabetes as compared with a population of women with normal glucose tolerance.[98]

According to the Pedersen hypothesis, maternal hyperglycemia results in fetal hyperglycemia and hyperinsulinemia, resulting in excessive fetal growth. Infants of mothers with gestational diabetes have an increase in fat mass as compared with fat-free mass.[102] This growth is disproportionate, with chest/head and shoulder/head ratios larger than those of infants of women with normal glucose tolerance. This factor may contribute to the higher rate of shoulder dystocia and birth trauma observed in these infants.[103] Excellent maternal glycemic control has been associated with a decline in the incidence of macrosomia.

In addition to an increased risk of birth trauma, fetal macrosomia in infants of women with abnormal glucose tolerance may be associated with significant long-term risks.[114] These children are at greater risk for obesity at ages 1 to 9 and in adolescence.

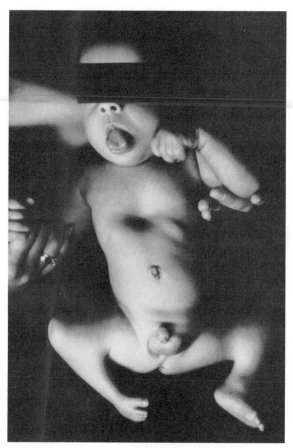

Figure 24–2. Infant of a diabetic mother with sacral agenesis. The mother of this infant presented with Class F diabetes at 26 weeks, in poor glycemic control. Ultrasound examination revealed absent lower lumbar spine and absent sacrum with hypoplastic lower extremities.

Hypoglycemia

Neonatal hypoglycemia, a blood glucose below 35 to 40 mg/dl during the first 12 hours of life, results from a rapid fall in plasma glucose concentrations following clamping of the umbilical cord. Presumably, prior poor maternal glucose control can result in fetal β-cell hyperplasia, leading to exaggerated insulin release following delivery. Hypoglycemia is particularly common in macrosomic new-

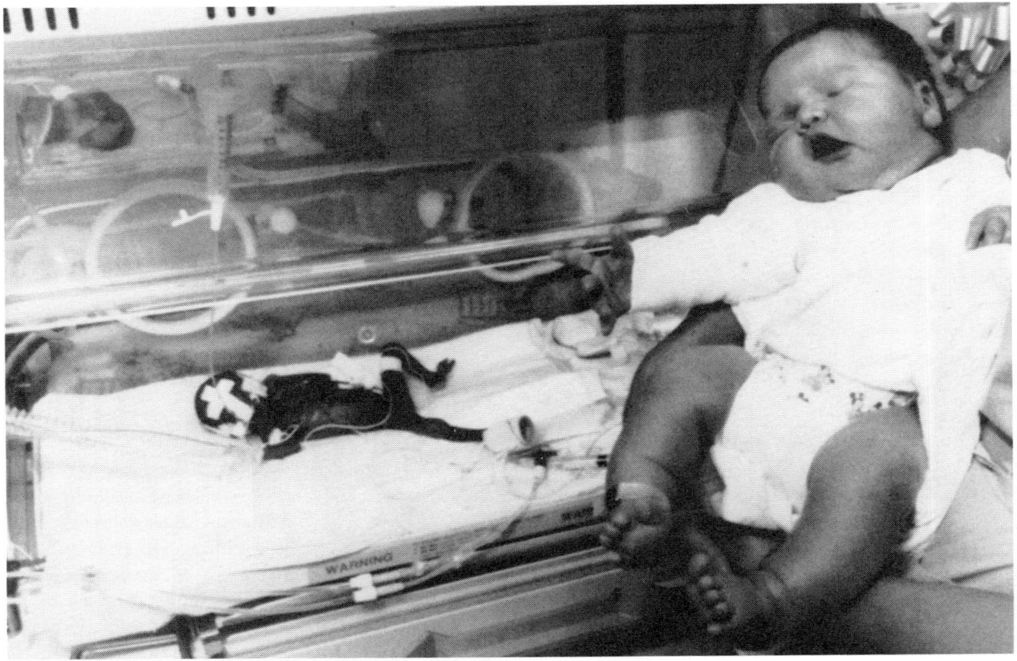

Figure 24–3. *See legend on opposite page*

borns, with rates exceeding 50 percent. With near physiologic control of maternal glucose levels during pregnancy, overall rates of 5 to 15 percent have been reported.[106,107] The degree of hypoglycemia may be influenced by at least two factors: (1) maternal glucose control during the latter half of pregnancy, and (2) maternal glucose control during labor and delivery. Maternal blood glucose levels greater than 90 mg/dl during delivery have been found to increase significantly the frequency of neonatal hypoglycemia.[116]

Respiratory Distress Syndrome

Hyperglycemia and hyperinsulinemia have been associated with delayed pulmonary maturation in the IDM. However, in well-controlled diabetic women delivered at term, the risk of RDS is no higher than that observed in the general population.[123,124]

Hyperbilirubinemia and Polycythemia

Hyperbilirubinemia is frequently observed in the IDM. Neonatal jaundice has been reported in as many as 53 percent of pregnancies complicated by diabetes and 38 percent of pregnancies with GDM.[128,129]

MATERNAL CLASSIFICATION AND RISK ASSESSMENT

Priscilla White[132] first noted that the patient's age at onset of diabetes, the duration of the disease, and the presence of vasculopathy significantly influenced perinatal outcome. Her pioneering work led to a classification system that has been widely applied to pregnant women with diabetes.[132] A modification of this scheme is presented in Table 24–7. Counseling a patient and formulating a plan of management requires assessment of both maternal and fetal risk. The White classification facilitates this evaluation.

Class A_1 diabetes mellitus includes those patients who have demonstrated carbohydrate intolerance during a 100-g 3-hour oral glucose

Figure 24–3. Two extremes of growth abnormalities in infants of diabetic mothers. The small growth-restricted infant on the left weighed 470 g and is the offspring of a woman with nephropathy and hypertension, delivered at 28 weeks' gestation. The neonate on the right is the 5,100- g baby of a woman with suboptimally controlled Class C diabetes.

Table 24–7. MODIFIED WHITE CLASSIFICATION OF PREGNANT DIABETIC WOMEN

	Diabetes			
	Onset	Duration	Vascular	Insulin
Class	*Age (yr)*	*(yr)*	*Disease*	*Need*
Gestational diabetes				
A1	Any	Any	0	0
A2	Any	Any	0	+
Pregestational diabetes				
B	>20	<10	0	+
C	10–19 or	10–19	0	+
D	<10 or	>20	+	+
F	Any	Any	+	+
R	Any	Any	+	+
T	Any	Any	+	+
H	Any	Any	+	+

Modified from White P: Pregnancy complicating diabetes. Am J Med 7:609, 1949.

tolerance test (OGTT); however, their fasting and 2-hour postprandial glucose levels are less than 95 mg/dl and 120 mg/dl, respectively. These patients are generally managed by dietary regulation alone. If the fasting value of the OGTT is elevated (>95 mg/dl) and/or 2-hour postprandial glucose levels exceed 120 mg/dl, patients are designated Class A_2. Insulin is most often required for these women.

International Workshop-Conferences on Gestational Diabetes sponsored by the American Diabetes Association in cooperation with the American College of Obstetricians and Gynecologists (ACOG) recommended that the term gestational diabetes rather than Class A diabetes be used to describe women with carbohydrate intolerance of variable severity with onset or recognition during the present pregnancy.[133,134] The term gestational diabetes fails to specify whether the patient requires dietary adjustment alone or treatment with diet and insulin. This distinction is important because those patients who are normoglycemic while fasting appear to have a significantly lower perinatal mortality rate.[135] Women with gestational diabetes who require insulin are at greater risk for a poor perinatal outcome than those controlled by diet alone.

Patients requiring insulin are designated by the letters B, C, D, R, F, and T. (Table 24–7).

In summary, risk assessment may be simplified by evaluating the patient's blood glucose and blood vessels. Patients with excellent glucose control and no blood vessel disease should do well. Those in poor control and with vasculopathy are at increased risk for fetal death, IUGR, preeclampsia, and preterm delivery.

Nephropathy

Class F describes the 5 to 10 percent of pregnant patients with underlying renal disease. This includes those with reduced creatinine clearance and/or proteinuria of at least 400 mg in 24 hours measured during the first 20 weeks of gestation. Two factors present prior to 20 weeks' gestation appear to be predictive of perinatal outcome in these women (e.g., preterm delivery, low birth weight, or preeclampsia): proteinuria greater than 3.0 g/24 h and serum creatinine greater than 1.5 mg/dl.

The management of the diabetic woman with nephropathy requires great expertise. Although controversial, some nephrologists recommend a modified reduction in protein intake for pregnant women with nephropathy. Control of hypertension in pregnant women with diabetic nephropathy is crucial to prevent further deterioration of kidney function and to optimize pregnancy outcome. Although debatable, some cautiously use diuretics when patients are extremely nephrotic, as this group may be prone to volume-dependent forms of hypertension. Angiotension-converting enzyme (ACE) inhibitors, which reduce intraglomerular pressure and improve proteinuria in nonpregnant diabetic patients, should be avoided during pregnancy, as these agents can affect fetal urine production resulting in oligohydramnios.

Several studies have failed to demonstrate a permanent worsening of diabetic renal disease as a result of pregnancy.[137–139] With improved survival of diabetic patients following renal transplantation, a small group of kidney recipients has now achieved pregnancy (Class T).

Retinopathy

Class R diabetes designates patients with proliferative retinopathy. Pregnancy does convey a greater than twofold independent risk for progression of existing retinopathy.[144] Progression to proliferative retinopathy during pregnancy rarely occurs in women with background retinopathy or those without any eye ground changes.[147] In contrast, most patients with untreated proliferative disease experienced worsening retinopathy during pregnancy. Ideally, women planning a pregnancy should have a comprehensive eye examination and treatment prior to conception. For those discovered to have proliferative changes during pregnancy, laser photocoagulation therapy with careful follow-up has helped maintain many pregnancies to a gestational age at which neonatal survival is likely.

Coronary Artery Disease

Class H diabetes refers to the presence of diabetes of any duration associated with ischemic myocardial disease. There is evidence that the small number of women who have coronary artery disease are at an increased risk for mortality during gestation.

DETECTION OF DIABETES IN PREGNANCY

It has been estimated that 4 to 5 percent of pregnancies are complicated by diabetes mellitus and that 90 percent of the cases represent women with GDM.[154] An increased prevalence of GDM is found in women of Hispanic, African, Native American, South or East Asian, and Pacific Island ancestry.[155] Women with GDM represent a group with significant risk for developing glucose intolerance later in life. Approximately, 50 percent of these patients will become diabetic in the 15 years following a pregnancy complicated by GDM.

GDM is a state restricted to pregnant women whose impaired glucose tolerance is discovered during pregnancy. Because, in most cases, patients with GDM have normal fasting glucose levels, some challenge of glucose tolerance must be undertaken.

Following the Fourth International Workshop-Conference in 1997, universal screening was recommended for women in ethnic groups with relatively high rates of carbohydrate intolerance during pregnancy and diabetes later in life.[159] If was recognized that certain features place women at low risk for GDM (see the box "Screening Strategy for Detection of GDM"), and it may not be cost-effective to screen this subgroup of women. Those at low risk include women who are not members of ethnic groups at increased risk for developing type 2 diabetes, those who have no previous history of abnormal glucose tolerance or poor obstetric outcomes usually associated with GDM, and those who have all of the following characteristics: age less than 25 years, normal body weight, and no family history of diabetes. Similarly, the ACOG first suggested that whereas selective screening for GDM may be appropriate in some clinical settings such as teen clinics (low-risk populations), universal screening may be more appropriate in other settings (high-risk populations).[160]

The screening test for GDM, a 50-g oral glucose challenge, may be performed in the fasting or fed state.[166,167] A plasma value of 140 mg/dl is commonly used as a threshold for performing a 3-hour OGTT.

Whereas most women can be screened for GDM at approximately 24 to 28 weeks' gestation, it is advisable to screen earlier in pregnancy those with strong risk factors such as morbid obesity, family history in first-degree relatives, or previous GDM.[168] If initial screening is negative, repeat testing is performed at 24 to 28 weeks. Utiliz-

Screening Strategy for Detection of GDM

Risk assessment for GDM should be ascertained at the first prenatal visit.

Low risk

    Blood glucose testing is not routinely required if all of the following characteristics are present:

        Member of an ethnic group with a low prevalence of GDM

        No known diabetes in first-degree relatives

        Age <25 years

        Weight normal before pregnancy

        No history of abnormal glucose metabolism

        No history of poor obstetric outcome

Average risk

    Perform blood glucose screening at 24 to 28 weeks using one of the following:

        Two-step procedure: 50-g GCT followed by a diagnostic OGTT in those meeting the threshold value in the GCT

        One-step procedure: diagnostic OGTT performed on all subjects

High risk

    Perform blood glucose testing as soon as feasible, using the procedures described above.

    If GDM is not diagnosed, blood glucose testing should be repeated at 24 to 28 weeks or at any time a patient has symptoms or signs suggestive of hyperglycemia.

Adapted from Fourth International Workshop-Conference on Gestational Diabetes Mellitus. Diabetes Care 21(Suppl 2): B161, 1998.

ing the plasma cut-off of 140 mg/dl, one can expect approximately 15 percent of patients with an abnormal screening value to have an abnormal 3-hour OGTT. Patients whose 1-hour screening value exceeds 190 mg/dl (10.5 mmol/L) rarely exhibit a normal OGTT.[169] In these women, it is preferable to check a fasting blood glucose level before administering a 100-g carbohydrate load. If the fasting glucose is 95 mg/dl or greater, the patient is treated for GDM.

The criteria for establishing the diagnosis of gestational diabetes are listed in Table 24–8. The U.S. National Diabetes Data Group (NDDG) criteria represent a calculated conversion of O'Sullivan's thresholds in whole blood. Carpenter and Coustan prefer to use another modification of these data that is supported by a comparison of the older Somogyi-Nelson method and current plasma glucose oxi-

Table 24–8. DETECTION OF GESTATIONAL DIABETES—UPPER LIMITS OF NORMAL

Screening Test (50-g) 1-Hour	Plasma (mg/dl) 140	
Oral GTT*	NDDG	Carpenter and Coustan[169]
Fasting	105	95
1-hour	190	180
2-hour	165	155
3-hour	145	140

*Diagnosis of gestational diabetes is made when any two values are met or exceeded.
NDDG, National Diabetes Data Group.
From the National Institutes of Health Diabetes Data Group: Classification and diagnosis of diabetes mellitus and other categories of glucose intolerance. Diabetes 28:1039, 1979.

dase assays.[170] These criteria have been recommended by the Fourth International Workshop-Conference on GDM. Several studies have confirmed that patients diagnosed using the less stringent Carpenter criteria experience as much perinatal morbidity as subjects diagnosed by the NDDG criteria.[171] Using either criteria, the patient must have a normal fasting value and two abnormal postprandial glucose determinations to be designated as Class A_1.

TREATMENT OF THE INSULIN-DEPENDENT PATIENT

As fetal glucose levels reflect those of the mother, it is not surprising that clinical efforts aimed at optimizing maternal control are considered paramount in the decline in perinatal death seen in pregnancies type 1 diabetics over the last few decades. Self-blood glucose monitoring combined with aggressive insulin therapy has made the maintenance of maternal normoglycemia (levels of 60 to 120 mg/dl) a therapeutic reality (Table 24–9). In most institutions, patients are taught to monitor their glucose control using glucose-oxidase–impregnated reagent strips and a meter.[172]

During pregnancy, intensive, individualized insulin therapy is an essential part of patient care. Insulin regimens have classically included multiple injections of insulin usually prior to breakfast,

Table 24–9. TARGET PLASMA GLUCOSE LEVELS IN PREGNANCY

Time	mg/dl
Before breakfast	60–90
Before lunch, supper, bedtime snack	60–105
Two hours after meals	≤120
2 A.M. to 6 A.M.	>60

the evening meal, and often bedtime, complemented by self-blood glucose monitoring and adjustments of insulin dose according to glucose profiles. Patients are instructed on dietary composition, insulin action, recognition and treatment of hypoglycemia, adjusting insulin dosage for exercise and sick days, as well as monitoring for hyperglycemia and potential ketosis. These principles form the foundation for intensive insulin therapy in which an attempt is made to simulate physiologic insulin requirements. Insulin administration is provided for both basal needs and meals, and rapid adjustments are made in response to glucose measurements. The treatment regimen generally involves three to four daily injections or the use of a continuous subcutaneous insulin infusion (CSII) device, the insulin pump. With either approach, frequent self-blood glucose monitoring is fundamental to achieve the therapeutic objective of physiologic glucose control. Glucose determinations are made in the fasting state and before lunch, dinner, and bedtime. Postprandial and nocturnal values are also helpful. Patients are instructed on an insulin dose for each meal and at bedtime if necessary. Meal-time insulin needs are determined by the composition of the meal, the premeal glucose measurement, and the level of activity anticipated following the meal. Basal or intermediate-acting insulin requirements are determined by periodic 2 A.M. to 4 A.M. glucose measurements as well as late afternoon values, which reflect morning neutral protamine Hagedorn (NPH) or Lente action. During pregnancy, diabetic women should develop the self-management skills that are essential to an intensive insulin therapy regimen. In patients who are not well controlled, a brief period of hospitalization is often necessary for the initiation of therapy.

Glycosylated hemoglobin measurements in each trimester can be used to assess glucose control in the previous 12 to 16 weeks. A hemoglobin A_{1c} level of 5 to 6 percent is desirable. The mean glucose represented by the hemoglobin A_{1c} level can be calculated using the "rule of 8's." A value of 8 percent equals 180 mg/dl, and each 1 percent increase or decrease represents ±30 mg/dl.

Insulin therapy must be individualized with dosage determinations tailored to diet and exercise. Beef and pork insulin have largely been replaced by semisynthetic human insulin preparations. Most recently, insulin lispro has been introduced. A rapid-acting insulin preparation, this insulin, which features reversal of proline and lysine at positions B28 and B29, remains in monomeric form, and is rapidly absorbed. Its action begins in 15 minutes and peaks in 2 to 3 hours. Because its duration of action is shorter than that of regular insulin, unexpected hypoglycemia hours after an injection is avoided. Insulin lispro is not yet approved for use in pregnancy, but it is a category B drug. While an early report raised some question regarding a possible association between insulin lispro and progression of retinopathy in pregnancy, recent experience suggests this is not the case.[173,174]

Insulin is generally administered in two to three injections. We prefer a three or four injection regimen, although most patients present taking a combination of intermediate-acting and short-acting insulin before dinner and breakfast. As a general rule, the amount of intermediate-acting insulin will exceed the short-acting component by a 2:1 ratio. Patients usually receive two thirds their total dose with breakfast and the remaining third in the evening as a combined dose with dinner or split into components with short acting insulin at dinner time and intermediate-acting insulin at bedtime in an effort to minimize periods of nocturnal hypoglycemia. These episodes frequently occur when the mother is in a relative fasting state while placental and fetal glucose consumption continue. Finally, some women may require a small dose of short-acting insulin before lunch, thus constituting a four-injection regimen.

There has now been considerable experience with open-loop CSII pump therapy during pregnancy. The pump is a battery-powered unit, which may be worn, like a pager, during most daily activities. These systems provide continuous short-acting insulin via a subcutaneous infusion. The basal infusion rate and bolus doses to cover meals are determined by frequent self-monitoring of blood glucose. The basal infusion rate is generally close to 1 unit/h.

Episodes of severe hypoglycemia are generally reduced with pump therapy.[176] When they occur, these events are usually secondary to errors in dose selection or failure to adhere to the required diet. The risk of nocturnal hypoglycemia, which is increased in the pregnant state, is reduced by lowering the basal rate from late evening until early morning. The basal rate can be programed to increase in the early morning hours to counteract the "dawn phenomenon."

Short-acting insulin is stored in the pump syringe. Infusion occurs at a basal rate, which can be fixed or altered for a specific time of day and duration. As noted above, the basal rate can be programmed for a lower rate at night. The size of preprandial boluses is based on the composition of each meal or snack. Approximately 60 percent of the total daily insulin dose is usually given as the basal rate and the remainder as premeal boluses infused. The largest bolus (30 to 35 percent) is administered with breakfast, followed by 25 percent before lunch and dinner and 15 to 20 percent before snacks.

Patients without any pancreatic reserve may have rapid elevations of blood glucose if there is pump failure or intercurrent infection. For this reason, many clinicians recommend that patients using a pump check their glucose level at 2 to 3 A.M. to detect hyperglycemia resulting from pump failure.

Diet therapy is critical to successful regulation of maternal diabetes. A program consisting of three meals and several snacks is used for most patients. Dietary composition should be 50 to 60 percent carbohydrate, 20 percent protein, and 25 to 30 percent fat with less than 10 percent saturated fats, up to 10 percent polyunsaturated fatty acids, and the remainder derived from monosaturated sources.[177] Caloric intake is established based on prepregnancy weight and weight gain during gestation. Weight reduction is not advised. Patients should consume approximately 35 kcal/kg ideal body weight. Obese women may be managed with an intake as low as 1,600 cal/ day, although if ketonuria develops, this allowance may be increased.

The presence of maternal vasculopathy should be thoroughly assessed early in pregnancy. The patient should be evaluated by an ophthalmologist familiar with diabetic retinopathy. Ophthalmologic examinations are performed during each trimester and repeated more often if retinopathy is detected. Baseline renal function is established by assaying a 24-hour urine collection for creatinine clearance and protein. An electrocardiogram, thyroid function studies, and a urine culture are also obtained.

Most patients are followed with outpatient visits at 1- to 2-week intervals. At each visit, control is assessed and adjustments in insulin dosage and diet are made. However, patients should be instructed to call at any time if periods of hypoglycemia (<50 mg/dl) or hyperglycemia (>200 mg/dl) occur. Family members should be instructed on how and when to administer a glucagon injection for the treatment of severe reactions.

KETOACIDOSIS

Diabetic ketoacidosis may develop in a pregnant woman with glucose levels barely exceeding 200 mg/dl (11.1 mmol/L). Thus, DKA may be diagnosed during pregnancy with minimal hyperglycemia accompanied by a fall in plasma bicarbonate and a pH value less than 7.30. Serum acetone is positive at a 1:2 dilution.

Management of DKA during Pregnancy

1. Laboratory assessment:
   Obtain arterial blood gases to document degree of acidosis present; measure glucose, ketones, electrolytes, at 1- to 2-hour intervals.

2. Insulin:
   Low-dose, intravenous (IV)
      Loading dose: 0.2–0.4 units/kg
      Maintenance: 2.0–10.0 units/h

3. Fluids:
   Isotonic NaCl
      Total replacement in first 12 h = 4–6 L
      L in first hour
      500–1,000 ml/h for 2–4 h
      250 ml/h until 80% replaced

4. Glucose:
   Begin 5% D/NS* when plasma level reaches 250 mg/dl (14 mmol/L)

5. Potassium:
   If initially normal or reduced, an infusion rate up to 15 to 20 mEq/h may be required; if elevated, wait until levels decline into the normal range, then add to IV solution in a concentration of 20–30 mEq/L

6. Bicarbonate:
   Add one ampule (44 mEq) to 1 L of 0.45 NS if pH is <7.10

---

*D/NS, dextrose in normal saline.

Early recognition of signs and symptoms of DKA will improve both maternal and fetal outcome. As in the nonpregnant state, clinical signs of volume depletion follow the symptoms of hyperglycemia, which include polydipsia and polyuria. Malaise, headache, nausea, and vomiting are common complaints. Diabetic ketoacidosis may present in an undiagnosed diabetic woman receiving β-mimetic agents to arrest preterm labor. Because of the risk of hyperglycemia and diabetic ketoacidosis in diabetic women receiving intravenous medications such as a terbutaline, magnesium sulfate has become the preferred tocolytic for cases of preterm labor in these cases. Administration of antenatal corticosteroids to accelerate fetal lung maturation can cause significant maternal hyperglycemia and precipitate DKA. These patients must be closely followed in an acute care setting for at least 48 to 72 hours after corticosteroids have been given.

An intravenous insulin infusion will usually be required and is adjusted on the basis of frequent capillary glucose measurements.

Treatment of any underlying cause for ketoacidosis, such as infection, should be instituted as well (see the box "Management of DKA during Pregnancy"). Diabetic ketoacidosis does represent a substantial risk for fetal compromise. Successful fetal resuscitation will often accompany correction of maternal acidosis. Every effort should therefore be made to correct maternal condition before intervening and delivering a preterm infant.

ANTEPARTUM FETAL EVALUATION

During the third trimester time period, when the risk of sudden intrauterine death increases, a program of fetal surveillance is initiated. Antepartum fetal monitoring tests are now used primarily to reassure the obstetrician and avoid unnecessary premature intervention. These techniques have few false-negative results, and in a patient who is well controlled and exhibits no vasculopathy or significant hypertension, reassuring antepartum testing allows the fetus to benefit from further maturation in utero.

Maternal assessment of fetal activity serves as a screening technique in a program of fetal surveillance. While the false-negative rate with maternal monitoring of fetal activity is low (~1 percent), the false-positive rate may be as high as 60 percent.

The nonstress test (NST) remains the preferred method to assess antepartum fetal well-being in the patient with diabetes mellitus.[182] If the NST is nonreactive, a biophysical profile (BPP) or contraction stress test is then performed (Fig. 24–4). Heart rate monitoring is begun early in the third trimester, usually by 32 weeks' gestation. If the NST is to be used as the primary method of antepartum heart rate testing, we prefer that it be done at least twice weekly once the patient reaches 32 weeks' gestation. In patients with vascular disease or poor control, in whom the incidence of abnormal tests and intrauterine deaths is greater, testing is often performed earlier and more frequently. The BPP or CST is often employed to evaluate the significance of a nonreactive NST result.

It is important to include not only the results of antepartum fetal testing but to weigh all the clinical features involving mother and fetus before a decision is made to intervene for suspected fetal distress, especially if this decision may result in a preterm delivery (Tables 24–10 and 24–11).

Ultrasound is a valuable tool in evaluating fetal growth, estimating fetal weight, and detecting hydramnios and malformations. A determination of maternal serum α-fetoprotein (MSAFP) at

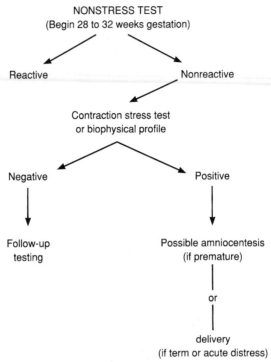

NONSTRESS TEST
(Begin 28 to 32 weeks gestation)

Reactive   Nonreactive

Contraction stress test
or biophysical profile

Negative   Positive

Follow-up
testing

Possible amniocentesis
(if premature)

or

delivery
(if term or acute distress)

Figure 24–4. Scheme for antepartum fetal testing in pregnancy complicated by diabetes mellitus.

approximately 16 weeks' gestation is often used in association with a detailed ultrasound study in an attempt to detect neural tube defects and other anomalies. A comprehensive ultrasound with fetal echocardiography is performed at approximately 20 weeks' gestation for the investigation of possible cardiac anomalies. Detailed cardiac imaging should be offered to all women with pregestational diabetes mellitus to assist in the detection of cardiac lesions, especially those of the great vessels and cardiac septum.

Ultrasound examinations may be repeated later in the third trimester to assess fetal growth. The detection of fetal macrosomia, the leading risk factor for shoulder dystocia, is important in the selection of patients who are best delivered by cesarean section. An increased rate of cephalopelvic disproportion and shoulder dystocia accompanied by significant risk of traumatic birth injury and asphyxia have been consistently associated with the vaginal delivery of large infants.

Table 24–10. ANTEPARTUM FETAL SURVEILLANCE IN LOW-RISK INSULIN-DEPENDENT DIABETES MELLITUS*

	Study
Ultrasonography at 4 to 6-week intervals	Yes
Maternal assessment of fetal activity, daily at 28 weeks	Yes
Nonstress test (NST) weekly at 28 weeks	Yes
	Twice weekly at 34 weeks
Contraction stress test or biophysical profile if NST nonreactive L/S, lung profile	Yes, if elective delivery planned prior to 39 weeks

*Low-risk pregestational diabetes mellitus: excellent control (60–120 mg/dl), no vasculopathy (classes B, C), no stillbirth.

TIMING AND MODE OF DELIVERY

Delivery should be delayed until fetal maturation has taken place, provided that the patient's diabetes is well controlled and antepartum surveillance remains normal. In our practice, elective induction of labor is often planned at 38 to 40 weeks' gestation in well-controlled patients without vascular disease. Patients with vascular disease are delivered prior to term only if hypertension worsens or fetal growth restriction mandates early delivery. Before elective delivery prior to

Table 24–11. ANTEPARTUM FETAL SURVEILLANCE IN HIGH-RISK PREGESTATIONAL DIABETES MELLITUS*

	Study
Ultrasonography at 4 to 6-week intervals intervals	Yes
Maternal assessment of fetal activity, daily at 28 weeks	Yes
Nonstress test (NST)	Minimum twice weekly
Contraction stress test or biophysical profile if NST nonreactive L/S, lung profile at 37–38 weeks	Yes

*High-risk pregestational diabetes mellitus: poor control (macrosomia, hydramnios), vasculopathy (classes D, F, R), prior stillbirth.

39 weeks' gestation, an amniocentesis may be performed to document fetal pulmonary maturity. There is much evidence that tests of fetal lung maturity have the same predictive value in diabetic pregnancies as they do in the normal population.[124]

When antepartum testing suggests fetal compromise, delivery must be considered. If amniotic fluid analysis yields a mature test result, delivery should be accomplished promptly. In the presence of presumed lung immaturity, the decision to proceed with delivery should be based on confirmation of deteriorating fetal condition by several abnormal tests. For example, if the NST as well as the BPP indicates fetal compromise, delivery is indicated. Finally, there remain several maternal indications for delivery including preeclampsia, worsening renal function, or deteriorating vision secondary to proliferative retinopathy.

The route of delivery for the diabetic patient remains controversial. Delivery by cesarean section usually is favored when fetal distress has been suggested by antepartum heart rate monitoring. If a patient reaches 38 weeks' gestation with a mature fetal lung profile and is at significant risk for intrauterine demise because of poor control or a history of a prior stillbirth, an elective delivery is planned. Cesarean delivery should be considered if the estimated fetal weight is ≥4,250 g.

During labor, continuous fetal heart rate monitoring is mandatory. Labor is allowed to progress as long as normal rates of cervical dilatation and descent are documented.

GLUCOREGULATION DURING LABOR AND DELIVERY

As neonatal hypoglycemia is in part related to maternal glucose levels during labor, it is important to maintain maternal plasma glucose levels within the physiologic normal range. The patient is given nothing by mouth after midnight of the evening before induction or elective cesarean delivery. The usual bedtime dose of insulin is administered or, for women receiving pump therapy, the infusion is continued overnight. Upon arrival to labor and delivery early in the morning, the patient's capillary glucose level is assessed with a bedside meter. Continuous infusion of both insulin and glucose are then administered based on maternal glucose levels (see the box "Insulin Management during Labor and Delivery"). Ten units of regular insulin may be added to 1,000 ml of solution containing 5 percent dextrose. An infusion rate of 100 to 125 ml/h (1 unit/h) will, in most cases, result in good glucose control. Insulin may also be infused from a syringe pump at a dose of 0.25 to 2.0 units/h, and adjusted to maintain normal

Insulin Management during Labor and Delivery

- Usual dose of intermediate-acting insulin is given at bedtime.
- Morning dose of insulin is withheld.
- Intravenous infusion of normal saline is begun.
- Once active labor begins or glucose levels fall below 70 mg/dl, the infusion is changed from saline to 5% dextrose and delivered at a rate of 2.5 mg/kg/min.
- Glucose levels are checked hourly using a portable meter allowing for adjustment in the infusion rate.
- Regular (short-acting) insulin in administered by intravenous infusion if glucose levels exceed 140 mg/dl.

Adapted from Jovanovic L, Peterson CM: Management of the pregnant, insulin-dependent diabetic woman. Diabetes Care 3:63, 1980.

glucose values. Glucose levels are recorded hourly, and the infusion rate is adjusted accordingly.

When cesarean delivery is to be performed, it should be scheduled for early morning. This simplifies intrapartum glucose control and allows the neonatal team to prepare for the care of the newborn. The patient is given nothing by mouth, and her usual morning insulin dose is withheld. If her surgery is not performed early in the day, one third to one half of the patient's intermediate-acting dose of insulin may be administered. Regional anesthesia is preferred because an awake patient permits earlier detection of hypoglycemia. Following surgery, glucose levels are monitored every 2 hours and an intravenous solution of 5 percent dextrose is administered.

After delivery, insulin requirements are usually significantly lower than were pregnancy or prepregnancy needs. The objective of "tight control" used in the antepartum period is relaxed for the first 24 to 48 hours. Patients delivered vaginally, who are able to eat a regular diet, are given one third to one half of their end-of-pregnancy dose of NPH insulin and short-acting insulin the morning of the first postpartum day. Frequent glucose determinations are used to guide insulin dosage. Most patients are stabilized on this regimen within a few days after delivery.

Women with diabetes are encouraged to breast-feed. The additional 500 kcal required daily are given as approximately 100 g of carbohydrate and 20 g of protein.[201] The insulin dose may be somewhat lower in lactating diabetic women. Hypoglycemia appears to be common in the first week following delivery and immediately after nursing.

MANAGEMENT OF THE PATIENT WITH GESTATIONAL DIABETES

The mainstay of treatment of GDM is nutritional counseling and dietary intervention. Women with GDM generally do not need hospitalization for dietary instruction and management. Once the diagnosis is established, patients are begun on a dietary program of 2,000 to 2,500 kcal daily.[202] This represents approximately 35 kcal/kg present pregnancy weight.

Once the patient with GDM is placed on an appropriate diet, surveillance of blood glucose levels is necessary to be certain that glycemic control has been established. Patients should perform daily measurements of fasting glucose and postprandial glucose levels after each meal.

Fasting capillary glucose should be maintained below 95 mg/dl and 1-hour postprandial glucose below 140 mg/dl or 2-hour postprandial glucose below 120 mg/dl.[212] If a patient repetitively exceeds these thresholds, then insulin or glyburide therapy is suggested.

Exercise has been recommended as an adjunctive treatment for GDM. Such an approach is also beneficial for nonpregnant type 2 diabetic patients in whom physical training increases insulin sensitivity. Three 20-minute aerobic exercise sessions weekly are recommended. Brisk walking is ideal.

Langer and his colleagues[216] have recently suggested that oral hypoglycemic therapy may be a suitable alternative to insulin treatment in women with GDM.[216] These investigators randomized 404 women to insulin versus glyburide and reported similar improvement in glycemia with both regimens. Most importantly, the frequency of macrosomia and neonatal hypoglycemia was similar in the two study groups. Further studies will be necessary to establish the safety of this regimen.

Patients with GDM who are well controlled are at low risk for an intrauterine death. For this reason, we do not routinely institute antepartum fetal heart rate testing in uncomplicated diet-controlled GDM patients unless the patient has a hypertensive disorder, history of a prior stillbirth, or suspected macrosomia.[217] Women in these categories as well as those who require insulin or glyburide treatment of GDM undergo twice-weekly heart rate testing at 32 weeks' gestation. Women with uncomplicated GDM do undergo fetal heart rate testing at 40 weeks' gestation.

Postpartum, women who have had GDM should be evaluated to determine if they have persistent carbohydrate intolerance. A fasting plasma glucose level can be obtained at the 6-week postpartum visit. Values of 110 mg/dl or less are normal; values above 110 mg/dl but below 126 mg/dl indicate impaired fasting glucose requiring close follow-up; and values of 126 mg/dl or more, if confirmed on repeat testing, indicate diabetes mellitus. Women with a prior history of GDM who have a normal fasting glucose should be tested annually to detect the onset of type 2 diabetes mellitus.

COUNSELING THE DIABETIC PATIENT

Anomalies of the cardiac, renal, and central nervous systems arise during the first 7 weeks of gestation, a time when it is most unusual for patients to seek prenatal care. Therefore, the management and counseling of women with diabetes in the reproductive age group should begin prior to conception. Unfortunately, it has been estimated that less than 20 percent of diabetic women in the United States obtain prepregnancy counseling.[182] A reduced rate of major congenital malformation in patients optimally managed before conception has been observed.

Glycosylated hemoglobin levels obtained during the first trimester may be used to counsel diabetic women regarding the risk for an anomalous infant. Overall, the risk of a major fetal anomaly may be as high as 1 in 4 or 1 in 5 when the glycosylated hemoglobin level is several percent above normal values. The risk for spontaneous abortion also appears to be increased with marked elevations in glycosylated hemoglobin. However, for diabetic women in good control, there appears to be no greater likelihood of miscarriage.[227]

With the increasing evidence that poor control is responsible for the congenital malformations seen in pregnancies complicated by diabetes, it is apparent that preconception counseling involving the patient and her family should be instituted.[224,228] Physicians who care for young women with diabetes must be aware of the importance of such counseling. At this time, the nonpregnant patient may learn techniques for self-glucose monitoring as well as the need for proper dietary management. Folic acid dietary supplementation at a dose of at least 0.4 mg daily should be prescribed, as there is increasing evidence that this vitamin may reduce the frequency of neural tube defects, although it has not specifically been studied in the diabetic population.[229,230] During counseling, questions may be answered regarding risk factors for complications and the plan for general management of diabetes in pregnancy. Planning for pregnancy should optimally be accomplished over several months. Glycosylated hemoglobin measurements are performed to aid in the timing of conception. The patient should attempt to achieve a glycosylated hemoglobin level of 7 percent prior to pregnancy.

CONTRACEPTION

There is no evidence that diabetes mellitus impairs fertility. Family planning is thus an important consideration for the diabetic woman. Barrier methods continue to be a safe and inexpensive method of birth control. The diaphragm, used correctly with a spermicide, has a failure rate of less than 10 percent. The intrauterine device may also be used by diabetic women without an increased risk of infection.[232]

Combined oral contraceptives (OCs) are the most effective reversible method of contraception, with failure rates generally less than 1 percent. Low-dose OCs to should probably be restricted to patients without serious vascular complications or additional risk factors such as a strong family history of myocardial disease. In these women, a monophasic preparation (progestin only) may be considered. In women receiving oral contraceptives, the lowest dose of estrogen and progesterone should be employed. Patients should have blood pressure monitoring after the first cycle and quarterly with baseline and follow-up lipid levels as well.[236] Despite the fact that carbohydrate metabolism may be affected by the progestin component of the pill, disturbances in diabetic control are actually uncommon with its use.

Key Points

➤ Pregnancy has been characterized as a diabetogenic state because of increased postprandial glucose levels in a late gestation.

➤ Both hepatic and peripheral (tissue) insulin sensitivity are reduced in normal pregnancy. As a result, a progressive increase in insulin secretion follows a glucose challenge.

➤ In women with gestational diabetes, the hormonal milieu of pregnancy may represent an unmasking of a susceptibility to the development of type 2 diabetes mellitus.

➤ According to the Pedersen hypothesis, maternal hyperglycemia results in fetal hyperglycemia and hyperinsulinemia, resulting in excessive fetal growth. Physiologic maternal glycemic control is associated with a reduced risk for fetal macrosomia.

➤ Congenital malformations occur with a two to sixfold increased rate in offspring of type 1 and type 2 diabetic women compared with the normal population. Impaired

Box continued on opposite page

Key Points *Continued*

glycemic control and the associated derangement in maternal metabolism appear to contribute to abnormal embryogenesis.

➤ Women with Class F (nephropathy) diabetes have an increased risk for preeclampsia and preterm delivery which correlates with their degree of renal impairment.

➤ Diabetic retinopathy may worsen during pregnancy, yet for women optimally treated with laser photocoagulation *prior* to pregnancy, significant deterioration of vision is uncommon.

➤ Screening for GDM is generally performed between 24–28 weeks gestation. Screening strategies include universal screening or limiting screening to women over age 25 with risk factors for developing type 2 diabetes mellitus.

➤ Treatment of the insulin-dependent woman during pregnancy requires intensive therapy consisting of frequent self blood glucose monitoring and aggressive insulin dosing by multiple injections or continous subcutaneous infusion (insulin pump).

➤ The cornerstone of treatment for GDM is dietary therapy. Insulin or glyburide are reserved for individuals who manifest significant fasting hyperglycemia or postprandial glucose elevations despite dietary intervention.

➤ Antepartum fetal assessment for both pregestational and GDM pregnancies is based on the degree of risk believed to be present in each case. Glycemic control, prior obstetric history, and the presence of vascular disease or hypertension are important considerations.

➤ Delivery should be delayed until fetal maturation has occurred, provided that diabetes is well controlled and fetal surveillance remains normal. The mode of delivery for the suspected large fetus remains controversial. In cases of suspected macrosomia, a low threshold for cesarean section has been recommended to prevent traumatic delivery.

➤ Women with type 1 and type 2 diabetes mellitus should seek prepregnancy consultation. Efforts to improve glycemic control prior to conception have been associated with a significant reduction in the rate of congenital malformations in the offspring of such women.

Other Endocrine Disorders

JORGE H. MESTMAN

PITUITARY DISEASES

Anterior Pituitary Insufficiency

Sheehan's syndrome or postpartum pituitary necrosis due to severe blood loss during delivery has been considered the most common cause of panhypopituitarism in women of childbearing age.[6] The classic clinical presentation of Sheehan's syndrome is severe bleeding during delivery or immediately postpartum in about 90 percent of patients; in more than 10 percent of patients no catastrophic event is elicited. In some cases, acute adrenal insufficiency with hypotension and shock results; in most cases, however, a more insidious onset occurs with lack of lactation following delivery, amenorrhea, loss of pubic and axillary hair or failure of pubic hair to grow back following cesarean delivery, anorexia and nausea, lethargy, weakness, and weight loss. The disease may be recognized in the few days or weeks following delivery or many years after the original event.[7] On physical examination, the findings depend on the severity and duration of the disease. Commonly, the skin has a waxy character with fine wrinkles about the eyes and mouth. There is some periorbital edema, and a decrease in pigmentation is often seen. Axillary and pubic hair becomes increasingly sparse. Atrophy of the breast tissue may be present. Even in those patients losing weight, cachexia is not a feature of the disease. Postural hypotension is not uncommon, patients complaining of dizziness on arising in the morning or when getting up from a sitting position. Normocytic anemia is common. Serum electrolytes may be within normal limits, unless severe vomiting is present. Most of the gastrointestinal and postural hypotension symptoms are due to secondary adrenal insufficiency, although the serum potassium remains normal because aldosterone production by the adrenal gland is not affected. This constellation of symptoms does not occur in every patient, and it is not unusual for the full-blown picture to take 10 to 20 years to develop. Occasionally, the diagnosis is made when the patient

673

develops acute adrenal insufficiency secondary to a stressful situation such as infection, trauma, or surgery.

The diagnosis is confirmed by the use of appropriate tests to investigate each of the pituitary hormones. Baseline or random determination of serum pituitary hormone concentrations is of little value, and dynamic tests to evaluate hypothalamic-pituitary hormonal reserve must be used.

Prolactinomas

Serum prolactin normally increases early in pregnancy, reaching values close to 140 ng/ml by the end of pregnancy.[28] Prolactinoma is the most common pituitary tumor diagnosed in women of childbearing age. Pituitary tumors are divided according to their size, into microadenomas, less than 10 mm in diameter, and macroadenomas; the latter are further classified according to suprasellar extension and invasion of adjacent structures. Serum prolactin concentrations correlate fairly well with the size of the tumor. Hyperprolactinemia may be diagnosed in the absence of an enlargement of the pituitary gland, known as idiopathic hyperprolactinemia. Hyperprolactinemia decreases gonadotropin-releasing hormone (GnRH) secretion, accounting for the infertility seen in these patients. However, high levels of serum prolactin in the presence of normal menses, normal fertility, and absence of a pituitary lesion have been reported.[29,30] Pregnancy outcome is excellent for both mother and infant.

Once the diagnosis of prolactinoma is confirmed, several types of therapy are available, the choice depending on tumor size, radiologic classification, local symptoms, and the patient's age and desire for pregnancy.[31]

Medical therapy with bromocriptine, a dopamine-receptor agonist, has been effective in producing ovulation in 80 to 90 percent of hyperprolactinemic women.[35] Most patients respond to doses between 2.5 and 5 mg/day, although occasionally a dose of 7.5 mg/day or more is needed. Bromocriptine is effective not only in normalizing prolactin levels but also in reducing the size of the tumor.[36,37] In women desiring a pregnancy, it is advisable to use mechanical contraception in the first few months of bromocriptine therapy, until normal menses have been established.

Once conception takes place, bromocriptine should be discontinued and the patient followed closely. For those women whose initial prolactin levels are over 200 ng/ml, or who have abnormal magnetic resonance imaging (MRI) scans with suprasellar extension, bromocriptine therapy during pregnancy should be continued.[39,40] Although the experience is limited to approximately 100 women who have used bromocriptine throughout gestation, no abnormalities have been noted in the infants, except for one with an undescended testicle and one with a talipes deformity.[31]

Complications during pregnancy are directly related to tumor size.[7,31,44-48] In patients with microadenomas, following induction of ovulation with bromocriptine, the reported incidence of headaches and visual field disturbances is between 1 and 4 percent. The incidence is close to 35 percent for patients with macroadenomas. However, if the pituitary macroadenoma is treated before pregnancy with either surgery or radiotherapy, the complication rate is about 4 percent. Complications may occur with equal frequency at any stage of pregnancy. Therefore, the management of patients with prolactinomas or any type of pituitary tumor in pregnancy depends on the size of the tumor and previous therapy. For patients with microadenomas, visual fields are indicated only if there are signs and symptoms of tumor enlargement; if the visual fields are abnormal, then an MRI scan of the pituitary gland is obtained. The determination of serum prolactin during gestation is not helpful in evaluating tumor growth. In the presence of any objective evidence of tumor enlargement, bromocriptine is resumed and continued throughout pregnancy at a dose of up to 20 mg/day. If after a few days there is no improvement, dexamethasone 4 mg every 6 hours is indicated. Surgery is performed in those complicated cases not responding to the above therapies.

Breast-feeding is not contraindicated in mothers with prolactinoma. There is no increase in prolactin secretion after suckling, and the mean value of prolactin is not increased compared with that of pregnancy.[50]

THYROID DISEASES

In early pregnancy, the maternal thyroid gland is challenged with an increased demand for thyroid hormone secretion, due mainly to three different factors: (1) the increase in thyroxine-binding globulin (TBG) due to the effect of estrogen on the liver, (2) the stimulatory effect of hCG on the TSH thyroid receptor, and (3) the supply of iodine available to the thyroid gland.

Active secretion of thyroid hormones by the fetal thyroid gland commences at about 18 weeks' gestation, although iodine uptake occurs between 10 and 14 weeks.[297] Transfer of thyroxine from the mother to the embryo occurs from early pregnancy. This maternal transfer continues until delivery, but only in significant amounts in the presence of fetal hypothyroidism.[300,301] Recent studies, that need to be confirmed, suggest that mild maternal thyroid deficiency in the first trimester could result in long-term neuropsychological damage to the offspring.[295,296]

The levels of maternal thyroid hormone concentrations, both total thyroxine (TT_4) and total triiodothyronine (TT_3) increase from early pregnancy as the result of an elevation in TBG and a reduced peripheral TBG degradation rate.[302] TBG reaches a plateau by 20 weeks' gestation and remains unchanged until delivery. In spite of these acute changes in total hormone concentration, the serum free fractions of both T_4 and T_3 remain within normal limits, unless there is a decreased supply of iodine to the mother or in the presence of abnormalities of the thyroid gland.[291]

Human chorionic gonadotropin is a weak thyroid stimulator, acting on the thyroid TSH receptor. It is estimated that a 10,000 IU/L increment in circulating hCG corresponds to a mean T_4 increment in serum of 0.1 ng/dl, and in turn to a lowering of TSH of 0.1 mU/L. In situations in which there is a high production of hCG, such as in cases of multiple pregnancies, hydatidiform mole, and hyperemesis gravidarum (HG), serum T_4 concentrations rise to levels seen in thyrotoxicosis with a transient suppression in serum TSH values.

Thyroid Function Tests

Measurement of serum TSH is the most practical, simple, and economic screening test for thyroid dysfunction. A high TSH value is consistent with the diagnosis of primary hypothyroidism, whereas a suppressed one, with few exceptions, is suggestive of hyperthyroidism (Fig. 24–5). In the presence of an abnormal serum TSH value, the determination of FT_4 or its equivalent free thyroxine index (FT_4I), is obtained for the assessment of thyroid function. A low TSH value and high concentrations of FT_4 or FT_4I is diagnostic of hyperthyroidism. There are special situations in which hyperthyroidism may be present in the presence of normal concentrations of FT_4. In such cases, a serum FT_3 or FT_3I determination should be obtained. High values are diagnostic of hyperthyroidism, the so-called T_3-toxicosis syndrome, sometimes seen in patients with an autonomous or "hot" thyroid nodule. Therefore, the use of a limited number of thyroid function tests (TFTs), properly ordered and interpreted, will allow the physician to assess thyroid function, and make the proper therapeutic decisions.[304]

The determination of TSH receptor antibodies (TSHRBAb or TRAb) is indicated in very special circumstances, in order to predict the possibility of fetal or neonatal thyroid dysfunction. These antibodies are immunoglobulins, usually of the IgG subclass, having different functional activity: stimulating (in most patients with Graves' disease) or blocking (in some patients with Hashimoto's thyroiditis, particularly in those without goiter) the TSH receptor of the thyroid gland. They do cross the placental barrier and may

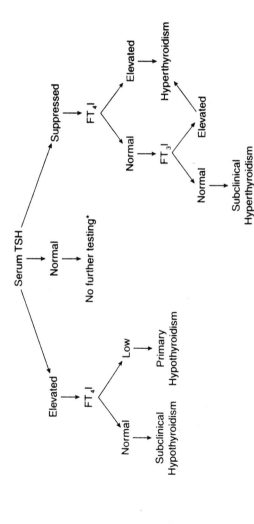

Figure 24–5. Algorithm for the diagnosis of thyroid disease. If there is clinical suspicion of secondary hypothyroidism, a determination of FT₄I is indicated. In this situation, the serum TSH is normal in the presence of low FT₄I. FT₄I, free thyroxine index or its equivalent, free thyroxine; FT₃I, free triiodothyronine index or its equivalent, free triiodothyronine; TSH, thyroid-stimulating hormone.

affect fetal thyroid function. Thyroid-stimulating immunoglobulins [TSIs], formerly known as long-acting thyroid-stimulating antibody (LATS), when present in high concentrations in the maternal serum may cause fetal or neonatal hyperthyroidism.[305] The chances for the offspring to be affected by these maternal antibodies are very low (up to 2 percent of mothers with autoimmune thyroid disease).

Goiter is commonly seen in pregnancy in areas of iodine deficiency. However, in the United States and other areas of the world with sufficient iodine intake, the thyroid gland does not clinically increase in size during pregnancy. Therefore, the detection of a goiter in pregnancy is an abnormal finding that needs careful evaluation. The most common cause of diffuse goiter is chronic autoimmune thyroiditis or Hashimoto's thyroiditis. Most patients are euthyroid and the diagnosis is made by the determination of thyroid antibodies, mainly thyroid peroxidase (TPO). Antibody concentration decreases during pregnancy, and increases in the postpartum period. High values in the first trimester of pregnancy are predictors of the syndrome of postpartum thyroid dysfunction.[307]

The indications for requesting TFTs are represented in the box "Indications for Thyroid Testing in Pregnancy." Whether routine thyroid screening in pregnant women is necessary remains a controversial issue, to be decided in the next few years, it is hoped, when more scientific information becomes available on the relationship of abnormal thyroid function early in pregnancy and neuropsychological and metabolic development of the offspring.

Prepregnancy Counseling

The physician may be faced with different clinical situations when counseling a woman contemplating pregnancy. They may be summarized as follows:

1. *Hyperthyroidism under treatment:* A choice of the three classic therapeutic options for hyperthyroidism treatment should be given: (1) long-term antithyroid drug therapy, (2) radioactive ^{131}I ablation, and (3) near total thyroidectomy. Potential side effects of antithyroid drugs on the fetus should be discussed. If the patient opts for ablation therapy, there is no long-term effect on the offspring of ^{131}I given to the future mother. However, it its customary to wait 6 months after the therapeutic dose is administered before pregnancy is contemplated. Surgery is another option, selected by some physicians and patients concerned about the potential side effects of antithyroid drugs or radioactive treatment. Regardless of the form of therapy chosen, it is important for the patient to be euthyroid at the time of conception.

2. *Previous ablation treatment for Graves' disease:* Two points are important: (1) the dose of thyroid replacement therapy needs to be increased in most women soon after conception[309,310]; and (2) in spite of euthyroidism, high maternal titers for TSI may be present, with the fetus being at risk of developing hyperthyroidism despite the mother being euthyroid.[311] Close follow-up during pregnancy and communication between the obstetrician and endocrinologist are essential.

3. *Previous treatment with ^{131}I for thyroid carcinoma:* Pregnancy does not affect the natural history of women previously treated for thyroid cancer. It appears reasonable for patients with thyroid carcinoma to wait 1 year after completion of radioactive treatment before conception.

4. *Treated hypothyroidism:* Women under treatment with thyroid hormone may require higher doses soon after conception.[309,310,313] As soon as the diagnosis of pregnancy is made, thyroid tests should be performed, and thyroid doses adjusted accordingly. Following delivery, the dose should be reduced to prepregnancy levels.

5. *Euthyroid chronic thyroiditis:* Patients with Hashimoto's thyroiditis are at greater risk of spontaneous abortions and the development of postpartum thyroiditis.[316,317] Thyroid tests are indicated in early pregnancy to detect elevations in TSH and assess the need for treatment with thyroid hormones or to adjust the dose in patients already on thyroid therapy.

Maternal – Placental – Fetal Interactions

Methimazole (MM) and propylthiouracil (PTU), drugs used for the treatment of hyperthyroidism, cross the placenta, and if given in inappropriate doses may produce fetal goiter and hypothyroidism.[320] Preparations containing iodine given in large doses or for prolonged periods of time are contraindicated in pregnancy, since accumulation by the fetal thyroid may induce goiter and hypothyroidism.[321]

Hyperthyroidism

Hyperthyroidism is diagnosed in pregnancy in about 0.1 to 0.4 percent of patients.[322,323] Classically, it has been stated that Graves' disease is the most common cause of hyperthyroxinemia in pregnancy, with other etiologies being uncommon. Transient hyperthyroidism due to inappropriate secretion or action of hCG is becoming recognized as the most common cause of hyperthyroidism in pregnancy.[324,325] Single toxic adenoma and multinodular toxic goiter are found in less than 10 percent of cases. Subacute thyroiditis is rarely seen during gestation.

Transient Hyperthyroidism of Hyperemesis Gravidarum

This disorder is characterized by severe nausea and vomiting, with onset between 4 to 8 weeks' gestation, requiring frequent visits to the emergency room and sometimes repeated hospitalizations for intravenous hydration. Weight loss of at least 5 kg, ketonuria, abnormal liver function tests, and hypokalemia are common findings, depending on the severity of vomiting and dehydration. Free thyroxine levels are elevated, sometimes up to four to six times the normal values, whereas FT_3 is elevated in up to 40 percent of affected women, values not as high as serum FT_4. The T_3/T_4 ratio is less than 20, as compared with Graves hyperthyroidism, where the ratio is over 20. Serum TSH is consistently suppressed.[324–328] In spite of the significant biochemical hyperthyroidism, signs and symptoms of hypermetabolism are mild or absent. Patients may complain of mild palpitations and heat intolerance, but perspiration, proximal muscle weakness, and frequent bowel movements are rare. On physical examination, ophthalmopathy and goiter are absent, a mild tremor of the outstretched fingers is occasionally seen, and tachycardia may be present due in part to dehydration. Significant in the medical history is the lack of hyperthyroid symptoms before conception, since patients with Graves' disease diagnosed for the first time during gestation give the history of hypermetabolic symptoms several months before pregnancy. Spontaneous normalization of hyperthyroxinemia parallels the improvement in vomiting and weight gain, with most of the cases resolving spontaneously between 14 and 20 weeks' gestation, although persistence of hyperthyroidism beyond 20 weeks' gestation has been reported in 15 to 25 percent of cases.[326,327] Suppressed serum TSH may lag for a few more weeks after normalization of free thyroid hormone levels. Antithyroid medications are not needed.

Graves' Disease

The natural course of hyperthyroidism due to Graves' disease in pregnancy is characterized by an exacerbation of symptoms in the first trimester and during the postpartum period and an amelioration of symptoms in the second half of pregnancy.

When hyperthyroidism is properly managed throughout pregnancy, the outcome for mother and fetus is good; however, maternal and neonatal complications for untreated or poorly controlled mothers are significantly increased.[339–342]

In the vast majority of patients in whom the diagnosis is made for the first time during pregnancy, hyperthyroid symptoms antedate conception. The clinical diagnosis of thyrotoxicosis may present difficulties during gestation, since many symptoms and signs are commonly seen in normal pregnancy, such as mild palpitations, heart rate between 90 and 100 beats/min, mild heat intolerance, shortness of breath on exercise, and warm skin. There are some clinical clues that increase the likelihood of the diagnosis of hyperthyroidism: presence of goiter, ophthalmopathy, proximal muscle weakness, tachycardia with a pulse rate over 100 beats/min, and weight loss or inability to gain weight in spite of a good appetite. Hyperthyroidism under poor control is frequently complicated by preeclampsia. The physician should suspect hyperthyroidism in the presence of systolic hypertension with an inappropriately low diastolic blood pressure and a wide pulse pressure, also seen in other conditions such as aortic insufficiency.

On physical examination, the thyroid gland is enlarged in almost every patient with Graves' disease. Indeed, the absence of a goiter makes the diagnosis unlikely. The gland is diffusely enlarged, between two and six times the normal size, varies from soft to firm, sometimes being irregular to palpation, and with one lobe being more prominent than the other one. A thrill may be felt or a bruit may be heard, indications of a hyperdynamic circulation. Examination of the eyes may reveal obvious ophthalmopathy, but in the majority of cases exophthalmos is absent or mild, with one eye slightly more prominent than the other.

Free thyroxine determination or the calculation of the free thyroxine index (using total thyroxine levels and a test for assessment of TBG, such as resin T_3 uptake) are standard tests in most clinical laboratories, with the result available in 24 to 48 hours. Almost every patient with Graves' disease will have an elevated FT_4 concentration. A suppressed TSH value in the presence of a high FT_4 or FT_4 index confirms the diagnosis of hyperthyroidism.[304] It must be kept in mind, however, that a suppressed serum TSH is present in about 15 percent of normal pregnant women in the first trimester of pregnancy.[291] In some unusual situations, the serum FT_4 may be at the upper limit of normal or be slightly elevated, in which case the determination of FT_3 and the FT_3 index will confirm the diagnosis of hyperthyroidism.

Fetal and neonatal complications are also related to maternal control of hyperthyroidism. Intrauterine growth restriction (IUGR), prematurity, stillbirth, and neonatal morbidity are the most common complications.

Treatment of hyperthyroidism is essential to prevent maternal, fetal, and neonatal complications. The goal of treatment is normalization of thyroid tests as soon as possible and to maintain euthyroidism with the minimum amount of antithyroid medication. Excessive amounts of antithyroid drugs crossing the placenta may affect the fetal thyroid, with the development of hypothyroidism with or without goiter. Patients should be monitored at regular intervals and the dose of their medications adjusted to keep the FT_4 in the upper one third of the range of normal.[345]

For this purpose, thyroid tests should be performed every 2 weeks at the beginning of treatment and every 2 to 4 weeks when euthyroidism is achieved. Patients with small goiters, a short duration of symptoms, and on minimal amounts of antithyroid medication will be able to discontinue antithyroid drugs by 34 weeks' gestation or beyond. It is not recommended to discontinue antithyroid therapy before 32 weeks' gestation, since in our experience relapses may occur in a significant number of patients.[354] In this country, the two antithyroid drugs available are PTU and methimazole (Tapazole). Both drugs are effective in controlling symptoms. To our knowledge, no studies have shown PTU to be superior to methimazole, both drugs having similar placental transfer kinetics.[355] Furthermore, when the efficacies of both drugs have been compared, euthyroidism was achieved with equivalent amounts of drugs and in the same period of time.[356,357] Neonatal outcomes were no different in both groups. Aplasia cutis, an unusual scalp lesion, occurred in a small group of patients taking methimazole,[358–360] but this is not a contraindication for its use in pregnancy.

The initial recommended dose of PTU is 100 to 450 mg/day, and methimazole 10 to 40 mg/day divided in two daily doses.[364] Methimazole is preferable in the outpatient setting, since it is given once or twice daily, allowing for improvement in patient compliance. PTU, due to its shorter half-life, should be given every 8 hours. In our experience, 10 mg of methimazole twice a day or 100 to 150 mg of PTU three times a day is an effective initial dose in most patients. Those with large goiters and longer duration of the disease may need larger doses at initiation of therapy. In patients with minimum symptoms, an initial dose of 10 mg of Tapazole daily or PTU 50 mg two or three times a day may be initiated. In most patients, clinical improvement is seen in 2 to 6 weeks, and improvement in thyroid tests occurs within the first 2 weeks of therapy, with normalization to chemical euthyroidism in 3 to 7 weeks.[356] Resistance to drug therapy is unusual, most likely due to poor patient compliance.[365] Once clinical improvement occurs, mainly weight gain and reduction in tachycardia, the dose of antithyroid medication may be reduced by half of the initial dose. The daily dose is adjusted every few weeks according to the clinical response and the results of thyroid tests. Serum TSH remains suppressed despite the normalization of thyroid hormone levels. Normalization of serum TSH is an indicator to reduce the dose of medication. We do not recommend adding thyroxine to antithyroid drug therapy in the management of Graves' disease in pregnancy. If there is an exacerbation of symptoms or worsening of the thyroid tests, the amount of antithyroid medication is doubled. The main concern of maternal drug therapy is the potential side effect on the fetus; mainly, goiter and hypothyroidism. In most studies this has been prevented by using doses no greater than 200 mg PTU or 20 mg methimazole in the last few weeks of gestation.[366]

Side effects of antithyroid drugs occur in 3 to 5 percent of treated patients.[368] The most common complications of both drugs are pruritus and skin rash. They usually resolve by switching to the other antithyroid medication. Agranulocytosis, a serious but unusual complication, has been reported in 1 in 300 patients receiving the drug.[369] It is manifested by fever, malaise, gingivitis, and sore throat. Agranulocytosis occurs in the first 12 weeks of therapy and appears to be related to the dose of medication.[370] Women should be made aware of the symptoms at the time the prescription is given, and advised to discontinue the drug and obtain a leukocyte count at once. Although some have recommended routine blood counts in patients on antithyroid therapy, it is not indicated.

β-Adrenergic blocking agents (propranolol 20 to 40 mg every 6 hours or atenolol 25 to 50 mg/day) are very effective in controlling hyperdynamic symptoms and are indicated for the first few weeks in symptomatic patients.[322] One situation in which β-adrenergic blocking agents may be very effective is in the treatment of severe hyperthyroidsm during labor.

[131]I therapy is contraindicated in pregnancy since, when given after 10 weeks' gestation, it produces fetal hypothyroidism.[373,374] A pregnancy test is mandatory in any woman of childbearing age before a therapeutic dose of ^{131}I is administered.

Excessive amounts of antithyroid drugs have induced fetal hypothyroidism and goiter. The diagnosis of goiter is made by ultrasonography, which shows hyperextension of the neck and a neck mass.

Breast-feeding should be permitted if the daily dose of PTU or methimazole is less than 150 to 200 mg/day, respectively. It is prudent to give the total dose in divided doses after each feeding. The infant should be followed with thyroid function tests.[378]

Assessment of fetal well-being with the use of ultrasonography, the nonstress test, and a biophysical profile is indicated for cases in poor metabolic control, in the presence of fetal tachycardia and/or IUGR, in pregnancies complicated by PIH or any other obstetrical or medical complications.

Hypothyroidism

Hypothyroidism in pregnancy is rarely diagnosed. However, subclinical hypothyroidism is more often encountered. Mild elevations in serum TSH are frequently detected in hypothyroid women on thyroid therapy soon after conception because of the increased demand for thyroid hormones in the first weeks of gestation.[309,310,398] The incidence of hypothyroidism, defined as any elevation in serum TSH above normal values, is between 0.19 and 2.5 percent.[399-403] The two most common etiologies of primary hypothyroidism are autoimmune thyroiditis (Hashimoto's thyroiditis) and postthyroid ablation therapy, surgical or ^{131}I treatment. Precent reports showed no increase in the incidence of congenital malformations, and perinatal mortality is only slightly elevated.[395-397]

Regàrdless of the etiology, primary hypothyroidism is classified as subclinical hypothyroidism (normal FT_4 and elevated TSH) and overt hypothyroidism (low FT_4 and elevated TSH).

The vast majority of patients with subclinical hypothyroidism are asymptomatic. Patients with overt hypothyroidism may complain of tiredness, cold intolerance, fatigue, muscle cramps, constipation, and deepening of the voice. On physical examination, the skin is dry and cold, deep tendon reflexes are delayed, and bradycardia may be detected as well as periorbital edema. A goiter is present in almost 80 percent of patients with chronic thyroiditis. The characteristic of the goiter is a diffuse enlargement, about two to three times the normal size, firm to palpation, painless, and with a rubbery consistency. In the other 20 percent, no goiter is found.

The diagnosis of hypothyroidism is confirmed by the determination of serum TSH and FT_4 or FT_4I. The degree of severity of the clinical symptoms varies with the chemical thyroid abnormalities, although there is not always good correlation between clinical and chemical parameters. Serum thyroid antibodies (thyroid peroxidase antibodies [anti-TPO] formerly known as antimicrosomal antibodies [AMAs]), are elevated in patients with autoimmune thyroiditis. The titer of antibodies does not correlate with the size of the goiter or the clinical severity of hypothyroidism.

As in the case of hyperthyroidism, the most common complications in hypothyroid pregnant women is PIH and low birth weight. The impact of maternal hypothyroidism on the intellectual development of the offspring has been the subject of recent reports.[295,296,408,409] These studies emphasize the importance of adjusting the dose of thyroxine in women under treatment for hypothyroidism soon after conception. Although we do not now support universal screening for hypothyroidism, we do recommend determination of thyroid tests early in pregnancy in those women at high risk for developing hypothyroidism (see the box "Indications for Thyroid Testing in Pregnancy").

Levothyroxine, or L-thyroxine, is the drug of choice for the treatment of hypothyroidism. It is important to normalize thyroid tests as soon as possible. An initial dose of 0.150 mg of levothyroxine is well tolerated by the majority of young hypothyroid patients. In those with severe hypothyroidism, there is a delay in the normalization of serum TSH, but normal serum FT4 values are achieved in the first two weeks of therapy. The maintenance dose required for most patients is between 0.125 and 0.250 mg of levothyroxine per day.

Indications for Thyroid Testing in Pregnancy

Family history of autoimmune thyroid disease
Women on thyroid therapy
Presence of goiter
Previous history of:
   High-dose neck radiation
   Therapy for hyperthyroidism
   Postpartum thyroid dysfunction
   Previous birth of an infant with thyroid disease
Type 1 diabetes mellitus

From Mestman JH: Thyroid diseases in pregnancy other than Graves' disease and postpartum thyroid dysfunction. Endocrinologist 9:924, 1999, with permission.

Patients on thyroid therapy before conception should have their TSH checked on their first visit and the amount of levothyroxine adjusted accordingly. The serum TSH should be repeated between 20 and 24 weeks and 28 and 32 weeks. Immediately after delivery, they should return to prepregnancy dosage.

Postpartum Thyroid Dysfunction

Thyroid dysfunction, hyper- and hypothyroidism, is recognized with increasing frequency in the 12 months following delivery, or following spontaneous or medically induced abortions. Most of the cases are due to intrinsic thyroid disease, with a few due to hypothalamic or pituitary lesions. Patients with autoimmune thyroid disease, chronic thyroiditis, and Graves' disease are most frequently affected.

Postpartum thyroiditis (PPT), a variant of Hashimoto's or chronic thyroiditis, is the most common cause of thyroid dysfunction in the postpartum period. The prevalence is between 5 and 10 percent of all women,[430,437–440] with the exception of women with type 1 diabetes, where the incidence is close to 30 percent.[441] The clinical diagnosis is not always obvious and the clinician should be concerned about nonspecific symptoms such as tiredness, fatigue, depression, palpitations, and irritability in women following the birth of their child or a miscarriage or abortion. Postpartum thyroiditis may also develop in women with negative antibodies.

PPT is characterized by symptoms of thyroid dysfunction, presenting in four different forms: (1) an episode of hyperthyroidism

(2 to 4 months), followed by hypothyroidism (4 to 6 months) and reverting to euthyroidism (after the seventh month); (2) an episode of hyperthyroidism (3 to 4 months) reverting to euthyroidism; (3) an episode of hypothyroidism (4 to 6 months) reverting to a euthyroid state; and (4) permanent hypothyroidism after the hypothyroid phase.

Since most cases of postpartum thyroid dysfunction recover spontaneously, treatment is indicated for symptomatic patients. In the presence of hyperthyroid symptoms, β-adrenergic-blocking drugs (propranolol 20 to 40 mg every 6 hours or atenolol 25 to 50 mg every 24 hours) are effective in controlling the symptoms. Antithyroid medications are not effective, because the hyperthyroxinemia is secondary to the release of thyroid hormones due to the acute injury to the gland (destructive hyperthyroidism). For hypothyroid symptoms, small amounts of levothyroxine 0.050 mg/day will control symptoms, allowing for a spontaneous recovery of thyroid function after discontinuation of the drug.

Key Points

➤ Hypopituitarism may present de novo in the second half of pregnancy, in the immediate postpartum period, or less commonly late postpartum. Severe hypoglycemia, responsive only to glucocorticoid therapy, is a characteristic feature. Lymphocytic hypophysitis with a normal or enlarged sella turcica on MRI appears to be the most common etiology.

➤ Hyperthyroidism due to Graves' disease needs to be differentiated in the first trimester of pregnancy from the syndrome of transient hyperthyroidism of hyperemesis gravidarum.

➤ Transient hyperthyroidism of hyperemesis gravidarum is the most common cause of hyperthyroxinemia in pregnancy; the cause is high or inappropriate levels of hCG.

➤ Both methimazole and PTU are used for the management of Graves' hyperthyroidism. The dosage should be adjusted frequently, aiming to use the minimum amount of drug that will keep the FT_4 at the upper limits of normal.

➤ Breast-feeding is not contraindicated in women on either methimazole or PTU, provided that the maximum daily dose is 200 mg of PTU and 20 mg of Tapazole.

Box continued on opposite page

Key Points *Continued*

➤ Hypothyroid women should have their thyroid tests checked early in pregnancy. An increase in dosage is needed in over 50 percent of patients.

➤ Postpartum thyroiditis affects between 5 and 10 percent of all women in the postpartum period. Women with chronic thyroiditis are at higher risk of developing the syndrome.

Hematologic Complications

PHILIP SAMUELS

PREGNANCY-ASSOCIATED THROMBOCYTOPENIA

Affecting approximately 4 percent of pregnancies, thrombocytopenia is the most frequent hematologic complication of pregnancy resulting in consultation. Hospital laboratories vary on their lower limit of a normal platelet count, but it is usually between 135,000 and 150,000/mm³. Platelet counts generally fall slightly, due to hemodilution and increased destruction, as gestation progresses, but should not fall below the normal range. In pregnancy, the vast majority of cases of mild to moderate thrombocytopenia are caused by gestational thrombocytopenia.[1] This form of thrombocytopenia has little chance of causing maternal or neonatal complications.[2] The obstetrician, however, is obliged to rule out other forms of thrombocytopenia that are associated with severe maternal or perinatal morbidity. The common and rare causes of thrombocytopenia in the gravida at term are shown in the box "Causes of Thrombocytopenia During Pregnancy."

Gestational Thrombocytopenia

Patients with gestational thrombocytopenia usually present with mild (platelet count = 100,000 to 149,000/mm³) to moderate (platelet count = 50,000 to 99,000/mm³) thrombocytopenia.[5] These patients usually require no therapy, and the fetus appears to be at little, if any, risk of being born with profound thrombocytopenia (platelet count <50,000/mm³) or a bleeding diathesis.

The decrease in platelet count, occurring in gestational thrombocytopenia, is not merely due to dilution of platelets with increasing blood volume. It appears to be due to an acceleration of the normal increase in platelet destruction that occurs during pregnancy.[1]

Causes of Thrombocytopenia During Pregnancy

Common causes
  Gestational thrombocytopenia
  Severe preeclampsia
  HELLP syndrome
  Immune thrombocytopenic purpura
  Disseminated intravascular coagulation

Rare causes
  Lupus anticoagulant/antiphospholipid antibody syndrome
  Systemic lupus erythematosus
  Thrombotic thrombocytopenic purpura
  Hemolytic uremic syndrome
  Type 2b von Willebrand's syndrome
  Folic acid deficiency
  Human immunodeficiency virus infection
  Hematologic malignancies
  May-Hegglin syndrome (congenital thrombocytopenia)

Immune Thrombocytopenic Purpura

Although it only affects 1 to 3 per 1,000 pregnancies, ITP has received much attention in the obstetrics literature because of the potential for profound neonatal thrombocytopenia in infants born to mothers with this condition.

In general, pregnancy has not been determined to cause ITP or to change its severity. Approximately 90 percent of women with ITP will have platelet-associated IgG.[21] Unfortunately, this is not specific for ITP, as studies have shown that these tests are??

Table 24–12 lists several studies in which all patients had true ITP and delineates the rates of profound neonatal thrombocytopenia. The neonatal morbidities included intraventricular hemorrhage, hemopericardium, gastrointestinal bleeding, and extensive cutaneous manifestations of bleeding.[3]

EVALUATION OF THROMBOCYTOPENIA DURING PREGNANCY AND THE PUERPERIUM

Before deciding on a course to follow in treating the patient with thrombocytopenia, the obstetrician must evaluate the patient and attempt to ascertain the etiology of her low platelet count. Important management decisions are dependent on arriving at an accurate diagnosis. A complete medical history, although time

Table 24–12. INCIDENCE OF PROFOUND NEONATAL THROMBOCYTOPENIA IN MOTHERS KNOWN TO HAVE IMMUNE THROMBOCYTOPENIC PURPURA

Reports	Total Patients with ITP	Infants with Platelet Count < 50,000/mm³	95% Confidence Interval
Karapatkin et al.[15]	19	6 (31.6%)	20.9%–52.5%
Burrows and Kelton[8]	60	3 (5%)	0%–10.5%
Noriega-Guerra et al.[13]	21	8 (38.1%)	17.3%–58.9%
Samuels et al.[3]	88	18 (20.5%)	12.0%–28.9%
Pooled (Crude)	188	35 (18.6%)	13%–24%

consuming, is critically important. It is essential to learn whether the patient has previously had a depressed platelet count or bleeding diathesis. It is also important to know whether these clinical conditions occur coincidentally with pregnancy. A complete medication history should be elicited, as certain medications, such as heparin, can result in profound maternal thrombocytopenia. The obstetric history should focus on whether there have been any maternal or neonatal bleeding problems in the past. Excessive bleeding from an episiotomy site or cesarean delivery incision site, a need for blood component therapy, easy bruising, or bleeding from intravenous sites during labor should alert the physician to the possibility of thrombocytopenia in the previous pregnancy. The obstetrician should also question whether the infant had any bleeding diathesis or if there was any problem following a circumcision. The obstetrician should also ask pertinent questions to determine whether severe preeclampsia or HELLP (Hemolysis, Elevated Liver Enzymes, Low Platelets) syndrome is the cause of her thrombocytopenia (see Chapter 23). Importantly, all thrombocytopenic pregnant women should be carefully evaluated for the presence of risk factors for human immunodeficiency virus (HIV) infection, as this infection can cause an ITP-like syndrome.

A thorough physical examination of the patient should also be performed. The physician should look for the presence of ecchymoses or petechiae. Blood pressure should be determined to ascertain whether the patient has impending preeclampsia. If the patient is developing HELLP syndrome, scleral icterus may be present. The eye grounds should be examined for evidence of arteriolar spasm or hemorrhage.

It is imperative that a peripheral blood smear be examined by an experienced hematologist or pathologist whenever a case of pregnancy-associated thrombocytopenia is diagnosed. This individual must determine if microangiopathic hemolysis is present. This specialist can also rule out platelet clumping, which will result in a factitious thrombocytopenia. Other laboratory evaluation should be performed as necessary to rule out preeclampsia and/or HELLP syndrome, as well as disseminated intravascular coagulopathy. If a diagnosis of ITP is entertained, appropriate platelet antibody testing should be performed.

THERAPY OF THROMBOCYTOPENIA DURING PREGNANCY

Gestational Thrombocytopenia

Gestational thrombocytopenia, the most common form encountered in the third trimester, requires no special therapy. The most important therapeutic issue is to refrain from therapies and testing that may lead to unnecessary intervention or iatrogenic preterm delivery. In patients with mild to moderate thrombocytopenia and no antenatal or antecedent history of thrombocytopenia, the patient should be treated like a normal pregnant patient. If the maternal platelet count drops below 50,000/mm^3, the patient may still have gestational thrombocytopenia, but there are not enough data on mothers with counts this low to determine if there are any maternal or fetal risks. These patients, therefore, should be treated as if they have de novo ITP. Although approximately 4 percent of patients have gestational thrombocytopenia, less than 1 percent of uncomplicated pregnant women will have gestational thrombocytopenia with platelet counts less than 100,000/mm^3.[8]

Immune Thrombocytopenic Purpura

Treatment of the gravida with ITP during pregnancy and the puerperium requires attention to both mother and fetus. Maternal therapy needs to be instituted only if there is evidence of a bleeding diathesis or to prevent a bleeding complication if surgery is anticipated. Again, there is usually no spontaneous bleeding unless the platelet count falls below 20,000/mm^3. Surgical bleeding does not usually occur until the platelet count is less than 50,000/mm^3. The conventional forms of raising a platelet count in the patient with ITP include glucocorticoid therapy, intravenous gammaglobulins, platelet transfusions, and splenectomy.

If the patient is having a bleeding diathesis or if the platelet count is below 20,000/mm^3, there is usually a need to raise the platelet count in a relatively short period of time. Although oral glucocorticoids can be used, intravenous glucocorticoids may work more rapidly. Hematologists have had the most experience with methylprednisolone. It can be given intravenously, and it has very little mineralocorticoid effect. The usual dose of methylprednisolone is 1.0 to 1.5 mg/kg of *total body weight* intravenously daily in divided doses. It usually takes about 2 days to see a response, but it may take up to 10 days to see a maximum response. Even though methylprednisolone has very little mineralocorticoid effect, there is some present, and it is important to follow the patient's electrolytes. There is little chance methylprednisolone will cause neonatal adrenal suppression because very little crosses the placenta. It is metabolized by placental 11-β-ol-dehydrogenase to an inactive 11-keto metabolite.

After the platelet count has risen satisfactorily using intravenous methylprednisolone, the patient can be switched to oral prednisone. The usual dose is 60 to 100 mg/day. It can be given in a single dose, but there is less gastrointestinal upset with divided doses. The physician can rapidly taper the dose to 30 or 40 mg/day, but slowly thereafter. The dose should be titrate to keep the platelet count around 100,000/mm³. If the physician begins therapy with oral prednisone, the usual initial daily dose is 1 mg/kg total body weight. The response rate to glucocorticoids is about 70 percent. It is important to realize that if the patient has been taking glucocorticoids for a period of at least 2 to 3 weeks, she may have adrenal suppression and should undergo increased doses of steroids during labor and delivery in order to avoid an adrenal crisis.

Although glucocorticoids are the mainstays of treating maternal thrombocytopenia, up to 30 percent of patients will not respond to these medications. In this instance, the next medication to use is intravenous immunoglobulin. This agent probably works by binding to the Fc receptors on reticuloendothelial cells and preventing destruction of platelets. The usual dose is 0.4 g/kg/day for 3 to 5 days. However, it may be necessary to use as much as 1 g/kg/day. The response usually begins in 2 to 3 days and usually peaks in 5 days. An alternate regimen is to give 1 g/kg once and observe the patient. Often this single dose will result in an adequate increase in platelets. The length of this response is variable, and the timing of the dose is extremely important. If the obstetrician wants a peak platelet count for delivery, he or she should institute therapy about 5 to 8 days before the planned delivery.

In midtrimester, splenectomy can also be used to raise the maternal platelet count. This procedure is reserved for those who do not respond to medical management, with the platelet count remaining below 20,000/mm³.

Platelet transfusions are indicated when there is clinically significant bleeding and while awaiting other therapies to become effective. Platelets can be given if the maternal platelet count is less than 50,000/mm³ during splenectomy, or during cesarean delivery if clinical bleeding is evident. They can be used before a vaginal delivery if the mother's platelet count is less than 20,000/mm³. Each "pack" of platelets will increase the platelet count by approximately 10,000/mm³. The half-life of these platelets is extremely short because the same antibodies and reticuloendothelial cell clearance rates that affect the mother's endogenous platelets will also affect the transfused platelets. However, if these platelets are transfused at the time the skin incision is made, it will allow enough hemostasis to carry out the surgical procedure.

There is no series large enough from which to draw adequate conclusions concerning mode of delivery of the profoundly thrombocytopenic fetus. Arguments have been made for both vaginal and cesarean delivery. In our series, 19.2 percent of untreated patients gave birth to profoundly thrombocytopenic infants compared with 22.7 percent of those receiving prednisone alone, 23 percent of those who had undergone a splenectomy and received prednisone, and 17.8 percent of those having undergone only splenectomy.

There are advantages of knowing whether a fetus is at risk of being born with a platelet count less than 50,000/mm. For example, the use of scalp electrodes and vacuum extractors are examples of interventions that may be avoided in the profoundly thrombocytopenic fetus. Nevertheless, cordocentesis is rarely indicated in patients with ITP.

In summary, the treatment of thrombocytopenia during gestation is dependent on the etiology. The obstetrician need not act on the mother's platelet count unless it is below 20,000/mm^3, or if it is below 50,000/mm^3 with evidence of clinical bleeding or if surgery is anticipated. In these cases, the treatment will depend upon the diagnosis. Furthermore, whether delivery needs to be expedited or can be delayed is also dependent on the etiology of thrombocytopenia. The fetal/neonatal platelet count need only be considered if the mother carries a true diagnosis of ITP or, in the case of presumed gestational thrombocytopenia, when the platelet count is less than 75,000/mm^3, as this may actually be de novo ITP. The key to managing these patients is to arrive at an accurate etiology for the thrombocytopenia and to approach the patient and her fetus rationally.

NEONATAL ALLOIMMUNE THROMBOCYTOPENIA

In neonatal alloimmune thrombocytopenia, a rare disorder, the mother lacks a specific platelet antigen and develops antibodies to this antigen. The disease is somewhat analogous to Rh isoimmunization, but involves platelets. If the fetus inherits this antigen from its father, maternal antibody can cross the placenta, resulting in severe neonatal thrombocytopenia. The mother, however, will have a normal platelet count. The most common antibodies noted in these patients are anti-PLA 1 and BAK antibodies.[57] After birth or in utero the child can be transfused with the mother's platelets, since she lacks the antigen that would lead to platelet destruction by circulating antibodies.

IRON DEFICIENCY ANEMIA

The first pathologic change to occur in iron deficiency anemia is the depletion of bone marrow, liver, and spleen iron stores (see Figure 24–6). The serum iron level falls, as does the percentage saturation of transferrin. The total iron-binding capacity rises, as this is a reflection of unbound transferrin. A falling hemoglobin and hematocrit follow. Microcytic hypochromic RBCs are released

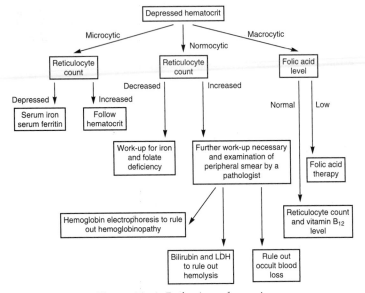

Figure 24–6. Evaluation of anemia.

into the circulation. If iron deficiency is combined with folate deficiency, normocytic and normochromic RBCs are observed on the peripheral blood smear.

Care must be taken when using laboratory parameters to establish the diagnosis of iron deficiency anemia during gestation. A serum iron concentration less than 60 mg/dl with less than 16 percent saturation of transferrin is suggestive of iron deficiency. An increase in iron-binding capacity, however, is not reliable, as 15 percent of pregnant women without iron deficiency will show an increase in this parameter.[67] Serum ferritin levels normally decrease mildly during pregnancy. A significantly reduced ferritin concentration is also indicative of iron deficiency anemia and is the best parameter with which to judge the degree of iron deficiency.

Iron prophylaxis is recommended. One 325-mg tablet of ferrous sulfate daily provides adequate prophylaxis. It contains 60 mg of elemental iron, 10 percent of which is absorbed. If the iron is not needed, it will not be absorbed and will be excreted in the feces.

In iron-deficient patients, one iron tablet three times daily is recommended. It should be taken 30 minutes before meals to allow maximum absorption. However, when taken in this manner, dyspepsia and nausea are more common. Vitamin C may increase the acid environment of the stomach and increase absorption. Therapy, therefore, must be individualized to maximize patient compliance. If isolated iron deficiency is present, one should see a dramatic reticulocytosis approximately 2 weeks after the initiation of therapy.

FOLATE DEFICIENCY

During pregnancy, folate deficiency is the most common cause of megaloblastic anemia, as vitamin B_{12} deficiency is extremely rare. The daily folate requirement in the nonpregnant state is approximately 50 μg, but this rises three- to fourfold during gestation.[85] Fetal demands increase the requirement, as does the decrease in the gastrointestinal absorption of folate during pregnancy.[86]

Clinical megaloblastic anemia seldom occurs before the third trimester of pregnancy. If the patient is at risk for folate deficiency or has mild anemia, an attempt should be made to detect this disorder before megaloblastosis occurs (see Fig. 24–6). Serum folate and RBC folate levels are the best tests for folate deficiency.[87]

Prenatal vitamins that require physician prescription contain 1 mg of folic acid. Most nonprescription prenatal vitamins contain 0.8 mg of folic acid. These amounts are more than adequate to prevent and treat folate deficiency. Women with significant hemoglobinopathies, patients ingesting anticonvulsant medications, women carrying a multiple gestation, and women with frequent conception may require more than 1 mg supplemental folate daily. If the patient is folic acid deficient, her reticulocyte count will be depressed. Within 3 days after the administration of sufficient folic acid, reticulocytosis usually occurs. In fact, folic acid deficiency should be considered when a patient has unexplained thrombocytopenia. The hematocrit level may rise as much as 1 percent per day after 1 week of folate replacement.

Iron deficiency is frequently associated with folic acid deficiency. If a patient with folate deficiency does not develop a significant reticulocytosis within 1 week after administration of sufficient replacement therapy, appropriate tests for iron deficiency should be performed.

HEMOGLOBINOPATHIES

The prevalences of the most common hemoglobinopathies are listed in Table 24–13.

Hemoglobin S

Hemoglobin S, an aberrant hemoglobin, is present in patients with sickle cell disease (hemoglobin SS) and sickle cell trait (hemoglobin AS). At low oxygen tensions, RBCs containing hemoglobin S assume a sickle shape. Sludging in small vessels occurs, resulting in microinfarction of the affected organs. Sickle cells have a life span of 5 to 10 days, compared with 120 days for a normal RBC. Sickling is triggered by hypoxia, acidosis, or dehydration.

Approximately 1 of 12 African-American adults in the United States is heterozygous for hemoglobin S and, therefore, has sickle cell trait (hemoglobin AS) and carries the affected gene. These individuals generally have 35 to 45 percent hemoglobin S and are asymptomatic. The child of two individuals with sickle cell trait has a 50 percent probability of inheriting the trait and a 25 percent probability of actually having sickle cell disease. One of every 625 African-American children born in the United States is homozygous for hemoglobin S, and the frequency of sickle cell disease among adult African-Americans is 1 in 708.[93] All at-risk patients should undergo hemoglobin electrophoresis at their first prenatal visit.

The traditional teaching is that women with sickle cell trait are not at increased risk for maternal and perinatal morbidity. However, recent data suggests that preeclampsia, decreased birth weight, and endometritis may all be increased in these patients.[95] This study indicates that our surveillance should be higher in patients with hemoglobin AS.

If a patient has hemoglobin AS, the spouse should be tested, and if both are carriers of a hemoglobinopathy, prenatal diagnosis should be offered. Prenatal diagnosis can be performed by DNA analysis with the polymerase chain reaction (PCR) and Southern blotting.[96,97]

Table 24–13. FREQUENCY OF COMMON HEMOGLOBINOPATHIES IN AFRICAN-AMERICAN ADULTS IN THE UNITED STATES

Hemoglobin Type	Frequency
Hemoglobin AS	1 in 12
Hemoglobin SS	1 in 708
Hemoglobin AC	1 in 41
Hemoglobin CC	1 in 4,790
Hemoglobin SC	1 in 757
Hemoglobin S/β-thalassemia	1 in 1,672

Painful vaso-occlusive episodes involving multiple organs are the clinical hallmark of sickle cell anemia. The most common sites for these episodes are the extremities, joints, and abdomen. Vaso-occlusive episodes can also occur in the lung, resulting in pulmonary infarction. Analgesia, oxygen, and hydration are the clinical foundations for treating these painful crises.

Many pregnancies complicated by sickle cell anemia are associated with poor perinatal outcomes. The rate of spontaneous abortion may be as high as 25 percent.[102-104] Perinatal mortality rates of up to 40 percent were reported in the past, but the current estimate is approximately 15 percent.[103-108] Much of this poor perinatal outcome is related to preterm birth. Approximately 30 percent of infants born to mothers with sickle cell disease have birth weights below 2,500 g.[108] Stillbirth rates of 8 to 10 percent have been described in patients with sickle cell anemia.[103] These fetal deaths happen not only during crises but also unexpectedly. Careful antepartum fetal testing must therefore be utilized, including serial ultrasonography to assess fetal growth.

Although maternal mortality is rare in patients with sickle cell anemia, maternal morbidity is great. Infections are common, occurring in 50 to 67 percent of women with hemoglobin SS. Most are urinary tract infections (UTIs), which can be detected by frequent urine cultures. Patients with hemoglobin AS are also at greater risk for a UTI and should be screened as well. Pulmonary infection and infarction are also common. Patients with sickle cell anemia should receive pneumococcal vaccine before pregnancy. Any infection demands prompt attention, because fever, dehydration, and acidosis will result in further sickling and painful crises. The incidence of pregnancy-induced hypertension is increased in patients with sickle cell anemia and may complicate almost one third of pregnancies in these patients.[106,111]

The care of the pregnant patient with sickle cell anemia must be individualized and meticulous. A folate supplement of at least 1 mg/day should be administered as soon as pregnancy is confirmed. Although hemoglobin and hematocrit levels are decreased, iron supplements need not be routinely given.

The role of prophylactic transfusions in the gravida with sickle cell anemia is controversial. This therapy, which replaces the patient's sickle cells with normal RBCs, can both improve oxygen-carrying capacity and suppress the synthesis of sickle hemoglobin. If one chooses to perform prophylactic transfusion, the goal is to maintain a percentage of hemoglobin A above 20 percent at all times and preferably above 40 percent, as well as to maintain the hematocrit above 25 percent. It has been recommended that prophylactic transfusion begin at 28 weeks' gestation. Buffy-coat-poor washed RBCs are used to reduce the risk of isosensitization.

Vaginal delivery is preferred for patients with sickle cell disease. Cesarean delivery should be reserved for obstetric indications. Patients should labor in the left lateral recumbent position and receive supplemental oxygen. Although adequate hydration should be maintained, fluid overload must be avoided. Conduction anesthesia is recommended, as it provides excellent pain relief and can be used for cesarean delivery, if necessary.

HEREDITARY THROMBOPHILIAS

Venous thrombosis is the third most common vascular disease in the nation.[161] Pregnant women are particularly susceptible to this disorder due to venous stasis caused by hormonally related relaxation of vascular smooth muscle as well as mechanical compression of pelvic veins leading to decreased venous return to the vena cava. There are also changes in clotting factors, as all factors except V, XI, and XIII increase during pregnancy. Furthermore, there is a decrease in fibrinolytic activity. Therefore, deep vein thrombosis (DVT), occurring in 0.4 per 1,000 pregnancies, is six times more frequent during gestation as in nonpregnant individuals. In pregnancy, deep venous thrombosis usually involves the deep femoral and pelvic veins. If inadequately treated, these thromboses may lead to chronic venous insufficiency and leg ulcerations. If untreated, 24 percent of DVTs will result in pulmonary embolus, which occurs in 0.5 to 3.0 per 1,000 pregnancies. Without therapy, recurrent emboli will occur in 33.3 percent of patients. The mortality rate from a pulmonary embolus is 15 percent in patients who are not treated for DVT, whereas the mortality rate is only 0.7 percent if prompt anticoagulation therapy is initiated. Therefore, prompt diagnosis and treatment are paramount.

Activated protein C resistance is responsible, at least in part, for about 40 percent of DVTs, fivefold more than any other single cause.[164] A single DNA point mutation at the activated protein C cleavage site on factor V, a substitution of arginine for glutamic acid at codon 506 (Arg506Gln), is responsible for 90 to 95 percent of activated protein C resistance.[165] This is known as the factor V_{Leiden} mutation. It is inheritable and fairly common. Homozygous and heterozygous forms exist. Heterozygous patients have a 5- to 10-fold clotting diathesis over the general population. Homozygotes, however, have a 50- to 100-fold increased risk.[166] It is unusual to find a homozygous patient that has not had thrombotic episodes prior to midlife. The frequency of this factor V_{Leiden} mutation varies with the population studied. The gene frequency in the United States is shown in the box "Population Frequency of Factor V_{Leiden} in the United States."

Individuals with these thrombophilic conditions do not always develop thromboses. There are also exogenous factors such as pregnancy that predispose individuals to thrombotic events. The recently discovered gene mutations that predispose an individual toward thrombosis can be tested using DNA techniques. These are reliable tests, and results are not affected by anticoagulation or the physiologic changes of pregnancy.

The prevalence of the factor V_{Leiden} mutation in an obstetric population in Utah was 3.4 percent, which is similar to the published rate for nonobstetric populations.[168] Whereas less than 1 percent of patients without the mutation experienced a thromboembolic event during pregnancy, 28 percent of those with the factor V_{Leiden} mutation experienced such an event.[168] Indeed, the factor V_{Leiden} mutation appears to be a significant cause of deep vein thrombosis during gestation.

The treatment of thrombosis during pregnancy consists of heparin therapy. If the patient has an active thrombosis, heparin can be dosed by a weight-based or non–weight-based regimen. The important component of this therapy is to check the APTT every 4 to 6 hours until the results are consistently about twice the control value. Obstetricians are increasingly using low-molecular-weight heparins. They are much more expensive, but may cause decreased heparin-induced thrombocytopenia and osteopenia. Monitoring the APTT is not necessary. Therefore, this therapy is more convenient for the patient. We have had the greatest experience using enoxaparin. The therapeutic dose is 1 mg/kg twice daily. Therapeutic levels can be ascertained by intermittent monitoring of activated factor X levels, as the pharmacokinetics of these drugs have not been reliably established in pregnancy.

Much research is needed concerning prophylactic anticoagulation in patients with factor V_{Leiden} mutation, patients with the thermolabile form of N^5,N^{10}-methylenetetrahydrofolate reductase, and patients with the prothrombin gene mutation. Because family members of patients with thrombotic events are being tested, we are identifying many patients who carry one of these genetic thrombophilias who have never experienced a sentinel event. We do not know if these individuals warrant prophylactic heparin during pregnancy, a time of hypercoagulability. It is our current practice to look for other risk factors such as diabetes mellitus, smoking, and obesity. We then have a long discussion concerning risks and benefits of prophylactic anticoagulation with the patient before a joint decision is made.

Population Frequency of Factor V_{Leiden} in the United States

U.S. Caucasians 5.7%
African-Americans 1.2%
Hispanic-Americans 2.2%
Asian-Americans 0.45%
Native-Americans 1.25%

Key Points

➤ Four percent of pregnancies will be complicated by maternal platelet counts of less than 150,000/mm³. The vast majority of these patients will have gestational thrombocytopenia with a benign course and will need no intervention.

➤ Surgical bleeding occurs if the platelet count falls below 50,000/mm³ and spontaneous bleeding occurs if the platelet count falls below 20,000/mm³.

➤ Glucocorticoids are the first-line medication used to raise a low platelet count.

➤ Iron deficiency anemia is the most common cause of anemia in pregnancy and serum ferritin is the single best test to diagnose it.

➤ If a patient with presumed iron deficiency does increase her reticulocyte count with iron therapy, she may also have a concomitant folic acid deficiency.

➤ Patients pregnant with twins, those on anticonvulsant therapy, those with a hemoglobinopathy, and those who conceive frequently need supplemental folic acid during gestation.

➤ Most hereditary hemoglobinopathies can be detected in utero and prenatal diagnosis should be offered to the patient early in pregnancy.

➤ As in the nonpregnant patient, analgesia, hydration, and oxygen are the key factors in treating pregnant women with sickle cell crisis.

➤ Patients with sickle cell disease are at high risk of having a fetus with growth restriction and adverse fetal outcomes. Therefore, they warrant frequent sonography and antepartum fetal evaluation.

➤ Factor V_{Leiden} mutation occurs in up to 5 percent of the population and is responsible for a significant proportion of the thrombotic disease seen in pregnancy.

Collagen Vascular Diseases

PHILIP SAMUELS

With the exception of rheumatoid arthritis, autoimmune diseases are associated with an increased risk of poor pregnancy outcome. Many have a predisposition for women in their childbearing years.[1] These diseases are characterized by the production of autoantibodies. Increasingly sensitive and specific laboratory tests have been developed to aid in the diagnosis of these disorders.

SYSTEMIC LUPUS ERYTHEMATOSUS

The course of SLE is characterized by chronic exacerbations and remissions. The prevalence of the disease in women 15 to 64 years of age is estimated to be 1 per 700,[2] but in black women of the same age group the prevalence is 1 per 245.[3] The diagnosis of SLE is based on a patient meeting at least four of the diagnostic criteria accepted by the American Rheumatism Association.

Clinical Manifestations

Approximately 80 percent of patients with SLE demonstrate skin lesions. These may include the classic malar (butterfly) rash, alopecia, or discoid lesions that are often discolored. Photosensitivity is common. Arthralgias with some arthritis will be evident in 90 percent of patients. Nephritis and neurologic or psychiatric features are found in approximately 50 percent of cases. Renal pathology is often not diagnosed until other symptoms arise.

The renal lesions of SLE include focal proliferative glomerulonephritis, membranous glomerulonephritis, mesangial nephritis, and diffuse proliferative glomerulonephritis.

Laboratory Diagnosis

More than 90 percent of patients with SLE will exhibit significant titers of antinuclear antibodies. In 80 to 90 percent of patients, an autoantibody directed against double-stranded DNA will be detected. Extractable nuclear antibodies can be subdivided into antibodies against ribonuclear protein (anti-RNP, anti-SM), anti-SSA (Ro), and anti-SSB (La). Anti-SSA and anti-SSB antibodies, which are found in 25 and 12 percent of patients with SLE, respectively, have been associated with fetal and neonatal heart block. Anti-SSA antibodies are generally associated with manifestations of neonatal lupus.

The Effects of Pregnancy on SLE

Pregnancy does not appear to affect or alter the long-term prognosis of patients with SLE.[4] Several studies, however, have documented increased flares of SLE during pregnancy and particularly during the puerperium.[4,5]

Although it remains debatable whether SLE is exacerbated by pregnancy, there is no dispute that there is a risk of major maternal morbidity and potentially of mortality in the gravida with SLE. Most maternal deaths occur during the puerperium as a result of pulmonary hemorrhage or lupus pneumonitis.[13,14] Most perinatologists advise their patients not to conceive during a time of increased lupus activity as this is associated with flares during pregnancy.[19] In general, a patient's disease should be quiescent for 5 to 7 months before conception.

Women with lupus nephritis must be aware that there is a small but significant risk of permanent deterioration of renal function during pregnancy. Poor pregnancy outcome is associated with active lupus nephropathy,[19] a serum creatinine level of at least 1.5 mg/dl, a BUN more than 50 mg/dl, and a creatinine clearance rate less than 50 ml/min.[19,21,26]

A lupus flare and preeclampsia present a difficult differential diagnosis, because they have similar signs and symptoms.[27] Both disorders often present with hypertension, edema, and proteinuria. To confound the issue, patients with lupus nephropathy are at an increased risk for developing superimposed preeclampsia during gestation. The treatment for preeclampsia is delivery, while the treatment for lupus nephritis is increased glucocorticoids and possibly azathioprine therapy. Complement levels (C3 and C4) are valuable in differentiating between heightened lupus activity and preeclampsia. In normal pregnancy, complement levels tend to rise. They are, therefore, high or normal in the SLE patient with pure preeclampsia. Conversely, these levels fall with an exacerbation of lupus.

The Effects of SLE on Pregnancy

Although fertility is not impaired, SLE can have an adverse effect on pregnancy outcome in each trimester.[29] There is an increase in the spontaneous abortion rate, with the estimated incidence between 16 and 36 percent.[11,18,30-33] The risk of miscarriage is not necessarily related to disease activity.

Preterm birth, IUGR, and fetal death are all increased in pregnancies complicated by SLE. Hypertension increases the risk of these adverse outcomes.

The lupus inhibitor and antiphospholipid antibodies have been associated with recurrent miscarriage. The diagnosis of the lupus inhibitor is often confusing. There is no single assay that is used to identify this phenomenon, and different assays have different sensitivities and specificities. Some clinicians and researchers rely solely on a prolongation of the activated partial thromboplastin time (aPTT) using platelet-poor plasma. A sensitive reagent must be used. Other commonly used tests include the tissue thromboplastin inhibition test (TTI), kaolin clotting time (KCT), dilute Russell viper venom time, platelet neutralization procedure, and the hexagonal antibody.

There is confusion concerning the difference between anticardiolipin antibodies and antiphospholipid antibodies. Antiphospholipid antibodies encompass many phospholipids, of which cardiolipin is only one. Nevertheless, the terms are often used interchangably in the obstetric literature.

In the absence of SLE, anticardiolipin antibodies can be associated with an increased risk for early preeclampsia, IUGR, and fetal death.[53,54] Patients with elevated anticardiolipin antibodies who have SLE are at significant risk to develop fetal distress in the second trimester with subsequent fetal death.

Although treatment with heparin and aspirin has become the standard for treating lupus inhibitor and antiphospholipid antibodies, the precise population to be treated remains somewhat debatable. Furthermore, the type and dose of heparin has not been firmly established. The role of low-dose aspirin alone also remains controversial. Because infarctions are often found in the placentas of patients with anticardiolipin antibodies, clinicians have begun using heparin therapy in this group. Heparin can result in heparin-induced thrombocytopenia, which can be life threatening. Danaparoid and r-hirudin (both heparinoids) have been used in such cases, as there is only a 10 to 20 percent cross-reactivity with heparin-associated antibodies.[71] There has been a great increase in the use of low-molecular-weight heparin in patients with antiphospholipid antibodies. The cost is greater than unfractionated heparin, but there is less heparin-induced thrombocytopenia and there may be less osteopenia associated with low molecular-weight heparin.

We currently individualize our therapy of patients with lupus inhibitor and antiphospholipid antibodies. We take the patient's history and laboratory results into account when making decisions regarding therapy. For the patient whom we feel truly has this syndrome, we usually prescribe low-dose aspirin and heparin. Low-dose unfractionated heparin needs to be given twice daily. In these patients, low-molecular-weight heparin can probably be given once daily. The true key in treating these patients is to make certain they understand the potential side effects of the prescribed medication regimen and that they undergo the proper fetal and maternal surveillance throughout pregnancy.

Neonatal Manifestations of SLE

Complete congenital heart block, an infrequent complication of SLE, can be diagnosed prenatally. In the mid-trimester, a fetal heart rate of about 60 bpm with no baseline variability is indicative of congenital heart block. The patient should immediately undergo fetal echocardiography to rule out associated congenital cardiac malformations. Affected fetuses usually show no evidence of congestive heart failure or hydrops. Nonetheless, they should be followed with serial ultrasonography every 1 to 2 weeks to ascertain if any evidence of anasarca has developed.

Infants born to mothers with SLE may exhibit erythematous skin lesions of the face, scalp, and upper thorax.[12,91,92] These lesions usually disappear by 12 months of age.

Surveillance

Because of the increased risk of miscarriage, stillbirth, preterm delivery, and IUGR, the obstetrician caring for the patient with SLE should maintain close maternal and fetal surveillance. Any patient with a history of SLE should undergo preconceptual counseling and should have tests performed for the presence of the lupus inhibitor, anticardiolipin antibodies, anti-SSA (Ro) antibodies, anti-SSB (La) antibodies, and anti-double stranded DNA antibodies. As previously described, these findings are associated with a poorer pregnancy outcome. If indicated, therapy should be initiated after fully informing the patient of risks and benefits to both her and the fetus. If anti-SSA or anti-SSB antibodies are present, fetal echocardiography should be performed in the second trimester to rule out complete congenital heart block. Because of the risks of IUGR and preterm birth, accurate gestational dating is imperative in the patient with SLE. Patients should also have an examination of their urine sediment and a 24-hour urine collection for creatinine clearance and total protein excretion in early pregnancy to determine if there is any renal involvement of their SLE.

At 28 weeks' gestation, weekly antepartum fetal heart rate testing should be initiated using the nonstress test. Antepartum fetal heart rate testing has been shown to improve fetal outcome in patients with SLE.[95] At 34 weeks, the frequency of testing should be increased to twice weekly.

Despite the sophisticated array of laboratory studies that are available to follow patients with SLE, the patient's clinical status remains of prime importance. There is no substitute for careful monitoring of maternal blood pressure and weight gain. These can be the earliest signs of superimposed preeclampsia, which is common in patients with SLE.[27,99] Twenty-four-hour urine collections for creatinine clearance and total protein excretion should be carried out every 1 to 2 months. Serum creatinine, BUN, and uric acid levels should be determined whenever these urine collections are performed. A rise in serum uric acid can be a sign of impending preeclampsia.

The timing of delivery is important and should be individualized. The obstetrician should strive for a vaginal delivery. If the patient is taking glucocorticoids or if there is any evidence of lupus exacerbation, peripartum steroids should be administered parenterally. In the patient who undergoes cesarean delivery, intravenous steroids should be continued for 48 hours postoperatively, because adequate gastrointestinal absorption cannot be guaranteed until normal bowel function returns. Steroids should be tapered slowly and with great care in the postpartum period to prevent an exacerbation of SLE.[24,100]

Key Points

> ➤ Systemic lupus erythematosus is associated with an increase in poor pregnancy outcome (i.e., from IUGR, stillbirth, and spontaneous abortion).

> ➤ The rate of pregnancy complications is decreased if patients with SLE have quiescent disease for 6 months prior to conception.

> ➤ Glucocorticoids are safe to use in pregnancy for the treatment of patients with SLE.

Box continued on following page

Key Points *Continued*

➤ The lupus inhibitor and anticardiolipin antibodies are found in 50 percent of patients with SLE. They are associated with an increased risk of pregnancy loss, including second- and third-trimester losses.

➤ Anti-SSA (Ro) and anti-SSB (La) antibodies are associated with complete congenital heart block and other manifestations of neonatal lupus.

➤ Low-dose heparin and low-dose aspirin are the therapies of choice for patients with lupus inhibitor/antiphospholipid antibodies who do not have active SLE.

Hepatic Disease

PHILIP SAMUELS

Liver dysfunction and disease occasionally complicate pregnancy. The most commonly seen problems include liver dysfunction associated with preeclampsia and hepatitis. These topics are covered in Chapters 23 and 25. This chapter focuses on acute fatty liver, intrahepatic cholestasis of pregnancy, and gallbladder disease associated with gestation (Table 24–14).

ACUTE FATTY LIVER

Acute fatty liver is a rare condition that has an incidence of between 1 in 6,692 and 1 in 15,900 pregnancies.[1-3] Since 1975, maternal survival has been reported as 72 percent, with neonatal survival slightly lower. The results are undoubtedly better now. These improved outcomes have been attributed to early recognition of the disorder followed by prompt delivery.[1,4-6] Usually beginning late in the third trimester, acute fatty liver often presents with nausea and vomiting,[1,6,8] followed by severe abdominal pain and headache. The right upper quadrant is generally tender, but the liver is not enlarged to palpation. Within a few days, jaundice appears, and the patient becomes somnolent and eventually comatose. Hematemesis and spontaneous bleeding result when the patient develops hypoprothrombinemia and disseminated intravascular coagulation (DIC). Oliguria, metabolic acidosis, and eventually anuria occur in approximately 50 percent of patients with acute fatty liver of pregnancy.[8] If the disease is allowed to progress, labor begins and the patient delivers a stillborn infant. During the immediate postpartum period, the mother becomes febrile, comatose and, without therapy, dies within a few days. DIC, renal failure, profound hypoglycemia, and occasionally pancreatitis are the most often cited immediate causes of death.[2,8,9]

The primary differential diagnoses in cases of acute fatty liver include fulminant hepatitis and the liver dysfunction associated

Table 24–14. DIFFERENTIAL DIAGNOSIS OF LIVER DISEASE IN PREGNANCY

	Serum Transaminase Levels (IU/L)	Bilirubin Level (mg/dl)	Coagulopathy	Histology	Other Features
Acute hepatitis B	>1,000	>5	-	Hepatocellular necrosis	Potential for perinatal transmission
Acute fatty liver	<500	<5	+	Fatty infiltration	Coma, renal failure, hypoglycemia
Intrahepatic cholestasis	<300	<5, mostly direct	-	Dilated bile canaliculi	Pruritus, increased bile acids
HELLP	>500	<5	+	Variable periportal necrosis	Hypertension, edema, thrombocytopenia

HELLP, *h*emolysis, *e*levated *l*iver enzymes, *l*ow *p*latelets; –, absent; +, present.

with the HELLP syndrome (*h*emolysis, *e*levated *l*iver enzymes, and *l*ow *p*latelet count) or preeclampsia (Table 24–14).[14–16]

Laboratory Diagnosis

In acute fatty liver of pregnancy, serum transaminase levels are elevated but usually remain below 500 IU/L.[5] In acute hepatitis, however, these levels are frequently above 1,000 IU/L. In liver dysfunction associated with preeclampsia or the HELLP syndrome, the transaminases are often in the same range as in acute fatty liver of pregnancy, but are occasionally higher. As a result of DIC, the prothrombin time and activated partial thromboplastin time (aPTT) are often prolonged. The prothrombin time is usually increased before the aPTT because it reflects the vitamin K–dependent clotting factors synthesized in the liver. A decreased fibrinogen level is accompanied by an elevation in fibrin degradation products, the D-dimer, and prothrombin.[1,2] Although the serum bilirubin level is elevated, it usually remains below 5 mg/dl and only rarely rises as high as 10 mg/dl, a level lower than one would expect in acute hepatitis. A liver biopsy specimen will reveal pericentral microvesicular fatty change.

Management

Once the diagnosis has been established, delivery should be accomplished as quickly as is safely possible.[35] Important supportive measures must first be undertaken to ensure maternal well-being. The patient's coagulopathy must be corrected with fresh frozen plasma. If more concentrated fibrinogen is needed, cryoprecipitate can be administered. Intravenous fluids containing adequate glucose should be given. This will prevent hypoglycemia, which can be fatal. If there is not a severe coagulopathy or the coagulopathy has been corrected, invasive hemodynamic monitoring may be instituted if necessary before delivery. This technique will allow the anesthesiologist and obstetrician to monitor the patient's fluid status.

Delivery soon after diagnosis is paramount. Vaginal delivery is preferable. Cesarean delivery, however, is warranted if it appears that delivery cannot be effected in a timely fashion, and the patient is deteriorating. If the patient's coagulopathy has been corrected, epidural anesthesia is the best choice. Spinal anesthesia can also be used. Regional anesthesia is preferable, because it allows adequate assessment of the patient's level of consciousness. General anesthesia should be avoided if possible because of the hepatotoxicity of some anesthetic agents. Narcotic doses must be adjusted, as these drugs are metabolized by the liver.

INTRAHEPATIC CHOLESTASIS OF PREGNANCY

Intrahepatic cholestasis is characterized by pruritus and mild jaundice usually occurring in the last trimester of pregnancy. It can, however, occur earlier in gestations. It has an uneven worldwide incidence of 1 in 1,000 to 1 in 10,000 deliveries.[39] Intrahepatic cholestasis tends to recur in subsequent pregnancies, but the severity may vary from one pregnancy to the next.

Clinical Manifestations

Patients with intrahepatic cholestasis usually begin having pruritus at night. It progresses, and the patient is soon experiencing bothersome pruritus continuously. Approximately 2 weeks later, clinical jaundice will develop in 50 percent of cases. The jaundice is usually mild, soon plateaus, and remains constant until delivery. The pruritus worsens with the onset of jaundice, and the patient's skin can become excoriated. The symptoms usually abate within 2 days after delivery. The differential diagnosis must include viral hepatitis and gallbladder disease.

Laboratory Findings

Serum alkaline phosphatase levels are increased 5- to 10-fold in intrahepatic cholestasis of pregnancy. Alkaline phosphatase, however, is normally increased in pregnancy. This is due to placental production of this enzyme. Upon fractionation, most of the alkaline phosphatase is hepatic in origin rather than placental. Serum 5'-nucleotidase levels are also increased. Bilirubin is elevated, but usually not above 5 mg/dl. Most is the direct, conjugated form. If intrahepatic cholestasis lasts for several weeks, liver dysfunction may result in decreased vitamin K reabsorption or decreased prothrombin production, leading to a prolongation of the prothrombin time. Serum transaminase levels are usually normal or moderately elevated, remaining well below the levels associated with viral hepatitis. Serum cholesterol and triglyceride levels may also be markedly elevated.

The serum bile acids (chenodeoxycholic acid, deoxycholic acid, and cholic acid) are increased. The levels are often more than 10 times the normal concentration. These acids are deposited in the skin and probably cause the extreme pruritus. The degree of pruritus, however, is not always related to the serum level of bile acids.[47] To make the diagnosis of intrahepatic cholestasis of pregnancy, the fasting levels of serum bile acids should be at least three times the upper limit of normal. Elevation of serum bile acids alone cannot be used to make the diagnosis. The patient must also have clinical symptoms.

Perinatal Outcome

The risk of preterm birth and fetal death may be increased in patients suffering from intrahepatic cholestasis of pregnancy.[51-54] Antepartum fetal heart rate testing and intense surveillance should be undertaken in gravidas with intrahepatic cholestasis of pregnancy. It may also be prudent to induce labor at term or when amniotic fluid studies indicate fetal lung maturity.[55]

Management

Treatment is aimed at reducing the intense pruritus. Diphenhydramine, hydroxyzine, and other antihistamines help only slightly. Cholestyramine is an anion-binding resin that interrupts the enterohepatic circulation, reducing the reabsorption of bile acids. A total of 8 to 16 g/day in three to four divided doses is often helpful in relieving pruritus. It is most effective if started as soon as the pruritus is noted, before it becomes severe. It often takes up to 2 weeks to work. Because cholestyramine also interferes with vitamin K absorption, the prothrombin time should be checked at least weekly. If prolonged, parenteral vitamin K should be administered. When the prothrombin time returns to normal, the frequency of injections can be decreased. Cholestyramine causes a sensation of bloating and often results in constipation. Cholestyramine also can interfere with the absorption of other ingested medications, including prenatal vitamins. If the patient cannot tolerate cholestyramine, antacids containing aluminum may be used to bind bile acids. These medications are usually not as effective as cholestyramine. Phenobarbital, in a dose of up to 90 mg daily given at bedtime, can be helpful. It is important to remember that phenobarbital must not be given within 2 hours of cholestyramine, or the phenobarbital will be bound and excreted without being absorbed. The key to treating pregnancy-induced cholestasis is to begin therapy as soon as the diagnosis is made. Dexamethasone has also been used with some success in treating pregnancy-induced cholestasis.

The two most recently studied medications for the treatment of intrahepatic cholestasis of pregnancy are S-adenyl-methionine (SAM-e) and ursodeoxycholic acid (UDCA). A combination of both drugs is more effective than either drug alone.[64] The dosage of UDCA is 14 to 16 mg/kg/day.[65,66]

Because of intolerable pruritus and the possible impact on perinatal outcome, delivery may be undertaken at term or as soon as fetal lung maturity has been documented. Jaundice usually disappears within 2 days after delivery. The patient should be counseled that the condition may recur during subsequent pregnancies.[40] It is also important to note that some patients may manifest symptoms of intrahepatic cholestasis when taking oral contraceptives.[41,68]

Key Points

➤ Acute fatty liver of pregnancy is a medical emergency requiring stabilization of the patient and timely delivery. Almost all cases will be complicated by disseminated intravascular coagulation.

➤ Liver transaminase levels in acute fatty liver of pregnancy are lower than what one would see in acute hepatitis.

➤ Profound hypoglycemia is a frequent concomitant of acute fatty liver and can cause death if untreated.

➤ Pregnancy-induced cholestasis usually occurs in the third trimester, causing intense pruritus and jaundice. Elevated serum bile acids are the best laboratory test for making the diagnosis in symptomatic patients.

Gastrointestinal Disease

MARK B. LANDON

PEPTIC ULCER DISEASE

The symptoms and complications of peptic ulcer seem to decrease during pregnancy. Several factors might improve the clinical course of patients with peptic ulcer disease during pregnancy. Patients with duodenal ulcer have higher levels of basal and stimulated acid secretion. The amelioration of symptoms during pregnancy may in part be secondary to progesterone-induced lower gastric acid output as well as increased mucus production. The latter may exert a protective effect on the intestinal mucosa. Plasma levels of placental histaminase increase dramatically during pregnancy and may be responsible for a decline in gastric acid output in patients who exhibit hyperacidity in the nonpregnant state.[3] Finally, pregnancy may favorably affect the gastric and duodenal mucosa's ability to regenerate as a result of increased levels of epidermal growth factor.[4]

Most physicians, when evaluating pregnant women with dyspepsia, attribute this complaint to gastric reflux in the lower esophagus. Heartburn is most often observed in the second and third trimesters. It usually responds to antacid therapy, and minimizing reflux by having the mother assume a semirecumbent position when she is supine. This regimen will often bring relief to patients with underlying peptic ulcer disease as well, and further diagnostic procedures are rarely needed. Duodenal ulcers produce either sharp or burning epigastric pain that is episodic following meals or it may awaken patients from sleep. Pain radiating to the back suggests posterior penetration. In patients with profound pain that is unresponsive to antacid regimens, panendoscopic examination of the stomach and upper duodenum may be performed. These procedures performed with appropriate analgesia are generally well tolerated during pregnancy.

The primary medical treatment for the symptomatic patient with peptic ulcer disease during pregnancy remains antacid therapy and diet. Administration of antacid 1 hour after meals and at bedtime usually provides relief of symptoms and promotes ulcer healing. In

715

refractory cases, a dose may be added at 3 hours after meals. It is important to be aware that potential side effects of antacid therapy exist. Patients with peptic ulcer disease should be maintained on a normal diet, avoiding caffeine, salicylates, ethanol, or any gastric stimulant that aggravates their condition. Because basal acid output may normally rise during evening hours, it follows that patients should avoid bedtime snacks.

H_2 antagonists continue to remain a second-line choice for therapy in pregnancy. If possible, these agents should be reserved for use during the second and third trimesters.[6] Cimetidine, ranitidine, and famotidine are category B medications.[7] The use of omeprazole, a powerful inhibitor of acid secretion, has been limited during pregnancy. Elective treatment of *H. pylori* with antibiotics and bismuth subsalicylate is generally recommended following delivery and breast-feeding.

ACUTE PANCREATITIS

There is a greater association of gallstones with the development of pancreatitis during gestation. Other causes for pancreatitis include hyperlipidemia, idiopathic factors, infection, previous surgery, preeclampsia, hyperparathyroidism, thiazide ingestion, and penetrating duodenal ulcer. The normal hypertriglyceridemia of pregnancy may be exaggerated in patients with hyperlipidemia, thereby inducing acute pancreatitis.[14] The clinical presentation of pancreatitis is not significantly altered in pregnancy.

In evaluating the pregnant patient with suspected pancreatitis, the differential diagnosis includes most causes of abdominal pain in young women. These are principally peptic ulcer disease including perforation, acute cholecystitis, biliary colic, and intestinal obstruction. Specific tests employed to corroborate the diagnosis of pancreatitis rely on the measurement of pancreatic enzymes, principally amylase. Elevated values should suggest pancreatitis, although they may be present with other conditions such as cholecystitis, intestinal obstruction, peptic ulcer disease, hepatic trauma, and ruptured ectopic pregnancy. Serum lipase levels should also be measured in suspected cases.

In most cases, acute pancreatitis resolves spontaneously within several days. However, in some 10 percent of cases, the illness is complicated and such patients are best managed in an intensive care environment. Pancreatic secretory activity should be reduced by keeping the patient NPO. Nasogastric suction is reserved for those with nausea and vomiting. Meperidine is the drug of choice for analgesia as, unlike morphine, it does not constrict the sphincter of Oddi. Fluid and electrolyte replacement, and serial laboratory assays of hemoglobin, white blood cell count, amylase, liver function enzymes, glucose, and calcium are essential. In advanced cases, hypocalcemia may be present, and calcium replacement is necessary. Patients who have been unable to eat for periods of greater than 1 week may benefit from intravenous alimentation.

Percutaneous aspiration of pancreatic exudate is important in refractory cases. This CT-guided procedure may be necessary to distinguish between sterile and infected pancreatic necrosis. For infected cases, surgical drainage of the pancreatic exudate is necessary.

INFLAMMATORY BOWEL DISEASE

The inflammatory bowel diseases, ulcerative colitis (UC) and Crohn's disease (CD), or regional enteritis, are idiopathic disorders that have their peak incidence in the reproductive age group. The prevalence of UC in the female population under 40 years of age is 40 to 100 per 100,000.[18] CD is considerably less common than UC with an incidence of 2 to 4 per 100,000. The average age of onset is between 20 and 30 years. CD, in contrast to UC, tends to run a more subacute and chronic course, with symptoms including fever, diarrhea, and cramping abdominal pain.[19] CD may be found anywhere from mouth to anus including the perineum. However, the distal ileum, colon, and anorectal region are most frequently involved.

Ulcerative Colitis

Patients with inactive UC at the start of pregnancy have the best prognosis in terms of perinatal and maternal outcome, while those whose UC has its onset in pregnancy or is active have the highest rate of complication. Overall, pregnancy outcome is good for most women with UC.

Crohn's Disease

Studies describing the effect of CD on pregnancy suggest minimal if any increased risk to both mother and fetus, although the rate of spontaneous abortion and preterm delivery may be higher in women with active CD. Overall, the risk of exacerbation during pregnancy is not higher than that in the nonpregnant population.[31]

Treatment of Inflammatory Bowel Disease During Pregnancy

The medical treatment of inflammatory bowel disease is not altered greatly by pregnancy. All patients should be followed closely so that the activity of their disease may be assessed and psychological support can be provided. Dietary counseling for patients with UC should emphasize proper nutritional intake. Patients with mild disease may respond to a low-roughage diet or the exclusion of milk products if they are lactose intolerant. Patients with CD often benefit from low-residue diets, presumably because the caliber of their small bowel may be limited by inflammation.

The initial therapy for inflammatory bowel disease during pregnancy is 5-aminosalicylic acid (5-ASA) products and corticosteroid therapy. The safety of both of these classes of medication has been well established in pregnancy. Sulfasalazine (Azulfidine) is most effective in maintaining remission and preventing further attacks. Patients who present early in pregnancy on sulfasalazine for a recent flare of their disease should probably be maintained on this therapy, as active colitis may develop if the drug is discontinued. The active metabolite of sulfasalazine, 5-ASA and its N-acetyl derivative, are also available for treatment.[35] Sulfasalazine and 5-ASA can be given safely to nursing mothers.[36] Steroids are indicated in patients who fail to respond to simple supportive measures.

Surgical Treatment

Although most acute episodes of inflammatory bowel disease respond to medical treatment, operative intervention will occasionally be necessary to treat perforation, obstruction, or patients unresponsive to standard therapies.

Ileostomy and colostomy function during pregnancy are normal in most cases. Complications from an episiotomy have been uncommon in patients previously operated on for UC. The higher rate of perineal involvement in patients with CD should warrant a thorough evaluation before contemplating vaginal delivery, especially for women with CD who have undergone a proctocolectomy.

Key Points

➤ Women with peptic ulcer disease usually have improvement in symptoms during pregnancy. Primary medical treatment for symptomatic cases is antacid therapy and diet. Secondary therapy is H_2 blockers.

Box continued on opposite page

Key Points *Continued*

➤ Most cases of pancreatitis during pregnancy are associated with gallstones. Conservative supportive care aimed at decreasing pancreatic secretion is generally successful.

➤ Women with active ulcerative colitis in early pregnancy usually have recurrent flare-ups during gestation and postpartum.

➤ The onset of ulcerative colitis or Crohn's disease during pregnancy is associated with increased miscarriage and fetal loss rates.

➤ Sulfasalazine (Azulfidine) and 5-ASA metabolite drugs may be safely used to treat inflammatory bowel disease during pregnancy and in lactating women.

Neurologic Disorders

PHILIP SAMUELS

SEIZURE DISORDERS

Affecting approximately 1 percent of the general population, seizure disorders are the most frequent major neurologic complication encountered in pregnancy. Seizure disorders may be divided into those that are acquired and those that are idiopathic.

In general, initial therapy is based on the type of seizure disorder experienced by the patient. There are, however, many crossovers, and patients may respond differently to each medication despite their seizure type. Furthermore, patients may be placed on a certain medication because they did not tolerate the side-effect profile of another anticonvulsant (Table 24–15). The obstetrician and neurologist must work closely together to guide the patient through her pregnancy and find the safest and most effective medical therapy for the patient. Through this cooperation, the vast majority of pregnant women with seizure disorders can have a successful pregnancy with minimal risk to mother and fetus.

Effects of Epilepsy on Reproductive Function

Contraception may present a challenge to women with epilepsy, and the use of oral contraceptives may require special adjustments because certain antiepileptic medications have been associated with contraceptive failure. Carbamazepine, phenobarbital, and phenytoin enhance the activities of hepatic microsomal oxidative enzymes.[1] This increased enzymatic activity may lead to rapid clearance of these hormones, which may allow ovulation to occur. Therefore, medicated patients taking low-dose oral con-traceptives may have more breakthrough bleeding[2] and may be at increased risk for unplanned pregnancy.[3,4] This rapid clearance does not appear to be induced by valproate or benzodiazepines.[1]

Table 24–15. COMMON SIDE EFFECTS OF ANTICONVULSANTS

Drug	Maternal Effects	Fetal Effects
Phenytoin	Nystagmus, ataxia, hirsutism, gingival hyperplasia, megaloblastic anemia	Possible teratogenesis and carcinogenesis, coagulopathy, hypocalcemia
Phenobarbital	Drowsiness, ataxia	Possible teratogenesis, coagulopathy, neonatal depression, withdrawal
Primidone	Drowsiness, ataxia, nausea	Possible teratogenesis, coagulopathy, neonatal depression
Carbamazepine	Drowsiness, leukopenia, ataxia, mild hepatotoxicity	Possible craniofacial and neural tube defects
Valproic acid	Ataxia, drowsiness, alopecia, hepatotoxicity, thrombocytopenia	Neural tube defects and possible craniofacial and skeletal defects
Ethosuximide	Nausea, hepatotoxicity, leukopenia, thrombocytopenia	Possible teratogenesis

Effect of Pregnancy on Epilepsy

Between 30 percent and 50 percent of patients will show an increase in seizure frequency during pregnancy. Patients with more frequent seizures tend to have exacerbations during pregnancy.[8] However, with a compliant patient and close surveillance, seizure frequency should remain the same or even improve in most epileptic patients during pregnancy.

Effects of Pregnancy on the Disposition of Anticonvulsant Medications

Levels of anticonvulsant medications can change dramatically during pregnancy, usually decreasing in total concentration as pregnancy progresses. Altered protein binding, delayed gastric emptying, nausea and vomiting, changes in plasma volume, and changes in the volume of distribution can affect the levels of anticonvulsant medications. Free levels of phenobarbital, carbamazepine, and phenytoin rise significantly throughout pregnancy while total levels fall. Therefore, the nonpregnant relationship between total drug and free (active) drug is not maintained. Free phenytoin levels, should be measured if possible. If free levels are unavailable, drug doses should be adjusted according to the total serum level and the clinical picture. If the patient has increased seizure activity, medication doses should be increased as long as the patient is not showing signs of toxicity. Likewise, if the medication level is low but the patient is seizure free, no adjustment in dosing is necessary.

All anticonvulsants interfere with folic acid metabolism. Patients on anticonvulsants may actually become folic acid deficient and develop macrocytic anemia. Folic acid deficiency has been associated with neural tube defects and other congenital malformations.[15,16] Because organogenesis occurs during the first weeks after conception, folic acid supplementation should be begun before pregnancy if possible. A dose of 4 mg daily is more than sufficient.

Neonatal hemorrhage, due to decreased vitamin K–dependent clotting factors (II, VII, IX, X), has been seen in infants born to mothers taking phenobarbital, phenytoin, and primidone.[18] Therefore, infants should be given 1 mg of vitamin K intramuscularly.

Effect of Epilepsy on Pregnancy

The majority of women with seizure disorders who become pregnant will have an uneventful pregnancy with an excellent outcome. Several complications may be more prevalent in the mother with epilepsy than in the general population including intrauterine growth restriction (IUGR), fetal death, and preeclampsia.

Effects of Anticonvulsant Medications on the Fetus

Anticonvulsant medications are associated with an increase in congenital malformations, but the magnitude of this risk and the association of certain anomalies with specific drugs remain debatable. A specific fetal hydantoin syndrome has been well characterized and includes growth and performance delays, craniofacial abnormalities (including clefting), and limb anomalies (including hypoplasia of nails and distal phalanges). Approximately 7 to 11 percent of infants exposed to phenytoin exhibit this recognizable pattern of malformations, while 31 percent of exposed fetuses had some aspects of the syndrome.

It remains of prime importance, to treat the patient with the medication that best controls her seizures. Patients treated with a single anticonvalsant have infants with a lower rate of anomalies than women on multiple drug regimens.

There is an association between neural tube defects and valproate exposure in utero. A 1.5 percent risk has been reported if the mother uses took valproate in the first trimester.

Carbamazepine was once thought to be safer than other anticonvulsant medications for use in pregnancy, but a pattern of minor craniofacial defects, fingernail hypoplasia, and developmental delay to now recognized in infants exposed in utero to carbamazepine. There is also a 1 percent risk of spina bifida in infants of mothers taking carbamazepine.

New antiepileptic drugs have been approved and are now being used in pregnant patients (Table 24–16). These newer medications work at the level of neurotransmitters such as γ aminobutyric acid (GABA) and also by blockade of sodium channels.

Table 24–16. NEWER ANTIEPILEPTIC AGENTS

Medication	Usual Dose (mg/day)	Doses/Day	Special Notes
Gabapentin	1,200–3,600	3	Not enzyme inducer Antacids interfere
Lamotrigine	300–500	1 or 2	Rash in 11.2% Half-life affected by meds
Topiramate	100–400	2	May interfere with O.C.s
Tiagabine	8–56	2 to 4	Does not interfere with O.C.s

Gabapentin is probably the most frequently used of these medications. It is only approved for use as an adjunct to other medications, but may soon have an indication for monotherapy. The usual maintenance dose is 900 to 2,400 mg daily in three divided doses, but doses up to 3,600 mg have been administered with only a minor increase in side effects. At present there are no studies of its safety in pregnancy.

Preconceptual Counseling for the Reproductive Age Woman with a Seizure Disorder

Although not always possible, it is preferable to counsel the patient with epilepsy before she becomes pregnant. The obstetrician must stress that the patient has greater than a 90 percent chance of having a successful pregnancy resulting in a normal newborn. The patient must be informed that if she has frequent seizures before conception, this pattern will probably continue. If she has frequent seizures, she should delay conception until control is better, even if this entails a change or addition of medication. The patient will need to take whatever medication(s) are necessary to achieve this goal throughout her pregnancy. If the patient has had no seizures during the past 2 to 5 years, an attempt may be made to withdraw her from anticonvulsant medications.

Care of the Patient During Pregnancy

Once the patient becomes pregnant, it is of the utmost importance to establish accurate gestational dating. This will prevent any confusion over fetal growth in later gestation. The patient's anticonvulsant level should be followed as needed and dosages adjusted accordingly to keep the patient seizure free. It is a common pitfall to monitor levels too frequently and adjust dosages in a likewise frequent manner. It is important to remember that it takes several half-lives for a medication to reach a steady state (Table 24–17). Drug levels should be drawn immediately before the next dose (trough levels) in order to assess if dosing is adequate. If the patient is showing signs of toxicity, a peak level may be obtained.

At approximately 16 weeks' gestation, the patient should undergo maternal serum marker screening in an attempt to detect neural tube defects. This, coupled with ultrasonography, gives a more than 90 percent detection rate for open neural tube defects. If the patient is difficult to scan or if she wants to be even more certain that there is no neural tube defect, an amniocentesis can be performed. This should be considered if the patient is taking valproate or carbamazepine, as these medications appear to carry almost the same risk as if the patient had a family history of a neural tube defect.[49,50,53]

Table 24–17. ANTICONVULSANTS COMMONLY USED DURING PREGNANCY

Drug	Therapeutic Level (mg/L)	Usual Nonpregnant Dosage	Half-Life
Carbamazepine	4–10	600–1,200 mg/day in three or divided doses (Two doses if extended-release forms are used)	Initially 36 h, chronic therapy 16 h
Phenobarbital	15–40	90–180 mg/day in two or three divided doses	100 h
Phenytoin	10–20, total; 1–2, free	300–500 mg/day in single or divided doses*	Avg 24 h
Primidone	5–15	750–1,500 mg/day in three divided doses	8 h
Valproic acid	50–100	550–2,000 mg/day in three or divided doses	Avg 13 h

*If a total dose of more than 300 mg is needed, dividing the dose will result in a more stable serum concentration.

At 18 to 22 weeks, the patient should undergo a comprehensive, targeted, ultrasound examination by an experienced obstetric sonographer to look for congenital malformations.

As previously noted, there appears to be an increased risk for intrauterine growth restriction for fetuses exposed in utero to anticonvulsant medications. If the patient's weight gain and fundal growth appear appropriate, regular ultrasound examinations for fetal weight assessment are probably unnecessary. If, however, there is a question of fundal growth or if the patient's habitus precludes adequate assessment of this clinical parameter, serial ultrasonography for fetal weight assessment can be performed.

In older and retrospective studies, there appears to be an increased risk of stillbirth in mothers taking anticonvulsant medications.[7,20-22] In a prospective study, however, this complication was not seen.[23] Non-stress testing, therefore, is not necessary in all mothers with seizure disorders. It should be limited to those who have other medical or obstetric complications that place the patient at increased risk of stillbirth.

If at all possible, the patient should be maintained on a single medication, and drug levels should be drawn at appropriate intervals to make certain that the patient is receiving enough medication. If the patient is taking phenytoin, free levels should be obtained if possible. It is best to use the lowest dose of a single medication possible that will keep the patient seizure free.

Labor and Delivery

Vaginal delivery is the route of choice for the mother with a seizure disorder. If the mother has frequent seizures brought on by the stress of labor, she may undergo cesarean delivery after stabilization. Seizures during labor may cause transient fetal bradycardia.[23]

Management of anticonvulsant medications during a prolonged labor presents a challenge. During labor, oral absorption of medications is erratic and, if the patient vomits, almost negligible. If the patient is taking phenytoin or phenobarbital, these medications may be administered parenterally. An anticonvulsant level should be obtained first to help ascertain the appropriate dosage. Phenobarbital may be given intramuscularly, and phenytoin may be given intravenously. Fosphenytoin, although expensive, is available and makes the administration of intravenous phenytoin much easier.

Carbamazepine is not manufactured in a parenteral form, although extended-release forms now exist. Oral administration may be attempted, but, if the patient has seizures or a pre-seizure aura, she may be loaded with a therapeutic dose of phenytoin to carry her through labor. The usual loading dose is 10 to 15 mg/kg administered intravenously at a rate no faster than 50 mg/min.

New Onset of Seizures in Pregnancy and the Puerperium

Occasionally, seizures will be diagnosed for the first time during pregnancy. This may present a diagnostic dilemma (Table 24–18).

Postpartum Period

The levels of anticonvulsant medications must be monitored frequently during the first few weeks postpartum, as they can rapidly rise. If the patient's medication dosages were increased during pregnancy, they will need to be decreased rather rapidly after delivery to prepregnancy levels. All of the major anticonvulsant medications cross into breast milk.[67,70] The use of these medications, however, is not a contraindication to breast-feeding.

All methods of contraception are available to women with idiopathic seizure disorders. The majority of women are able to take oral contraceptives without any adverse side effects.[71] Oral contraceptive failures are more common in women taking anticonvulsants.

MIGRAINE

Headaches are extremely common in women, and the majority of migraine headaches occur in women of childbearing age. Migraine symptoms tend to improve during pregnancy[73–75] Most patients experience either complete remission or a significant percent reduction in headaches during pregnancy.

Supportive therapy is recommended for patients who experience migraine attacks during gestation. Both narcotic and nonnarcotic analgesics can be used as necessary. The use of nonsteroidal anti-inflammatory agents should be avoided if possible in late pregnancy. When pain is severe, parenteral narcotics and appropriate anti-emetic therapy may be used. β-Blockers, calcium channel blockers, tricyclic anti-depressants, and fluoxetine have been successfully used for migraine prophylaxis during pregnancy. Ergotamine is best avoided during pregnancy. Sumatriptan, should only be used if the physician feels that the potential benefits clearly outweigh the potential of increased risk for preterm birth and IUGR. In a review by O'Quinn and colleagues, there were no untoward effects in 76 first-trimester exposures to sumatriptan.[81] Using logistic regression, Olesen and colleagues[82] compared 34 sumatriptan exposures to 89 migraine controls and 15,995 healthy women. They found the risk of preterm birth was elevated (odds ratio 6.3). They also found the risk of IUGR was greater.[82] They do state that they did not control for disease severity.

Table 24–18. DIFFERENTIAL DIAGNOSIS OF PERIPARTUM SEIZURES

	Blood Pressure	Proteinuria	Seizures	Timing	CSF	Other Features
Eclampsia	+++	+++	+++	Third trimester	Early: RBC, 0–1,000; protein, 50–150 mg/dl Late: grossly bloody	Platelets normal or ↓ RBC normal
Epilepsy	Normal	Normal to +	+++	Any trimester	Normal	Low anticonvulsant levels
Subarachnoid hemorrhage	+ to +++ (labile)	0 to +	+	Any trimester	Grossly bloody	
Thrombotic thrombocytopenic purpura	Normal to +++	++	++	Third trimester	RBC 0–100	Platelets ↓ RBC fragmented
Amniotic fluid embolus	Shock	−	+	Intrapartum	Normal	Hypoxia, cyanosis Platelets ↓ → RBC normal
Cerebral vein thrombosis	+	−	++	Postpartum	Normal (early)	Headache Occasional pelvic phlebitis

Table continued on following page

Table 24–18. DIFFERENTIAL DIAGNOSIS OF PERIPARTUM SEIZURES *Continued*

	Blood Pressure	Proteinuria	Seizures	Timing	CSF	Other Features
Water intoxication	Normal	–	++	Intrapartum	Normal	Oxytocin infusion rate >45 mU/min Serum Na <124 mEq/L
Pheochromocytoma	+++ (labile)	+	+	Any trimester	Normal	Neurofibromatosis
Autonomic stress syndrome of high paraplegics	+++ with labor pains	–	–	Intrapartum	Normal	Cardiac arrhythmia
Toxicity of local anesthetics	Variable	–	++	Intrapartum	Normal	

Modified from Donaldson JO: Peripartum convulsions. *In* Donaldson JO (ed): Neurology of Pregnancy. Philadelphia, WB Saunders, 1989, p 312.

CARPAL TUNNEL SYNDROME

The median nerve and flexor tendons pass through the carpal tunnel, which has little room for expansion. If the wrist is extremely flexed or extended, the volume of the carpal tunnel is reduced. In pregnancy, weight gain and edema further restrict the tunnel and predispose to the carpal tunnel syndrome. Compression of the median nerve leads to pain, numbness, and/or tingling in the distribution of the median nerve in the hand and wrist. This includes the thumb, index finger, long finger, and radial side of the ring finger on the palmar aspect. In severe cases, weakness and decreased motor function can occur.

Supportive and conservative therapies are usually adequate for the treatment of carpal tunnel syndrome. Symptoms usually subside in the postpartum period as total body water returns to normal.[127] Splints placed on the dorsum of the hand, which keep the wrist in a neutral position and maximize the capacity of the carpal tunnel, often provide dramatic relief. The splints are usually worn during the night. Local injections of glucocorticoids may also be used in severe cases.

Key Points

➤ Idiopathic seizures affect approximately 1 percent of the general population and are the most frequent neurologic complication of pregnancy.

➤ Prepregnancy counseling is imperative in the patient with a seizure disorder, and preconceptual folic acid therapy should be implemented under the direction of an obstetrician and a neurologist.

➤ Those with seizures occurring less than once each month will have the best control during pregnancy.

➤ The anticonvulsant medication that best controls the patient's seizures should be used during pregnancy.

➤ Because of the changes in plasma volume, drug distribution, and metabolism that occur during pregnancy, anticonvulsant levels should be checked frequently and dosages adjusted accordingly.

Box continued on following page

Key Points *Continued*

➤ Patients taking anticonvulsants have an increased risk of giving birth to an infant with both major and minor anomalies, but this risk is probably less than 10 percent. Therefore, the majority of patients with epilepsy will give birth to healthy infants.

➤ Carbamazepine and valproate are associated with neural tube defects, and these patients should receive 4 mg folic acid daily before and during early pregnancy.

➤ The vasoconstrictor drugs used to treat migraines should be avoided during pregnancy and lactation.

➤ Carpal tunnel syndrome is common in pregnancy and usually responds to conservative splinting and/or glucocorticoid injection. Surgery can be safely undertaken if indicated during pregnancy.

Malignant Diseases and Pregnancy

LARRY J. COPELAND AND MARK B. LANDON

While cancer is the second most common cause of death for women in their reproductive years, only about 1 in 1,000 pregnancies[1] is complicated by cancer. A successful outcome is dependent on a cooperative multidisciplinary approach. The malignancies most commonly encountered in the pregnant patient are, in descending order, breast cancer, cervical cancer, melanoma, ovarian cancer, thyroid cancer, leukemia, lymphoma, and colorectal cancer.[3]

CHEMOTHERAPY DURING PREGNANCY

Drug Effects on the Fetus

Delayed Effects

In summary, the risks of exposing a fetus to chemotherapy correlate highly with the gestational age at the time of the exposure. Most organogenesis occurs between 3 and 8 weeks of embryonic life, and it is during this time that major morphologic abnormalities are most likely to occur from exposure to any chemotherapeutic agent. Second- and third-trimester chemotherapy exposure does not appear to carry a significantly increased risk of major fetal anomalies. Disruption of the ductal system may increase the rate of mastitis. Breast-feeding is contraindicated in women receiving chemotherapy, since significant levels can be found in breast milk.

PREGNANCY FOLLOWING CANCER TREATMENT

With improved survival rates for many childhood and adolescent malignancies, one must be prepared to offer prenatal counseling to the young woman who presents with a personal cancer history. Issues

> **Counseling Issues for Pregnancy Following Cancer Treatment**
>
> 1. What is the risk of recurrence of the malignancy?
> 2. If a recurrence was diagnosed, depending on the most likely sites, what would be the nature of the probable treatment? How would such treatment compromise both the patient and the fetus?
> 3. Will prior treatments—pelvic surgery, radiation to pelvis or abdomen, or chemotherapy—affect fertility or reproductive outcome?
> 4. Will the hormonal milieu of pregnancy adversely affect an estrogen-receptor–positive tumor?

worthy of review and in need of clarification for the obstetrician and the patient are listed in the box "Counseling Issues for Pregnancy Following Cancer Treatment."

CANCER DURING PREGNANCY

General Considerations

The risk of having a coincident malignant tumor during pregnancy is approximately 0.1 percent. Approximately one third of recorded maternal deaths are secondary to a coexisting malignancy. Delays in diagnosis of the cancer during pregnancy are common for a number of reasons: (1) many of the presenting symptoms of cancer are often attributed to the pregnancy; (2) many of the physiologic and anatomic alterations of pregnancy can compromise the physical examination; (3) many serum tumor markers (β-human chorionic gonadotropin [hCGs], α-fetoprotein, CA 125, and others) are increased during pregnancy; and (4) our ability to perform either imaging studies or invasive diagnostic procedures is often altered during pregnancy.

Since the gestational age is significant when evaluating the risks of treatments, it is important to determine gestational age accurately. An early ultrasound evaluation may be useful in this regard.

BREAST CANCER

The predicted number of breast cancer cases in women in the United States for the year 2000 is 184,200, and the predicted number of related deaths is 41,200.[34] Approximately 2 to 3 percent of all breast cancers in women under age 40 occur concurrent with pregnancy or lactation, and approximately 1 in 1,360 to 3,330 pregnancies is complicated by breast cancer.[35]

Paradoxically, carriers of BRCA1 and BRCA2 mutations may have an increased risk of developing breast cancer by having children.[38]

Diagnosis and Staging

Breast abnormalities should be evaluated in the same manner as if the patient were not pregnant. The most common presentation of breast cancer in pregnancy is a painless lump discovered by the patient. Despite the striking physiologic breast changes of pregnancy, including nipple enlargement and increases in glandular tissue resulting in engorgement and tenderness, breast cancer should be screened for during pregnancy. Since the breast changes become more pronounced in later pregnancy, it is important to perform a thorough breast examination at the initial visit. Diagnostic delays are often attributed to physician reluctance to evaluate breast complaints or abnormal findings in pregnancy. While bilateral serosanguinous discharge may be normal in late pregnancy, masses require prompt and definitive evaluation.

Mammography in pregnancy is controversial. While the radiation exposure to the fetus is negligible,[41] the hyperplastic breast of pregnancy is characterized by increased tissue density, making interpretation more difficult.[42]

Fine-needle aspiration (FNA) of a mass for cytologic study is recommended. FNA is reliable for a diagnosis of carcinoma (false-positive results are rare), but if a solid mass is negative for tumor it should be evaluated by excisional biopsy. Similar to the nonpregnant patient, approximately 20 percent of breast biopsies performed in pregnancy reveal cancer. Tissue biopsies should be submitted for estrogen receptor (ER) and progesterone receptor (PR) analyses. Consistent with the fact that these patients are young, the majority are receptor negative.[43]

Prior to proceeding with treatment, the patient requires staging. All draining lymph nodes should be evaluated. The contralateral breast must be carefully assessed. Laboratory tests should include baseline liver function tests and serum tumor markers, carcinoembryonic antigen (CEA), and CA 15-3. CA 15-3 appears to be a useful tumor marker for monitoring breast cancer in pregnancy.[44] A chest x-ray is indicated and, if the liver function tests are abnormal, the liver can be evaluated by ultrasound. With precautions of good hydration and insertion of a urinary bladder catheter, a bone scan can be performed in pregnancy. In a symptomatic patient, radiographs of the specific symptomatic bones are advised.

Breast cancers in pregnancy are histologically identical to the nonpregnant patient of the same age. Because inflammatory breast cancer can be mistaken for mastitis, a biopsy of breast tissue should be performed when a breast suspected of being infected is incised and drained.

Treatment

The usual criteria for breast-preserving therapy versus modified radical mastectomy pertain to the patient with breast cancer, stages I to III.[46] However, the option of lumpectomy, axillary node dissection, and irradiation is complicated by the presence of the pregnancy. Consideration should be given to the delay of irradiation until after delivery. At present, a harmful effect of continuing pregnancy has not been demonstrated in most published series.

Prognosis

As with any malignant disease, the prognosis best correlates with the anatomic extent of disease at the time of diagnosis. The presence and extent of nodal involvement is especially predictive of prognosis in both nonpregnant and pregnant patients. In the pregnant patient, the 5-year survival rate is 82 percent for patients with three or fewer positive nodes and 27 percent if greater than three nodes contain tumor.[45] Pregnancy, probably due to the associated delays in diagnosis, appears to increase the frequency of nodal disease, with 60 to 85 percent of patients exhibiting axillary nodal disease at diagnosis.[45,64]

When controlled for age and stage, pregnancy does not seem to affect prognosis adversely.[40,63,65,66] Some have suggested a worse prognosis if the cancer is diagnosed in the second trimester.[65]

Subsequent Pregnancy

While the consensus is that subsequent pregnancies do not adversely affect survival, there are recommendations regarding the timing of a subsequent pregnancy.[67,68] It is generally advised that women with node-negative disease wait for 2 to 3 years, and this interval should be extended to 5 years for patients with positive nodes.[69] It has been advised that patients should undergo a complete metastatic work-up prior to a subsequent pregnancy.

CERVICAL CANCER

Approximately 3 percent of all invasive cervical cancers occur during pregnancy. Cervical cancer is the most common gynecologic malignancy associated with pregnancy, occurring in approximately 1 per 2,200 pregnancies.[127-129] While some have suggested that the survival of patients with cervical cancer associated with pregnancy is compromised,[148] most reports indicate that the prognosis is not altered.[127-129,148,149]

All pregnant patients should be evaluated on their initial obstetric visit with visualization of the cervix and cervical cytology, including an endocervical brush. The general principles of screening for cervical neoplasia apply to the pregnant patient. The Papanicolaou smear is used to screen the normal-appearing cervix. If the cervix appears friable, cervical cytology alone may not be sufficient to alert the physician to the presence of a malignant tumor. False-negative cervical cytology is at increased risk in pregnancy due to excess mucus and bleeding from cervical eversion. Therefore, it is necessary to obtain a biopsy to ensure that tissue friability is not secondary to tumor. Also, an ulcerative or exophytic lesion must have histologic sampling performed. While approximately one third of pregnant patients with cervical cancer are asymptomatic at the time of diagnosis, the most common symptoms are vaginal bleeding or discharge.

The diagnosis of cervical cancer is commonly made postpartum rather than during pregnancy and, while stage IB disease is the most commonly diagnosed stage, all stages are represented in significant numbers. Both patient and physician factors, including lack of prenatal care, failure to obtain cervical cytology or to biopsy gross cervical abnormalities, false-negative cytology, and failure to evaluate abnormal cytology or vaginal bleeding properly, contribute to the delays in diagnosis.

Cervical cytology suggestive of a squamous intraepithelial lesion or a report of atypical glandular cells during pregnancy requires appropriate clinical evaluation (Fig. 24–7). The colposcopic evaluation of the pregnant cervix is altered by the physiologic changes of pregnancy and, since most practicing physicians will diagnose invasive cervical cancer associated with pregnancy only once or twice in their careers, it may be prudent to consult a gynecologic oncologist. While colposcopy during pregnancy is usually enhanced by the physiologic eversion of the lower endocervical canal, vascular changes and redundant vagina may alter or obscure normal visualization. During pregnancy, failure to visualize the entire transformation zone and squamocolumnar junction is uncommon. While endocervical curettage is not generally recommended during pregnancy, lesions involving the lower endocervical canal can often be directly visualized and

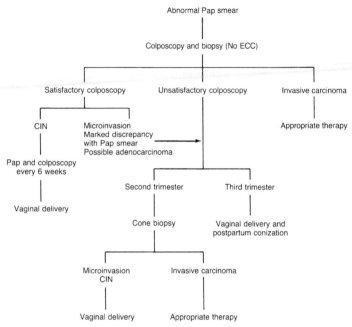

Figure 24–7. Suggested protocol for evaluation of abnormal cervical cytology in pregnancy. ECC, endocervical curettage; CIN, cervical intraepithelial neoplasia. (From Hacker NF, Berek JS, Lagasse LD, et al: Carcinoma of the cervix associated with pregnancy. Obstet Gynecol 59:735, 1982, with permission.)

biopsied. While the pregnant cervix is hypervascular, serious hemorrhage from an outpatient biopsy is uncommon, and the risk of bleeding is offset by the risk of missing an early invasive cancer. Following a coloposcopic evaluation with appropriate tissue sampling, most patients with preinvasive lesions can be followed with repeat colposcopy at 6- to 8-week intervals to delivery.[130,131]

Patients then require a careful and complete colposcopic evaluation 6 weeks' postpartum. Cone biopsy during pregnancy, when necessary, should ideally be performed during the second trimester to reduce the risks of first-trimester abortion and rupture of membranes or premature labor in the third trimester.[132–134] Complications from conization of the pregnant cervix are common. Therapeutic conization for intraepithelial squamous lesions is contraindicated during pregnancy. Diagnostic cone biopsy in pregnancy is reserved for patients whose colposcopic-directed biopsy has shown superficial invasion (suspect microinvasion) or in other situations where an invasive lesion is suspected but cannot be confirmed by biopsy. When a cone biopsy is necessary during pregnancy, one should keep in mind the anatomic alteration of the cervix secondary to pregnancy. A shallow disk-like cone is usually satisfactory to clarify the diagnosis with a minimum of morbidity. It should be kept in mind that patients who have had a conization during pregnancy are at higher risk for residual disease. Therefore, close follow-up is essential.

Following the diagnosis of invasive cervical cancer, a staging evaluation is indicated. The standard cervical staging is clinical and usually based on the results of physical examination, cystoscopy, proctoscopy, chest x-ray, and intravenous pyelogram. CT scan or, in some centers, lymphangiography is often performed to identify lymph node metastasis. In the pregnant patient, the standard staging evaluation is modified. The chest radiograph is performed with abdominal shielding. Sonography is used to detect hydronephrosis and, if additional retroperitoneal imaging is desired for the evaluation of lymphadenopathy, consideration should be given to using MRI.

Invasive, Early-Stage Disease

Since the definitive treatment of invasive cervical cancer is not compatible with pregnancy continuation, the clinical question that must be addressed is when to conclude the pregnancy so that therapy can be completed. Considering this requirement, treatment options will be influenced by gestational age, tumor stage and metastatic evaluation, and maternal desires and expectations regarding the pregnancy. The management of early invasive cervical cancer (stages IB and IIA) in the young patient is usually by radical hysterectomy, pelvic lymphadenectomy, and aortic lymph node sampling.[136] The primary advantage over radiation therapy for these patients is preservation of ovarian function. For the patient with a high probability of having a poor prognostic lesion and therefore requiring postoperative irradiation, consideration can be given to performing a unilateral or bilateral oophoropexy at the time of the hysterectomy. The ovarian suspension should be intraperitoneal, as retroperitoneal placement seems to predispose to subsequent ovarian cyst formation. In the first trimester, this surgery is usually carried out with the fetus in utero. In the third trimester, the radical hysterectomy and pelvic lymphadenectomy are performed after completion of a high classic cesarean delivery. Delays in therapeutic intervention have not been reported to increase recurrence rates for patients with small-volume stage I disease.[138] While the pelvic vessels are large, the dissection is enhanced by more easily defined tissue planes.[139,140]

Second-trimester situations are more problematic. Serious consideration should be given to administering one to three cycles of platinum-based chemotherapy and thereby allowing an additional 7 to 15 weeks of fetal maturation. In one study, maturation from 26 to

27 weeks' gestation compared with 34 to 35 weeks increased fetal viability from 67 percent to 97 percent.[141] Neoadjuvant chemotherapy approach (chemotherapy prior to either surgery or irradiation) would unlikely compromise and may enhance the overall efficacy of treatment. Also, having passed the primary interval of organogenesis, it is unlikely that serious fetal sequelae will occur secondary to the chemotherapy. Certainly in terms of general fetal salvage and outcome, the risk of extreme prematurity would far outweigh the risk of the chemotherapy expo. While this management of second-trimester cervical cancer presentations seems logical, there is scant information about this treatment approach. However, neoadjuvant chemotherapy with vincristine and platinum-based chemotherapy for ovarian cancers has been reported with no fetal sequelae identified.[20]

Invasive, Locally Advanced Disease

The management of the patient with more advanced local disease is based on treatment with chemotherapy and irradiation, both external beam to treat the regional nodes and shrink the central tumor and brachytherapy to complete the delivery of a tumoricidal dose to the cervix and adjacent tissues.[136]

OVARIAN CANCER

While adnexal masses are frequently encountered in pregnancy, only 2 to 5 percent are malignant ovarian tumors.[151,152] Ovarian cancer occurs in approximately 1 in 18,000 to 1 in 47,000 pregnancies.[153,154]

While the three major categories of ovarian tumors—epithelial, germ cell, and stromal—occur during pregnancy, there is a disproportionate number of patients with germ cell tumors compared with the nonpregnant patient. Germ cell tumors account for 45 percent; 37.5 percent are epithelial tumors, 10 percent are stromal tumors, and 7.5 percent are categorized as miscellaneous. This distribution is undoubtedly skewed by the reporting bias associated with rare tumors. The majority of epithelial ovarian tumors complicating pregnancy are of low grade (grade 1 or low malignant potential) or early stage, not uncommonly both low grade and stage I.

Management of the adnexal mass in pregnancy is the subject of some controversy. The risks of surgical intervention may favor a conservative approach.[156] Serial sonograms may be of some value in determining the nature and biologic potential of the tumor. If the clinical presentation is consistent with torsion, rupture, or hemorrhage, immediate surgical intervention is indicated. Prompt surgical exploration is also performed for the mass associated with ascites or when there is evidence of metastatic disease. Since surgical exploration during pregnancy is associated with an increase in pregnancy loss and neonatal morbidity, it is ideal to delay surgical intervention until term or after delivery. A number of opposing risks require consideration prior to following a conservative approach. The risk of greatest concern is that a delay of surgical intervention could permit a malignant ovarian tumor to spread, resulting in a decreased opportunity for cure. However, considering the rarity of advanced-stage poorly differentiated epithelial tumors in this age group, this risk is relatively small. There does appear to be an increased probability that an adnexal mass during pregnancy will undergo torsion or rupture,[157,158] and surgical intervention for these events is associated with higher fetal loss than an elective procedure.[151,159] While ovarian tumors may be the cause of obstructed labor,[151] this is uncommon. Serial sonographic evaluations will identify the rare tumor that remains pelvic as the gestation progresses. Since most ovarian masses relocate to the abdomen as the pregnancy advances, other explanations should be considered for persistent pelvic masses, including pelvic kidney, uterine fibroids, and colorectal or bladder tumors.

When a malignant ovarian tumor is encountered at laparotomy, surgical intervention should be similar to that for the nonpregnant patient. If the patient is preterm and the tumor appears confined to one ovary, consideration should be given to limiting the staging to removal of the ovary, cytologic washings, and a thorough manual exploration of the abdomen and pelvis. The potential benefit of more extensive staging, including aortic node sampling, may be offset by higher pregnancy loss or neonatal morbidity. Prior to surgery, a comprehensive discussion with the patient should guide the extent of surgery if metastatic disease, especially a high-grade epithelial lesion, is encountered. Depending on the gestational age and the patient's desires, limited surgery followed by chemotherapy and additional extirpative surgery following delivery must be offered in select cases. Preoperative serum tumor markers are of limited value during pregnancy secondary to the physiologic increases in hCG, α-fetoprotein, and CA 125.

Virilizing ovarian tumors during pregnancy are most commonly secondary to theca-lutein cysts, and their evaluation and management should be conservative.

FETAL-PLACENTAL METASTASIS

Metastatic spread of a maternal primary tumor to the placenta or fetus is rare. Malignant melanoma is the most frequently reported tumor metastatic to the placenta. Hematologic malignancies are the second most common tumor to spread to the placenta. Placental and fetal dissemination of lymphomas have been reported.[202-205]

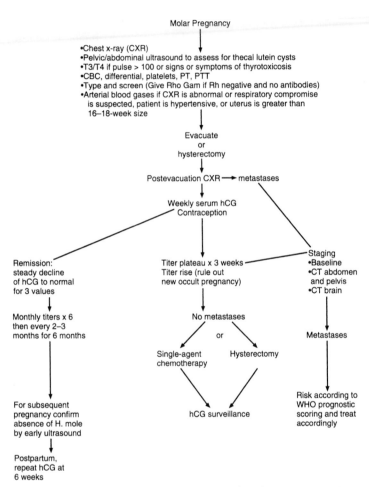

Figure 24–8. Algorithm for the management of molar pregnancy. (From Copeland LJ: Gestational trophoblastic neoplasia. *In* Copeland LJ [ed]: Textbook of Gynecology. 2nd ed. Philadelphia, WB Saunders Company, 2000, p 1414, with permission.)

GESTATIONAL TROPHOBLASTIC DISEASE AND PREGNANCY-RELATED ISSUES

Hydatidiform Mole (Complete Mole)

The incidence of hydatidiform mole has great geographic variability. In the United States it occurs in approximately 1 in 1,000 to 1 in 1,500 pregnancies. The two clinical risk factors that carry the highest risk of a molar pregnancy are (1) the extremes of the reproductive years (age 50 or older carries a relative risk of over 500)[211] and (2) the history of a prior hydatidiform mole (the risk for development of a second molar pregnancy is 1 to 2 percent,[212–214] and the risk of a third after two is approximately 25 percent).[215] Patients with these risk factors should have an ultrasound evaluation of uterine contents in the first trimester. Most patients are diagnosed either by ultrasound while asymptomatic or by ultrasound for the evaluation of vaginal spotting or cramping symptoms.

The safest technique of evacuating a hydatidiform mole is with the suction aspiration technique. Oxytocin should not be initiated until the patient is in the operating room and evacuation is imminent in order to minimize the risk of embolization of trophoblastic tissue. The alternative management for the elderly patient who requests concurrent sterilization is hysterectomy. Following either evacuation or hysterectomy, weekly β-hCG is drawn until the hCG titer is within normal limits for 3 weeks. The titers are then observed at monthly intervals for 6 to 12 months. Figure 24–8 illustrates an algorithm for molar pregnancy management.[216]

For the patient with a complete molar pregnancy, the risk of requiring chemotherapy for persistent GTD is approximately 20 percent. Clinical features that increase this risk include delayed hemorrhage, excessive uterine enlargement, theca-lutein cysts, serum hCG greater than 100,000 mIU/ml, and maternal age over 40. It is obviously particularly important not to misinterpret a rising β-hCG due to a new intervening pregnancy as persistent GTD.

Key Points

➤ Since many of the common complaints of pregnancy are also early symptoms of metastatic cancer, pregnant women with cancer are at risk for delays in diagnosis and therapeutic intervention.

Box continued on following page

Key Points *Continued*

➤ The safest interval for most cancer therapies in pregnancy is the second trimester, thereby avoiding induction of teratogenic risks or miscarriage in the first trimester and avoiding neonatal morbidity associated with preterm delivery in the third trimester.

➤ Antimetabolites and alkylating agents present the greatest hazard to the developing fetus.

➤ Diagnostic delays of breast cancer in pregnancy are often attributed to physician reluctance to properly evaluate breast complaints or abnormal findings in pregnancy.

➤ If a mother is exposed to cytotoxic drugs within 1 month of delivery, the newborn should be monitored closely for evidence of granulocytopenia or thrombocytopenia.

➤ After stratifying for stage and age, patients with pregnancy-associated cervical carcinoma have survival rates similar to the nonpregnant patient.

➤ Since most malignant ovarian tumors found in pregnancy are either germ cell tumors or low-grade, early-stage epithelial tumors, the therapeutic plan will usually permit continuation of the pregnancy and preservation of fertility.

Dermatologic Disorders

ROXANNE STAMBUK AND ROY COLVEN

SPECIFIC DERMATOLOGIC CONDITIONS ASSOCIATED WITH PREGNANCY

See Table 24–19.

Pruritus

Pruritus is a common symptom in pregnancy, occurring in 3 to 14 percent of all women.[34]

Intrahepatic cholestasis is one of the most common causes of pregnancy-related pruritus. Intrahepatic cholestasis leads to increased levels of serum bile salts, and increased deposition of bile salts in the skin leads to itching.[32,34] Cholestatic pruritus occurs in the second or third trimester of pregnancy.[36] The pregnant patient experiences itch mainly on the palms and soles, although the itch can become generalized. There are no primary skin lesions. Changes on the skin are secondary from excoriations.[31] Liver function tests demonstrating increased serum levels of hepatic transaminases and bilirubin confirm the diagnosis of cholestasis.[37] Although the maternal prognosis is good, cholestasis has been associated with increased risks for the fetus, with risks of fetal prematurity and fetal death.

Pemphigoid Gestationis

Pemphigoid gestationis is a rare, pruritic, autoimmune, bullous skin disease that occurs during the second and third trimesters of pregnancy and the puerperium.[38] The term *pemphigoid gestationis* supercedes the older term, *herpes gestationis,* because it does not involve the herpes viruses and because of its antigenic and clinical similarity to bullous pemphigoid. It affects only female patients and occurs only in the presence of placental tissue. The disease occurs in 1 per 1,700 pregnancies.[32,38,39] The occurrence during the third

Table 24–19. SPECIFIC INFLAMMATORY DERMATOSES OF PREGNANCY

Disease	Onset	Degree of Pruritus	Types of Lesions	Distribution	Increased Incidence of Fetal Morbidity or Mortality
Pemphigoid gestationis	First month to postpartum	Moderate to severe	Erythematous papules, vesicles bullae	Abdomen, extremities, generalized	Unresolved
Prurigo gestationis	Fourth to ninth month	Moderate	Excoriated papules	Extensor surfaces of extremities	No
Impetigo herpetiformis	First to ninth month	Minimal	Pustules	Genitalia, medial thighs umbilicus, breasts, axillas	Yes
Polymorphic eruption of pregnancy	Third trimester	Severe	Erythematous urticarial papules and plaques	Abdomen, thighs, buttocks, occasionally arms and legs	No
Pruritic folliculitis of pregnancy	Third trimester	Moderate	Erythematous papules or pustules	Shoulder, back, arms, chest, abdomen	No
Cholestasis of pregnancy	Third trimester	Moderate to severe	None or excoriations	Generalized	Unresolved

trimester of pregnancy and the recurrence of pemphigoid gestationis with menstruation and with oral contraceptive use strongly implicates a hormonal influence. The increased frequency of certain histocompatibility locus antigens (HLA) in women with pemphigoid gestationis suggests a genetic predisposition. A circulating IgG1 autoantibody with complement-fixing capability, previously referred to as the *herpes gestationis factor* (HG factor), incites the pathology of pemphigoid gestationis.[44,45]

Clinically, pemphigoid gestationis typically presents with severely pruritic erythematous, urticarial, or hive-like, papules and plaques around the umbilicus (Fig. 24–9). Within days to weeks, the eruption spreads to involve the trunk, back, buttocks, forearms, palms, and soles, usually sparing the face, scalp, and mucosa. Within 2 to 4 weeks of the onset of the disease, vesicles and tense serum-filled bullae develop either at the margins of the edematous, erythematous plaques or de novo in clinically uninflamed skin. Sometimes vesicles and bullae do not develop, adding confusion to the diagnosis.[38] The lesions tend to heal without scarring if secondary infection does not ensue.

Pemphigoid gestationis usually presents during the second or third trimester, with a mean of 21 weeks' gestation, although patients may present with recurring crops of blisters at any time during pregnancy. It occurs for the first time during the early postpartum period in 20 percent of patients.[38] Pemphigoid gestationis usually recurs and may be more severe with an earlier onset in subsequent pregnancies.

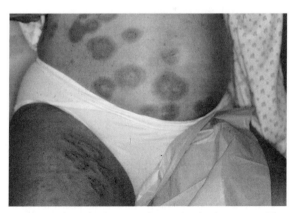

Figure 24–9. Pemphigoid gestationis during the third trimester. This patient developed erythematous urticarial superficial plaques on the thighs and abdomen that progressed to bullae formation. Biopsy revealed a heavy linear complement deposition at the basement membrane zone, consistent with pemphigoid gestationis.

One can easily make a presumptive diagnosis of pemphigoid gestationis in a pregnant woman with a typical distribution of vesicles and bullae. Skin biopsy, including a sample processed for direct immunofluorescence (DIF), confirms the diagnosis. This confirmation distinguishes pemphigoid gestationis from polymorphic eruption of pregnancy, which does not recur with subsequent pregnancies. Distinguishing these two diseases enables counseling of the patient about the recurrence risk in future pregnancies.

Histology reveals intercellular epidermal edema, with basal keratinocyte necrosis, and occasionally eosinophils and lymphocytes along the dermal–epidermal junction. Immunopathology of these specimens demonstrates the third component of complement in a linear band of fluorescence along the basement membrane zone between the epidermis and dermis.[44]

Treatment is aimed at controlling pruritus, suppressing formation of new vesicles and bullae, and preventing secondary infection of skin lesions. Topical steroids and antihistamines may be used initially if the symptoms are mild. Most patients, however, will require systemic corticosteroid therapy. Prednisone dosages start at 40 to 60 mg/day. With improvement of clinical symptoms and no new bullae formation, the dose can then be tapered to 10 to 20 mg/day if clinical improvement is noted. Azathioprine, dapsone and, rarely, plasmapheresis have been employed in cases that fail to respond to corticosteroids.[38] For postpartum patients who experience a flare of pemphigoid gestationis requiring continued steroids, prednisone doses of 20 mg/day still allow safe breast-feeding.

Pemphigoid gestationis appears to increase the risk for IUGR and prematurity. For this reason, fetal growth should be carefully evaluated.

The HG factor, crosses the placenta, binds with the basement membrane of the amnion,[55] and deposits in fetal skin.[38] Transient newborn pemphigoid gestationis has been reported in up to 5 percent of newborns.[43,54] Neonatal pemphigoid gestationis is usually mild and presents with erythematous papules or frank bullae.[56] This process generally resolves within a short period of time.[56,57]

Polymorphic Eruption of Pregnancy

In the past, a severe pruritic eruption seen during the third trimester of pregnancy[58] was labeled *pruritic urticarial papules and plaques of pregnancy* (PUPPP). Today, the preferred term is *polymorphic eruption of pregnancy* (PEP) The incidence of PEP ranges from 1 in 240 to 1 in 200 pregnancies.[31,58]

The etiology and pathogenesis are unknown.[59] The majority of women affected by PEP are primigravidae with prominent striae or have uterine distention with twins or hydramnios.[32,35] A provoca-

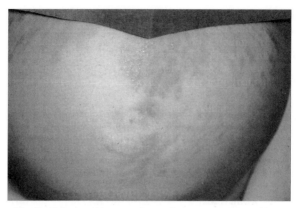

Figure 24–10. Polymorphic eruption of pregnancy (pruritic urticarial papules and plaques of pregnancy [PUPPP] syndrome). Erythematous urticarial plaques and small papules erupted on the abdomen of this patient pregnant with conjoined female twins during the third trimester.

tive new hypothesis proposes that fetal male DNA acting as a skin antigen precipitates PEP.[62]

The lesions of PEP typically begin in the abdominal striae distensae of primigravidas during the third trimester (Fig. 24–10). Lesions initially present as 1- to 2-mm erythematous papules, surrounded by a narrow pale halo of vasoconstriction, that coalesce into urticarial plaques.[63] Small vesicles also can develop on the plaques. Lesions usually spread to the thighs and may involve the buttocks and arms. In contrast to pemphigoid gestationis, the periumbilical area is often spared in PEP. The face is also spared. Most patients experience intense pruritus that improves rapidly following delivery and resolves 1 to 2 weeks postpartum. The mean onset of skin lesions is 36 weeks' gestation; PEP rarely commences postpartum.[63] In general, PEP does not recur with subsequent pregnancies. In contrast to pemphigoid gestationis, PEP shows no specific immunofluorescence pattern from skin biopsies.

As with pemphigoid gestationis, the main goal of therapy is symptomatic relief of the intense pruritus.[63] High-potency topical steroids generally effect a response in the vast majority of women, though some will require systemic steroids.[63] Antipruritic drugs such as hydroxyzine or diphenhydramine also may help. Fortunately, for these patients, delivery brings relief of both symptoms and lesions.[58] In some women, the severe pruritus will warrant induction of labor once fetal lung maturity is ensured.[66]

Key Points

➤ Pregnancy is associated with several physiologic changes of the skin that may concern the pregnant woman. These include hyperpigmentation, mild hirsutism, hair loss, striae distensae, and vascular changes.

➤ During pregnancy, some nevi may increase in size, and new nevi may develop. This may necessitate the need to perform a biopsy if one suspects melanoma.

➤ Pruritus is a common symptom in pregnancy and usually resolves postpartum; infrequently, it is due to a serious dermatologic disease. In addition to evaluating the pregnant woman for dermatologic diseases that occur unassociated with pregnancy, the health care provider must evaluate for pregnancy-specific dermatologic diseases.

➤ The most common pregnancy-specific causes of pruritic rashes are polymorphic eruption of pregnancy, prurigo gestationis, and cholestasis of pregnancy.

➤ Rare dermatologic conditions associated with pregnancy are pemphigoid gestationis, pruritic folliculitis of pregnancy, and impetigo herpetiformis.

➤ The only dermatologic diseases of pregnancy that have been shown to cause fetal morbidity are pemphigoid gestationis and impetigo herpetiformis. Antepartum testing for fetal well-being should be utilized in these women. Transient newborn pemphigoid gestationis has also been reported.

➤ Pemphigoid gestationis can be difficult to clinically distinguish from polymorphic eruption of pregnancy. Skin biopsies with immunofluorescence studies differentiates the two disorders.

➤ The treatment for pemphigoid gestationis is aimed at controlling symptoms. Most patients will require systemic corticosteroid therapy.

➤ Topical steroid therapy generally induces a response in the vast majority of women with polymorphic eruption of pregnancy, but some will require systemic steroids. The main goal of therapy is symptomatic relief of the intense pruritus. In some women, the pruritus will be significant enough to warrant induction of labor once fetal lung maturity is ensured.

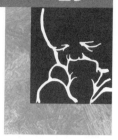

Maternal and Perinatal Infection

PATRICK DUFF

This chapter reviews the major maternal and perinatal infections that the obstetrician confronts in clinical practice. The first portion of the chapter focuses primarily on bacterial infections of the lower and upper genital tract. The second portion considers the infections that pose special risks to the fetus. The principal features of these infections are summarized in Tables 25–1 and 25–2.

VAGINAL INFECTIONS

Bacterial Vaginosis

Epidemiology

Bacterial vaginosis (BV) is responsible for approximately 45 percent of cases of vaginitis. It is a polymicrobial infection, and the predominant pathogens are anaerobes, *Gardnerella vaginalis, Mobiluncus* species, and genital mycoplasmas.[1] BV usually results from disturbances in the normal vaginal ecosystem caused by hormonal changes, pregnancy, or antibiotic administration. The principal feature of this alteration in vaginal flora is a marked decrease in the lactobacilli species that produce lactic acid and a corresponding increase in anaerobic organisms. In some instances, BV can result from sexual contact with an infected partner. In contrast to trichomoniasis and candidiasis, symptomatic BV in pregnancy has been associated with several serious maternal complications, including preterm labor, preterm premature rupture of membranes, chorioamnionitis, and puerperal endometritis.[2-4]

Diagnosis

The most prominent clinical manifestation of BV is a thin, gray, homogeneous, malodorous vaginal discharge. Vulvar or vaginal pruritus is uncommon, and the vaginal pH is characteristically greater than 4.5. When vaginal secretions are mixed with several drops of

Text continued on page 759

Table 25–1. ETIOLOGY, DIAGNOSIS, AND MANAGEMENT OF MAJOR OBSTETRIC INFECTIONS

Condition	Microbiology	Confirmatory Diagnostic Test	Treatment*
Vaginal infection			
Bacterial vaginosis	*Gardnerella vaginalis,* *Mobiluncus* species, anaerobes, mycoplasmas	Saline preparation Vaginal pH Amine test	Topical or oral clindamycin or metronidazole
Candidiasis	*Candida albicans, C. tropicalis, C. glabrata*	KOH preparation	Topical antifungal cream
Trichomoniasis	*Trichomonas vaginalis*	Saline preparation	Oral metronidazole
Endocervical infection			
Gonorrhea	*Neisseria gonorrhoeae*	Endocervical culture	Oral cefixime or intramuscular ceftriaxone
Chlamydia	*Chlamydia trachomatis*	Endocervical culture Antigen detection	Oral erythromycin, azithromycin, or amoxicillin
Urinary tract infection			
Urethritis	*N. gonorrhoeae*	Culture of urethral discharge	Oral cefixime or intramuscular ceftriaxone
	C. trachomatis	Culture of urethral discharge or antigen detection	Oral erythromycin, azithromycin, or amoxicillin

Asymptomatic bacteriuria or cystitis	E. coli, Klebsiella pneumoniae, Proteus species	Urinalysis Culture	Sulfisoxazole, nitrofurantoin monohydrate macrocrystals, trimethoprim-sulfamethoxazole DS
Pyelonephritis	As above	As above	Intravenous cefazolin and/or gentamicin or aztreonam
Chorioamnionitis	Group B streptococci, coliforms, anaerobes	Clinical examination Amniotic fluid leukocyte esterase, glucose, Gram's stain, and culture	Intravenous penicillin or ampicillin plus gentamicin; add clindamycin or metronidazole if cesarean delivery is required
Puerperal endometritis	Group B streptococci, coliforms, anaerobes	Clinical examination	Intravenous clindamycin plus gentamicin or extended spectrum cephalosporin or penicillin or carbapenem

*See text for detailed prescribing information.

Table 25–2. SUMMARY OF ETIOLOGY, DIAGNOSIS, AND MANAGEMENT OF MAJOR PERINATAL INFECTIONS

Condition	Complications		Diagnosis		Management*	
	Maternal	Fetal/ Neonatal	Maternal	Fetal/ Neonatal	Maternal	Fetal/ Neonatal
CMV	Chorioretinitis, pneumonia in immunocompromised patient	Congenital infection	Detection of antibody	Amniocentesis— culture amniotic fluid Ultrasound	Ganciclovir for severe infection	Consider pregnancy termination when mother has primary infection
Group B streptococci	UTI Chorioamnionitis Endometritis Wound infection Preterm labor PROM	Sepsis Pneumonia Meningitis	Culture	Culture	Intrapartum antibiotic prophylaxis	Treatment with ampicillin or penicillin

Hepatitis						
A	Rare	None	Detection of antibody	N/A	Prevention—hepatitis A vaccine Supportive care	Administer immune globulin to neonate if mother acutely infected at delivery
B	Chronic liver disease	Neonatal infection	Detection of surface antigen	N/A	Prevention—HBIG + HBV for susceptible household contacts	HBIG + HBV immediately after delivery
C	Chronic liver disease	Neonatal infection	Detection of antibody	N/A	Supportive care Interferon	Nonimmunoprophylaxis available
D	Chronic liver disease	Neonatal infection	Detection of antigen and antibody	N/A	Supportive care	HBIG + HBV immediately after delivery
E	Increased mortality	None	Detection of antibody	N/A	Supportive care	None

Table continued on following page

Table 25–2. SUMMARY OF ETIOLOGY, DIAGNOSIS, AND MANAGEMENT OF MAJOR PERINATAL INFECTIONS *Continued*

Condition	Complications		Diagnosis		Management*	
	Maternal	Fetal/Neonatal	Maternal	Fetal/Neonatal	Maternal	Fetal/Neonatal
Herpes simplex	Disseminated infection in immunocompromised patient	Neonatal infection	Clinical examination, culture, PCR	Clinical examination, culture	Acyclovir, valacyclovir, or famciclovir for severe infection	Cesarean delivery when mother has over infection
HIV infection	Opportunistic infection, malignancy	Congenital or perinatal infection	Detection of antibody or antigen	Same	Combination chemotherapy	Combination chemotherapy for prevention of vertical transmission
Parvovirus infection	Rare	Anemia hydrops	Detection of antibody	Ultrasound	Supportive care	Intrauterine transfusion for severe anemia

Rubella	Rare	Congenital infection	Detection of antibody	Ultrasound	Prevention—vaccination prior to pregnancy Supportive care	Pregnancy termination for affected fetus
Rubeola	Otitis media, pneumonia, encephalitis	Abortion, preterm delivery	Detection of antibody	N/A	Prevention—vaccination prior to pregnancy Supportive care	N/A
Syphilis	Aortitis Neurosyphilis	Congenital infection	Darkfield examination or serology	Ultrasound	Penicillin	Penicillin

Table continued on following page

Table 25-2. SUMMARY OF ETIOLOGY, DIAGNOSIS, AND MANAGEMENT OF MAJOR PERINATAL INFECTIONS *Continued*

	Complications		Diagnosis		Management*	
Condition	Maternal	Fetal/ Neonatal	Maternal	Fetal/ Neonatal	Maternal	Fetal/ Neonatal
Toxoplasmosis	Chorioretinitis, CNS infection	Congenital infection	Detection of antibody	Amniocentesis— detection of toxoplasma DNA by nucleic acid probe	Sulfadiazine Pyrimethamine Spiramycin	Treatment of mother prior to delivery prior reduces risk of fetal infection
Varicella	Pneumonia Encephalitis	Congenital infection	Clinical examination, decision of antibody	Ultrasound	VZIG, acyclovir for prophylaxis or treatment	VZIG, acyclovir for prophylaxis or treatment of neonate

UTI, urinary tract infection; CMV, cytomegalovirus; PROM, premature rupture of membranes; HBIG, hepatitis B immune globulin; HBV, hepatitis B vaccine; PCR, polymerase chain reaction; HIV, human immunodeficiency virus; CNS, central nervous system; DNA, deoxyribonucleic acid; VZIG, varicella zoster immune globulin.
*See text for detailed discussion of patient management.

a 10 percent potassium hydroxide (KOH) solution, a pungent fishy odor is produced ("whiff test" or amine test). On microscopic examination of a saline preparation, the normal lactobacilli flora is largely replaced by multiple small bacilli and cocci. Motile, comma-shaped *Mobiluncus* species, and clue cells are present. Culture of vaginal secretions is not indicated in routine clinical practice.[1]

Treatment

Symptomatic patients with BV should be treated.[5-7] In addition, asymptomatic patients who are at increased risk of preterm delivery (e.g., history of prior preterm birth) also should be screened for BV and treated if positive. The value of *routine* screening of asymptomatic, low-risk patients has *not* been confirmed.

The drug of choice for treating BV in pregnancy is oral metronidazole (250 mg three times daily for 7 days). For patients who are unable to tolerate metronidazole, clindamycin (300 mg orally [PO] twice daily for 7 days) can be used.

Candidiasis

Epidemiology

Candidiasis is responsible for approximately 25 to 30 percent of all cases of vaginitis. Several conditions predispose to symptomatic moniliasis, including recent antibiotic or corticosteroid therapy, diabetes, use of oral contraceptives, pregnancy, and immunodeficiency states.

Diagnosis

Infected patients usually report vaginal and vulvar pruritus and a white, curd-like vaginal discharge. The vaginal mucosa and vulva may be erythematous and edematous, and punctate, erythematous satellite lesions may be present on the lateral aspect of the vulva and medial aspect of the thighs.[9]

The simplest test for confirmation of this diagnosis is microscopic examination of a KOH preparation for hyphae, pseudohyphae, and budding yeast.

Treatment

For uncomplicated candida infections, topical therapy for 3 to 7 days with agents such as miconazole, terconazole, clotrimazole, and butoconazole is usually highly effective. Treatment of women with persistent or recurrent infection is more problematic. These patients should be counseled about preventive measures such as avoidance of bubble baths, use of cotton undergarments, and close attention to perineal hygiene.[9,10] In particularly refractory cases, administration of systemic antimicrobials such as ketoconazole or fluconazole should be considered because of their greater activity against reservoirs of yeast in the gastrointestinal tract.[11-13] In pregnancy, fluconazole appears to have a more favorable toxicity profile. The appropriate oral dose of this compound for treatment of a refractory infection is 150 mg in a single dose.

Trichomoniasis

Epidemiology

Trichomoniasis is a sexually transmitted disease caused by the protozoan *Trichomonas vaginalis*. *Trichomonas* is responsible for approximately 25 percent of cases of vaginitis. It is an extremely contagious infection. Trichomoniasis is not commonly associated with serious maternal or neonatal complications.

Diagnosis

The usual symptoms of trichomoniasis are vaginal pruritus, superficial dyspareunia, frequency, dysuria, and a malodorous, yellow-green, frothy vaginal discharge. On physical examination, the vaginal mucosa is typically erythematous, and punctate hemorrhages may be present on the cervix ("strawberry cervix").

The most useful test for rapid confirmation of infection is direct visualization of the flagellated organisms in a saline preparation (wet mount). The sensitivity of this test is 60 to 80 percent.

Treatment

Metronidazole is the only antibiotic with uniform activity against *T. vaginalis*. Treatment efficacy is 95 percent or higher if the patient is compliant and her sexual partner is treated concurrently.

Metronidazole can be given in three oral dosage regimens: a single dose of 2 g; 250 mg three times daily for 7 days, or 500 mg twice daily for 7 days. The former dosage schedule improves compliance and reduces expense.[8]

ENDOCERVICAL INFECTIONS

Chlamydia

Epidemiology

Chlamydia trachomatis is the most common sexually transmitted pathogen in Western nations. The organism can cause localized infection of the urethra, endocervix, and rectum. Infants delivered to infected women may develop either conjunctivitis and/or pneumonia. The former complication occurs in up to 50 percent of infants delivered to infected mothers; the latter affects 3 to 18 percent of infants.[17,18]

Diagnosis and Clinical Management

Rapid identification tests such as nucleic acid probes are sufficiently sensitive to justify their clinical use for identification of chlamydia infection. In high-risk populations, the sensitivity and specificity of the newest tests exceed 90 percent.[17,19]

Although tetracycline and doxycycline have the greatest activity against *C. trachomatis*, these drugs should not be used in pregnancy because of their harmful effects on fetal teeth. The agent of choice is azithromycin, 1,000 mg (powder formulation) PO in a single dose.[21] Amoxicillin (500 mg PO three times a day for 7 days) also is an acceptable alternative.[22]

A test of cure should be performed approximately 2 weeks after therapy is completed. In addition, infected patients should be screened for other sexually transmitted diseases such as gonorrhea, syphilis, hepatitis B, and human immunodeficiency virus infection. Neonates delivered to infected mothers should receive prophylaxis with tetracycline or erythromycin ophthalmic preparations and observed for evidence of an ensuing respiratory tract infection.

Gonorrhea

Epidemiology

Gonorrhea is caused by the gram-negative, intracellular diplococcus, *Neisseria gonorrhoeae*. The infection is transmitted primarily by sexual contact. Gonorrhea also may be transmitted perinatally from mother to infant and cause serious ophthalmic injury *(ophthalmia neonatorum)*.

In pregnant women, gonorrhea may be manifested as an asymptomatic to mildly symptomatic localized infection of the urethra, endocervix, and/or rectum. Local infection may increase the risk of preterm labor and preterm premature rupture of membranes and predispose to intrapartum and postpartum infection. Gonorrhea also may present as a moderately severe pharyngitis or as a disseminated infection.[17]

Diagnosis and Management

The most reliable test for confirmation of gonococcal infection is culture of the organism on selective agar such as Thayer-Martin medium.

The drugs of choice for treating *localized* gonococcal infection in pregnancy are ceftriaxone (125 intramuscularly [IM] in a single dose) and cefixime (400 mg PO once). The former drug is the preferred agent for treatment of *disseminated* infection and should be administered in a dose of 1 g intravenously (IV) or IM every 24 hours until a clinical response has been achieved.[8,17] Patients who are allergic to β-lactam antibiotics may be treated with a single 2-g IM dose of spectinomycin.[8] Treatment of the neonate with either silver nitrate or tetracycline ophthalmic preparations is effective in preventing most cases of ophthalmia neonatorum.

Patients who test positive for gonorrhea should be screened for other sexually transmitted diseases. Because of the uniformly excellent activity of ceftriaxone and cefixime against *N. gonorrhoeae,* tests of cure are not *routinely* indicated when patients are treated with these agents. However, patients with persistent symptoms and/or signs of infection should be carefully reevaluated.

URINARY TRACT INFECTIONS

Acute Urethritis

Acute urethritis (acute urethral syndrome) is usually caused by one of three organisms: coliforms (principally *Escherichia coli*), *Neisseria gonorrhoeae,* or *Chlamydia trachomatis.*

Affected patients typically experience frequency, urgency, and dysuria. On microscopic examination, the urine usually has white blood cells (WBCs), but bacteria are not consistently present. Urine cultures may have low colony counts of coliform organisms, and cultures of the urethral discharge may be positive for gonorrhea and chlamydia. A rapid diagnostic test, such as a nucleic acid probe, may be used in lieu of culture for *C. trachomatis.*[24]

Most patients with acute urethritis warrant empiric treatment before the results of urine or urethral cultures are available. Infections caused by coliforms will usually respond to the antibiotics described below for treatment of asymptomatic bacteriuria and cystitis. If gonococcal infection is suspected, the patient should be treated as described above.

Asymptomatic Bacteriuria and Acute Cystitis

The prevalence of asymptomatic bacteriuria in pregnancy is 5 to 10 percent, and the vast majority of cases antedate the onset of pregnancy. The frequency of acute cystitis in pregnancy is 1 to 3 percent.

E. coli is responsible for 80 to 90 percent of cases of *initial* infections and 70 to 80 percent of recurrent cases. *Klebsiella pneumoniae* and *Proteus* species also are important pathogens, particularly in patients who have a history of recurrent infection.

Approximately 3 to 7 percent of infections will be caused by gram-positive organisms such as group B streptococci, enterococci, and staphylococci.[24,25]

All pregnant women should have a urine culture at their first prenatal appointment to detect preexisting asymptomatic bacteriuria. If the culture is negative, the likelihood of the patient subsequently developing an *asymptomatic* infection is 5 percent or less. If the culture is positive (defined as $\geq 10^5$ colonies/ml urine from a midstream clean-catch specimen), prompt treatment is necessary to prevent ascending infection.[25]

Patients with acute cystitis usually have symptoms of frequency, dysuria, urgency, suprapubic pain, hesitancy, and dribbling. Gross hematuria may be present, but high fever and systemic symptoms are uncommon. In symptomatic patients, the leukocyte esterase and nitrate tests will usually be positive. When a urine culture is obtained, a catheterized sample is preferred because it minimizes the probability that urine will be contaminated by vaginal flora. With a catheterized specimen, a colony count greater than or equal to 10^2/ml is considered indicative of infection.[26]

Asymptomatic bacteriuria and acute cystitis characteristically respond well to short courses of oral antibiotics. Single dose therapy is not as effective in pregnant women as in nonpregnant patients. However, a 3-day course of treatment appears to be comparable to a 7- to 10-day regimen for an initial infection.[24] The longer courses of therapy are most appropriate for patients with recurrent infections. Table 25-3 lists several antibiotics of value for treatment of asymptomatic bacteriuria and cystitis.

When sensitivity tests are available (e.g., in patients with asymptomatic bacteriuria), they may be used to guide antibiotic selection. Because of theoretical concerns about their effect on protein binding of bilirubin, sulfonamide drugs should probably be avoided near the time of delivery.

For patients who have an initial infection and experience a prompt response to treatment, a urine culture for test of cure is probably unnecessary.[29] Cultures during, or immediately after, treatment are indicated for patients who have a poor response to therapy or who have a history of recurrent infection. During subsequent clinic appointments, the patient's urine should be screened for nitrites and leukocyte esterase. If either of these tests is positive, repeat urine culture and retreatment are indicated.[30]

Acute Pyelonephritis

The incidence of pyelonephritis in pregnancy is 1 to 2 percent.[25] The vast majority of cases develop as a consequence of undiagnosed or inadequately treated lower urinary tract infection.

Table 25–3. ANTIBIOTICS FOR TREATMENT OF ASYMPTOMATIC BACTERIURIA AND ACUTE CYSTITIS

Drug	Strength of Activity	Oral Dose × 3 Days	Relative Cost
Amoxicillin	Some *E. coli,* most *Proteus* species, group B streptococci, entero-cocci, some staphylococci	875 mg bid	Low
Amoxicillin-clavulanic acid (Augmentin)	Most gram-negative aerobic bacilli and gram-positive cocci	875 mg bid	High
Ampicillin	Some *E. coli,* most *Proteus* species, group B streptococci, enterococci, some staphylococci	250–500 mg qid	Low
Cephalexin (Keflex)	Most *E. coli,* most *Klebsiella* and *Proteus* species, group B streptococci, staphylococci	250 mg qid	Low

Nitrofurantoin monohydrate macrocrystals—sustained–release preparation (Macrobid)	Most gram-negative aerobic bacilli	100 mg bid	Moderate
Sulfisoxazole (Gantrisin)	Most gram-negative aerobic bacilli	2 g ×1 dose, then 1 g qid	Low
Trimethoprim-sulfamethoxazole–double strength (Bactrim-DS, or Septra-DS)	Most gram-negative aerobic bacilli	800 mg/160 mg bid	Low

bid, twice daily; qid, four times daily.
Modified from Duff P: Urinary tract infections. Prim Care Update Obstet Gynecol 1:12, 1994.

Approximately 75 to 80 percent of cases of pyelonephritis occur on the right side. *E. coli* is again the principal pathogen.[25,27] *Klebsiella pneumoniae* and *Proteus* species also are important causes of infection, particularly in women with recurrent episodes of pyelonephritis.[27] Highly virulent gram-negative bacilli, such as *Pseudomonas, Enterobacter,* and *Serratia* are unusual isolates except in immunocompromised patients.

The usual clinical manifestations of acute pyelonephritis in pregnancy are fever, chills, flank pain and tenderness, frequency, urgency, hematuria, and dysuria. Patients also may have signs of preterm labor, septic shock, and adult respiratory distress syndrome (ARDS). Urinalysis is usually positive for white cell casts, red blood cells, and bacteria.

Pregnant patients with pyelonephritis may be considered for outpatient therapy if their disease manifestations are mild, they are hemodynamically stable, and they have no evidence of preterm labor. If an outpatient approach is adopted, the patient should be treated with agents that have a high level of activity against the common uropathogens. Acceptable oral agents include amoxicillin (875 mg)-clavulanic acid (125 mg), one tablet twice daily or trimethoprim-sulfamethoxazole-DS (one tablet twice daily for 7 to 10 days). Alternatively, a visiting home nurse may be contracted to administer a parenteral agent, such as ceftriaxone (2 g IM or IV once daily).

Pregnant patients who appear to be moderately to severely ill or who show any signs of preterm labor should be hospitalized for intravenous antibiotic therapy. They should receive appropriate supportive treatment and be monitored closely for complications such as sepsis, ARDS, and preterm labor. One of the best choices for empiric intravenous antibiotic therapy is cefazolin (1 to 2 g every 8 hours).[27] If the patient is critically ill or is at high risk for a resistant organism, a second antibiotic, such as gentamicin (1.5 mg/kg every 8 hours) or aztreonam (500 mg to 1 g every 8 to 12 hours) should be administered, along with cefazolin, until the results of susceptibility tests are available.

Once antibiotic therapy is initiated, approximately 75 percent of patients defervesce within 48 hours. The two most likely causes of treatment failure are a resistant microorganism or obstruction.

Once the patient has begun to defervesce and her clinical examination has improved, she may be discharged from the hospital. Oral antibiotics should be prescribed to complete a total of 7 to 10 days of therapy.

Approximately 20 to 30 percent of pregnant patients with acute pyelonephritis will develop a recurrent urinary tract infection later in pregnancy.[25] The most cost-effective way to reduce the frequency of recurrence is to administer a daily prophylactic dose of an antibiotic, such as sulfisoxazole (1 g) or nitrofurantoin monohydrate macrocrystals (100 mg). Patients receiving prophylaxis should have their urine screened for bacteria at each subsequent clinic appointment.

CHORIOAMNIONITIS

Epidemiology

Chorioamnionitis (amnionitis, intra-amniotic infection) occurs in approximately 1 to 5 percent of term pregnancies.[32] In patients with preterm delivery, the frequency of clinical or subclinical infection may approach 25 percent.[33] Chorioamnionitis is usually an ascending infection caused by organisms that are part of the normal vaginal flora. The principal pathogens are *Bacteroides* and *Prevotella* species, *E. coli,* anaerobic streptococci, and group B streptococci.[34] The most important clinical risk factors are young age, low socioeconomic status, nulliparity, extended duration of labor and ruptured membranes, multiple vaginal examinations, and preexisting infections of the lower genital tract.[32]

Diagnosis

The diagnosis of chorioamnionitis can be established on the basis of the clinical findings of maternal fever and maternal and fetal tachycardia, in the absence of other localizing signs of infection. In more severely ill patients, uterine tenderness and purulent amniotic fluid may be present.[32] The differential diagnosis of chorioamnionitis includes upper respiratory infection, bronchitis, pneumonia, pyelonephritis, viral syndrome, and appendicitis.

Laboratory confirmation of the diagnosis of chorioamnionitis is not routinely necessary in term patients who are progressing to delivery. However, in preterm patients who are being evaluated for tocolysis or corticosteroids, laboratory assessment may be of value. Table 25–4 summarizes the abnormal laboratory findings that may be present in infected patients.[32,35–40]

Management

Both the mother and infant may experience serious complications when chorioamnionitis is present. Bacteremia occurs in 3 to 12 percent of infected women. When cesarean delivery is required, up to 8 percent of women develop a wound infection, and approximately

Table 25-4. DIAGNOSTIC TESTS FOR CHORIOAMNIONITIS

Test	Abnormal Finding	Comment
Maternal white blood cell (WBC) count[32]	≥15,000 cells/mm^3 with preponderance of leukocytes	Labor and/or corticosteroids may result in elevation of WBC count.
Amniotic fluid glucose[35-37]	≤10 to 15 mg/dl	Excellent correlation with positive amniotic fluid culture and clinical infection.
Amniotic fluid interleukin-6[38]	≥7.9 ng/ml	Excellent correlation with positive amniotic fluid culture and clinical infection.
Amniotic fluid leukocyte esterase[39]	≥1 + reaction	Good correlation with positive amniotic fluid culture and clinical infection.
Amniotic fluid Gram's stain[32]	Any organism in an oil immersion field	Allows identification of particularly virulent organism such as group B streptococci; however, the test is very sensitive to inoculum effect. In addition, it cannot identify pathogens such as mycoplasmas.
Amniotic fluid culture[32]	Growth of aerobic or anaerobic microorganism	Results are not immediately available for clinical management.
Blood cultures[32,40]	Growth of aerobic or anaerobic microorganism	Will be positive in 5–10% of patients. However, will usually not be of value in making clinical decisions unless patient is at increased risk for bacterial endocarditis, is immunocompromised, or has a poor response to initial treatment.

1 percent develop a pelvic abscess. Fortunately, maternal death due to infection is exceedingly rare.[32]

Five to 10 percent of neonates delivered to mothers with chorioamnionitis have pneumonia or bacteremia. The predominant organisms responsible for these infections are group B streptococci and *E. coli.* Mortality due to infection ranges from 1 to 4 percent in term neonates but may approach 15 percent in preterm infants.

To prevent maternal and neonatal complications, parenteral antibiotic therapy should be initiated as soon as the diagnosis of chorioamnionitis is made, unless delivery is imminent. Three separate investigations have demonstrated that mother–infant pairs who receive prompt intrapartum treatment have better outcomes than patients treated after delivery.[41–43] The principal benefits of early treatment include decreased frequency of neonatal bacteremia and pneumonia and decreased duration of maternal fever and hospitalization.

The most extensively tested intravenous antibiotic regimen for treatment of chorioamnionitis is the combination of ampicillin (2 g every 6 hours) or penicillin (5 million units every 6 hours) plus gentamicin (1.5 mg/kg every 8 hours).[15,32] In patients who are allergic to β-lactam antibiotics, either vancomycin (500 mg every 6 hours or 1 g every 12 hours), erythromycin (1 g every 6 hours), or clindamycin (900 mg every 8 hours) can be substituted for ampicillin.

If a patient with chorioamnionitis requires cesarean delivery, a drug with activity against anaerobic organisms should be added to the antibiotic regimen, either clindamycin (900 mg every 8 hours) or metronidazole (500 mg every 12 hours). Extended spectrum cephalosporins, penicillins, and carbapenems also provide excellent coverage against the bacteria that cause chorioamnionitis.

Parenteral antibiotics should be continued until the patient has been afebrile and asymptomatic for approximately 24 hours. Once an adequate clinical response has been achieved, antibiotics may be discontinued and the patient discharged. A course of oral antibiotics administered as an outpatient is rarely indicated.[15,32,44]

There are two principal exceptions to the above rule. First, a patient with a documented staphylococcal bacteremia may require a longer period of intravenous therapy and, subsequently, an extended course of oral antibiotics. Second, the patient who has a vaginal delivery and then experiences a rapid defervescence may be a suitable candidate for a short course of oral antibiotics administered as an outpatient. In this situation, amoxicillin (875 mg)-clavulanic acid (125 mg), one tablet twice daily for 2–3 days, provides effective coverage.

Patients with chorioamnionitis are at increased risk for dysfunctional labor. Affected patients need careful monitoring during labor to ensure that uterine contractility is optimized. In addition, the fetus also needs close surveillance. Fetal heart rate abnormalities such as tachycardia and decreased variability occur in most cases.

PUERPERAL ENDOMETRITIS

Epidemiology

The frequency of puerperal endometritis in women having vaginal delivery is approximately 1 to 3 percent; in women having a scheduled cesarean prior to the onset of labor and rupture of membranes, 5 to 15 percent; and in women having a cesarean delivery after an extended period of labor and ruptured membranes, 30 to 35 percent without antibiotic prophylaxis and 15 to 20 percent with prophylaxis.

Endometritis is a polymicrobial infection caused by microorganisms that are part of the normal vaginal flora. These bacteria gain access to the upper genital tract, peritoneal cavity and, occasionally, the bloodstream as a result of vaginal examinations during labor and manipulations during surgery. The most common pathogenic bacteria are group B streptococci, anaerobic streptococci, aerobic gram-negative bacilli (predominantly *E. coli, Klebsiella pneumoniae,* and *Proteus* species), and anaerobic gram-negative bacilli (principally *Bacteroides* and *Prevotella* species).

The principal risk factors for endometritis are cesarean delivery, young age, low socioeconomic status, extended duration of labor and ruptured membranes, and multiple vaginal examinations. In addition, preexisting infection or colonization of the lower genital tract (gonorrhea, group B streptococci, bacterial vaginosis) also predisposes to ascending infection.[46]

Clinical Presentation and Diagnosis

Affected patients typically have a fever of 38 °C or higher within 36 hours of delivery. Associated findings include malaise, tachycardia, lower abdominal pain and tenderness, uterine tenderness, and discolored, malodorous lochia.

The initial differential diagnosis of puerperal fever should include endometritis, atelectasis, pneumonia, viral syndrome, pyelonephritis, and appendicitis. Endometrial cultures are of primary value in evaluating patients who have a poor initial response to antibiotic treatment. When these cultures are obtained, they should be collected with a double-lumen instrument to prevent contamination by lower genital tract flora.[47] Blood cultures also are indicated in such patients and in those who are immunocompromised or at increased risk for bacterial endocarditis.[46]

Management

Patients who have mild to moderately severe infections, particularly after vaginal delivery, can be treated with short intravenous courses of single agents such as the extended spectrum cephalosporins and penicillins or carbapenem antibiotics such as imipenem-cilastatin and meropenem. Combination antibiotic regimens should be considered for more severely ill patients, particularly those who are indigent and in poor general health and those who have had cesarean deliveries.

Once antibiotics are begun, approximately 90 percent of patients will defervesce within 48 to 72 hours. When the patient has been afebrile and asymptomatic for approximately 24 hours, parenteral antibiotics should be discontinued, and the patient should be discharged. As a general rule, an extended course of oral antibiotics is not necessary following discharge.[48]

Patients who fail to respond to the antibiotic therapy outlined above usually have one of two problems, a drug-resistant organism or a wound infection. Table 25–5 lists possible weaknesses in

Table 25–5. TREATMENT OF RESISTANT MICROORGANISMS IN PATIENTS WITH PUERPERAL ENDOMETRITIS

Initial Antibiotic(s)	Principal Weakness in Coverage	Modification of Therapy
Extended spectrum cephalosporins	Some aerobic and anaerobic gram-negative bacilli Enterococci	Change treatment to clindamycin or metronidazole plus penicillin or ampicillin plus gentamicin
Extended spectrum penicillins	Some aerobic and anaerobic gram-negative bacilli	As above
Clindamycin plus gentamicin or aztreonam	Enterococci Some anaerobic gram-negative bacilli	Add ampicillin or penicillin* Consider substitution of metronidazole for clindamycin

*Ampicillin alone is highly active against enterococci. Penicillin *plus* gentamicin work synergistically to provide excellent coverage against this organism.
From Duff P: Antibiotic selection for infections in obstetric patients. Semin Perinatol 17:367, 1993, with permission.

coverage of selected antibiotics and indicates the appropriate change in treatment.

When changes in antibiotic therapy do not result in clinical improvement and no evidence of wound infection is present, the differential diagnosis should be expanded (Table 25–6[46]).

Table 25–6. DIFFERENTIAL DIAGNOSIS OF PERSISTENT PUERPERAL FEVER

Condition	Diagnostic Test(s)	Treatment
Resistant microorganism	Endometrial culture Blood culture	Modify antibiotic therapy
Wound infection	Physical examination Needle aspiration Ultrasound	Incision and drainage Antibiotics
Pelvic abscess	Physical examination Ultrasound CT MRI	Drainage Antibiotics
Septic pelvic vein thrombophlebitis	Ultrasound CT MRI	Heparin anticoagulation Antibiotics
Recrudescence of connective tissue disease	Serology	Corticosteroids
Drug fever	Inspection of temperature graph WBC–identify eosinophilia	Discontinue antibiotics
Mastitis	Physical examination	Modify antibiotic treatment to provide coverage of staphylococcal organisms

From Duff P: Antibiotic selection for infections in obstetric patients. Semin Perinatol 17:367, 1993, with permission.

Prevention of Puerperal Endometritis

Prophylactic antibiotics are clearly of value in reducing the frequency of postcesarean endometritis, particularly in women having surgery after an extended period of labor and ruptured membranes.[50] The most appropriate agent for prophylaxis is a limited spectrum (first-generation) cephalosporin, such as cefazolin, administered in an intravenous dose of 1 g immediately after the neonate's umbilical cord is clamped. A second dose is indicated approximately 8 hours after the first dose in high-risk patients, especially when operating time is prolonged beyond 1 hour.

Patients who have an immediate hypersensitivity to β-lactam antibiotics pose a special problem. One alternative is to administer metronidazole, 500 mg IV. Another alternative is to administer a single dose of clindamycin (900 mg) plus gentamicin (1.5 mg/kg). Although these antibiotics are commonly used for treatment of overt infections, their administration is still warranted in penicillin-allergic patients who are at high risk for postoperative infection.

SERIOUS SEQUELAE OF PUERPERAL INFECTION

Wound Infection

Wound infection after cesarean delivery occurs in approximately 3 to 5 percent of patients with endometritis.[46] The major risk factors for wound infection are listed in the box "Principal Risk Factors for Postcesarean Wound Infection." The principal causative organisms are *Staphylococcus aureus,* aerobic streptococci, and aerobic and anaerobic bacilli.[51]

The diagnosis of wound infection always should be considered in patients who have a poor clinical response to antibiotic therapy for endometritis.[46] Clinical examination characteristically shows erythema, induration, and tenderness at the margins of the abdominal incision. When the wound is probed with either a cotton-tipped applicator or fine needle, pus usually exudes. Gram's stain and culture of the wound exudate are not routinely needed.

When pus is present in the incision, the wound must be opened and drained completely. Antibiotic therapy should be modified to provide coverage against staphylococci. Nafcillin (2 g IV every 6 hours) would be a suitable drug for this purpose. In a patient who is allergic to β-lactam antibiotics, vancomycin (1 g IV every 12 hours) is an acceptable alternative.[44]

> **Principal Risk Factors for Postcesarean Wound Infection**
>
> - Poor surgical technique
> - Low socioeconomic status
> - Extended duration of labor and ruptured membranes
> - Preexisting infection such as chorioamnionitis
> - Obesity
> - Type 1 (insulin-dependent) diabetes
> - Immunodeficiency disorder
> - Corticosteroid therapy
> - Immunosuppressive therapy

Once the wound is opened, a careful inspection should be made to be certain that the fascial layer is intact. If it is disrupted, surgical intervention will be necessary to reapproximate the fascia. Otherwise, the wound should be irrigated two to three times daily with a solution such as warm saline, a clean dressing should be maintained, and the incision should be allowed to heal by secondary intention. Antibiotics should be continued until the base of the wound is clean and all signs of cellulitis have resolved. Patients usually can be treated at home once the acute signs of infection have subsided.

Necrotizing fasciitis is an uncommon but extremely serious complication of abdominal wound infection.[52] This condition is most likely to occur in patients with diabetes, cancer, or an immunosuppressive disorder. Multiple bacterial pathogens, particularly anaerobes, have been isolated from patients with necrotizing fasciitis.

Necrotizing fasciitis should be suspected when the margins of the wound become discolored, cyanotic, and devoid of sensation. When the wound is opened, the subcutaneous tissue is easily dissected free of the underlying fascia, but muscle tissue is not affected. If the diagnosis is uncertain, a tissue biopsy should be performed and examined by frozen section.

Necrotizing fasciitis is a life-threatening condition and requires aggressive medical and surgical management. Broad-spectrum antibiotics with activity against all potential aerobic and anaerobic pathogens should be administered. Intravascular volume should be maintained with infusions of crystalloid, and electrolyte abnormalities should be corrected. Finally, and most importantly, the wound must be debrided and all necrotic tissue removed. In many instances, the dissection must be quite extensive and may be best managed in conjunction with an experienced surgeon.[52]

Pelvic Abscess

With the advent of modern antibiotics, pelvic abscesses after cesarean or vaginal delivery have become extremely rare. When present, abscess collections are typically located in the anterior or posterior cul de sac, most commonly the latter, or the broad ligament. The usual bacteria isolated from abscess cavities are coliforms and anaerobic gram-negative bacilli, particularly *Bacteroides* and *Prevotella* species.[54]

Patients with an abscess typically experience a persistent fever despite initial therapy for endometritis. In addition, they usually have malaise, tachycardia, lower abdominal pain and tenderness, and a palpable pelvic mass anterior, posterior, or lateral to the uterus. The peripheral WBC count is usually elevated, and there is a shift toward immature cell forms. Ultrasound, computed tomographic (CT) scan, and magnetic resonance imaging (MRI) may be used to confirm the diagnosis of pelvic abscess.[55]

Patients with a pelvic abscess require surgical intervention to drain the purulent collection and antibiotics with excellent activity against coliform organisms and anaerobes.[54] One regimen that has been tested extensively in obstetric patients with serious infections is the combination of penicillin (5 million units IV every 6 hours) or ampicillin (2 g IV every 6 hours) plus gentamicin (1.5 mg/kg IV every 8 hours or 7 mg/kg of ideal body weight every 24 hours) plus clindamycin (900 mg IV every 8 hours) or metronidazole (500 mg IV every 12 hours). If a patient is allergic to β-lactam antibiotics, vancomycin (500 mg IV every 6 hours or 1 g IV every 12 hours) can be substituted for penicillin or ampicillin. Aztreonam (1 to 2 g IV every 8 hours) also can be used in lieu of gentamicin when the patient is at risk for nephrotoxicity. Alternatively, the single agents imipenem-cilastatin (500 mg IV every 6 hours) or meropenem (1 g every 8 hours) provide excellent coverage against the usual pathogens responsible for an abscess. Antibiotics should be continued until the patient has been afebrile and asymptomatic for a minimum of 24 to 48 hours.[46]

Septic Pelvic Vein Thrombophlebitis

Like pelvic abscess, septic pelvic vein thrombophlebitis is extremely rare. Septic pelvic vein thrombophlebitis occurs in two distinct forms.[57] The most commonly described disorder is acute thrombosis of one (usually the right) or both ovarian veins (*ovarian vein syndrome*).[58] Affected patients typically develop a moderate temperature elevation in association with lower abdominal pain in the first 48 to 96 hours postpartum.

On physical examination, the patient's pulse is usually elevated. Tachypnea, stridor, and dyspnea may be evident if pulmonary embolization has occurred. The abdomen is tender, and bowel sounds are often decreased or absent. Most patients demonstrate voluntary and involuntary guarding, and 50 to 70 percent have a tender, rope-like mass originating near one cornua and extending laterally and cephalad toward the upper abdomen. The principal conditions that should be considered in the differential diagnosis of ovarian vein syndrome are pyelonephritis, nephrolithiasis, appendicitis, broad ligament hematoma, adnexal torsion, and pelvic abscess.

The second presentation of septic pelvic vein thrombophlebitis is termed *enigmatic fever*.[59] Initially, affected patients have clinical findings suggestive of endometritis and receive systemic antibiotics. Subsequently, they experience subjective improvement, with the exception of temperature instability. They do not appear to be seriously ill, and positive findings are limited to persistent fever and tachycardia. Disorders that should be considered in the differential diagnosis of enigmatic fever are drug fever, viral syndrome, collagen vascular disease, and pelvic abscess.

The diagnostic tests of greatest value in evaluating patients with suspected septic pelvic vein thrombophlebitis are CT scan and MRI. These tests are most sensitive in detecting large thrombi in the major pelvic vessels. In some cases, the ultimate diagnosis may depend on the patient's response to an empiric trial of heparin.[60,61]

Patients with septic pelvic vein thrombophlebitis should be treated with therapeutic doses of intravenous heparin.[57,60] The dose of heparin should be adjusted to maintain the activated partial thromboplastin time (aPTT) at approximately 2 times normal or to achieve a serum heparin concentration of 0.2 to 0.7 IU/ml. Therapy should be continued for 7 to 10 days. Long-term anticoagulation with oral agents is probably unnecessary unless the patient has massive clotting throughout the pelvic venous plexus or has sustained a pulmonary embolism. Patients should be maintained on broad-spectrum antibiotics throughout the period of heparin administration.

Once medical therapy is initiated, the patient should have objective evidence of a response within 48 to 72 hours. If no improvement is noted, surgical intervention may be necessary.[57,60]

CYTOMEGALOVIRUS INFECTION

Epidemiology

CMV is not highly contagious and, therefore, close personal contact is required for infection to occur. *Horizontal transmission* may result from receipt of an infected organ or blood, from sexual contact, or from contact with contaminated saliva or urine. *Vertical transmission* may occur as a result of transplacental infection, exposure to contaminated genital tract secretions during delivery, or breast-feeding. The incubation period of the virus ranges from 28 to 60 days, with a mean of 40 days.[70-72]

In addition to acquiring infection from young children, adolescents and adults may develop infection as a result of sexual contact.

Clinical Manifestations

Most adults with either primary or recurrent CMV are asymptomatic. Symptomatic patients typically have findings suggestive of mononucleosis.

Diagnosis of Infection

The diagnosis of CMV infection can be confirmed by isolation of virus in tissue culture. The highest concentration of CMV is usually present in urine, seminal fluid, saliva, and breast milk. Use of the polymerase chain reaction (PCR) permits identification of viral antigen within 24 hours.[80-83]

Serologic methods also are helpful in establishing the diagnosis of CMV infection, provided that the reference laboratory is skilled in performing such tests. In the acute phase of infection, virus-specific immunoglobulin M (IgM) antibody is present in serum. IgM titers usually decline rapidly over a period of 30 to 60 days, but they can remain elevated for several months. There is no absolute immunoglobulin G (IgG) titer that clearly will differentiate acute from recurrent infection. However, a fourfold or greater change in the IgG titer is consistent with recent acute infection.[70]

Congenital and Perinatal Infection

Approximately 50 to 80 percent of adult women in the United States have serologic evidence of past CMV infection. Unfortunately, the presence of antibody is not perfectly protective against vertical transmission; thus, pregnant women with both recurrent and primary infection pose a special risk to their fetus. Fetal and neonatal CMV infection may occur at three distinct times: antepartum, intrapartum, and postpartum. Antepartum or congenital infection is the greatest risk to the fetus.

Congenital (Antepartum) Infection

Congenital CMV infection results from hematogenous dissemination of virus across the placenta. Dissemination may occur with both primary and recurrent (reactivated) infection but is much more likely in the former setting. The overall risk of congenital infection is greatest when maternal infection occurs in the third trimester, but the probability of severe fetal injury is highest when maternal infection occurs in the first trimester.

Of fetuses with congenital infection, 5 to 18 percent will be overtly symptomatic at birth. The most common clinical manifestations are hepatosplenomegaly, intracranial calcifications, jaundice, growth restriction, microcephaly, chorioretinitis, and hearing loss. Approximately 30 percent of severely infected infants die. Eighty percent of the survivors have severe neurologic morbidity, ocular abnormalities, or sensorineural hearing loss.[86,87] Approximately 85 to 90 percent of infants delivered to mothers with primary infection will be asymptomatic at birth. Ten to 15 percent subsequently develop hearing loss, chorioretinitis, or dental defects within the first 2 years of life.

Overall, approximately 1 percent of infants (40,000) born in the United States each year have congenital CMV infection. Approximately 3,000 to 4,000 infants are symptomatic at birth, and an additional 4,000 to 6,000 subsequently have neurologic or developmental problems in the first years of life. CMV infection is now the principal cause of hearing deficits in children.

Perinatal (Intrapartum and Postpartum) Infection

Perinatal infection may occur *during delivery* as a result of exposure to infected genital tract secretions. Infants rarely have serious sequelae if infection is acquired during delivery.[86,89]

Perinatal infection also may develop as a *result of breast-feeding*. Fortunately, serious sequelae did not occur in infected infants.

Diagnosis of Fetal Infection

In recent years, much attention has focused on analysis of amniotic fluid and fetal serum as a means to diagnose congenital infection. Amniotic fluid culture or nucleic acid probe for viral antigen are superior in confirming the diagnosis of congenital CMV infection.

Although identification of virus in amniotic fluid appears to be the most sensitive and specific test for diagnosing congenital infection, it does not necessarily identify the *severity* of fetal injury. Detailed sonography can be invaluable in providing information about severity of fetal impairment. The principal sonographic findings suggestive of serious fetal injury include microcephaly, ventriculomegaly, intracerebral calcifications, hydrops, growth restriction, and oligohydramnios.[92]

Treatment and Prevention

At the present time, a vaccine for CMV is not available. Antiviral agents such as ganciclovir and foscarnet have moderate activity against CMV, but their use is limited primarily to treatment of severe infections in immunocompromised patients. Accordingly, obstetrician–gynecologists should focus most of their attention on educating patients about preventive measures.

One of the most important interventions is helping patients understand that CMV infection can be a sexually transmitted disease. Another important intervention is educating health care workers, day-care workers, elementary school teachers, and mothers of young children about the importance of simple infection control measures such as handwashing and proper cleansing of environmental surfaces. Obstetricians and pediatricians must be consistently aware of the importance of transfusing only CMV-free blood products to fetuses, neonates, pregnant women, and immunocompromised patients, and screening potential donors of organs and semen for CMV infection.[71] Finally, health care workers must adhere to the principles of universal precautions when treating patients and handling potentially infected body fluids.[84]

Routine prenatal screening for CMV infection is not recommended.

GROUP B STREPTOCOCCAL INFECTION

Epidemiology

Group B streptococcus is one of the most important causes of early-onset neonatal infection. The prevalence of neonatal group B streptococcal infection is 1 to 2 per 1,000 live births, and approximately 10,000 to 12,000 cases of neonatal streptococcal septicemia occur each year in the United States.[97,98]

Neonatal group B streptococcal infection can be divided into *early-onset* and *late-onset* infection. Approximately 80 to 85 percent of cases of neonatal group B streptococcal infection are early in onset and result almost exclusively from vertical transmission from a colonized mother. Early-onset infection presents primarily as a severe pneumonia and/or overwhelming septicemia. In preterm infants, the mortality from early-onset group B streptococcal infection approaches 25 percent. In term infants, the mortality is lower, averaging approximately 5 percent. Late-onset neonatal group B streptococcal infection occurs as a result of both vertical and horizontal transmission. It is typically manifested by bacteremia, meningitis, and pneumonia. The mortality from late onset infection is approximately 5 to 10 percent.

Major risk factors for early-onset infection include preterm labor, especially when complicated by preterm premature rupture of membranes (PROM); intrapartum maternal fever (chorioamnionitis); prolonged rupture of membranes, defined as greater than 12–18 hours; and previous delivery of an infected infant.[97,99,100] Approximately 25 percent of pregnant women have at least one risk factor for group B streptococcal infection. The neonatal attack rate in colonized patients is 40 to 50 percent in the presence of a risk factor, and 5 percent or less in the absence of a risk factor. In infected infants, neonatal mortality approaches 30 to 35 percent when a maternal risk factor is present but is 5 percent or less when a risk factor is absent.[97–99]

Maternal Complications

Group B streptococcus is a major cause of chorioamnionitis and postpartum endometritis. It also may cause postcesarean wound infection. Group B streptococci also are responsible for approximately 2 to 3 percent of lower urinary tract infections in pregnant women, a risk factor for preterm labor. Investigations have confirmed the association between group B streptococcal colonization and preterm labor and preterm PROM.

Diagnosis

The "gold standard" for the diagnosis of group B streptococcal infection is bacteriologic culture. Todd-Hewitt broth or selective blood agar is the preferred medium. Specimens for culture should be obtained from the lower vagina, perineum, and perianal area, using a simple cotton swab. Although the rapid diagnostic tests have reasonable sensitivity in identifying heavily colonized patients, they had poor sensitivity in identifying lightly and moderately colonized patients, limiting their usefulness in clinical practice.

Prevention of Group B Streptococcal Infection

Several strategies have been proposed for the prevention of neonatal group B streptococcal infection.[98–106] Each strategy has had major imperfections. Centers for Disease Control and Prevention (CDC) guidelines recommend universal culturing of all patients at 35 to 37 weeks. Samples should be obtained from the lower vagina, perineum, and perianal area and cultured in selective media such as Todd-Hewitt broth. Patients who are colonized should receive intrapartum prophylaxis with one of the antibiotic regimens

Table 25–7. ANTIBIOTICS WITH ACTIVITY AGAINST GROUP B STREPTOCOCCI

Drug	Dose for Intrapartum Prophylaxis
Ampicillin	2 g initially, then 1 g q4h
Penicillin	5 million units initially, then 2.5 million units q4h
Erythromycin	500 mg q6h
Clindamycin	900 mg q8h
Vancomycin	500 mg q6h

listed in Table 25–7. If culture results are unavailable (e.g., a patient with preterm labor or a patient who failed to register for prenatal care), the patient should receive intrapartum prophylaxis if she has a recognized risk factor for early-onset neonatal group B streptococcal infection. Ideally, antibiotics should be administered at least four hours prior to delivery.

HEPATITIS

Hepatitis A

Hepatitis A is responsible for approximately 30 to 35 percent of cases of hepatitis in the United States. Individuals at particular risk for hepatitis A are those who have recently immigrated from, or traveled to, developing nations of the world where the disease is endemic.[111]

The incubation period of hepatitis A ranges from 15 to 50 days, with a mean of 28 to 30 days. The highest concentration of viral particles is in fecal material. The virus is not normally excreted in urine or other body fluids. The characteristic physical findings of acute hepatitis A are jaundice, hepatic tenderness, darkened urine, and acholic stools.

The most useful diagnostic test for hepatitis A is detection of IgM-specific antibody. IgM antibody usually is detectable 25 to 30 days following the initial exposure and persists in the serum for up to 6 months. IgG antibody is detectable within 35 to 40 days of exposure and persists indefinitely, thus conferring lifelong immunity. In addition, the serum concentration of alanine aminotransferase (ALT), aspartate aminotransferase (AST), and bilirubin are usually moderately to markedly elevated.

Fortunately, acute hepatitis A is usually a self-limited illness, and only supportive care is required for the vast majority of patients. Recovery is typically complete within 4 to 6 weeks. Sexual and household contacts should receive immunoprophylaxis with a single intramuscular dose of immune globulin, 0.02 ml/kg within 2 weeks of exposure. In addition, they also should receive the formalin-inactivated hepatitis A vaccine, in a single intramuscular dose of 0.06 ml. The vaccine is highly immunogenic and is safe for use in pregnancy.[115,116]

As a general rule, unless the pregnant mother becomes severely ill, hepatitis A does not pose a serious risk to the fetus. Perinatal transmission of infection rarely occurs, and a chronic carrier state does not exist. An infant delivered to an acutely infected mother should receive immune globulin to prevent horizontal transmission of infection after delivery.[114]

Hepatitis B

Approximately 40 to 45 percent of all cases of hepatitis in the United States are caused by hepatitis B virus. The virus has three major structural antigens: surface antigen (HBsAg), core antigen (HBcAg), and e antigen (HBeAg). Transmission of hepatitis B occurs primarily as a result of parenteral injection, sexual contact, and perinatal exposure.[114]

Following an acute infection caused by hepatitis B virus, less than 1 percent of patients develop fulminant hepatitis and die. Eighty-five to 90 percent experience complete resolution of their physical findings and develop protective levels of antibody. Ten to 15 percent of patients become chronically infected. Of these, 15 to 30 percent subsequently develop chronic active or persistent hepatitis or cirrhosis.

The diagnosis of *acute* hepatitis B is confirmed by detection of the surface antigen and IgM antibody to the core antigen. Identification of HBeAg is indicative of an exceptionally high viral inoculum and active viral replication. Patients who have *chronic* hepatitis B infection have persistence of the surface antigen in the serum and liver tissue.

Infected women also may transmit infection to their fetus. Perinatal transmission occurs primarily as a result of the infant's exposure to infected blood and genital secretions during delivery. In the absence of immunoprophylaxis for the neonate, perinatal transmission occurs in 10 to 20 percent of women who are seropositive for HBsAg. The frequency of perinatal transmission increases to almost 90 percent in women who are seropositive for both HBsAg and HBeAg.[114,115,119]

A combination of passive and active immunization is highly effective in preventing both horizontal and vertical transmission of hepatitis B infection. All individuals who have had household or sexual exposure to another person with hepatitis B infection should be tested to determine if they have antibody to the virus. If they are seronegative, they should immediately receive immunoprophylaxis with hepatitis B immune globulin (HBIG), 0.06 ml/kg IM. They then should receive the hepatitis B vaccination series. Similarly, infants who are delivered to seropositive mothers should receive HBIG, 0.5 ml IM, immediately after birth. They then should begin the hepatitis B vaccination series within 12 hours of birth.

In view of the extremely favorable results of immunoprophylaxis, the CDC recently recommended universal hepatitis B vaccination for all infants.[120] Dosage recommendations vary depending on the mother's serostatus. Infants born to seronegative mothers require only the vaccine. Infants born to seropositive mothers should receive both the vaccine and hepatitis B immune globulin. Therefore, obstetricians must continue to screen *all* of their patients for hepatitis B at some point during pregnancy.

Hepatitis C

The principal risk factors for hepatitis C are intravenous drug abuse, transfusion, and sexual intercourse.[122] Approximately 50 percent of infected patients develop biochemical evidence of hepatic dysfunction. Of these, about 20 percent subsequently develop chronic active hepatitis or cirrhosis.[114] Approximately 75 percent of patients with hepatitis C are asymptomatic. The diagnosis of hepatitis C infection is confirmed by identification of anti-C antibody.

In a general obstetric population, the prevalence of hepatitis C is 1 to 3 percent. The principal risk factors that identify an obstetric patient at high risk for hepatitis C include concurrent STDs such as hepatitis B and HIV infection, multiple sexual partners, history of recent multiple transfusions, and history of intravenous drug abuse.[125] The frequency of perinatal transmission is highly variable. In women who are co-infected with human immunodeficiency virus and/or who have high serum concentrations of hepatitis C RNA, the transmission rate may be as high as 40 percent. In other patients, the rate of transmission is less than or equal to 10 percent.[122,126]

At the present time, a vaccine for hepatitis C is not available. Passive immunization with immunoglobulin (0.06 ml/kg IM) should be administered following percutaneous exposure to a person with hepatitis C.

HERPES SIMPLEX VIRUS INFECTION

Epidemiology

Herpes simplex virus (HSV), a double-stranded DNA virus, is transmitted by direct, intimate contact. Following the initial infection, the virus remains dormant in neuronal ganglia and may reactivate at later times. Two strains of the virus have been identified: HSV-1 and HSV-2. The former causes primarily oropharyngeal infection and the latter, genital tract infection. Approximately 0.5 to 1.0 percent of women have an overt herpetic infection during pregnancy. About 400 cases of neonatal herpes occur annually in the United States.

HSV infections are classified as *primary, nonprimary first episode,* and *recurrent* on the basis of historical and clinical findings and serologic testing.[137-140] Table 25–8 summarizes the criteria for each diagnosis. Approximately 20 to 40 percent of Americans are seropositive for HSV. Up to 80 percent of these individuals do not have a history of an overt primary infection.

Clinical Manifestations

The onset of HSV infection is usually heralded by a prodrome of neuralgias, paresthesias, and hypesthesias, followed by an eruption of painful vesicles in either the orolabial area or genitalia. The vesicles typically rupture, forming a shallow-based ulcer, and then form a dry crust. Some vesicles become secondarily infected and evolve into frank pustules. Ultimately, the vesicles heal without scarring.[137,138]

Table 25–8. CLASSIFICATION OF HERPES SIMPLEX VIRUS INFECTION

Classification	Criteria
Primary	First clinical infection
	No preexisting antibody
Nonprimary, first episode	No history of genital tract infection
	Positive antibody for the other strain of the virus (HSV1 or HSV2)
Recurrent	Prior history of clinical infection
	Positive antibody for the same strain of virus causing the present infection

Table 25–9. COMPARISON OF PRIMARY VERSUS RECURRENT HERPES SIMPLEX VIRUS INFECTION

	Type of Infection	
Stage of Illness	**Primary**	**Recurrent**
Incubation period and/or prodrome (days)	2–10	1–2
Vesicle, pustule (days)	6	2
Wet ulcer (days)	6	3
Dry crust (days)	8	7
Total	22–30	13–14

In patients experiencing a primary HSV infection, vesicles may be present for up to 3 weeks. Systemic symptoms may be moderately severe, and local complications such as urinary retention may occur. In recurrent infections, overt vesicles are fewer in number and less painful and typically persist for less than or equal to 14 days. Table 25–9 compares the incubation period and clinical features of primary and recurrent HSV infection.[137]

Diagnosis

Serology is useful in classifying the initial herpetic episode as *primary* versus *nonprimary first episode*.[137,138] However, serologic testing is rarely indicated in patients who experience recurrent HSV infection.

Until the advent of PCR, viral isolation in tissue culture was considered the gold standard for confirmation of diagnosis. Viral isolation is usually possible within 72 to 96 hours of inoculation of the tissue culture. The highest rate of isolation is achieved when clinical specimens are obtained from fresh vesicles or pustules. Vesicular fluid should be aspirated with a fine needle into a tuberculin syringe. Ulcers should be scraped vigorously with a wooden spatula or cotton-tipped applicator.[137,138]

Obstetric and Perinatal Complications

Severe primary HSV infection has been associated with spontaneous abortion, preterm delivery, and intrauterine growth restriction (IUGR). The greatest risk to the fetus occurs when overt HSV infection is present at the time of labor. In this situation, the principal mechanism of infection is direct contact with infected vesicles during the process of vaginal birth. The frequency of neonatal infection clearly is dependent on whether the mother has a primary or recurrent HSV infection. In the setting of a primary infection, the viral inoculum in the genital tract is high, and maternal antibody is not present. Approximately 40 percent of neonates delivered vaginally to such women will become infected. In the absence of antiviral chemotherapy, almost half of these infants die, and 35 to 40 percent experience severe neurologic morbidity such as chorioretinitis, microcephaly, mental retardation, seizures, and apnea. In women who have recurrent *symptomatic* HSV infection, the risk of neonatal infection following vaginal delivery is 5 percent or less. In women who have a history of recurrent HSV infection but no prodromal symptoms or overt lesions, the risk of neonatal infection with vaginal delivery is less than or equal to 1 in 1,000.[137,138,140,143–145]

Neonatal HSV infection may appear as a localized abscess at the site of attachment of a scalp electrode or as isolated mucocutaneous lesions. In its more severe forms, neonatal HSV infection may present as widely disseminated mucocutaneous lesions, visceral infection, meningitis, and encephalitis. In such instances, mortality may approach 50 to 60 percent, and up to half of the survivors may have persistent morbidity.[137,138,140,142,143,146]

Management during Pregnancy

The following simplified guidelines have now been recommended by the Infectious Diseases Society for Obstetrics and Gynecology and endorsed by the American College of Obstetricians and Gynecologists.[138,144] At the time of the patient's initial prenatal appointment, she should be questioned about a prior history of HSV infection. If her history is positive, she should be screened for other STDs such as gonorrhea, chlamydia, syphilis, hepatitis B and C, and HIV infection. When the patient ultimately is admitted for delivery, she should be asked about prodromal symptoms and examined thoroughly for cervical, vaginal, and vulvar lesions. If no prodromal symptoms or overt lesions are present, vaginal delivery should be anticipated. If symptoms or lesions are present, cesarean delivery should be performed. Cesarean secton is indicated even in the presence of ruptured membranes, since operative delivery significantly decreases the size of the viral inoculum to which the infant is exposed.

Mothers with symptomatic infection do not need to be isolated from their infants or other patients. They should wash their hands carefully before handling the infant and shield the baby from any contact with vesicular lesions. Breast-feeding is permissible as long as no skin lesions are present on the breast.

Prophylactic treatment with oral acyclovir (400 mg twice daily) or valacyclovir (1,000 mg daily) may be appropriate in women with frequent recurrent infections in pregnancy, particularly near term.[151,152] Acyclovir is classified by the FDA as a pregnancy category C drug. To date, the Acyclovir Registry has reported no increase in the frequency of adverse effects in infants exposed in utero to this antiviral agent.[153,154] Valaclovir and famciclovir are classified as pregnancy category B.

HUMAN IMMUNODEFICIENCY VIRUS INFECTION

Epidemiology

At the present time, almost 500,000 Americans have AIDS, or have died from AIDS. An additional 1 million are infected with the virus but are not yet in the terminal stage of their illness. In the United States, approximately 15 to 20 percent of all cases of HIV infection occur in women. Almost 75 percent of infected women are black or Hispanic. In women, the two most important mechanisms of HIV infection are intravenous drug abuse and heterosexual contact with a high-risk male. In the general obstetric population in the United States, the frequency of HIV infection is approximately 1 per 1,000. However, in some inner city populations, the prevalence of infection is as high as 1 to 1.5 percent.[158-160]

Clinical Manifestations

Symptomatic patients with HIV infection typically have fever, malaise, fatigue, anorexia, nausea, vomiting, diarrhea, weight loss, and generalized lymphadenopathy. Opportunistic infections, of course, are the hallmark of HIV infection.[162] Among the most common are *Pneumocystis carinii* pneumonia, mycobacterium avium complex, pulmonary tuberculosis, toxoplasmosis, candidiasis, and cytomegalovirus infection. Genital herpes; hepatitis B, C, and D; and syphilis are common concurrent sexually transmitted diseases.

Diagnosis

The diagnosis of HIV infection may be confirmed by direct culture of virus from peripheral blood lymphocytes and monocytes. The diagnosis also can be established by detection of viral antigen by PCR. Infected patients usually have a decreased number of CD4 cells and an inverted CD4:CD8 ratio. Serum immunoglobulin levels also are elevated.[164]

The principal diagnostic test at present is identification of virus-specific antibody.[164] The initial serologic screening test should be an enzyme immunoassay (EIA). This test is highly sensitive, inexpensive, and readily suited for screening large numbers of patients. If the initial EIA test is positive, the test should be repeated. If the second test is positive, a confirmatory Western blot assay or immunofluorescent antibody assay (IFA) should be performed. The Western blot test detects specific viral antigens and is considered positive when any two of the following three antigens are identified: p24 (viral core), gp-41 (envelope), and gp-120/160 (envelope). If a patient has two positive EIAs, followed by a confirmatory Western blot or IFA, the likelihood of a false-positive test is less than 1 in 10,000.[165,166]

Perinatal Transmission

Approximately 90 percent of all cases of HIV infection in children are due to perinatal transmission. Perinatal transmission may occur as a result of hematogenous dissemination, but it is most likely to result from intrapartum exposure to infected maternal blood and genital tract secretions.[157,159] The frequency of vertical transmission of HIV infection varies from a low of 5 to 10 percent to a high of 50 to 60 percent. The average in most investigations has been 20 to 30 percent.[167,168]

Obstetric Complications

Infected women appear to be at increased risk for several major complications: preterm delivery, preterm PROM, IUGR, increased perinatal mortality, and postpartum endometritis. Pregnancy per se probably does not significantly accelerate the progression of HIV infection.[157,159]

Management

All obstetric patients should be offered voluntary screening for HIV infection at the time of their first prenatal appointment. Selective screening only in patients presumed to be high risk will fail to identify approximately 50 percent of seropositive women.[169] Infected women should be counseled about the risk of perinatal transmission of infection and about potential obstetric complications. They should then be offered the option of pregnancy termination. In addition, arrangements should be made for patients to obtain assistance from appropriate support personnel such as social workers, nutritionists, and psychologists.

Infected patients should be screened for other sexually transmitted diseases such as gonorrhea, chlamydia, herpes, hepatitis B and C, and syphilis. They should be tested for antibody to cytomegalovirus and toxoplasmosis because both of these infections can cause severe chorioretinitis and central nervous system disease, and both are amenable to treatment with antimicrobial agents. Patients also should have a tuberculin skin test. In addition, patients should receive vaccinations for hepatitis A and B, pneumococcal infection, and viral influenza. Finally, a Papanicolaou smear should be done to determine if cervical intraepithelial neoplasia is present. They also should have periodic assays for CD4 count and viral load (HIV RNA-PCR) to assess the state of their immune system and the progression or remission of their disease.

Patients with HIV infection should receive treatment with antiviral chemotherapy. The rationale for treatment is twofold: prevention of perinatal transmission of HIV infection and improvement in the course of the mother's disease. Until recently, treatment guidelines in pregnancy focused primarily on the first objective and were based on the landmark study of the AIDS Clinical Trials Group (ACTG) Protocol 076.[170] This study, conducted in the United States and France, included a select group of obstetric patients: asymptomatic woman beyond the first trimester of pregnancy who had CD4 counts greater than 200/mm^3 and who had not previously been treated with zidovudine. Women were randomized to receive placebo or zidovudine (100 mg PO five times daily) during the antepartum period. Patients then received intravenous zidovudine during labor, in a loading dose of 2 mg/kg over 1 hour, followed by 1 mg/kg/h throughout labor. Following delivery, infants in the treatment group received oral zidovudine (2 mg/kg every 6 hours) for six weeks postpartum. The study was discontinued when interim data analysis revealed the frequency of perinatal transmission was 25.5 percent in the placebo arm versus 8.3 percent in the active treatment arm, representing a 67 percent reduction in the risk of vertical transmission ($p = 0.00006$).

In addition to these new findings related to intrapartum chemoprophylaxis, several treatment trials in nonpregnant patients have demonstrated a distinct advantage for multiagent regimens compared to monotherapy with respect to suppression of viral load, elevation of CD4 count, improvement in quality of life, and prolongation of disease-free interval. Accordingly, there is a growing consensus that these new treatment options should be offered to pregnant women as well.[174]

Table 25–10 lists the drugs most commonly used for treatment of HIV infection in pregnant women. Pending new information from ongoing trials, a reasonable approach is treatment with

Table 25–10. AGENTS MOST COMMONLY USED FOR TREATMENT OF HIV INFECTION IN PREGNANT WOMEN

Agent	Usual Adult Dose	Remarks	Cost of 30-Day Treatment
Nucleoside analogs			
Lamivudine (3TC, Epivir)	150 mg bid	Adverse effects are similar to those of zidovudine, but are less frequent. Drug is eliminated by renal excretion.	$230.00
Zidovudine (Retrovir)	300 mg bid	Main adverse effect is marrow suppression.	$287.00
Nonnucleoside reverse transcriptase inhibitors			
Nevirapine (Viramune)	200 mg bid	Most common adverse effect is rash. If the rash is extensive, the drug should be permanently discontinued. Hepatitis is a rare side effect.	$248.00
Protease inhibitors			
Indinavir (Crixivan)	800 mg q8h	Well tolerated. Most serious adverse effect is nephrolithiasis. Most common side effect is GI upset. Less expensive than Ritonavir.	$450.00
Nelfinavir (Viracept)	750 mg tid or 1250 mg in am and 1000mg in pm	Clinical efficacy data are limited. Most common adverse effects are diarrhea, fatigue, poor concentration.	$557.00

GI, gastrointestinal.

two nucleoside reverse transcriptase inhibitors and a protease inhibitor.[174] In view of the favorable results of the ACTG 076 study, one of the nucleosides should be zidovudine, administered in a dose of 300 mg orally, twice daily. Lamivudine (150 mg PO twice daily) also has an exceptionally good safety and efficacy profile. These two agents can be administered in a convenient combination formulation, Combivir, twice daily. Of the current protease inhibitors, the one with the best combination of safety, efficacy, and expense is nelfinavir (750 mg PO three times daily). In addition to specific antiviral chemotherapy, patients also should receive prophylaxis against the most common opportunistic infections.

When the physician is delivering the HIV-positive patient, every effort must be made to avoid instrumentation that would increase the neonate's exposure to infected maternal blood and secretions. Specifically, whenever feasible, the fetal membranes should be left intact until delivery. In addition, application of the fetal scalp electrode and scalp pH sampling should be avoided.

Elective cesarean appears to be indicated to reduce perinatal transmission for the following patients: those receiving no antiviral treatment, those receiving monotherapy alone, and those receiving combination chemotherapy but who have detectable viral loads. Women receiving optimal combination chemotherapy who have undetectable viral loads should be advised that it is uncertain whether elective cesarean delivery offers an additional protective effect against perinatal transmission.[178]

In the postpartum period, the mother should be advised to avoid any contact between her body fluids and an open area on the skin or mucous membranes of the neonate. She also should be cautioned against breast-feeding. Finally, infected patients should be urged to use secure contraception and adopt responsible sexual practices to prevent spread of infection to their partners.

PARVOVIRUS INFECTION

Epidemiology

Human parvovirus B19 is transmitted by respiratory droplets and infected blood components, and the incubation period is 4 to 20 days. Serum and respiratory secretions become positive for the virus several days before clinical symptoms develop. Once symptoms appear, respiratory secretions and serum are usually free of the virus.[180,181] Prevalence of antibody to parvovirus increases with age. In adolescents and adults, the seroprevalence increases to more than 60 percent.[180,181]

Clinical Manifestations

The most common clinical presentation of parvovirus infection is *erythema infectiosum* or *fifth disease*. This illness typically occurs in elementary school and day-care populations in the late winter and early spring. Patients usually have low-grade fever, malaise, adenopathy, and polyarthritis affecting the hands, wrists, and knees. In addition, they have a characteristic pruritic, erythematous "slapped cheek" rash on the face and a finely reticulated erythematous rash on the trunk and extremities. Erythema infectiosum is a self-limited illness, and serious long-term sequelae rarely occur.[180,181]

The second major clinical presentation of parvovirus infection is *transient aplastic crisis*, resulting from viral infection of the bone marrow, with resultant destruction of red blood cell precursors. Full recovery without sequelae is the usual outcome.

Fetal Infection

The risk that a susceptible mother will acquire infection from an infected household member is 50 to 90 percent.[180-182] The risk of transmission in a day-care setting or classroom is lower, ranging from 20 to 30 percent.[182-184] Published information regarding subsequent risk of transmission to the fetus is based on one principal end point, namely, fetal hydrops. Hydrops appears to result primarily from viral infection of fetal erythroid stem cells, leading to an aplastic anemia and high-output congestive heart failure. The risk of fetal infection is greatest when maternal illness occurs in the first trimester, as noted in Table 25–11.

Diagnosis of Maternal Infection

The mainstay of laboratory diagnosis is serologic testing. IgM-specific antibody is usually positive by the third day after symptoms develop.

Table 25–11. ASSOCIATION BETWEEN GESTATIONAL AGE AT TIME OF EXPOSURE AND RISK OF FETAL PARVOVIRUS INFECTION

Time of Exposure (Weeks' Gestation)	Frequency of Severely Affected Fetuses (%)
1–12	19
13–20	15
>20	6

Table 25-12. INTERPRETATION OF SEROLOGIC TESTS FOR MATERNAL PARVOVIRUS INFECTION

Condition	Maternal Antibody	
	IgM	IgG
Susceptible	−	−
Immune—infection > 120 days ago	−	+
Infection within 7 days	+	−
Infection within 7–120 days	+	+

It typically disappears within 30 to 60 days, but may persist for up to 120 days. IgG antibody is detectable by the seventh day of illness and persists for life.[180–182] Table 25–12 summarizes the interpretation of serologic tests for parvovirus.

Diagnosis of Fetal Infection

The most valuable test for diagnosis of fetal parvovirus infection is ultrasound. Severely affected fetuses typically have evidence of hydrops. Since the incubation period of the virus may be longer in the fetus than in the child or adult, the patient should be followed with serial ultrasound examinations for 8 to 10 weeks after her acute illness. If the fetus shows no signs of hydrops during this observation period, additional diagnostic studies are unnecessary. If hydropic changes appear and the fetus is at an appropriate gestational age, cordocentesis is indicated (see below).[180–182,188]

Maternal Management

Following a documented exposure to parvovirus, the mother should immediately have a serologic test to determine if she is immune or susceptible to the virus. If preexisting IgG antibody is present, the patient can be reassured that second infections are extremely unlikely and that her fetus is not at risk. If the patient is susceptible, she should have a repeat serologic test in approximately 3 weeks to determine if she has seroconverted. If seroconversion is detected, serial ultrasound examinations should be performed over the ensuing 8 to 10 weeks to evaluate fetal well-being.

No antiviral agent or vaccine is presently available for treatment of parvovirus infection, but patients with erythema infectiosum rarely need more than simple supportive care. Isolation of patients with erythema infectiosum is not of value in reducing transmission of infection, since spread by respiratory droplets has already occurred by the time the patient has clear signs of clinical disease.

Fetal Management

If fetal hydrops is documented by ultrasound, cordocentesis should be performed if technically feasible. Fetal blood should be collected for determination of hematocrit and detection of IgM-specific antibody.[188] If severe anemia is present, intrauterine transfusion should be performed.[191] Although the long-term prognosis for the neonate is excellent, there are reports of infants who have had neurologic injury and/or prolonged anemia as a result of congenital parvovirus infection.[192]

RUBELLA

Epidemiology

Rubella occurs primarily in young children and adolescents. The disease is most common in the springtime. With licensure of an effective rubella vaccine in 1969, the frequency of this infection has declined by almost 99 percent.[197] The persistence of this infection appears to be due to failure to vaccinate susceptible individuals rather than to lack of immunogenicity of the vaccine.

The rubella virus enters the host through the upper respiratory tract. The incubation period is approximately 2 to 3 weeks. The virus is present in blood and nasopharyngeal secretions for several days before appearance of the characteristic rash. The virus is also shed from the nasopharynx for several days after appearance of the exanthem. Therefore, the patient can be contagious for an extended period of time.[196,199]

Antibody against rubella does not normally appear in the serum until after the rash has developed. Acquired immunity to rubella is usually lifelong. Second infections have occurred after both natural primary infections and vaccination. However, recurrent infections generally are not associated with serious illness, viremia, or congenital infection.

Clinical Manifestations

Most children and adults with rubella have mild constitutional symptoms such as malaise, headache, myalgias, and arthralgias. The principal clinical manifestation of this illness, of course, is a widely disseminated, nonpruritic, erythematous, maculopapular rash. Postauricular adenopathy and mild conjunctivitis also are common. These clinical manifestations usually are short-lived and typically resolve within 3 to 5 days.

Diagnosis

The diagnosis of rubella can usually be established on the basis of the patient's physical examination. If necessary, serologic tests can be used to confirm the diagnosis. IgM antibody usually reaches a peak 7 to 10 days after the onset of illness and then declines over a period of 4 weeks. The serum concentration of IgG antibody usually rises more slowly, but antibody levels persist throughout the lifetime of the individual. Enzyme immunoassay and latex agglutination tests are the most rapid and convenient methods for screening for antibody to rubella.

Congenital Rubella Syndrome

Approximately 10 to 20 percent of women in the United States remain susceptible to rubella and, hence, their fetuses are at risk for serious injury should the mother become infected during pregnancy.

The rubella virus crosses the placenta by hematogenous dissemination, and the frequency of congenital infection is critically dependent on the time of exposure to the virus.[196,201,202] Approximately 50 percent of infants exposed to the virus within 4 weeks of conception will manifest signs of congenital infection. When maternal infection occurs in the second 4-week period after conception, approximately 25 percent of fetuses will be infected. When infection develops in the third month, approximately 10 percent of fetuses will be infected. When maternal infection occurs beyond this point in time, less than 1 percent of babies will be infected.

Of anomalies associated with the congenital rubella syndrome, the four most common abnormalities are deafness (affecting 60 to 75 percent of fetuses), eye defects (10 to 30 percent), CNS anomalies (10 to 25 percent), and cardiac malformations (10 to 20 percent). The most common cardiac abnormality associated with congenital rubella is patent ductus arteriosus, although supravalvular pulmonic stenosis is perhaps the most pathognomonic. Other possible abnormalities include microcephaly, mental retardation, pneumonia, IUGR hepatosplenomegaly, hemolytic anemia, and thrombocytopenia.[201,202] Detailed ultrasound examination is the best test to determine if serious fetal injury has occurred.

A variety of tests have been proposed for the diagnosis of congenital rubella syndrome. Cordocentesis can be performed to determine the total serum IgM concentration in fetal blood and to detect virus-specific antibody. However, fetal immunoglobulin production usually cannot be detected prior to 19 to 22 weeks of gestation. Some authors have proposed chorionic villus sampling (CVS) as a diagnostic test because placental tissue infected with rubella virus produces a cytopathic effect when grown in tissue culture. Viral antigen also can be identified rapidly in tissue culture by RNA-DNA hybridization techniques, and amniotic fluid can be cultured for rubella virus. Unfortunately, although the tests outlined above can demonstrate that rubella virus is present in the fetal compartment, they do not indicate the degree of fetal injury.

The prognosis for infants with congenital rubella syndrome is guarded. Approximately 50 percent of affected individuals have to attend schools for the hearing impaired. An additional 25 percent of infected children require at least some special schooling because of hearing impairment, and only 25 percent are able to attend mainstream regular schools.

Obstetric Management

If preconception serologic testing demonstrates they are susceptible, women should be vaccinated with rubella vaccine prior to conception.[196] When preconception counseling is not possible, all obstetric patients should have a test for rubella at the time of their first prenatal appointment. Women who are susceptible to rubella should be counseled to avoid exposure to other individuals who may have viral exanthems.

If a susceptible patient subsequently has exposure to rubella, serologic tests should be obtained to determine whether acute infection has occurred. If acute infection is documented, patients should be counseled about the risk of congenital rubella syndrome. Obviously, specific counseling should be based on the time in gestation when maternal infection occurred. The diagnostic tests for detection of in utero infection should be reviewed. Patients should be offered the option of pregnancy termination based on the assessed risk of serious fetal injury.[199]

Susceptible patients who are fortunate enough to escape infection during pregnancy should be vaccinated immediately postpartum. Approximately 95 percent of patients who receive rubella vaccine seroconvert. Antibody levels persist for at least 18 years in more than 90 percent of vaccinees.

There are few adverse effects of vaccination, even in adults. Breast-feeding is not a contraindication to vaccination. In addition, the vaccine can be administered in conjunction with other immune globulin preparations such as Rh-immune globulin.

Women who receive rubella vaccine should practice secure contraception for a minimum of 3 months after vaccination. The maximum theoretical risk of congenital rubella resulting from rubella vaccine in early pregnancy is 1 to 2 percent.

SYPHILIS

Epidemiology

Syphilis is caused by the spirochete *Treponema pallidum.* Infection occurs primarily as a result of sexual contact. The organism penetrates mucosal barriers and is highly contagious. Infection develops in 10 percent of contacts after a single exposure and in 70 percent after multiple exposures.[215,216] Syphilis also may be transmitted perinatally, with devastating consequences for the fetus.

The prevalence of syphilis in the United States has increased dramatically in recent years, coincident with the upsurge in cases of HIV infection and the growing epidemic of drug abuse. The greatest increase has been in females, aged 15 to 24 years, and a disproportionate number of cases have occurred in blacks and Hispanics living in urban areas.[215,216]

Clinical Manifestations and Staging

Syphilis may be divided into four *clinical* categories: primary, secondary, tertiary, and neurosyphilis. In addition, syphilis may present as a latent infection. Latent syphilis is subdivided into early latent (<1 year duration) and late latent infection (>1 year).[215–217] The incubation period of syphilis ranges from 10 to 90 days. At the end of this period, the characteristic raised, painless chancre appears. In women, the chancre is usually on the cervix or vaginal wall and may not be apparent except on close inspection. The chancre usually heals in 3 to 6 weeks even without specific antimicrobial treatment. The principal disorders that must be considered in the differential diagnosis of primary syphilis are HSV infection, chancroid, trauma, scabies, and carcinoma.

Patients who receive either no treatment, or inadequate treatment, may develop secondary syphilis 2 to 6 months after their primary infection. The principal clinical manifestation of this stage of the infection is a generalized maculopapular rash that is most obvious on the palms of the hands and soles of the feet. This rash may be confused with disseminated gonococcal infection, measles, rubella, scabies, psoriasis, and drug eruption. Other findings associated with secondary syphilis include mucous patches, shallow, painless ulcerations in the oropharynx; and condylomata lata, grayish, raised papules that appear on the vulva and near the anus. In addition, bone tenderness, iritis, alopecia, and generalized lymphadenopathy also may be present. The lesions of secondary syphilis usually resolve spontaneously in 3 to 6 weeks, even without treatment. Untreated patients then enter a latent phase of their illness. In this phase, infected women pose only a small risk of horizontal transmission of infection to their sexual partner. However, vertical transmission to the fetus still may occur.[215-217]

Approximately one third of patients with untreated secondary disease ultimately develop tertiary syphilis after an interval of several years. Tertiary syphilis is distinguished by three principal findings: gumma formation, cardiac lesions, and central nervous system abnormalities (neurosyphilis).

Diagnosis

T. pallidum cannot be cultured. It can be identified from overt lesions such as the chancre by darkfield microscopy and fluorescent antibody staining. However, most cases of infection, particularly those in the latent stage, are diagnosed by serology. The initial screening test for syphilis should be a nontreponemal assay such as the Venereal Disease Research Laboratories (VDRL) test or rapid plasma reagin (RPR) test. Several factors can cause biologically false-positive (BFP) test results such as collagen vascular disease, bacterial and viral infections, multiple myeloma, advanced cancer, chronic liver disease, IV drug use, multiple blood transfusions, and pregnancy. Accordingly, a positive screening test must be confirmed by a specific treponemal assay such as the fluorescent treponemal antibody absorption test (FTA-ABS) or microhemagglutination assay (MHATP). Biologic false-positive treponemal tests have been reported in patients with Lyme disease, leprosy, malaria, mononucleosis, and collagen vascular disease.

Lumbar puncture is indicated when neurosyphilis is suspected and in all patients who are co-infected with syphilis and HIV. Cerebrospinal fluid (CSF) abnormalities include a mononuclear pleocytosis (10 to 400 cells/mm^3), elevated protein (>45 mg/dl), and a positive VDRL test.[215-217]

Virtually all patients will have a positive serologic test within 4 weeks of their primary infection. With appropriate antibiotic treatment, quantitative nontreponemal tests usually decrease fourfold within 3 months in patients with primary or secondary syphilis. When this decline does not occur, patients should be reevaluated and considered for a second course of treatment. Antibody titers may decline more slowly in patients with more advanced stages of disease. Specific treponemal tests typically remain positive for life even after adequate treatment, although 13 to 24 percent of patients may ultimately become seronegative.[215-217] Ideally, patients should be followed with quantitative titers for up to 12 to 18 months after their initial infection to determine if they become seronegative.

Perinatal Complications

Syphilis in pregnancy may be associated with an increased risk of fetal demise, IUGR, and preterm delivery.[218] It also may accelerate the course of HIV infection in pregnant women. However, the most frequent (and potentially ominous) complication of syphilis in pregnancy is congenital infection. *T. pallidum* can cross the placenta and infect the fetus *at any stage of gestation.* Up to one third of fetuses with congenital syphilis are stillborn.[4] The frequency of vertical transmission varies primarily with the stage of maternal disease, as noted in Table 25–13.

The prenatal diagnostic test with the greatest potential for identifying the severely infected fetus is ultrasound. Ultrasound findings suggestive of in utero infection include placentomegaly, IUGR, microcephaly, hepatosplenomegaly, and hydrops.

Treatment

The treatment of syphilis in pregnancy is summarized in Table 25–14.[215-217] Clearly, penicillin is the drug of choice for this infection because of its proven ability to prevent congenital infection in most cases. Patients who have a previous history of an allergic reaction to penicillin should be skin tested to determine if their allergy persists.[215-217] In point of fact, approximately 10 percent of patients who report a history of severe allergy to penicillin remain allergic throughout life. They can be reliably identified by testing with major and minor penicillin determinants. If allergy is

Table 25–13. FREQUENCY OF VERTICAL TRANSMISSION OF SYPHILIS

Stage of Maternal Infection	Approximate Frequency of Congenital Syphilis
Primary	50%
Secondary	50%
Early latent	40%
Late latent	10%
Tertiary	10%

Table 25–14. RECOMMENDATIONS FOR TREATMENT OF SYPHILIS IN PREGNANCY

Stage of Disease	Principal Treatment	Alternate Treatment if Allergic To Penicillin*
Primary, secondary, or latent syphilis <1 year's duration	Benzathine penicillin G, 2.4 million units IM × 1†	Erythromycin 500 mg PO qid × 15 days Ceftriaxone 250 mg IM qd × 10 days
Latent syphilis >1 year's duration or cardiovascular syphilis	Benzathine penicillin G, 2.4 million units IM weekly × 3	Erythromycin 500 mg qid × 30 days
Neurosyphilis	Aqueous crystalline penicillin G, 3–4 million units q4h × 10–14 days, followed by benzathine penicillin G, 2.4 million units IM × 1 or Aqueous procaine penicillin G, 2.4 million units IM daily with probenecid, 500 mg PO qid, both for 10–14 days, followed by benzathine penicillin G, 2.4 million units IM × 1	No regimen of proven value other than penicillin

*These regimens should be administered only if desensitization to penicillin is unsuccessful.
†In patients who are concurrently infected with HIV, treat as outlined below for late latent or tertiary syphilis. Patients also should have a lumbar puncture to determine if neurosyphilis is present.

confirmed, patients should be desensitized with either oral or intravenous regimens.[215,217,220] Desensitization can usually be completed within 4 hours. It is best accomplished in consultation with an allergist and performed in an area of the hospital with immediate access to emergency resuscitative equipment. Alternative antibiotic regimens are not of proven value for prevention of congenital syphilis or treatment of advanced stages of disease. Accordingly, they should be used only if desensitization is unsuccessful.

Almost half of the pregnant women receiving penicillin for treatment of syphilis may develop uterine contractions and decreased fetal movement as a result of a Jarisch-Herxheimer reaction. The reaction was particularly likely in those patients who had primary and secondary syphilis, and the abnormalities typically appeared 2 to 8 hours after treatment and resolved within 24 hours. There are no reliable clinical or laboratory assessments that predict which patients will develop the Jarisch-Herxheimer reaction, and no specific treatment is available.

TOXOPLASMOSIS

Epidemiology

Toxoplasma gondii is a protozoan that has three distinct forms: trophozoite, cyst, and oocyst. The life cycle of *T. gondii* is dependent on wild and domestic cats, which are the only host for the oocyst. The oocyst is formed in the cat intestine and subsequently excreted in the feces. Mammals, such as cows, then ingest the oocyst, which is disrupted in the animal's intestine, releasing the invasive trophozoite. The trophozoite then is disseminated throughout the body, ultimately forming cysts in brain and muscle.

Human infection occurs when infected meat is ingested or when food is contaminated by cat feces. Infection rates are highest in areas of poor sanitation and crowded living conditions. Stray cats and domestic cats that eat raw meat are most likely to carry the parasite. The cyst is destroyed by heat. For this reason, meat should be cooked thoroughly before consumption.

Approximately 40 to 50 percent of adults in the United States have antibody to this organism. The frequency of seroconversion during pregnancy is 5 percent or less. Clinically significant congenital toxoplasmosis occurs in approximately 1 in 8,000 pregnancies.

Clinical Manifestations

The ingested organism invades across the intestinal epithelium and spreads hematogenously throughout the body. Clinical manifestations of infection are the result of direct organ damage and the subsequent immunologic response to parasitemia and cell death.

Most infections in humans are asymptomatic. Even in the absence of symptoms, however, patients may have evidence of multiorgan involvement, and clinical disease can follow a long period of asymptomatic infection. Symptomatic toxoplasmosis usually presents as an illness similar to mononucleosis.[222,223]

Because immunity to *T. gondii* is cell-mediated, patients with HIV infection and those treated with chronic immunosuppressive therapy after organ transplantation are particularly susceptible to new or reactivated infection.

Diagnosis

The diagnosis of toxoplasmosis can be confirmed by serologic and histologic methods. Serologic tests that suggest an acute infection include detection of IgM-specific antibody, demonstration of an extremely high IgG antibody titer, and documentation of IgG seroconversion from negative to positive.[222,223] Because serologic assays for toxoplasmosis are not well standardized, when initial laboratory tests appear to indicate that an acute infection has occurred, repeat serology should be performed in a well-recognized reference laboratory.

Congenital Toxoplasmosis

Congenital infection can occur if a woman develops *acute* toxoplasmosis during pregnancy. Chronic or latent infection is unlikely to cause fetal injury except perhaps in an immunosuppressed patient. Approximately 40 percent of neonates born to mothers with acute toxoplasmosis show evidence of infection. Congenital infection is most likely to occur when maternal infection develops in the third trimester. Less than half of affected infants are symptomatic at birth. The clinical manifestations of congenital toxoplasmosis are quite varied.

The most valuable tests for antenatal diagnosis of congenital toxoplasmosis are ultrasound, cordocentesis, and amniocentesis. Ultrasound findings suggestive of infection include ventriculomegaly, intracranial calcifications, microcephaly, ascites, hepatosplenomegaly, and IUGR. Fetal blood samples can be tested for IgM-specific antibody after 20 weeks of gestation. Fetal blood and amniotic fluid can be inoculated into mice, and the organism can subsequently be recovered from the blood of infected animals. *T. gondii* can also be identified in amniotic fluid using a PCR test.

Management

Toxoplasmosis in the immunocompetent adult is usually an asymptomatic or self-limited illness and does not require treatment. However, treatment is indicated when acute toxoplasmosis occurs during pregnancy. Treatment of the mother clearly has been shown to reduce the risk of congenital infection and decrease the late sequelae of infection.[224,225] Pyrimethamine is not recommended for use during the first trimester of pregnancy because of possible teratogenicity. Sulfonamides can be used alone, but single-agent therapy appears to be less effective than combination therapy. In Europe, spiramycin has been used extensively in pregnancy with excellent success.[224,225] It is available for treatment in the United States through the CDC.

In the management of the pregnant patient, *prevention* of acute toxoplasmosis is of paramount importance. Pregnant women should be advised to avoid contact with stray cats or cat litter. They should always wash their hands after preparing meat for cooking and should never eat raw or rare meat. Fruits and vegetables also should be washed carefully to remove possible contamination by oocysts.

VARICELLA

Epidemiology

Natural varicella infection occurs primarily during early childhood. Less than 10 percent of cases occur in individuals greater than 10 years of age; however, older patients account for more than 50 percent of all fatalities due to varicella. Varicella is transmitted by direct contact and respiratory droplets. The virus is highly infectious, and approximately 95 percent of susceptible household contacts become infected following exposure. The incubation period is 10 to 14 days. Patients are infectious from 1 day before the outbreak of the rash until all of the cutaneous lesions have dried and crusted over. Immunity to varicella is usually lifelong.[228]

Herpes zoster infection occurs as a result of reactivation of latent virus infection in a patient who already has had varicella. Because of the presence in the host of virus-specific antibody, herpes zoster is usually a much less serious disorder than varicella and rarely poses a major risk to either the mother or her baby unless the former is immunocompromised.

Clinical Manifestations

The usual clinical manifestations of varicella are fever, malaise, and a skin rash. The characteristic skin lesions usually begin as pruritic macules that appear in crops. The macules progress to papules, then to vesicles, and finally to crusts. The lesions initially appear on the trunk and then spread centripetally to the extremities.

In adults, two life-threatening sequelae may develop: encephalitis and pneumonia. The former occurs in 1 percent or less of pregnant women; the latter may develop in up to 20 percent of patients. Prior to the development of acyclovir, the mortality associated with varicella pneumonia in pregnancy approached 40 percent.[228,229]

Diagnosis

The diagnosis of varicella is usually made by clinical examination alone. Serologic assays are of primary value in assessing a patient's susceptibility to varicella immediately following exposure. The two most useful antibody assays are the fluorescent antimembrane antibody test (FAMA) and ELISA. Both assays show sustained elevations, usually lifelong, following natural infection.[228,230]

Management of Maternal Infection

The optimal approach to maternal varicella infection is *prevention.* All women of reproductive age should be assessed for immunity to varicella, ideally before they attempt pregnancy. Susceptible patients, particularly those who are likely to be exposed to varicella either at home or in the workplace, should be offered the new varicella vaccine. Vaccine recipients should use effective contraception for 3 months after immunization. The vaccine is contraindicated in patients who are pregnant.

Patients should be questioned about varicella immunity at the time of their first prenatal appointment. If she is uncertain about prior infection, an IgG varicella serology should be performed. If the serology is positive, the patient can be reassured that she is immune and that she and her fetus are not at risk should subsequent exposure occur. If the serology is negative, the patient should be counseled to avoid exposure to individuals who may have varicella or herpes zoster.

Unfortunately, however, the more common situation that the obstetrician encounters is a pregnant patient who has been exposed acutely to an individual who "may have had chickenpox." The clinician's first step in the approach to this situation is to verify that the index patient actually has varicella. If infection is confirmed, the pregnant woman should then be questioned about immunity to varicella. If immunity cannot be documented by history, an IgG varicella serology should be obtained, and the result should be reviewed within 24 to 48 hours of exposure. If the serology is positive, the patient can be reassured that her fetus is not at risk. If the serology is negative, the patient should receive varicella-zoster immune globulin (VZIG). This preparation is 60 to 80 percent effective in preventing infection if given within 72 to 96 hours of exposure. The dose of VZIG is one vial (125 units) per 10 kg of actual body weight, up to a maximum of 5 vials. In problematic cases, if waiting for the varicella serology will delay administration of VZIG for more than 96 hours after exposure, the immunization should be given without confirmatory serology.[228,232,233] Acyclovir also is effective in preventing varicella when given prophylactically. The appropriate dose is 800 mg PO five times daily for 5 to 7 days.[234]

Patients who receive VZIG, as well as those who present for care too late for passive immunoprophylaxis, should be counseled about the clinical signs and symptoms of varicella. In particular, they must be advised to report immediately if early manifestations of varicella encephalitis or pneumonia develop. If serious sequelae occur, the patient should be admitted to the hospital for intravenous therapy with acyclovir. The recommended dose of acyclovir is 500 mg/m^2 every 8 hours, and treatment should be continued until the patient's systemic symptoms have resolved and the cutaneous lesions have begun to crust.

Congenital Infection

Congenital varicella results primarily from hematogenous dissemination of virus across the placenta. Congenital infection may lead to spontaneous abortion, intrauterine fetal demise, and varicella embryopathy. The latter disorder is manifested by multiple abnormalities such as cutaneous scars, limb hypoplasia, muscle atrophy, malformed digits, psychomotor retardation, microcephaly, cortical atrophy, cataracts, chorioretinitis, and microophthalmia.[228] The frequency of varicella embryopathy associated with infection in the first 20 weeks of gestation is 1 to 2 percent.

Ultrasonography is the preferred diagnostic modality. Sonographic findings suggestive of fetal varicella include polyhydramnios, hydrops, hyperechogenic foci in the abdominal organs (particularly the liver), cardiac malformations, limb deformities, microcephaly, and IUGR.[228]

Neonatal Infection

The final major complication of varicella infection in pregnancy is *neonatal varicella*. Infection of the neonate occurs in 10 to 20 percent of infants whose mothers have acute varicella within the period from 5 days before to 2 days after delivery.[228] Infection usually results from hematogenous dissemination of virus across the placenta at a time when no maternal antibody is present to provide passive immunity to the fetus.

The clinical course of neonatal varicella can be variable in progression and severity. The infant usually becomes symptomatic within 5 to 10 days of delivery. Some neonates have only scattered skin lesions and no systemic signs of illness. Others have a biphasic course, initially presenting with a cluster of skin lesions, followed by more widespread dissemination. Still others have a more severe acute illness associated with extensive cutaneous lesions and visceral infection. The most common life-threatening complication is pneumonia. In reports published before the widespread availability of acyclovir, the mortality associated with neonatal varicella was 20 to 30 percent.[228]

To prevent neonatal varicella, an effort should be made to delay delivery until 5 to 7 days after the onset of maternal illness. If delay is not possible, the neonate should receive VZIG (one vial, 125 units) immediately after birth. An important additional preventive measure is isolation of the infant from the mother until all vesicular lesions likely to come in contact with the infant have crusted over.[228,233]

Key Points

➤ Vaginal infections occur commonly in pregnancy. Moniliasis is best treated with topical antifungal compounds such as miconazole, terconazole, or chlortrimazole. Metronidazole is the only antibiotic with uniform efficacy against trichomonas. Clindamycin and metronidazole, administered either orally or topically, are effective for treatment of bacterial vaginosis.

➤ Urinary tract infections in pregnancy are caused primarily by *E. coli, Klebsiella pneumoniae,* and *Proteus* species. Pyelonephritis is a particularly serious infection in pregnancy because it may be complicated by preterm labor, bacteremia, and ARDS.

➤ Chorioamnionitis and puerperal endometritis are caused by multiple aerobic and anaerobic organisms. Antibiotic therapy should be directed against group B streptococci, aerobic gram-negative bacilli, and *Bacteroides* and *Prevotella* species.

➤ Primary maternal CMV infection during pregnancy is associated with a 40 percent risk of fetal infection. Ten to 15 percent of infected infants are severely affected at birth. Ultrasonography and amniotic fluid viral culture are the best methods for diagnosing fetal infection.

Box continued on opposite page

Key Points *Continued*

➤ All pregnant women should be screened for hepatitis B infections. Infants delivered to seropositive mothers should receive both hepatitis B immune globulin (HBIG) and hepatitis B vaccine shortly after birth.

➤ HSV infection may be classified as *primary, initial, non-primary,* and *recurrent. Primary infection* poses the major risk of perinatal transmission. Women with prodromal symptoms or visible lesions should be delivered by cesarean section; asymptomatic women may deliver vaginally.

➤ All pregnant women should be screened for HIV infection. Prophylactic treatment of seropositive women with combination chemotherapy significantly reduces the risk of perinatal transmission of infection and prolongs maternal survival.

➤ Maternal parvovirus infection may result in fetal hydrops. Intrauterine transfusion may be a lifesaving intervention for the hydropic fetus.

➤ Primary maternal toxoplasmosis poses a serious risk of fetal infection. Fetal infection is best diagnosed by DNA analysis of amniotic fluid. Spiramycin is effective in treating both maternal and fetal infection.

➤ Varicella in pregnancy presents serious risk to both the mother and her infant. Susceptible women exposed to varicella should be treated with VZIG. Neonates delivered to mothers with acute varicella also should receive immunoprophylaxis with VZIG. Following delivery, susceptible women should be vaccinated with the new live virus vaccine, provided they are willing to use effective contraception for 3 months.

Appendices: Obstetric Ultrasound Measurement Tables

With Obstetric Doppler

Compiled by:

Pamela M. Foy, BS, RDMS
Clinical Coordinator of Ultrasound Services
Department of Obstetrics and Gynecology
The Ohio State University Hospitals
Columbus, Ohio

First Trimester

Appendix 1. CROWN–RUMP LENGTH MEASUREMENT

Gestational Age (weeks)	Mean Predicted Crown–Rump Length (mm)	Gestational Age (weeks)	Mean Predicted Crown–Rump Length (mm)
6.3	6.7	10.1	34
6.4	7.4	10.3	35.5
6.6	8.0	10.4	36.9
6.7	8.7	10.6	38.4
6.9	9.5	10.7	39.9
7.0	10.2	10.9	41.4
7.1	11.0	11.0	43
7.3	11.8	11.1	44.6
7.4	12.6	11.3	46.2
7.6	13.5	11.4	47.8
7.7	14.4	11.6	49.5
7.9	15.3	11.7	51.2
8.0	16.3	11.9	52.9
8.1	17.3	12.0	54.7
8.3	18.3	12.1	56.5
8.4	19.3	12.3	58.3
8.6	20.4	12.4	60.1
8.7	21.5	12.6	62
8.9	22.6	12.7	63.9
9.0	23.8	12.9	65.9
9.1	25.0	13.0	67.8
9.3	26.2	13.1	69.3
9.4	27.4	13.3	71.8
9.6	28.7	13.4	73.9
9.7	30.0	13.6	76.0
9.9	31.3	13.7	78.1
10.0	32.7	13.9	80.2
		14.0	82.4

From Robinson HP, Fleming JEE: A critical evaluation of sonar crown-rump length measurements. Br J Obstet Gynaecol 82:702, 1975, with permission.

Appendix 2. GESTATIONAL SAC MEASUREMENT

Gestational Age (weeks)	Mean Predicted Gestational Sac (mm)	Gestational Age (weeks)	Mean Predicted Gestational Sac (mm)
5.0	10	8.8	36
5.2	11	8.9	37
5.3	12	9.0	38
5.5	13	9.2	39
5.6	14	9.3	40
5.8	15	9.5	41
5.9	16	9.6	42
6.0	17	9.7	43
6.2	18	9.9	44
6.3	19	10.0	45
6.5	20	10.2	46
6.6	21	10.3	47
6.8	22	10.5	48
6.9	23	10.6	49
7.0	24	10.7	50
7.2	25	10.9	51
7.3	26	11.0	52
7.5	27	11.2	53
7.6	28	11.3	54
7.8	29	11.5	55
7.9	30	11.6	56
8.0	31	11.7	57
8.2	32	11.9	58
8.3	33	12.0	59
8.5	34	12.2	60
8.6	35		

From Hellman LM, Kobayashi M, Fillisti L et al: Growth and development of the human fetus prior to the twentieth week of gestation. Am J Obstet Gynecol 103:789, 1969, with permission.

Second- and Third-Trimester

Appendix 3. TRANSVERSE CEREBELLAR DIAMETER

Gestational Age (weeks)	Cerebellum (mm) by Percentile				
	10	25	50	75	90
15	10	12	14	15	16
16	14	16	16	16	17
17	16	17	17	18	18
18	17	18	18	19	19
19	18	18	19	19	22
20	18	19	20	20	22
21	19	20	22	23	24
22	21	23	23	24	24
23	22	23	24	25	26
24	22	24	25	27	28
25	23	21.5	28	28	29
26	25	28	29	30	32
27	26	28.5	30	31	32
28	27	30	31	32	34
29	29	32	34	36	38
30	31	32	35	37	40
31	32	35	38	39	43
32	33	36	38	40	42
33	32	36	40	43	44
34	33	38	40	41	44
35	31	37	40.5	43	47
36	36	29	43	52	55
37	37	37	45	52	55
38	40	40	48.5	52	55
39	52	52	52	55	55

From Goldstein I, Reece EA, Pilu G et al: Cerebellar measurements with ultrasonography in the evaluation of fetal growth and development. Am J Obstet Gynecol 156:1065, 1987, with permission.

Appendix 4. COMPOSITE BIPARIETAL DIAMETER (BPD)

BPD (mm)	Gestational Age (weeks)			BPD (mm)	Gestational Age (weeks)		
	10 %ile	50 %ile	90 %ile		10 %ile	50 %ile	90 %ile
20	12	12	12	61	22.6	24.2	25.8
21	12	12	12	62	23.1	24.6	26.1
22	12.2	12.7	13.2	63	23.4	24.9	26.4
23	12.4	13	13.6	64	23.8	25.3	26.8
24	12.6	13.2	13.8	65	24.1	25.6	27.1
25	12.9	13.5	14.1	66	24.5	26	27.5
26	13.1	13.7	14.3	67	25	26.4	27.8
27	13.4	14	14.6	68	25.3	26.7	28.1
28	13.6	14.3	15	69	25.8	27.1	28.4
29	13.9	14.5	15.2	70	26.3	27.5	28.7
30	14.1	14.8	15.5	71	26.7	27.9	29.1
31	14.3	15.1	15.9	72	27.2	28.3	29.4
32	14.5	15.3	16.1	73	27.6	28.7	29.8

Table continued on following page

Appendix 4. COMPOSITE BIPARIETAL DIAMETER (BPD) *Continued*

BPD (mm)	Gestational Age (weeks)			BPD (mm)	Gestational Age (weeks)		
	10 %ile	50 %ile	90 %ile		10 %ile	50 %ile	90 %ile
33	14.7	15.6	16.5	74	28.1	29.1	30.1
34	15	15.9	16.8	75	28.5	29.5	30.5
35	15.2	16.2	17.2	76	29	30	31
36	15.4	16.4	17.4	77	29.2	30.3	31.4
37	15.6	16.7	17.8	78	29.6	30.8	32
38	15.9	17	18.1	79	29.9	31.1	32.5
39	16.1	17.3	18.5	80	30.2	31.6	33
40	16.4	17.6	18.8	81	30.7	32.1	33.5
41	16.5	17.9	19.3	82	31.2	32.6	34
42	16.6	18.1	19.8	83	31.5	33	34.5
43	16.8	18.4	20.2	84	31.9	33.4	35.1
44	16.9	18.8	20.7	85	32.3	34	35.7
45	17	19.1	21.2	86	32.8	34.3	36.2
46	17.4	19.4	21.4	87	33.4	35	36.6

47	17.8	19.7	21.6	88	33.9	35.4	37.1
48	18.2	20	21.8	89	34.6	36.1	37.6
49	18.6	20.3	22	90	35.1	36.6	38.1
50	19	20.6	22.2	91	35.9	37.2	38.5
51	19.3	20.9	22.5	92	36.7	37.8	38.9
52	19.5	21.2	22.9	93	37.3	38.8	39.3
53	19.8	21.5	23.2	94	37.9	39	40.1
54	20.1	21.9	23.7	95	38.5	39.7	40.9
55	20.4	22.2	24	96	39.1	40.6	41.5
56	20.7	22.5	24.3	97	39.9	41	42.1
57	21.1	22.8	24.5	98	40.5	41.8	43.1
58	21.5	23.2	24.9				
59	21.9	23.5	25.1				
60	22.3	23.8	25.5				

From Kurtz A, Wapner R, Kurtz R et al: Analysis of biparietal diameter as an accurate indicator of gestation age. J Clin Ultrasound 8:319, 1980, with permission.

Appendix 5. HEAD AND ABDOMINAL CIRCUMFERENCE: HC/AC RATIO

Gestational Age (Weeks)	Head Circumference HC (mm)			Abdominal Circumference AC (mm)			HC/AC Ratio		
	-2SD	Mean	+2SD	-2SD	Mean	+2SD	-2SD	Mean	+2SD
12	51	70	89	31	56	81	1.12	1.22	1.31
13	65	89	103	44	69	94	1.11	1.21	1.30
14	79	98	117	56	81	106	1.11	1.20	1.30
15	92	111	130	68	93	118	1.10	1.19	1.29
16	105	124	143	80	105	130	1.09	1.18	1.28
17	118	137	156	92	117	142	1.08	1.18	1.27
18	131	150	169	104	129	154	1.07	1.17	1.26
19	144	163	182	116	141	166	1.06	1.16	1.25
20	156	175	194	127	152	177	1.06	1.15	1.24
21	168	187	206	139	164	189	1.05	1.14	1.24
22	180	199	218	150	175	200	1.04	1.13	1.23
23	191	210	229	161	186	211	1.03	1.12	1.22

24	202	221	240	172	197	220	1.02	1.12	1.21
25	213	232	251	183	208	233	1.01	1.11	1.20
26	223	242	261	194	219	244	1.00	1.10	1.19
27	233	252	271	204	229	254	1.00	1.09	1.18
28	243	262	281	215	240	265	0.99	1.08	1.18
29	252	271	290	225	250	275	0.98	1.07	1.17
30	261	280	299	235	260	285	0.97	1.07	1.16
31	270	289	308	245	270	295	0.96	1.06	1.15
32	278	297	316	255	280	305	0.95	1.05	1.14
33	285	304	323	265	290	315	0.95	1.04	1.13
34	293	312	331	275	300	325	0.94	1.03	1.13
35	299	318	337	284	309	334	0.93	1.02	1.12
36	306	325	344	293	318	343	0.92	1.01	1.11
37	311	330	349	302	327	352	0.91	1.01	1.10
38	319	336	355	311	336	361	0.90	1.00	1.09
39	322	341	360	320	345	370	0.89	0.99	1.08
40	326	345	364	329	354	379	0.89	0.98	1.08

From Hadlock FP et al: Appl Radiol, 12:28, 1983, with permission.

Appendix 6. NORMAL VALUES FOR THE ARM

Gestational Age (Weeks)	Humerus (mm) by Percentile			Ulna (mm) by Percentile			Radius (mm) by Percentile		
	5	50	95	5	50	95	5	50	95
12		9			7			7	
13	6	11	16	5	10	15	6	10	14
14	9	14	19	8	13	18	8	13	17
15	12	17	22	11	16	21	11	15	20
16	15	20	25	13	18	23	13	18	22
17	18	22	27	16	21	26	14	20	26
18	20	25	30	19	24	29	15	22	29
19	23	28	33	21	26	31	20	24	29
20	25	30	35	24	29	34	22	27	32
21	28	33	38	26	31	36	24	29	33
22	30	35	40	28	33	38	27	31	34
23	33	38	42	31	36	41	26	32	39
24	35	40	45	33	38	43	26	34	42
25	37	42	47	35	40	45	31	36	41

26	39	44	49	37	42	47	32	37	43
27	41	46	51	39	44	49	33	39	45
28	43	48	53	41	46	51	33	40	48
29	45	50	55	43	48	53	36	42	47
30	47	51	56	44	49	54	36	43	49
31	48	53	58	46	51	56	38	44	50
32	50	55	60	48	53	58	37	45	53
33	51	56	61	49	54	59	41	46	51
34	53	58	63	51	56	61	40	47	53
35	54	59	64	52	57	62	41	48	54
36	56	61	65	53	58	63	39	48	57
37	57	62	67	55	60	65	45	49	53
38	59	63	68	56	61	66	45	49	54
39	60	65	70	57	62	67	45	50	54
40	61	66	71	58	63	68	46	50	55

From Jeanty P: Fetal limb biometry (letter). Radiology 147:602, 1983, with permission.

Appendix 7. NORMAL VALUES FOR THE LEG

Gestational Age (Weeks)	Femur (mm) by Percentile			Tibia (mm) by Percentile			Fibula (mm) by Percentile		
	5	50	95	5	50	95	5	50	95
12	4	8	13		7			6	
13	6	11	16		10			9	
14	9	14	18	7	12	17	6	12	19
15	12	17	21	9	15	20	9	15	21
16	15	20	24	12	17	22	13	18	23
17	18	23	27	15	20	25	13	21	28
18	21	25	30	17	22	27	15	23	31
19	24	28	33	20	25	30	19	26	33
20	26	31	36	22	27	33	21	28	36
21	29	34	38	25	30	35	24	31	37
22	32	36	41	27	32	38	27	33	39
23	35	39	44	30	35	40	28	35	42
24	37	42	46	32	37	42	29	37	45
25	40	44	49	34	40	45	34	40	45

26	42	47	51	37	42	47	36	42	47
27	45	49	54	39	44	49	37	44	50
28	47	52	56	41	46	51	38	45	53
29	50	54	59	43	48	53	41	47	54
30	52	56	61	45	50	55	43	49	56
31	54	59	63	47	52	57	42	51	59
32	56	61	65	48	54	59	42	52	63
33	58	63	67	50	55	60	46	54	62
34	60	65	69	52	57	62	46	55	65
35	62	67	71	53	58	64	51	57	62
36	64	68	73	55	60	65	54	58	63
37	65	70	74	56	61	67	54	59	65
38	67	71	76	58	63	68	56	61	65
39	68	73	77	59	64	69	56	62	67
40	70	74	79	61	66	71	59	63	67

From Jeanty P: Fetal limb biometry (letter). Radiology 147:602, 1983, with permission.

Appendix 8. ESTIMATED FETAL WEIGHT (g) BASED ON BIPARIETAL DIAMETER (BPD) AND ABDOMINAL CIRCUMFERENCE

BPD (mm)	Abdominal Circumference (mm)																
	155	160	165	170	175	180	185	190	195	200	205	210	215	220	225	230	235
31	224	234	244	255	267	279	291	304	318	332	346	362	378	395	412	431	450
32	231	241	251	263	274	286	299	312	326	340	355	371	388	406	423	441	461
33	237	248	259	270	282	294	307	321	335	349	365	381	397	415	433	452	472
34	244	255	266	278	290	302	316	329	344	359	374	391	408	425	444	463	483
35	251	262	274	285	298	311	324	338	353	368	384	401	418	436	455	475	495
36	259	270	281	294	306	319	333	347	362	378	394	411	429	447	466	486	507
37	266	278	290	302	315	328	342	357	372	388	404	422	440	458	478	496	519
38	274	286	298	310	324	337	352	368	382	398	415	432	451	470	490	510	532
39	282	294	306	319	333	347	361	376	392	409	426	444	462	482	502	523	545
40	290	303	315	328	342	356	371	386	403	419	437	455	474	494	514	536	558
41	299	311	324	338	352	366	381	397	413	430	448	467	486	506	527	549	572
42	308	320	333	347	361	376	392	408	424	442	460	479	498	519	540	562	585
43	317	330	343	357	371	387	402	419	436	453	472	491	511	532	554	576	600
44	326	339	353	367	382	397	413	430	447	465	484	504	524	545	567	590	614
45	335	349	363	377	393	408	425	442	459	478	497	517	538	559	581	605	629
46	345	359	373	386	404	420	436	454	472	490	510	530	551	573	596	620	644
47	355	369	384	399	415	431	448	466	484	503	524	544	565	588	611	635	660

48	366	380	395	410	426	443	460	478	497	517	537	558	580	602	626	650	676
49	376	391	406	422	438	455	473	491	510	530	551	572	594	617	641	666	692
50	387	402	418	434	451	468	486	505	524	544	565	587	610	633	657	683	709
51	399	414	430	446	463	481	499	518	538	559	580	602	625	649	674	699	726
52	410	426	442	459	476	494	513	532	552	573	595	618	641	665	690	717	744
53	422	438	455	472	489	508	527	547	567	589	611	634	657	682	708	734	762
54	435	451	468	485	503	522	541	561	582	604	627	650	674	699	725	752	780
55	447	464	481	499	517	536	556	577	598	620	643	667	691	717	743	771	799
56	461	477	495	513	532	551	571	592	614	636	660	684	709	735	762	789	818
57	474	491	509	527	547	566	587	608	630	653	677	701	727	753	780	809	838
58	488	505	524	542	562	582	603	625	647	670	695	719	745	772	800	829	858
59	502	520	539	558	578	598	619	642	664	688	713	738	764	792	820	849	879
60	517	535	554	573	594	615	636	659	682	706	731	757	784	811	840	870	900
61	532	550	570	590	610	632	654	677	700	725	750	777	804	832	861	891	922
62	547	566	586	606	627	649	672	695	719	744	770	797	824	853	882	913	945
63	563	583	603	624	645	667	690	714	738	764	790	817	845	874	904	935	967
64	580	600	620	641	663	686	709	733	758	784	811	838	867	896	927	958	991

Table continued on following page

Appendix 8. ESTIMATED FETAL WEIGHT (g) BASED ON BIPARIETAL DIAMETER (BPD) AND ABDOMINAL CIRCUMFERENCE *Continued*

BPD (mm)	Abdominal Circumference (mm)																
	155	160	165	170	175	180	185	190	195	200	205	210	215	220	225	230	235
65	597	617	638	659	682	705	728	753	778	805	832	860	889	919	950	982	1015
66	614	635	656	678	701	724	748	773	799	826	853	882	911	942	973	1006	1039
67	632	653	675	697	720	744	769	794	820	848	876	905	935	965	997	1030	1065
68	651	672	694	717	740	765	790	816	842	870	898	928	958	990	1022	1056	1090
69	670	691	714	737	761	786	811	838	865	893	922	952	983	1015	1048	1082	1117
70	689	711	734	758	782	807	833	860	888	916	946	976	1008	1040	1074	1108	1144
71	709	732	755	779	804	830	856	883	912	941	971	1002	1033	1066	1100	1135	1171
72	730	763	777	801	827	853	880	907	936	965	996	1027	1060	1093	1128	1163	1200
73	751	775	799	824	850	876	904	932	961	991	1022	1054	1087	1121	1156	1192	1229
74	773	797	822	847	874	901	928	957	987	1017	1049	1081	1114	1149	1184	1221	1259
75	796	820	845	871	898	925	954	983	1013	1044	1076	1109	1143	1178	1214	1251	1289
76	819	844	870	896	923	951	980	1009	1040	1072	1104	1137	1172	1207	1244	1281	1320
77	843	868	894	921	949	977	1007	1037	1068	1100	1133	1167	1202	1238	1275	1313	1352
78	868	894	920	947	975	1004	1034	1065	1096	1129	1162	1197	1232	1269	1306	1345	1385
79	893	919	946	974	1003	1032	1062	1094	1126	1159	1193	1228	1264	1301	1339	1378	1418
80	919	946	973	1002	1031	1061	1091	1123	1156	1189	1224	1259	1296	1333	1372	1412	1453

81	946	973	1001	1030	1060	1090	1121	1153	1187	1221	1256	1292	1329	1367	1406	1446	1488
82	974	1001	1030	1059	1089	1120	1152	1185	1218	1253	1288	1325	1363	1401	1441	1482	1524
83	1002	1030	1059	1089	1120	1151	1183	1217	1251	1286	1322	1359	1397	1436	1477	1518	1561
84	1032	1060	1090	1120	1151	1183	1216	1249	1284	1320	1356	1394	1433	1473	1513	1555	1599
85	1062	1091	1121	1151	1183	1216	1249	1283	1318	1355	1392	1430	1469	1510	1551	1594	1637
86	1093	1122	1153	1184	1216	1249	1283	1318	1354	1390	1428	1467	1507	1548	1589	1633	1677
87	1125	1155	1186	1218	1250	1284	1318	1353	1390	1427	1465	1505	1545	1586	1629	1673	1717
88	1157	1188	1220	1252	1285	1319	1354	1390	1427	1465	1504	1543	1584	1626	1669	1714	1759
89	1191	1222	1254	1287	1321	1356	1391	1428	1465	1503	1543	1583	1625	1667	1711	1756	1802
90	1226	1258	1290	1324	1358	1393	1429	1456	1504	1543	1583	1624	1666	1709	1753	1799	1845
91	1262	1294	1327	1361	1396	1432	1468	1506	1544	1584	1624	1666	1708	1752	1797	1843	1890
92	1299	1332	1365	1400	1435	1471	1508	1546	1586	1626	1667	1709	1752	1796	1841	1886	1936
93	1337	1370	1404	1439	1475	1512	1550	1588	1628	1668	1710	1753	1796	1841	1887	1934	1982
94	1376	1410	1444	1480	1516	1554	1592	1631	1671	1712	1755	1798	1842	1887	1934	1982	2030
95	1416	1450	1486	1522	1559	1597	1635	1675	1716	1758	1800	1844	1889	1935	1982	2030	2080
96	1457	1492	1528	1565	1602	1641	1680	1720	1762	1804	1847	1892	1937	1984	2031	2080	2130
97	1500	1535	1572	1609	1647	1686	1726	1767	1809	1852	1895	1940	1986	2033	2082	2131	2181
98	1544	1580	1617	1654	1693	1733	1773	1815	1857	1900	1945	1990	2037	2085	2133	2183	2234
99	1589	1625	1663	1701	1740	1781	1822	1864	1907	1951	1996	2042	2089	2137	2186	2237	2288
100	1635	1672	1710	1749	1789	1830	1871	1914	1958	2002	2048	2094	2142	2191	2241	2292	2344

Table continued on following page

Appendix 8. ESTIMATED FETAL WEIGHT (g) BASED ON BIPARIETAL DIAMETER (BPD) AND ABDOMINAL CIRCUMFERENCE Continued

BPD (mm)	Abdominal Circumference (mm)																	
	240	245	250	255	260	265	270	275	280	285	290	295	300	305	310	315	320
31	470	491	513	536	559	584	610	638	666	696	726	759	793	828	865	903	943
32	481	502	525	548	572	597	624	651	680	710	742	774	809	844	882	921	961
33	493	514	537	560	585	611	638	666	693	725	757	790	825	861	899	938	979
34	504	526	549	573	596	624	652	680	710	740	773	806	841	878	916	956	996
35	517	539	562	587	612	638	666	695	725	756	789	823	858	896	934	975	1017
36	529	552	575	600	626	653	681	710	740	772	805	840	876	913	953	993	1036
37	542	565	589	614	640	667	696	725	756	788	822	857	893	931	971	1012	1056
38	554	578	602	626	654	682	711	741	772	805	839	874	911	950	990	1032	1076
39	568	592	616	642	669	697	727	757	789	822	856	892	930	969	1009	1052	1096
40	581	606	631	657	684	713	743	773	806	839	874	911	949	988	1029	1072	1117
41	595	620	645	672	700	729	759	790	828	857	892	929	968	1008	1049	1093	1138
42	609	634	660	688	716	745	776	807	841	875	911	948	987	1028	1070	1114	1159
43	624	649	676	703	732	762	793	825	859	893	930	968	1007	1048	1091	1135	1181
44	639	665	692	719	749	779	810	843	877	912	949	987	1027	1069	1112	1157	1204
45	654	680	708	736	765	796	828	861	896	932	969	1008	1048	1090	1134	1179	1226
46	670	696	724	753	783	814	846	880	915	951	989	1028	1069	1112	1156	1202	1249
47	686	713	741	770	801	832	865	899	934	971	1010	1049	1091	1134	1178	1225	1273

48	702	730	758	788	819	851	884	919	954	992	1031	1071	1113	1156	1201	1248	1297
49	719	747	776	806	837	870	903	938	975	1013	1052	1093	1135	1179	1225	1272	1322
50	736	765	794	824	856	889	923	959	996	1034	1074	1115	1158	1203	1249	1297	1347
51	754	783	812	843	876	909	944	980	1017	1056	1096	1138	1181	1226	1273	1322	1372
52	772	801	831	863	895	929	964	1001	1039	1078	1119	1161	1205	1251	1298	1347	1398
53	790	820	851	883	916	950	986	1023	1061	1101	1142	1185	1229	1276	1323	1373	1425
54	809	839	870	903	936	971	1007	1045	1084	1124	1166	1209	1254	1301	1349	1399	1452
55	828	859	891	924	958	993	1030	1068	1107	1148	1190	1234	1279	1327	1376	1426	1479
56	848	879	911	945	979	1015	1052	1091	1131	1172	1215	1259	1305	1353	1402	1454	1507
57	869	900	933	966	1001	1038	1075	1114	1155	1197	1240	1285	1332	1380	1430	1482	1535
58	889	921	954	989	1024	1061	1099	1139	1180	1222	1266	1311	1358	1407	1458	1510	1564
59	911	943	977	1011	1047	1085	1123	1163	1205	1248	1292	1338	1386	1435	1486	1539	1594
60	932	965	999	1035	1071	1109	1148	1189	1231	1274	1319	1366	1414	1464	1515	1569	1624
61	955	988	1023	1058	1095	1134	1173	1214	1257	1301	1346	1393	1442	1493	1545	1599	1655
62	977	1011	1046	1083	1120	1159	1199	1241	1284	1328	1374	1422	1471	1522	1575	1630	1686
63	1001	1035	1071	1107	1145	1185	1226	1268	1311	1356	1403	1451	1501	1552	1606	1661	1718
64	1025	1059	1096	1133	1171	1211	1253	1295	1339	1385	1432	1481	1531	1583	1637	1693	1751
65	1049	1084	1121	1159	1198	1238	1280	1323	1368	1414	1462	1511	1562	1615	1669	1725	1784
66	1074	1110	1147	1185	1225	1266	1308	1352	1397	1444	1492	1542	1594	1647	1702	1759	1817
67	1100	1136	1174	1213	1253	1294	1337	1381	1427	1474	1523	1574	1626	1679	1735	1792	1852
68	1126	1163	1201	1241	1281	1323	1367	1411	1458	1505	1555	1606	1658	1713	1769	1827	1887
69	1153	1190	1229	1269	1310	1353	1397	1442	1489	1537	1587	1639	1692	1747	1803	1862	1922
70	1181	1219	1258	1298	1340	1383	1427	1473	1521	1570	1620	1672	1726	1781	1839	1898	1959

Table continued on following page

Appendix 8. ESTIMATED FETAL WEIGHT (g) BASED ON BIPARIETAL DIAMETER (BPD) AND ABDOMINAL CIRCUMFERENCE *Continued*

BPD (mm)	Abdominal Circumference (mm)																
	240	245	250	255	260	265	270	275	280	285	290	295	300	305	310	315	320
71	1209	1247	1287	1328	1370	1414	1459	1505	1553	1603	1654	1706	1761	1817	1875	1934	1996
72	1238	1277	1317	1358	1401	1445	1491	1538	1586	1636	1688	1741	1796	1853	1911	1971	2044
73	1267	1307	1348	1390	1433	1478	1524	1571	1620	1671	1723	1777	1832	1890	1948	2009	2072
74	1297	1338	1379	1421	1465	1511	1557	1605	1655	1706	1759	1813	1869	1927	1987	2048	2111
75	1328	1369	1411	1454	1499	1544	1592	1640	1690	1742	1795	1850	1907	1965	2025	2087	2151
76	1360	1401	1444	1487	1533	1579	1627	1676	1727	1779	1833	1888	1945	2004	2065	2127	2192
77	1393	1434	1477	1522	1567	1614	1663	1712	1764	1816	1871	1927	1985	2044	2105	2168	2233
78	1426	1468	1512	1557	1603	1650	1699	1749	1801	1855	1910	1966	2025	2085	2146	2210	2275
79	1460	1503	1547	1592	1639	1687	1737	1787	1840	1894	1949	2006	2065	2126	2188	2252	2318
80	1495	1538	1583	1629	1676	1725	1775	1826	1879	1934	1990	2048	2107	2168	2231	2296	2362
81	1531	1575	1620	1666	1714	1763	1814	1866	1919	1975	2031	2089	2149	2211	2275	2340	2407
82	1567	1612	1657	1704	1753	1803	1854	1906	1960	2016	2073	2132	2193	2255	2319	2385	2462
83	1605	1650	1696	1744	1793	1843	1895	1948	2002	2059	2116	2176	2237	2300	2364	2431	2499

84	1643	1689	1735	1784	1833	1884	1936	1990	2045	2102	2160	2220	2282	2345	2410	2477	2546
85	1682	1728	1776	1825	1875	1926	1979	2033	2089	2146	2205	2266	2328	2392	2457	2525	2594
86	1722	1769	1817	1866	1917	1969	2022	2077	2134	2192	2251	2312	2375	2439	2505	2573	2643
87	1764	1811	1859	1909	1960	2013	2067	2122	2179	2238	2298	2359	2423	2488	2554	2623	2693
88	1806	1854	1903	1953	2005	2058	2113	2169	2226	2285	2346	2408	2472	2537	2604	2673	2744
89	1849	1897	1947	1998	2050	2104	2159	2216	2274	2333	2394	2457	2521	2587	2655	2725	2796
90	1893	1942	1992	2044	2097	2151	2207	2264	2322	2382	2444	2507	2572	2639	2707	2777	2849
91	1938	1988	2039	2091	2144	2199	2256	2313	2372	2433	2496	2559	2624	2691	2760	2830	2903
92	1984	2035	2086	2139	2193	2248	2305	2363	2423	2484	2547	2611	2677	2744	2814	2885	2958
93	2032	2083	2135	2188	2242	2298	2356	2414	2475	2536	2599	2664	2731	2799	2869	2940	3014
94	2080	2132	2184	2238	2293	2350	2407	2467	2527	2590	2653	2719	2786	2854	2925	2997	3070
95	2130	2182	2235	2289	2345	2402	2460	2520	2582	2644	2709	2774	2842	2911	2982	3054	3129
96	2181	2233	2287	2342	2398	2456	2515	2575	2637	2700	2765	2831	2899	2969	3040	3113	3188
97	2233	2286	2340	2396	2452	2510	2570	2631	2693	2757	2822	2889	2958	3028	3099	3173	3248
98	2286	2340	2395	2451	2508	2567	2627	2688	2751	2815	2881	2948	3017	3088	3160	3234	3309
99	2341	2395	2450	2507	2565	2624	2684	2746	2810	2874	2941	3009	3078	3149	3222	3296	3372
100	2397	2452	2507	2564	2623	2682	2743	2806	2870	2935	3002	3070	3140	3211	3285	3359	3436

Table continued on following page

Appendix 8. ESTIMATED FETAL WEIGHT (g) BASED ON BIPARIETAL DIAMETER (BPD) AND ABDOMINAL CIRCUMFERENCE *Continued*

BPD (mm)	\multicolumn{16}{c}{Abdominal Circumference (mm)}
	325	330	335	340	345	350	355	360	365	370	375	380	385	390	395	400
31	985	1029	1075	1123	1173	1225	1279	1336	1396	1458	1523	1591	1661	1735	1812	1893
32	1004	1048	1094	1143	1193	1246	1301	1358	1418	1481	1546	1615	1686	1761	1838	1920
33	1022	1067	1114	1163	1214	1267	1323	1381	1441	1504	1570	1639	1711	1786	1865	1946
34	1041	1087	1134	1183	1235	1289	1345	1403	1464	1528	1595	1664	1737	1812	1891	1973
35	1061	1107	1154	1204	1256	1311	1367	1426	1488	1552	1619	1689	1762	1838	1918	2001
36	1080	1127	1175	1226	1278	1333	1390	1450	1512	1577	1645	1715	1789	1865	1945	2029
37	1101	1147	1196	1247	1300	1356	1413	1474	1536	1602	1670	1741	1815	1893	1973	2057
38	1121	1168	1218	1269	1323	1379	1437	1498	1561	1627	1696	1768	1842	1920	2001	2086
39	1142	1190	1240	1292	1346	1402	1461	1523	1586	1653	1722	1794	1870	1948	2030	2115
40	1163	1212	1262	1315	1369	1426	1485	1548	1612	1679	1749	1822	1898	1977	2059	2145
41	1185	1234	1285	1338	1393	1451	1511	1573	1638	1706	1776	1849	1926	2005	2088	2174
42	1207	1256	1308	1361	1417	1475	1536	1599	1664	1733	1804	1878	1954	2035	2118	2205
43	1229	1279	1331	1385	1442	1500	1562	1625	1691	1760	1832	1906	1984	2064	2148	2236
44	1252	1303	1355	1410	1467	1526	1588	1652	1718	1788	1860	1935	2013	2094	2179	2267
45	1275	1326	1380	1435	1492	1552	1614	1679	1746	1816	1889	1964	2043	2125	2210	2298
46	1299	1351	1404	1460	1518	1579	1641	1706	1774	1845	1918	1994	2073	2156	2241	2330
47	1323	1375	1430	1486	1545	1605	1669	1734	1803	1874	1948	2024	2104	2187	2273	2363

48	1348	1401	1455	1512	1571	1633	1697	1763	1832	1904	1976	2055	2136	2219	2306	2396
49	1373	1426	1482	1539	1599	1661	1725	1792	1861	1934	2009	2086	2167	2251	2339	2429
50	1399	1452	1508	1566	1626	1689	1754	1821	1891	1964	2040	2118	2200	2284	2372	2463
51	1425	1479	1535	1594	1655	1718	1783	1851	1922	1995	2071	2150	2232	2317	2406	2498
52	1451	1506	1563	1622	1683	1747	1813	1882	1953	2027	2103	2183	2266	2351	2440	2532
53	1478	1533	1591	1651	1713	1777	1843	1913	1984	2059	2136	2216	2299	2386	2475	2568
54	1506	1562	1620	1680	1742	1807	1874	1944	2016	2091	2169	2250	2333	2420	2510	2604
55	1534	1590	1649	1710	1773	1838	1906	1976	2049	2124	2203	2284	2368	2456	2546	2640
56	1562	1619	1678	1740	1803	1869	1938	2008	2082	2158	2237	2319	2403	2491	2582	2677
57	1591	1649	1709	1770	1835	1901	1970	2041	2115	2192	2272	2354	2439	2528	2619	2714
58	1621	1679	1739	1802	1866	1934	2003	2075	2150	2227	2307	2390	2475	2564	2657	2752
59	1651	1710	1770	1834	1899	1966	2037	2109	2184	2262	2342	2426	2512	2602	2694	2790
60	1682	1741	1802	1866	1932	2000	2071	2144	2219	2298	2379	2463	2550	2640	2733	2829
61	1713	1773	1835	1899	1965	2034	2105	2179	2255	2334	2416	2500	2588	2678	2772	2869
62	1745	1805	1868	1932	1999	2069	2140	2215	2291	2371	2453	2538	2626	2717	2811	2909
63	1777	1838	1901	1967	2034	2104	2176	2251	2328	2408	2491	2577	2665	2757	2851	2949
64	1810	1872	1935	2001	2069	2140	2213	2288	2366	2446	2530	2616	2705	2797	2892	2991
65	1844	1906	1970	2037	2105	2176	2250	2326	2404	2485	2569	2656	2745	2838	2933	3032
66	1878	1941	2006	2073	2142	2213	2287	2364	2443	2524	2609	2696	2786	2879	2975	3075
67	1913	1976	2042	2109	2179	2251	2326	2403	2482	2564	2649	2737	2827	2921	3018	3117
68	1949	2012	2078	2147	2217	2290	2365	2442	2522	2605	2690	2778	2869	2964	3061	3161
69	1985	2049	2116	2184	2255	2329	2404	2482	2563	2646	2732	2821	2912	3007	3104	3205
70	2022	2087	2154	2223	2295	2368	2444	2523	2604	2688	2774	2863	2955	3050	3149	3250

Table continued on following page

Appendix 8. ESTIMATED FETAL WEIGHT (g) BASED ON BIPARIETAL DIAMETER (BPD) AND ABDOMINAL CIRCUMFERENCE *Continued*

BPD (mm)	\multicolumn{16}{c}{Abdominal Circumference (mm)}															
	325	330	335	340	345	350	355	360	365	370	375	380	385	390	395	400
71	2059	2125	2193	2262	2334	2409	2485	2564	2646	2730	2817	2907	2999	3095	3193	3295
72	2098	2164	2232	2302	2375	2450	2527	2607	2689	2773	2861	2951	3044	3140	3239	3341
73	2137	2203	2272	2343	2416	2491	2569	2649	2732	2817	2905	2996	3089	3186	3285	3386
74	2176	2244	2313	2384	2458	2534	2612	2693	2776	2862	2950	3041	3135	3232	3332	3435
75	2217	2285	2354	2426	2501	2577	2656	2737	2821	2907	2996	3088	3182	3279	3380	3483
76	2258	2326	2397	2469	2544	2621	2700	2782	2866	2953	3042	3134	3229	3327	3428	3531
77	2300	2369	2440	2513	2588	2666	2746	2828	2912	3000	3090	3182	3277	3376	3477	3581
78	2343	2412	2484	2557	2633	2711	2792	2874	2959	3047	3137	3230	3326	3425	3526	3631
79	2386	2456	2528	2603	2679	2757	2838	2921	3007	3095	3186	3279	3376	3475	3576	3681
80	2431	2501	2574	2649	2725	2804	2886	2969	3056	3144	3235	3329	3426	3525	3627	3733
81	2476	2547	2620	2695	2773	2852	2934	3018	3105	3194	3286	3380	3477	3577	3679	3785
82	2522	2594	2667	2743	2821	2901	2983	3068	3155	3244	3336	3431	3529	3629	3732	3838

83	2569	2641	2715	2791	2870	2950	3033	3118	3206	3296	3388	3483	3581	3682	3785	3891
84	2617	2689	2764	2841	2920	3001	3084	3169	3257	3348	3441	3536	3634	3735	3839	3945
85	2665	2739	2814	2891	2970	3052	3135	3221	3310	3401	3494	3590	3688	3790	3894	4000
86	2715	2789	2864	2942	3022	3104	3188	3274	3363	3454	3548	3644	3743	3845	3949	4056
87	2765	2840	2916	2994	3074	3157	3241	3328	3417	3509	3603	3700	3799	3901	4005	4113
88	2817	2892	2968	3047	3128	3210	3295	3383	3472	3565	3659	3756	3855	3958	4063	4170
89	2869	2944	3021	3101	3182	3265	3351	3438	3528	3621	3716	3813	3913	4015	4120	4228
90	2923	2998	3076	3155	3237	3321	3407	3495	3585	3678	3773	3871	3971	4074	4179	4287
91	2977	3053	3131	3211	3293	3377	3464	3552	3643	3736	3832	3930	4030	4133	4239	4347
92	3032	3109	3187	3268	3350	3435	3522	3611	3702	3795	3891	3989	4090	4193	4299	4408
93	3089	3166	3245	3326	3409	3494	3581	3670	3761	3855	3951	4050	4151	4254	4361	4469
94	3146	3224	3303	3384	3468	3553	3641	3738	3822	3916	4013	4111	4213	4316	4423	4532
95	3205	3283	3362	3444	3528	3614	3701	3791	3884	3978	4075	4174	4275	4379	4486	4595
96	3264	3343	3423	3505	3589	3675	3763	3854	3946	4041	4138	4237	4339	4443	4550	4659
97	3325	3404	3484	3567	3651	3738	3826	3917	4010	4105	4202	4302	4404	4508	4615	4724
98	3387	3466	3547	3630	3715	3802	3890	3981	4074	4170	4267	4367	4469	4573	4680	4790
99	3450	3529	3611	3694	3779	3866	3956	4047	4140	4236	4333	4433	4536	4640	4747	4857
100	3514	3594	3676	3759	3845	3932	4022	4113	4207	4303	4400	4501	4603	4708	4815	4924

From Shepard MJ, Richards VA, Berkowitz RL et al: An evaluation of two equations for predicting fetal weight by ultrasound. Am J Obstet Gynecol 142:47, 1982, with permission.

Appendix 9. ESTIMATED FETAL WEIGHT (g) BASED ON ABDOMINAL CIRCUMFERENCE AND FEMUR LENGTH (FL)

FL (mm)	Abdominal Circumference (mm)																				
	200	205	210	215	220	225	230	235	240	245	250	255	260	265	270	275	280	285	290	295	300
40	663	691	720	751	783	816	851	887	925	964	1006	1048	1093	1139	1188	1239	1291	1346	1403	1463	1525
41	680	709	738	769	802	836	871	907	946	986	1027	1070	1115	1162	1211	1262	1315	1371	1429	1489	1551
42	697	726	757	788	821	855	891	928	967	1007	1049	1093	1138	1186	1235	1287	1340	1396	1454	1515	1578
43	715	745	776	808	841	875	912	949	988	1029	1071	1116	1162	1209	1259	1311	1365	1422	1480	1541	1605
44	734	764	795	827	861	896	933	971	1010	1051	1094	1139	1185	1234	1284	1336	1391	1448	1507	1568	1632
45	753	783	815	847	882	917	954	993	1033	1074	1118	1163	1210	1259	1309	1362	1417	1474	1534	1596	1660
46	772	803	835	868	903	939	976	1015	1056	1098	1142	1187	1235	1284	1335	1388	1444	1501	1561	1623	1688
47	792	823	856	889	924	961	999	1038	1079	1122	1166	1212	1260	1310	1361	1415	1471	1529	1589	1652	1717
48	812	844	877	911	947	984	1022	1062	1103	1146	1191	1237	1286	1336	1388	1442	1498	1557	1618	1681	1746
49	833	865	899	933	969	1007	1046	1086	1128	1171	1216	1263	1312	1363	1415	1470	1527	1585	1647	1710	1776
50	855	887	921	956	993	1031	1070	1111	1153	1197	1243	1290	1339	1390	1443	1498	1555	1615	1676	1740	1806
51	877	910	944	980	1016	1055	1095	1136	1179	1223	1269	1317	1367	1418	1471	1527	1584	1644	1706	1770	1837
52	899	933	967	1004	1041	1080	1120	1162	1205	1250	1296	1344	1395	1447	1500	1556	1614	1674	1737	1801	1868
53	922	956	992	1028	1066	1105	1146	1188	1232	1277	1324	1373	1423	1476	1530	1586	1645	1705	1768	1833	1900
54	946	981	1016	1053	1091	1131	1172	1215	1259	1305	1352	1401	1452	1505	1560	1617	1675	1736	1799	1865	1933
55	971	1005	1041	1079	1118	1158	1199	1242	1287	1333	1381	1431	1482	1535	1591	1648	1707	1768	1832	1897	1966
56	995	1031	1067	1105	1144	1185	1227	1271	1316	1362	1411	1461	1513	1566	1622	1679	1739	1801	1864	1931	1999
57	1021	1057	1094	1132	1172	1213	1255	1299	1345	1392	1441	1491	1544	1598	1654	1712	1772	1834	1898	1964	2033
58	1047	1084	1121	1160	1200	1242	1285	1329	1375	1422	1472	1523	1575	1630	1686	1744	1805	1867	1932	1999	2068
59	1074	1111	1149	1188	1229	1271	1314	1359	1406	1454	1503	1555	1608	1663	1719	1778	1839	1902	1966	2034	2103

60	1102	1139	1178	1217	1258	1301	1345	1390	1437	1485	1535	1587	1641	1696	1753	1812	1873	1936	2002	2069	2139
61	1130	1168	1207	1247	1289	1331	1376	1421	1469	1518	1568	1620	1674	1730	1788	1847	1908	1972	2038	2105	2175
62	1160	1198	1237	1278	1319	1363	1408	1454	1501	1551	1602	1654	1709	1765	1823	1882	1944	2008	2074	2142	2212
63	1189	1228	1268	1309	1351	1395	1440	1487	1535	1585	1636	1689	1744	1800	1858	1919	1981	2045	2111	2180	2250
64	1220	1259	1299	1341	1384	1428	1473	1520	1569	1619	1671	1724	1779	1836	1895	1956	2018	2082	2149	2218	2289
65	1251	1291	1332	1373	1417	1461	1507	1555	1604	1655	1707	1760	1816	1873	1932	1993	2056	2121	2188	2256	2328
66	1284	1324	1365	1407	1451	1496	1542	1590	1640	1691	1743	1797	1853	1911	1970	2031	2094	2160	2227	2296	2367
67	1317	1357	1399	1441	1486	1531	1578	1626	1676	1728	1780	1835	1891	1949	2009	2070	2134	2199	2267	2336	2408
68	1351	1391	1433	1477	1521	1567	1615	1663	1713	1765	1819	1873	1930	1988	2048	2110	2174	2240	2307	2377	2449
69	1385	1427	1469	1513	1558	1604	1652	1701	1752	1804	1857	1913	1970	2028	2089	2151	2215	2281	2348	2418	2490
70	1421	1463	1506	1550	1595	1642	1690	1740	1791	1843	1897	1953	2010	2069	2130	2192	2256	2322	2391	2461	2533
71	1458	1500	1543	1588	1633	1681	1729	1779	1830	1883	1938	1994	2051	2110	2171	2234	2299	2365	2433	2504	2576
72	1495	1538	1581	1626	1673	1720	1769	1819	1871	1924	1979	2035	2093	2153	2214	2277	2342	2408	2477	2547	2620
73	1534	1577	1621	1666	1713	1761	1810	1861	1913	1966	2021	2078	2136	2196	2258	2321	2386	2453	2521	2592	2665
74	1573	1616	1661	1707	1754	1802	1852	1903	1955	2009	2065	2122	2180	2240	2302	2365	2431	2498	2566	2637	2710
75	1614	1657	1702	1749	1796	1845	1895	1946	1999	2053	2109	2166	2225	2285	2347	2411	2476	2543	2612	2683	2756
76	1655	1699	1745	1791	1839	1888	1939	1990	2043	2098	2154	2211	2270	2331	2393	2457	2523	2590	2659	2730	2803
77	1698	1742	1788	1835	1883	1933	1983	2035	2089	2144	2200	2258	2317	2378	2440	2504	2570	2638	2707	2778	2851
78	1741	1786	1833	1880	1928	1978	2029	2082	2135	2191	2247	2305	2365	2426	2488	2553	2618	2686	2755	2827	2899
79	1786	1832	1878	1926	1975	2025	2076	2129	2183	2238	2295	2353	2413	2474	2537	2602	2668	2735	2805	2876	2949
80	1832	1878	1925	1973	2022	2073	2124	2177	2232	2287	2344	2403	2463	2524	2587	2652	2718	2785	2855	2926	2999
81	1879	1926	1973	2021	2071	2121	2173	2227	2281	2337	2394	2453	2513	2575	2638	2702	2769	2837	2906	2977	3050
82	1928	1974	2022	2070	2120	2171	2224	2277	2332	2388	2446	2504	2565	2626	2690	2754	2821	2889	2958	3029	3102
83	1978	2024	2072	2121	2171	2223	2275	2329	2384	2440	2498	2557	2617	2679	2743	2807	2874	2942	3011	3082	3155

Table continued on following page

835

Appendix 9. ESTIMATED FETAL WEIGHT (g) BASED ON ABDOMINAL CIRCUMFERENCE AND FEMUR LENGTH (FL) *Continued*

FL (mm) 300	Abdominal Circumference (mm)																			
	200	205	210	215	220	225	230	235	240	245	250	255	260	265	270	275	280	285	290	295
40	1590	1658	1729	1802	1879	1959	2042	2129	2220	2314	2413	2515	2622	2734	2850	2972	3098	3230	3367	3511
41	1617	1685	1756	1830	1907	1987	2071	2158	2249	2344	2442	2545	2652	2764	2880	3002	3128	3260	3397	3540
42	1644	1712	1783	1858	1935	2016	2100	2187	2279	2373	2472	2575	2683	2794	2911	3032	3159	3290	3427	3570
43	1671	1740	1812	1886	1964	2045	2129	2217	2308	2404	2503	2606	2713	2825	2942	3063	3189	3321	3458	3600
44	1699	1768	1840	1915	1993	2075	2159	2247	2339	2434	2533	2637	2744	2856	2973	3094	3220	3352	3488	3630
45	1727	1797	1869	1944	2023	2105	2189	2278	2370	2465	2565	2668	2776	2888	3004	3125	3251	3383	3519	3661
46	1756	1826	1898	1974	2053	2135	2220	2309	2401	2497	2596	2700	2807	2919	3036	3157	3283	3414	3550	3692
47	1785	1855	1928	2004	2084	2166	2251	2340	2432	2528	2628	2732	2840	2952	3068	3189	3315	3446	3582	3723
48	1814	1885	1959	2035	2115	2197	2283	2372	2464	2560	2660	2764	2872	2984	3100	3221	3347	3478	3613	3754
49	1845	1916	1990	2066	2146	2229	2315	2404	2497	2593	2693	2797	2905	3017	3133	3254	3380	3510	3645	3786
50	1875	1947	2021	2098	2178	2261	2347	2437	2530	2626	2726	2830	2938	3050	3166	3287	3412	3542	3677	3818
51	1906	1978	2053	2130	2210	2294	2380	2470	2563	2659	2760	2864	2972	3084	3200	3320	3445	3575	3710	3850
52	1938	2010	2085	2163	2243	2327	2413	2503	2597	2693	2794	2898	3006	3117	3234	3354	3479	3608	3743	3882
53	1970	2043	2118	2196	2277	2360	2447	2537	2631	2728	2828	2932	3040	3152	3268	3388	3513	3642	3776	3915
54	2003	2076	2151	2229	2311	2395	2482	2572	2665	2762	2863	2967	3075	3186	3302	3422	3547	3676	3809	3948
55	2036	2109	2185	2264	2345	2429	2516	2607	2700	2797	2898	3002	3110	3221	3337	3457	3581	3710	3843	3981
56	2070	2143	2220	2298	2380	2464	2552	2642	2736	2833	2933	3038	3145	3257	3372	3492	3616	3744	3877	4015
57	2104	2178	2254	2333	2415	2500	2587	2678	2772	2869	2970	3074	3181	3293	3408	3527	3651	3779	3911	4048
58	2139	2213	2290	2369	2451	2536	2624	2714	2808	2905	3006	3110	3218	3329	3444	3563	3686	3814	3946	4082
59	2175	2249	2326	2405	2488	2573	2660	2751	2845	2942	3043	3147	3254	3366	3480	3599	3722	3849	3981	4117

60	2211	2286	2363	2442	2525	2610	2698	2789	2883	2980	3080	3184	3292	3403	3517	3636	3758	3885	4016	4151
61	2248	2323	2400	2480	2562	2647	2736	2827	2921	3018	3118	3222	3329	3440	3554	3673	3795	3921	4052	4186
62	2285	2360	2438	2518	2600	2686	2774	2865	2959	3056	3157	3260	3367	3478	3592	3710	3832	3957	4087	4222
63	2323	2398	2476	2556	2639	2725	2813	2904	2998	3095	3195	3299	3406	3516	3630	3747	3869	3994	4124	4257
64	2362	2437	2515	2595	2678	2764	2852	2943	3037	3134	3235	3338	3445	3555	3668	3785	3906	4031	4160	4293
65	2401	2477	2555	2635	2718	2804	2892	2983	3077	3174	3274	3378	3484	3594	3707	3824	3944	4069	4197	4329
66	2441	2517	2595	2675	2759	2844	2933	3024	3118	3215	3315	3418	3524	3633	3746	3863	3983	4106	4234	4366
67	2481	2557	2636	2716	2800	2885	2974	3065	3159	3256	3355	3458	3564	3673	3786	3902	4021	4144	4271	4402
68	2523	2599	2677	2758	2841	2927	3016	3107	3200	3297	3397	3499	3605	3714	3826	3941	4060	4183	4309	4439
69	2564	2641	2719	2800	2884	2969	3058	3149	3242	3339	3438	3541	3646	3754	3866	3981	4100	4222	4347	4477
70	2607	2683	2762	2843	2927	3012	3101	3192	3285	3381	3481	3583	3688	3796	3907	4022	4140	4261	4386	4514
71	2650	2727	2806	2887	2970	3056	3144	3235	3328	3424	3523	3625	3730	3838	3948	4062	4180	4300	4425	4552
72	2694	2771	2850	2931	3014	3100	3188	3279	3372	3468	3567	3668	3772	3880	3990	4104	4220	4340	4464	4591
73	2739	2816	2895	2976	3059	3145	3233	3323	3416	3512	3610	3712	3816	3922	4032	4145	4261	4381	4503	4629
74	2785	2861	2940	3021	3105	3190	3278	3369	3461	3557	3655	3756	3859	3966	4075	4187	4303	4421	4543	4668
75	2831	2908	2987	3068	3151	3236	3324	3414	3507	3602	3700	3800	3903	4009	4118	4230	4344	4462	4583	4708
76	2878	2955	3034	3115	3198	3283	3371	3461	3553	3648	3745	3845	3948	4053	4161	4272	4387	4504	4624	4747
77	2926	3003	3081	3162	3245	3331	3418	3508	3600	3694	3791	3891	3993	4098	4205	4316	4429	4545	4665	4787
78	2974	3051	3130	3211	3294	3379	3466	3555	3647	3741	3838	3937	4039	4143	4250	4360	4472	4588	4706	4827
79	3024	3100	3179	3260	3343	3427	3514	3604	3695	3789	3885	3984	4085	4188	4295	4404	4515	4630	4748	4868
80	3074	3151	3229	3310	3392	3477	3564	3653	3744	3837	3933	4031	4131	4234	4340	4448	4559	4673	4790	4909
81	3125	3202	3280	3360	3443	3527	3614	3702	3793	3886	3981	4079	4179	4281	4386	4493	4604	4716	4832	4950
82	3177	3253	3332	3412	3494	3578	3664	3752	3843	3935	4030	4127	4226	4328	4432	4539	4648	4760	4875	4992
83	3230	3306	3384	3464	3546	3630	3716	3803	3893	3985	4080	4176	4275	4376	4479	4585	4693	4804	4918	5034

From Hadlock FP, Harrist RB, Carpenter RJ et al: Sonographic estimation of fetal weight. Radiology 150:535, 1984, with permission.

Appendix 10. BIRTH WEIGHT FOR U.S. SINGLE LIVE BIRTHS IN 1991

Gestational Age (weeks)	Percentile (g)				
	5th	10th	50th	90th	95th
20	249	275	412	772	912
21	280	314	433	790	957
22	330	376	496	826	1023
23	385	440	582	882	1107
24	435	498	674	977	1223
25	480	558	779	1138	1397
26	529	625	899	1362	1640
27	591	702	1035	1635	1927
28	670	798	1196	1977	2237
29	772	925	1394	2361	2553
30	910	1085	1637	2710	2847

31	1088	1278	1918	2986	3108
32	1294	1495	2203	3200	3338
33	1513	1725	2458	3370	3536
34	1735	1950	2667	3502	3697
35	1950	2159	2831	3596	3812
36	2156	2354	2974	3668	3888
37	2357	2541	3117	3755	3956
38	2543	2714	3263	3867	4027
39	2685	2852	3400	3980	4107
40	2761	2929	3495	4060	4185
41	2777	2948	3527	4094	4217
42	2764	2935	3522	4098	4213
43	2741	2907	3505	4096	4178
44	2724	2885	3491	4096	4122

From Alexander GR, Himes JH, Kaufman RB et al: A United States national reference for fetal growth. Obstet Gynecol 87:163, 1996, with permission.

Appendix 11. TENTH PERCENTILE BIRTH WEIGHT BY GENDER FOR U.S. SINGLE LIVE BIRTHS IN 1991

Gestational Age (weeks)	Birth Weight (g)	
	Male	Female
20	270	256
21	328	310
22	388	368
23	446	426
24	504	480
25	570	535
26	644	592
27	728	662
28	828	760
29	956	889
30	1117	1047
31	1308	1234
32	1521	1447
33	1751	1675
34	1985	1901
35	2205	2109
36	2407	2300
37	2596	2484
38	2769	2657
39	2908	2796
40	2986	2872
41	3007	2891
42	2998	2884
43	2977	2868
44	2963	2853

From Alexander GR, Himes JH, Kaufman RB et al: A United States national reference for fetal growth. Obstet Gynecol 87:163, 1996, with permission.

Appendix 12. ESTIMATED FETAL WEIGHT IN TWIN GESTATIONS

Gestational Age (Weeks)	Fetal Weight (g)			
	5th %	25th %	50th %	75th %
16	132	141	154	189
17	173	194	215	239
18	214	248	276	289
19	223	253	300	333
20	232	259	324	378
21	275	355	432	482
22	319	452	540	586
23	347	497	598	684
24	376	543	656	783
25	549	677	793	916
26	722	812	931	1049
27	755	978	1087	1193
28	789	1145	1244	1337
29	900	1266	1395	1509
30	1011	1387	1546	1682
31	1198	1532	1693	1875
32	1385	1677	1840	2068
33	1491	1771	2032	2334
34	1597	1866	2224	2601
35	1703	2093	2427	2716
36	1809	2321	2631	2832
37	2239	2540	2824	3035
38	2669	2760	3017	3239

From Yarkoni S, Reece EA, Holford T: Estimated fetal weight in the evaluation of growth in twin gestations: A perspective longitudinal study. Obstet Gynecol 69:636, 1987, with permission.

Appendix 13. AMNIOTIC FLUID INDEX VALUES IN NORMAL PREGNANCY

	Amniotic Fluid Index Percentile Values (mm)					
Week	2.5th	5th	50th	95th	97.5th	n
16	73	79	121	185	201	32
17	77	83	127	194	211	26
18	80	97	133	202	220	17
19	83	90	137	207	225	14
20	86	93	141	212	230	25
21	88	95	143	214	233	14
22	89	97	145	216	235	14
23	90	98	146	218	237	14
24	90	98	147	219	238	23
25	89	97	147	221	240	12
26	89	97	147	223	242	11
27	85	95	146	226	245	17
28	86	94	146	228	249	25
29	84	92	145	231	254	12
30	82	90	145	234	258	17
31	79	88	144	238	263	26
32	77	86	144	242	269	25
33	74	83	143	245	274	30
34	72	81	142	248	278	31
35	70	79	140	249	279	27
36	68	77	138	249	279	39
37	66	75	135	244	275	36
38	65	73	132	239	269	27
39	64	72	127	226	255	12
40	63	71	123	214	240	64
41	63	70	116	194	216	162
42	63	69	110	175	192	30

From Moore TR, Cayle JE: The amniotic fluid index in normal human pregnancy. Am J Obstet Gynecol 171:218, 1990, with permission.

Obstetric Doppler

Appendix 14. UMBILICAL ARTERY RESISTANCE INDEX (RI) AND SYSTOLIC-TO-DIASTOLIC (S/D) RATIO

Gestational Age (weeks)	5th Percentile		50th Percentile		95th Percentile	
	RI	S/D	RI	S/D	RI	S/D
16	0.70	3.33	0.80	5.00	0.90	10.00
17	0.69	3.23	0.79	4.76	0.89	9.09
18	0.68	3.13	0.78	4.55	0.88	8.33
19	0.67	3.03	0.77	4.35	0.87	7.69
20	0.66	2.94	0.76	4.17	0.86	7.14
21	0.65	2.86	0.75	4.00	0.85	6.67
22	0.64	2.78	0.74	3.85	0.84	6.25
23	0.63	2.70	0.73	3.70	0.83	5.88
24	0.62	2.63	0.72	3.57	0.82	5.56
25	0.61	2.56	0.71	3.45	0.81	5.26
26	0.60	2.50	0.70	3.33	0.80	5.00
27	0.59	2.44	0.69	3.23	0.79	4.76
28	0.58	2.38	0.68	3.13	0.78	4.55
29	0.57	2.33	0.67	3.03	0.77	4.35
30	0.56	2.27	0.66	2.94	0.76	4.17
31	0.55	2.22	0.65	2.86	0.75	4.00
32	0.54	2.17	0.64	2.78	0.74	3.85
33	0.53	2.13	0.63	2.70	0.73	3.70
34	0.52	2.08	0.62	2.63	0.72	3.57
35	0.51	2.04	0.61	2.56	0.71	3.45
36	0.50	2.00	0.60	2.50	0.70	3.33
37	0.49	1.96	0.59	2.44	0.69	3.23
38	0.47	1.89	0.57	2.33	0.67	3.03
39	0.46	1.85	0.56	2.27	0.66	2.94
40	0.45	1.82	0.55	2.22	0.65	2.86
41	0.44	1.79	0.54	2.17	0.64	2.78
42	0.43	1.75	0.53	2.13	0.63	2.70

From Kofinas AD, Espeland MA, Penry M et al: Uteroplacental Doppler flow velocity waveform indices in normal pregnancy: a statistical exercise and the development of appropriate reference values. Am J Perinatol 9:98, 1990, with permission.

Index

Note: Page numbers followed by the letter b refer to boxed material; those followed by the letter f refer to figures, and those followed by t refer to tables.